OXFORD CLINICAL NEPHROLOGY SERIES

Polycystic Kidney Disease

Oxford Clinical Nephrology Series

Editorial Board

Professor J. Stewart Cameron, Professor David N. S. Kerr, Professor Leon
G. Fine, and Dr Christopher G. Winearls

Prevention of progressive chronic renal failure
Edited by A. Meguid El Nahas, Netar P. Mallick, and Sharon Anderson
Analgesic and NSAID-induced kidney disease
Edited by J. H. Stewart
Dialysis amyloid
Edited by Charles van Ypersele and Tilman B. Drüeke
Infections of the kidney and urinary tract
Edited by W. R. Cattell
Polycystic kidney disease
Edited by Michael L. Watson and Vicente E. Torres

*To subscribe to this series, see subscription information and order form at the back of this
book.*

Polycystic Kidney Disease

Edited by

MICHAEL L. WATSON

Medical Renal Unit, Royal Infirmary
Edinburgh, Scotland

and

VICENTE E. TORRES

Mayo Clinic
Rochester, Minnesota, USA

Oxford   New York   Tokyo
OXFORD UNIVERSITY PRESS
1996

Oxford University Press, Walton Street, Oxford OX2 6DP

Oxford   New York
Athens   Auckland   Bangkok   Bombay
Calcutta   Cape Town   Dar es Salaam   Delhi
Florence   Hong Kong   Istanbul   Karachi
Kuala Lumpur   Madras   Madrid   Melbourne
Mexico City   Nairobi   Paris   Singapore
Taipei   Tokyo   Toronto
and associated companies in
Berlin   Ibadan

Oxford is a trade mark of Oxford University Press

Published in the United States
by Oxford University Press Inc., New York

A catalogue record for this book is available from the British Library

Library of Congress Cataloging in Publication Data
Polycystic kidney disease / edited by Michael L. Watson and Vicenta E. Torres.
p.   cm. — (Oxford clinical nephrology series)
Includes bibliographical references and index.
ISBN 0–19–262578–0 (hardback)
1. Polycystic kidney disease.   I. Watson, Michael L. (Leonard)
II. Torres, Vicente E.   III. Series.
[DNLM: 1. Kidney, Polycystic.   WJ 358 P782 1996]
RC918.P58P65   1996
616.6'1—dc20
DNLM/DLC
for Library of Congress   95–31363
CIP

ISBN 0 19 262578 0

Typeset by EXPO Holdings, Malaysia
Printed in Great Britain by St Edmundsbury Press Ltd, Bury St Edmunds
and bound by Bookcraft (Bath) Ltd, Midsomer Norton, Avon

PREFACE

The cystic degeneration of the kidneys, once it reaches the point where it can be recognized or suspected during life, is an illness without cure. (Rayer 1841)

Thus we are led to the study of the pathogenesis of the bulky polycystic kidney: a much debated and long disputed issue, as proven by the number of works which it has elicited; but that today, owing to recent histological research it may perhaps be amenable to receiving a solution. (Lejars 1888)

Original descriptions of polycystic kidney disease are difficult to trace with confidence. Hippocrates (460BC) mentions diseases of the kidney in many passages of his works, and indeed he recommends incisions to be made in cases of abscess in order to furnish an outlet for pus. Calculi may well have been removed in some of these operations; given the lack of imaging techniques it would be surprising if some patients with pain associated with polycystic kidney disease did not have the same treatment. Hippocrates describes four diseases of the kidney. The first two fit descriptions of renal calculus associated with ureteric obstruction, the third and fourth types are less easy to classify, but by a stretch of the imagination the fourth type might encompass polycystic kidney disease:

The fourth disease arises from the gall and mucus chiefly in summer time and also after sexual excess. The patient feels pain in the side, in the groin, and in the inguinal region and in the muscles; he cannot lie on the healthy side, suffers fearful pain, and feels as if something were torn in the side. The feet and ankles are always cold, urine is passed with difficulty on account of the mucus and if the urine is allowed to stand a sediment is left like flour. If gall predominates the urine is slightly red, and if mucus, white and thick. The symptoms may last a year, and suffering during that time becomes more acute. If a swelling appears during suppuration, it should be cut. A purgative and warm bath should be given in the treatment of the disease, and the patient should be kept warm.

Hippocrates was unusual in promoting the use of surgical incisions, but the willingness to operate on patients with kidney problems was not widely accepted, one suspects because results were poor. Galen, for example, describes many aspects of disease of the kidney but makes no mention of surgery as a means of treatment. Aetius (6th century) describes some of the causes of bleeding from the kidneys: 'according as it arises in those who have lifted a heavy weight, or have jumped vigorously, or have fallen from a height, or undergone some other similar violent shock'. How many of these patients would, one wonders, would have had cysts present on an ultrasound scan?

For many centuries, however, the approach to medicine remained philosophical and although there are passing references to possible cystic kidneys, it was not until the rapid expansion of pathological anatomy in the early nineteenth century that good descriptions of polycystic kidneys were made. The atlas by Cruveilhier, *Anatomie pathologique de corps humain* (1829–35) and the treatise by Rayer, *Traité des maladies des reins* published in 1841, have some fine illustrations of 'cystic transformation' (Cruveilhier) or 'degeneration' (Rayer) of the kidneys (Figs 1 and 2). In the atlas by Cruveilhier, there is also an illustration of a liver containing many cysts (Fig. 3). In 1856, Dr Bristowe presented

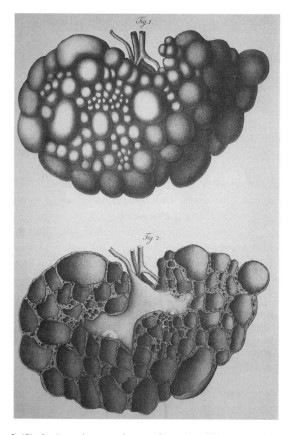

Fig. 1 'Figure 1 (*) depicts the exterior surface of a kidney transformed into a countless multitude of cysts. The uneven bumps on this surface pertain to as many cysts, well differentiated one from the other. Most of them contained fluid once clear as spring water, while being cloudy, blackish, blurry, yellowish in others.' 'Figure 2 depicts a cut of the same kidney: we see the unequal capacity of these different cysts, which are moulded one on top of the other and separated by partitions of different thickness, which are also pitted by small cavities or cysts at a rudimentary stage. Even though at first the kidney matter seems to have disappeared completely, nonetheless, on close inspection some vestiges can be found in the intermediate partitions, which convinces me that urinary secretion had not stopped completely.' '*Anatomical specimen given by Dr. Martin author of the lithography.' From *Anatomie pathologique du corps humain* by Jean Cruveilhier (1829–35). (Courtesy of the library of the Mayo Clinic, Rochester, Minnesota.)

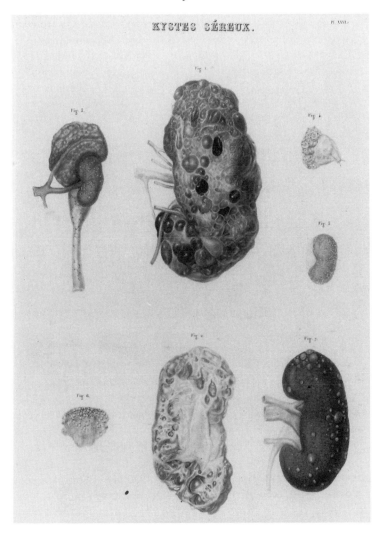

Fig. 2 'This figure depicts serous cysts of the cortical matter of the kidneys.' From *Traité des maladies des reins* by Pierre Rayer (1841). (Courtesy of the library of the Royal College of Physicians, Edinburgh.)

at the Pathological Society of London a case of cystic liver and kidney disease, although he was unsure as to how the two were related (Bristowe 1856). This presentation stimulated Dr Wilks to present, two weeks later, a similar case that had lain on the shelves of the Museum of Guy's Hospital, London for an undisclosed number of years (Wilks 1856). Many other cases of cystic kidneys and liver were subsequently reported, but for most of the nineteenth century these entities remained autopsy findings. It is towards the end of the nineteenth century that Lejars, in his doctoral thesis published in 1888, introduces the term 'polycystic kidneys', insists on the bilaterality of the cystic changes, and con-

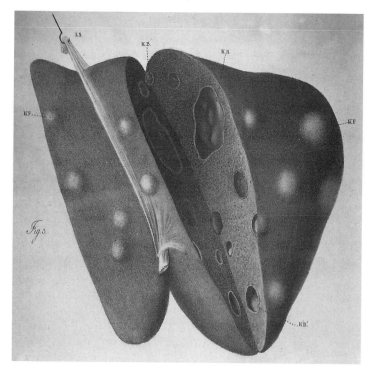

Fig. 3 'Biliary cysts. This liver had a multitude of scattered cysts of variable capacity some of which raise the surface and others are located within the substance of the organ. These cysts, totally isolated from the biliary ducts, contain a fluid of a yellow colour.' From *Anatomie Pathologique du Corps Humain* by Jean Cruveilhier (1829–35). (Courtesy of the library of the Mayo Clinic, Rochester, Minnesota.)

cludes that polycystic kidney disease is not only an anatomico-pathological entity but also a defined clinical entity with a characteristic symptomatology and susceptible of being clinically diagnosed', (Fig. 4). This view was reinforced by Osler in a series of case reports (Osler 1902). By the early twentieth century, this increased clinical awareness, the development of successful surgery of renal tumours (Newman 1901), and the advent of X-ray imaging techniques resulting in the development of retrograde pyelography (Voelcker and Lichtenberg 1906) and excretory urography (Lichtenberg and Swick 1929; Binz 1937) set the scene for a long series of clinical studies, many of them from the Mayo Clinic (Braasch 1916; Schacht 1931; Braasch and Schacht 1933; Walters and Braasch 1934; Rall and Odell 1949; Comfort *et al.* 1952; Simon and Thompson 1955), which culminated with the landmark comprehensive review of Dalgaard in 1957. The hereditary nature of polycystic kidney disease was first described by Steiner in 1899 and later clearly demonstrated by Cairns in 1925 and by Dalgaard in 1957.

Descriptions of polycystic kidneys in newborn and infants date back to the eighteenth century and are quoted by Rayer in 1841; but widened portal spaces with increased connective tissue and proliferation of bile ducts showing cystic

FACULTÉ DE MÉDECINE DE PARIS

Année 1888   THÈSE   No.

POUR LE

DOCTORAT EN MÉDECINE

Présentée et soutenue le Jeudi 15 Mars 1888, à 1 heure

Par Félix LEJARS

Né à Unverre (Eure-et-Loir), le 30 janvier 1863

Ancien interne lauréat des Hôpitaux

Prosecteur à la Faculté.

DU

GROS REIN POLYKYSTIQUE

DE L'ADULTE

Président : M. VERNEUIL, professeur.

Juges { MM. POLAILLON, professeur.

BOUILLY et JALAGUIER, agrégés

PARIS

G. STEINHEIL, ÉDITEUR

2, Rue Casimir-Delavigne, 2

1888

Fig. 4   Title page of the doctoral thesis by Félix Lejars (1888). (Courtesy of the library of the Mayo Clinic, Rochester, Minnesota.)

dilatation in infants with polycystic kidneys were not described until the turn of the nineteenth century (Couvelaire 1899; Bunting 1906). The term 'congenital hepatic fibrosis' was first used by Parker in 1956 in his description of six cases at the Berhnard Baron Institute of Pathology, the London Hospital, four of which also had associated polycystic disease of the kidneys. In 1934, Marquardt concluded from the literature and pedigrees published nine years earlier by Cairns that the mode of the inheritance of polycystic kidneys in non-viable infants was autosomal recessive (Marquardt 1934).

Early descriptions of acquired renal cystic disease also date back to the nineteenth century. In the paper to the London Royal Medical and Surgical Society in 1847, Simon reported that renal cysts form as a consequence of tubular obstruction caused by a variety of kidney diseases, including subacute inflammation. He went on to suggest that the clear fluid in the cysts represented an attempt by cyst epithelial cells 'to withdraw from the blood, if they cannot eliminate from the body, the materials which fill them' (Simon 1847). In 1882, Sabourin also described the partial cystic degeneration of the kidney in a case of Bright's disease and proposed that as a result of this process the epithelium of the convoluted tubules in the renal cortex regresses to a stage of undifferentiated cells.

Theories on the origin of polycystic kidneys were not in short supply during the nineteenth century. Virchow originated the urinary retention theory based on obstruction of the tubular lumen, either by uric acid crystals (1869) or in later publications as a consequence of connective tissue proliferation resulting from pyelonephritis or papillitis (1892). Neoplasia as an explanation has always been attractive, with early descriptions of renal cystic disease as a result of hamartomatous or cystadenomatous proliferation (Sturm 1875; Brigidi and Severi 1880). Following the description by Kupffer of the dual origin of the renal tubules (1865), views that polycystic kidneys resulted from errors of embryonic development prevailed, such as a lack of union between the metanephric blastema and the ureteric bud (Hilderbrand 1894), or a failure to involute of the metanephric nephrons induced by the first division of the ureteric bud (Kampmeier 1923). Opinions on the origin of cystic livers have in general passed through the same stages of inflammation, neoplasm, and embryonic maldevelopment (Moschcowitz 1906). Even when histological (Lambert 1947), microdissection (Osathanondh and Potter 1964), and functional studies (Bricker and Patton 1955; Gardner 1969) made Hildebrand's and Kampmeier's hypothesis untenable, the basic idea of abnormal embryogenesis was perpetuated by Potter's observation of an abnormal branching of the collecting ducts in autosomal dominant polycystic kidney disease (Osathanondh and Potter 1964). More recently, Potter's hypothesis was challenged by microdissection studies of early polycystic kidneys that failed to confirm an abnormal branching but demonstrated a great number of diverticula in all segments of the nephron, thought to be precursors of macroscopic cysts (Baert 1978).

Despite innumerable papers published on the pathology and clinical aspects of polycystic kidney disease during the nineteenth and most of the twentieth centuries, there has been until recently little hope to change Rayer's opinion that 'the cystic degeneration of the kidneys is an illness without remedy'. In the last 15 years, however, the rate of acquisition of knowledge on the genetics, pathophysiology, and natural history of cystic kidneys has been phenomenal and provides ground to believe the premature opinion of Lejars that 'thanks to recent research the pathogenesis of polycystic kidney disease may finally be solved'. This book draws on the experience of geneticists, molecular biologists, physiologists, and clinicians to provide a state-of-the-art review of the investigation and rapidly changing knowledge of polycystic kidney disease.

Edinburgh						M. L. W.
Rochester, Minnesota					V. E. T.
July 1995

References

Baert, L. (1978). Hereditary polycystic kidney disease (adult form); A micro-dissection study of two cases at an early stage of the disease. *Kidney International*, **13**, 519–25.

Binz, A. (1937). Gesichte des Uroselectans. *Urol. Nephrol.* **31**, 73–84.

Braasch, W. F. and Schacht, F. W. (1933). Pathological and clinical data concerning polycystic kidneys. *Surgery, Gynaecology and Obstetrics*, **57**, 467–75.

Braasch, W. F. (1916). Clinical data of polycystic kidney. *Surgery, Gynaecology and Obstetrics*, **23**, 697–702.

Bricker, N. S. and Patton, J. F. (1955). Cystic disease of the kidney: A study of dynamics and chemical composition of cystic fluid. *American Journal of Medicine*, **13**, 207–19.

Brigidi, D. V. and Severi, A. (1880). Contributo alla patogenesi delle cisti renali. *Sperimentale*, **46**, 1.

Bristowe, F. (1856). Cystic disease of the liver, associated with similar disease of the kidneys. *Transactions of the Pathological Society of London*, **7**, 229–34.

Bunting, C. H. (1906). Congenital cystic kidney and liver with familial tendency. *Journal of Experimental Medicine*, **8**, 271.

Cairns, H. W. B. (1925). Heredity in polycystic disease of the kidneys. *Quarterly Journal of Medicine*, **18**, 359–70.

Comfort, M. W., Gray, H. K., Dahlin, D. C., and Whitesell, F. B. (1952). Polycystic disease of the liver: A study of 24 cases. *Gastroenterology*, **20**, 60.

Couvelaire, A. (1899). Sur la dégénérescence kystique congénitale des organes glandulaires et en particulier des reins et du foie. *Annales de gynécologie et obstétriques*, **52**, 453.

Cruveilhier, J. (1829–35). *Anatomie pathologique du corps humain*, Vol. 1. Paris.

Dalgaard, O. Z. (1957). Bilateral polycystic disease of the kidneys: A follow-up study of 284 patients and their families. *Acta Medica Scandinavica*, **158**, S328.

Gardner, K. D. (1969). Composition of fluid in twelve cysts of a polycystic kidney. *New England Journal of Medicine*, **281**, 985–88.

Hilderbrand (1894). Weiterer Beitrag zur pathologischen Anatomie der Nierengeschwülste. *Archiv für Klinische Chirurgie*, **48**, 343.

Kampmeier, O. F. (1923). A hitherto unrecognized mode of origin of congenital renal cysts. *Surgery, Gynaecology, and Obstetrics*, **36**, 208–16.

Kupffer, C. (1865). Untersuchungen über die Entwickelung des Harnund Geschlechtssystems. *Archiv fül mikroskopische Anatomie I*, 233–38.

Lambert, P. P. (1947). Polycystic disease of the kidney: A review. *Archives of Pathology*, **44**, 34–58.

Lichtenberg, A. and Swick, M. (1929). Klinische Prüfung des Uroselectans. *Klin. Wochenschr.* **8**, 2089–94.

Lejars, F. (1888). *Du gros rein polykystique de l'adulte*. Steinhei, Paris.

Marquardt, W. (1934). *Cystenniere, Cystenleber and Cystenpankreas*. Tübingen.

Moschovwitz, E. (1906). Non-parasitic cysts (congenital) of the liver, with a study of aberrant-like ducts. *Am. J. Med. Sci.* **131**, 674–99.

Newman, A. (1901). History of renal surgery. *Lancet*, **1**, 649–51.

Osathanondh, V. and Potter, E. L. (1964). Pathogenesis of polycystic kidneys. Historical survey. *Archives of Pathology*, **77**, 459–65.

Osler, W. (1902). On the diagnosis of bilateral cystic kidney. *American Medicine*, **3**, 463–4.

Parker, R. G. (1956). Fibrosis of the liver as a congenital anomaly. *Journal of Pathology and Bacteriology*, **71**, 35a.

Rall, J. E. and Odel, H. M. (1949). Congenital polycystic disease of the kidney: review of the literature and data on 207 cases. *American Journal of Medical Science*, **218**, 399–407.

Rayer, P. (1841). Atlas in *Traité des maladies des reins. Paris.*

Sabourin, C. (1882). Etude de la dégénérescence kystique du foie et des reins. *Arch. de Physiol. Norm. et Path.* **2s**(X), 63–76.

Schacht, F. W. (1931). Hypertension in cases of congenital polycystic kidney. *Archives of Internal Medicine*, **1931, 47**, 500–9.

Simon, H. B. and Thompson, G. J. (1955). Congenital renal polycystic disease. *JAMA*, **159**, 657–62.

Simon, J. (1847). Subacute inflammation of the kidney. *Medico-Churigical Transactions*, **30**, 141–64.

Steiner, (1899). Ueber grosscystische Degeneration der Nieren und der Leber. *Deutsche medizinische Wochenschrift*, **25**, 677–8.

Sturm, P. (1875). Ueber das Adernon der Niere und über die Beziechung desselben zu einigen andern Neubildungen der Niere. *Arch. der Heilkunde* **16**, 193.

Virchow, R. (1869). Ueber Hydrops renum cysticus congenitus. *Archiv für Pathologische Anatomie*, **46**, 506.

Virchow, R. (1892). Diskussion über den Vortrage des Herrn A. Ewald: Zur totalen cystechen Degeneration der Nieren. *Klinische Wochenschrift*, **29**, 104.

Voelker, F. and Lichtenberg, A. (1906). Pyelographie (Röntgenographic des Nierenbeckens nach Kollargol-Jüllung). *München Med. Wschr.* **53**, 105–7.

Walters, W. and Braasch, W. F. (1934). Surgical aspects of polycystic kidneys. Report of 85 surgical cases. *Surgery, Gynaecology and Obstetrics*, **58**, 647.

Wilks, S. (1856). Cystic disease of the liver and kidney. *Transactions of the Pathological Society of London* **7**, 235–7.

CONTENTS

CONTRIBUTORS

Ellis D. Avner Rainbow Babies' and Children's Hospital and University Hospitals of Cleveland, Cleveland, Ohio, USA

Robert Bacallao Northwestern Memorial Hospital, Chicago, Illinois, USA

Willaim M. Bennett Oregon Health Sciences University, Portland, Oregon, USA

M. H. Breuning University of Leiden, Leiden, The Netherlands

James P. Calvet University of Kansas Medical Center, Kansas City, Kansas, USA

Frank A. Carone Northwestern Memorial Hospital,Chicago, Illinois, USA

Arlene B. Chapman University of Colorado Health Sciences Center, Denver, Colorado, USA

Dominique Chauveau Hôpital Necker, Paris, France

Eric P. Cohen Medical College of Wisconsin, Milwaukee, Wisconsin, USA

Benjamin D. Cowley Jr University of Kansas Medical Center, Kansas City, Kansas, USA

Bruce Culleton The Health Sciences Centre, Memorial University of Newfoundland, Newfoundland, Canada

Lawrence W. Elzinga Oregon Health Sciences University, Portland, Oregon, USA

Patricia A. Gabow University of Colorado Health Sciences Center, Denver, Colorado, USA

Vincent H. Gattone II University of Kansas Medical Center, Kansas City, Kansas, USA

Gregory Germino The Johns Hopkins Hospital, Baltimore, Maryland, USA

Jared J. Grantham University of Kansas Medical Center, Kansas City, Kansas, USA

Lisa M. Guay-Woodford University of Alabama at Birmingham, Birmingham, Alabama, USA

Sheila G. Jowsey Mayo Clinic, Rochester, Minnesota, USA

Yashpal S. Kanwar Northwestern Memorial Hospital, Chicago, Illinois, USA

Bernard F. King Mayo Clinic, Rochester, Minnesota, USA

Anne M. Macnicol University of Edinburgh Royal Infirmary, Edinburgh, Scotland, UK

Roberto Mangoo-Karim University of Kansas Medical Center, Kansas City, Kansas, USA

Patricia Martin Mayo Clinic, Rochester, Minnesota, USA

Jane S. Matsumoto Mayo Clinic, Rochester, Minnesota, USA

Ruth A. MacDonald Children's Hospital and Medical Center, Seattle, Washington, USA

Virginia Michels Mayo Clinic, Rochester, Minnesota, USA

Patrick S. Parfrey The Health Sciences Centre, Memorial University of Newfoundland, Newfoundland, Canada

D. J. M. Peters University of Leiden, Leiden, The Netherlands

Yves Pirson Clinique Universitaire St Luc UCL, Brussels, Belgium

Eberhard Ritz Klinikum Universität Heidelberg, Heidelberg, Germany

Joseph W. Segura Mayo Clinic, Rochester, Minnesota, USA

Lawrence P. Sullivan University of Kansas Medical Center, Kansas City, Kansas, USA

Vicente E. Torres Mayo Clinic, Rochester, Minnesota, USA

Rüdiger Waldherr Klinikum Universität Heidelberg, Heidelberg, Germany

Michael L. Watson University of Edinburgh Royal Infirmary, Edinburgh, Scotland, UK

Patricia D. Wilson The Johns Hopkins Hospital, Baltimore, Maryland, USA

Alan F. Wright Western General Hospital, Edinburgh, Scotland, UK

Min Ye University of Kansas Medical Center, Kansas City, Kansas, USA

Martin Zeier Klinikum Universität Heidelberg, Heidelberg, Germany

Klaus Zerres Institut für Humangenetik, Bonn, Germany

Horst Zincke Mayo Clinic, Rochester, Minnesota, USA

PART I

Cystic renal disease:
experimental models and pathology

1
Principles of molecular biology as applied to the study of disease

James P. Calvet

Introduction

Advances in molecular biology over the past decade have created a considerable expansion in our knowledge about basic cell function, and with it an overwhelming proliferation of terms, procedures, and protocols. Despite this, however, a large number of experimental techniques in molecular biology have become standardized and are now commonplace in the laboratories of a wide range of basic and clinical investigators.

This chapter provides an introduction to the molecular basis of gene expression. It reviews our present knowledge of gene structure and expression, and covers some of the procedures being used to investigate gene products and the regulation of gene activity. An attempt has been made to provide basic aspects of only the more frequently utilized techniques, as they are currently being used in a number of research laboratories. Additional information may be obtained from the cited references and the following books, chapters, and manuals (Glover 1985; Hames and Higgins 1985; Berger and Kimmel 1987; Sambrook *et al.* 1989; Calvet 1990; Ausubel *et al.* 1994).

Basic aspects

Genes are discrete chromosomal regions that encode information for the synthesis of protein (or for RNA molecules, such as ribosomal RNA, or transfer RNA as the end-products). Chromosomal DNA is composed of two strands that are complementary to each other, based on the principle that A (adenosine) pairs with T (thymidine), and G (guanosine) pairs with C (cytidine). There are approximately 3 billion such base pairs (bp) in the human genome. Genes are also associated with regulatory elements, which allow them to respond to *trans*-acting proteins (transcription factors) that regulate which genes are active and the degree to which they are active in a particular developmental or metabolic setting.

Gene transcription gives rise to messenger RNA (mRNA) molecules that represent complementary copies of one of the two DNA strands of the double helix (Fig. 1.1). The coding strand is copied into RNA according to the same rules

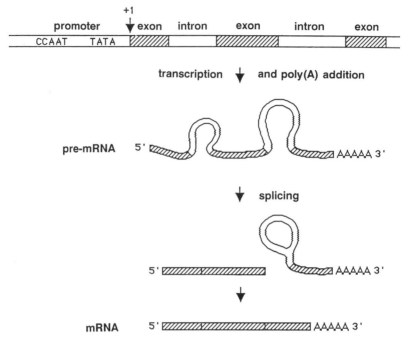

Fig. 1.1 *Gene structure and expression*. The alternating exon–intron–exon structure of a eukaryotic gene is shown at the top. The promoter region containing the CCAAT and TATA sequence elements is upstream of the transcribed region of the gene, which begins at the +1 nucleotide. The primary RNA transcript contains information encoded by exons (cross-hatched) and introns (open). After capping at the 5′ end and polyadenylation at the 3′ end, the intron sequences are removed from the mRNA precursor. Adapted from Calvet (1990).

governing DNA base-pairing, except that U (uridine) is used in RNA instead of T. mRNA has a protein-coding region within it that begins with the initiating AUG methionine codon and ends with one of three termination codons, UAA, UAG, or UGA. Upstream (toward the 5′ end) of the AUG is a 5′ untranslated region and downstream (toward the 3′ end) of the termination codon is a 3′ untranslated region. The very 5′ end of the mRNA has a methylated guanosine residue, termed a cap, which is added co- or post-transcriptionally. The sequence context immediately flanking the AUG and structural features in the 5′ untranslated region are important for determining the efficiency of initiation of protein synthesis (Kozak 1991*a,b*, 1994). The very 3′ end has a stretch of approximately 150–200 adenosine residues, also added post-transcriptionally, which comprises the poly(A) tail. Virtually all mRNAs have 5′ caps and 3′ poly(A) tails, and because of their additional 5′ and 3′ untranslated sequences, can be considerably longer than would be expected from the sizes of the proteins they encode.

All of the 64 possible combinations of three nucleotide (triplet) codons containing any of the four bases at each position (4 × 4 × 4 = 64) are utilized in protein synthesis. Each codon (with the exception of the three used for termination) specifies a unique amino acid. Since there are only 20 amino acids, it follows that some are specified by more than one codon. The AUG initiation codon determines the start site for protein synthesis and establishes the reading frame. From that point on, every codon is read (or translated) sequentially in a 5′ to 3′ direction, directing the tRNAs to incorporate the appropriate amino acids into the growing polypeptide chain. A nucleotide sequence flanked by an AUG codon at one end and a termination codon at the other end is called an open reading frame (ORF) because it has the potential to be translated into protein. In practice, open reading frames are important to look for when sequencing DNA, since gene regions encoding proteins can often be recognized this way. As such, it is possible to find and sequence a gene, and then to translate it to predict the amino acid sequence of its protein end-product without knowing ahead of time very much or anything about the gene or the encoded protein.

Estimates have suggested that the human genome contains at least 50,000 and perhaps as many as 100,000 genes (Fields *et al.* 1994). The differential expression of these genes is responsible for the diversity of cellular specialization that goes into producing an organism or individual. Cells are different from one another because of the proteins they make. These proteins are a reflection of gene activity, and of other processes that regulate the levels of individual species of mRNA. The amount of a particular protein being synthesized is often a function of the level of its mRNA, and thus, it is frequently possible to determine what a cell is doing by examining at its population of mRNAs. As will be discussed below, it is now possible by using recombinant DNA techniques to identify differentially expressed genes (without knowing ahead of time what you are looking for) by identifying differences in the levels of mRNAs between different cell types, or in the same cell under different conditions.

Gene structure and expression

Transcriptional controls

All genes have a minimum set of regulatory sequences that permits a basal level of RNA synthesis. In addition, there can be other regulatory elements that allow genes to be up-regulated or down-regulated, or to be controlled in a developmental or tissue-specific manner. Genes frequently employ both positively and negatively acting regulatory proteins that sense and respond to signaling molecules responsible for controlling their activities (Schleif 1988; Johnson and McKnight 1989; Pabo and Sauer 1992). These regulatory proteins are *trans*-acting factors, so named because they move on and off the DNA elements they recognize. The DNA sequences to which the *trans*-acting factors bind are called *cis*-acting elements.

There are three classes of *cis*-acting regulatory elements for eukaryotic genes. Two of these lie upstream of the point at which transcription is initiated in what might be called the promoter region (Fig. 1.1). The third type, the so-called 'enhancer sequences', can lie anywhere in the vicinity of the gene. The *cis*-acting elements adjacent to eukaryotic genes regulate transcriptional rates (both up and down) when associated with their corresponding trans-acting factors. Most genes appear to have some combination of one, two, or all three types of *cis*-acting elements (Dynan and Tjian 1985). Thus, transcriptional regulation in eukaryotes appears to be mediated by control regions that are composed of different combinations of promoter and enhancer elements, usually arranged in tandem, that seem to allow different regulatory factors to function co-ordinately (Maniatis *et al.* 1987). An initiation complex is thought to form by the interactions of *trans*-acting factors with their DNA elements, and with each other via protein–protein interactions, to facilitate the stable binding of RNA polymerase to the appropriate sequence region to initiate transcription (Ptashne 1988; Conaway and Conaway 1991, 1993).

The three classes of *cis*-acting elements appear to have somewhat different functions. Just upstream of the point at which initiation takes place (designated the +1 site) there is often a sequence between approximately –25 and –30 (nucleotides upstream of the +1 site are given negative numbers) that helps to determine the exact start site for transcription. This element usually conforms to the sequence TATAAA, or something very close to it, and as a result is named the TATA box (Sawadogo and Roeder 1985). It is now known to interact with the TATA binding protein, TFIID (Conaway and Conaway 1991, 1993). Further upstream, usually around –50 to –150, is a region that can contain one or several sequence elements that are required for maximal expression. There can be a variety of elements in that region that are more or less specific to certain classes of genes. One of these elements, which has the consensus sequence CCAAT, is shared by a large number of genes. It is known to be the binding site for a *trans*-acting factor called either CTF (for CCAAT transcription factor) or NF-1 (for nuclear factor-1) (Jones *et al.* 1987), which can stimulate transcription approximately 10–2-fold. Another element found in this region, which has the consensus sequence GGGCGG (called the GC box), is known to be the binding site for the promoter-specific transcription factor, Sp1 (Kadonaga *et al.* 1986).

Enhancers can be responsible for both basal-level and tissue-specific gene expression (Khoury and Gruss 1983; Atchison 1988). They differ from promoter elements by being able to function in a characteristic position-independent fashion, and by being located upstream, downstream, or even within a gene (in one of the introns). Enhancers can also function at considerable distances from genes (up to several kilobases). The *trans*-acting factor AP-1 (for activator protein-1) is an enhancer-binding protein that regulates a number of genes, and is responsible for either basal level expression or induced expression, depending on the gene (Angel *et al.* 1987; Lee *et al.* 1987). The glucocorticoid receptor is another enhancer-binding protein, which interacts with the glucocorticoid response element (GRE) located adjacent to hormone-responsive genes. Target cells, defined as such because they contain glucocorticoid receptor, are triggered by the binding of hormone and receptor in the cytoplasm. This interaction activates the receptor molecules, permitting them to bind to the GREs in the nucleus and to stimulate gene transcription (Lucas and Granner 1992; Tsai and O'Malley 1994). Other steroid-responsive elements and their corresponding receptors together, all comprise the steroid/thyroid receptor or nuclear factor superfamily.

Transcription factors are thought to regulate cellular events by being activated by signalling mechanisms. It is currently thought that, in many cases, inducers of gene transcription exert their effects by the modification (e.g. phosphorylation) of the relevant transcription factors, to affect their DNA-binding or transcriptional activation via signalling pathways to the nucleus (Davis 1994; Daum *et al.* 1994).

Intron–exon structure

Although some genes are relatively simple units, most genes have a very complex structure, being composed of alternating exons and introns (Sharp 1994). Exons are gene regions that encode RNA sequence information ending up in the mature mRNA product. Introns are stretches of DNA within genes, lying between exons, that are transcribed along with exons as segments of the primary transcript. They are removed during RNA processing and as a result are not found in the final mRNA product (Fig. 1.1).

There appears to be little size constraint on introns and exons; however, exons are often quite small relative to introns. Thus, a gene with a fairly small protein coding region and with only one (or no) intron can be very compact in size (on the order of hundreds of base pairs in length), whereas a gene with a large number of relatively long introns can be spread out over a considerable distance (frequently tens of thousands of base pairs). A case in point are the type IV collagen genes, which have been shown to contain over 50 introns (Hudson *et al.* 1993; Takami *et al.* 1994). Even more remarkable is the dystrophin gene, which, when mutated, is the cause of Duchenne–Becker muscular dystrophy. This gene is on the order of 2.4 Mb (2 400 000 base pairs) in length and has 79 exons (Roberts *et al.* 1993).

Most introns lie within protein-coding regions of genes, and because of this, their transcripts have to be removed to generate functional, translatable mRNAs. The process by which introns are removed is called splicing (Wassarman and Steitz 1992; Sharp 1994).This is actually a two-step reaction: first, the 5′ end of the intron is cleaved and simultaneously ligated to the branch site nucleotide within the intron (giving rise to a lariat structure as an intermediate in the reaction), and secondly, the 3′ end of the intron is cleaved and the exon fragments are ligated together. Splicing signals are present at every exon–intron (5′) and intron–exon (3′) border. These are relatively short sequences that designate the 5 and 3′ ends of introns, and precisely specify the sites for this two-step cleavage and ligation reaction.

Each intron has to be removed with absolute fidelity. If even a single nucleotide is inappropriately added or deleted during the splicing of any of the introns within the coding region of a precursor, the translational reading frame of the resulting mRNA would be altered and the mRNA would be incapable of producing a proper protein. (Either a termination codon would be encountered by the translational apparatus, causing premature termination, or a completely abnormal amino acid sequence would be generated, giving rise to a totally unrelated polypeptide. In fact, both of these would probably happen.) The thalassaemias have been particularly instructive in this regard (Orkin and Kazazian 1984). These are caused by mutations in the α- or β-globin genes and these mutations affect the levels (rather than functions) of the globin chains. Almost every conceivable kind of genetic defect has been discovered in thalassaemia patients, including point mutations in the critical splice site sequences that block normal splicing, and point mutations in intron or exon sequences that actually create new splice sites from sequences that resemble, but do not normally function in splicing. With this latter class of mutations, a choice of two alternative splice sites (one normal and one abnormal) is presented to the cell. Some but not all of the gene transcripts are spliced correctly, resulting in decreased levels (rather than a complete absence) of the globin chain.

Alternative cleavage and splicing

For most genes there is only one pathway of messenger RNA production. This constitutive (or required) pathway generates a single-species of mRNA from a single gene. Other genes follow a more complex pathway of messenger RNA production (Leff *et al.* 1986; Andreadis *et al.* 1987). In these cases, a single gene is capable of producing alternative primary transcripts, or alternative mRNA species from a single primary transcript (Fig. 1.2). These mRNA species usually have some sequence information in common, and as a result produce different but related protein isoforms.

Sequence differences can be generated at either end or within an mRNA. A gene, for example, can have two promoters, and as a result can produce two different 5′ exons. The mouse α-amylase gene is an example (Young *et al.* 1981). In this case, the two promoters are regulated in a tissue-specific fashion, one utilized in the salivary gland and the other utilized in the liver. Cleavage near the 3′ end of the primary transcript gives rise to the site at which the poly(A) tail is added to form the mature 3′ end of the mRNA (Wahle and Keller 1992). Pre-mRNAs can have alternative cleavage (and polyadenylation) sites that will result in the inclusion or exclusion of sequence information at the 3′ end. An example is the immunoglobulin-μ heavy chain (IgM) gene where alternative cleavage sites are chosen depending on the state of maturation of the immunocyte (Alt *et al.* 1980; Rogers *et al.* 1980; Early *et al.* 1980).

The internal exons of primary transcripts can also be alternatively spliced. There are cases where a sequence that functions as an exon in one pre-mRNA molecule, is removed in another (e.g. αA-crystallin, King and Piatigorski 1984). In other situations, adjacent exons are alternatively spliced in a mutually exclusive manner (e.g. troponin T, Breitbart *et al.* 1987) (Fig. 1.2, top). More complex

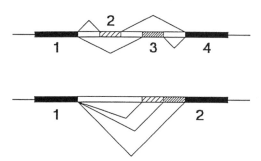

Fig. 1.2 *Alternative RNA processing.* Two motifs are shown for generating different but related products from a single gene. Constitutively expressed exons are black, introns are open, and alternatively expressed sequences are hatched. Spliced ends are connected by brackets. (Top) exon selection can be mutually exclusive. When exon 2 is spliced to exons 1 and 4, exon 3 is excluded; when exon 3 is spliced to exons 1 and 4, exon 2 is excluded. (Bottom) an exon can have several ends. Modified from Calvet (1990).

cases also exist, in which exons can be spliced together utilizing several different splice sites at one end or the other of introns (e.g. fibronectin, Schwarzbauer *et al.* 1983) (Fig. 1.2, bottom). The gene for the muscle protein, troponin T, has 18 exons. Eleven of the exons are constitutively spliced, five are alternatively spliced (in every possible combination), and two are spliced in a mutually exclusive fashion. The extraordinary result is that 64 different developmentally regulated protein isoforms are produced from a single troponin T gene (Breitbart *et al.* 1987).

mRNA stability

The steady-state levels of mRNAs depend not only on their rates of synthesis and processing, but also on their rates of decay (Decker and Parker 1994). Individual mRNAs are known to have different cytoplasmic half-lives that range from only minutes to as long as days, or even weeks (Brawerman 1987). Short half-lives allow mRNAs to be expressed transiently and to respond quickly to enviromental signals. Long half-lives allow mRNAs to accumulate to high levels. Protein synthetic capacity can be significantly amplified by stabilizing mRNAs, since mRNAs that exist for longer periods of time can continue to produce protein.

Constitutively expressed mRNAs (that produce the so-called housekeeping proteins required of all cells) are now thought to be regulated primarily by mRNA stability (Raghow 1987). Other mRNAs are known to be stabilized in response to hormones (e.g. vitellogenin mRNA, Brock and Shapiro 1983), cAMP (e.g. phosphoenolpyruvate carboxykinase mRNA, Hod and Hanson 1988), and growth factors (e.g. type I procollagen mRNA, Raghow *et al.* 1987; EGF receptor mRNA, Jinno *et al.* 1988).

The poly(A) tail appears to contribute to mRNA stability, and may be involved in the process of regulation (Wormington 1993; Sachs and Wahle 1993; Decker and Parker 1994). Several mRNAs appear to be regulated by sequences in either the 5′ to 3′ untranslated region (Raghow *et al.* 1987). These regions operate as *cis*-acting RNA elements, and function is response to *trans*-acting, RNA-binding regulatory factors. One example is a class of transiently expressed mRNAs, including the c-fos and c-myc proto-oncogenes, interferon, and the lymphokine, GM-CSF (Shaw and Kamen 1986; Clemens 1987). These mRNAs have short half-lives, and share an AU-rich sequence motif in their 3′ untranslated regions. The possibility that these mRNAs are under the control of a *trans*-acting factor is suggested by the observation that they are stabilized by the protein synthesis inhibitor, cycloheximide,which is thought to block the synthesis of a labile regulatory protein, thereby reducing its amount.

Recombinant DNA manipulation

Restriction enzymes

Recombinant DNA techniques involve the joining of DNA molecules from different sources to create novel combinations of genetic material. The purpose of doing is to facilitate the handling of large, complex genomes by breaking them down into much smaller fragments. Among the most useful of the tools used to manipulate DNA are the restriction enzymes (Arber 1979; Smith 1979; Nathans 1979). The unique property of these enzymes is that they can cleave DNA in a sequence-specific fashion, and thus will reproducibly generate a specific and characteristic set of fragments from any source of DNA. These enzymes provide the most basic instrument for isolating a gene, because they can utilize nucleotide sequence information to cut out and remove a gene from its chromosomal site. Restriction enzymes are essential for recombinant DNA purposes because they generate specific DNA fragments that can be joined with other DNA fragments cut with the same enzyme (or enzymes that produce compatible ends), to create novel DNA sequence combinations.

Hundreds of restriction enzymes having different specificities have now been purified and are commercially available (Brooks 1987; Roberts 1988). These enzymes are isolated from bacteria, where they are used for the protection of the bacterial cell from invasion by foreign DNA. By convention, restriction enzymes are named after the genus and species of the bacteria from which they were isolated (e.g. EcoRI is isolated from *Escherichia coli* and PstI is isolated from *Providencia stuartii*). Most restriction enzymes used for recombinant DNA purposes recognize specific 4-base, 5-base, or 6-base symmetrical DNA sequences. The cleavage sites on the two DNA strands may be directly opposite from one another, giving rise to blunt-ended double-stranded molecules, or may be staggered with respect to one another, giving rise to overhanging or protruding ends of 2–4 nucleotides at the cut sites. While both types of ends can be used in forming recombinant molecules, the overhanging complementary ends produced by staggered cuts are particularly useful because they allow different DNA molecules having identical ends to anneal with each other prior to joining.

The frequency with which restriction sites can be found in DNA depends on the particular sequence. As an approximation, 4-, 5-, and 6-base cutters would find their sites on average every 256, 1024, and 4096 base pairs (bp) in a random stretch of DNA. In practical terms, this means that a 4-base cutter may have 10 or so sites in a gene that is approximately 3000 bp in length, whereas a 6-base cutter may or may not have a site in that gene. In addition, there are so-called rare cutters which have 8 bp recognition sequences. These sites would be found on average every 65 536 bp and thus are very useful for making large pieces of DNA for chromosome analysis. Since the recognition sites for hundreds of restriction enzymes are known (Roberts 1988), it is possible using a computer program to predict where these enzymes will cleave a particular nucleotide sequence.

If the desired gene (or gene piece) is not flanked by restriction sites that are convenient for a particular cloning protocol, the sites can be supplied artifically (Wu *et al.* 1987). The recognition sequences are synthesized as short double-stranded oligonucleotides that can be added to the ends of the DNA fragment and then cut with the appropriate restriction enzyme, giving rise to overhanging cohesive ends that will facilitate the joining of other, similarly cut DNA molecules. Thus, one can make use of the convenience of restriction enzyme technology by furnishing the appropriate restriction sites in order to clone virtually any DNA molecule of interest.

Host–vector systems

Genes are purified by getting the sequence of interest into a DNA vector and propagating the recombinant molecule in a bacterial host (Glover 1985). There are two main types of vectors (which suit different purposes). Plasmids are small, circular DNAs that can replicate autonomously in bacteria, and in essence behave as mini-chromosomes. Bacteriophage (or phage) are bacterial viruses that can carry recombinant DNA sequences and are propagated as viruses. In both cases, the vector DNA is cut with an appropriate restriction enzyme, the foreign DNA (having ends compatible with those of the vector) is annealed with the vector DNA, and a recombinant molecule is constructed by ligating the ends of these DNA molecules together with the enzyme, DNA ligase. DNA ligase requires phosphorylated 5′ ends; thus to prevent recircularization of the vector alone (without an insert) the vector is frequently treated with phosphatase (the phosphates for ligation are supplied by the insert). Alternatively, the vector is cut with two different restriction enzymes leaving incompatible ends. These recombinant molecules are then put into a host, where they replicate into a large number of identical copies of the original recombinant molecule.

Recombinant plasmids are introduced into bacteria by transformation. Under certain conditions bacteria will take up DNA molecules, especially if the DNA is a closed circle. In practice, a culture of bacteria is made ready and mixed with the recombinant plasmids. DNA is taken up by perhaps 1 in 10^6 cells, and begins to replicate by making use of the DNA replication enzymes of the host. The transformed cells are easily identified because plasmids contain antibiotic resistance genes which are expressed when the plasmid takes up residence in the host. The bacteria are plated on antibiotic-containing agar plates, and the so-called transformants are grown up as isolated colonies. A bacterial cell is transformed by only one recombinant plasmid (because the process is an infrequent event statistically). Thus, all of the replicated copies of that original plasmid in the initial transformant and all of the plasmid copies in all the cells in the bacterial colony derived from that initial, transformed bacterial cell are identical. The DNA is said to be cloned. Once a colony has grown, it is then a relatively simple matter to transfer it to broth and to grow virtually unlimited quantities of a pure recombinant plasmid.

Recombinant bacteriophage are propagated by a somewhat different procedure. After construction of the chimeric DNA molecule, a functional virus particle is assembled *in vitro* by incubating the DNA with a packaging mixture containing all the necessary viral proteins. The packaged phage are then used to infect a culture of bacteria. Most cells will not get infected, and those that do will be infected with only one virus particle. These are then plated out on a lawn of bacteria on agar and allowed to grow. As the virus replicates and lyses its original host cell, its progeny invade surrounding cells which, in turn, lyse and spread the infection outward from the initial, infected cell. This creates a small clear area, or plaque, on the culture plate, which contains the countless identical progeny of the original recombinant. The cloned bacteriophage from this plaque can then be isolated and used to start as many large-scale preparations as necessary.

An example of a popular and well-designed plasmid cloning vector is pBR322. It is approximately 4.3 kilobases (kb) in size, has a number of unique restriction sites, contains an origin of DNA replication, and has two drug-resistant genes (for ampicillin and tetracycline). In general, DNA molecules of greater than approximately 10–15 kb are not handled well in pBR322. Since many eukaryotic genes are considerably larger than this, plasmids can have their limitations, and for cloning larger DNA molecules it may be preferable to use a phage vector. Lambda bacteriophage is frequently used for these purposes. As such, a number of lambda derivatives have been engineered to meet various cloning needs. The lambda Charon vectors (Williams and Blattner 1979), for example, have been used frequently for the construction of genomic libraries. This virus has a genome size of approximately 49 kb and a region (containing genes that are dispensible for vegetative growth of the virus) that can be removed and replaced with foreign DNA of approximately 15–20 kb in size. It is possible to clone even larger pieces of DNA by using a hybrid phage–plasmid vector called a cosmid (Collins and Hohn 1979; Lau and Kan 1983), which combines some of the more useful features of the two. This construct has the origin of replication and selectable drug-resistance genes of the plasmid, and the packaging (or cos) sequences of the bacteriophage. This relatively small plasmid, which can accept DNA molecules of up to 35–45 kb, can be packaged into a pseudo-virus particle and introduced into cells by transduction (infection), rather than transformation.

A number of plasmids and phages have been designed to express foreign DNA inserts as RNA transcripts and as protein products. If an RNA transcript of a particular DNA sequence is desired, for example, to use as a radioactively labelled hybridization probe or as a synthetic mRNA to be translated into protein, the DNA sequence can be cloned into one of the SP6 or T7/T3 transcription vectors. These are derivatives of pBR322 that contain promoters for bacteriophage RNA polymerase adjacent to a short, so-called multiple cloning region that has a number of convenient restriction sites for placing DNA inserts. Once cloned, the purified recombinant plasmid can be transcribed *in vitro*, for example, with purified SP6 bacteriophage RNA polymerase to produce relatively short (approximately 100–300 nucleotides), high specific-activity radioactive probes (Melton *et al.* 1984), or relatively long (several kb) unlabelled mRNA products (Krieg and Melton 1984). For additional convenience, vectors have a multiple cloning region flanked by an SP6 promoter on one side and a T7 bacteriophage promoter on the other side, or alternatively, T7 and T3 bacteriophage promoters. By choosing two different restriction sites (within the multiple cloning region) that correspond to the different, cut ends of a DNA fragment to be cloned, one can insert the DNA into the vector with a predicted orientation. Transcription of the fragment with one of the two RNA polymerases will give rise to a sense strand RNA product (e.g. an mRNA). Transcription with the other RNA polymerase will give rise to an antisense product (e.g. a hybridization probe to detect the complementary mRNA).

Expression of cloned genes as proteins in bacteria and in eukaryotic cells has been used to select transformants and to screen libraries, to analyse the *in vivo* functions of genes, and to produce large amounts of recombinant proteins. Plasmid and phage vectors (e.g. pUC, pGEM, and lambda gt11) that contain the *E. coli* β-galactosidase gene have been developed to facilitate selection and screening (Helfman *et al.* 1987; Jendrisak *et al.* 1987). The β-galactosidase gene has a multiple cloning site placed within it for cloning a foreign piece of DNA. Proper functioning of this gene in *E. coli* can be monitored by reaction of a dye (X-gal) that indicates the presence of β-galactosidase enzyme. However, insertion of foreign DNA into the β-galactosidase gene interrupts the coding sequence and prevents its expression. Thus, plasmid colonies or phage plaques that contain recombinants appear white or clear, in contrast to those that lack recombinants, which appear blue.

The production of recombinant proteins in bacteria (Shatzman and Rosenberg 1987) requires that a gene sequence be cloned adjacent to a strong promoter so that high levels of mRNA can be obtained. It is also advantageous to make use of a promoter that can be regulated in the cell so that the production of the protein can be delayed until the bacterial culture has reached its optimum density. This latter point is important since eukaryotic proteins are often toxic to bacterial cells, especially if they are synthesized in large amounts. Proteins produced in bacteria in high concentrations often form inclusion bodies and are sometimes difficult to get into solution for purification. It should also be recognized that post-translational modifications, such as proteolytic processing, phosphorylation, and glycosylation, will not occur with eukaryotic proteins synthesized in bacteria, thus perhaps compromising their biological activity. Some of these problems can be circumvented by expressing recombinant proteins in eukaryotic cells. For example, the baculovirus expression systems (Miller 1988), in which recombinant viruses are grown in cultured insect cells or in insect larvae, have proven to be particularly useful for the high-level expression (synthesis, modification, targeting, and/or secretion) of many eukaryotic proteins, in part because of their very strong polyhedrin and p10 promoters, and the fact that these promoters are active very late in the virus life cycle, allowing production of the recombinant proteins at a time that does not interfere with viral replication.

Eukaryotic expression vectors for analysis of gene regulation and protein function make use of plasmid constructs and viruses that provide an efficient means of introducing genes into cells and of expressing them once they are there (Cullen 1987; Rosenthal 1987). A typical vector may have plasmid sequences that include a bacterial origin of DNA replication and a selectable drug-resistance marker so that the eukaryotic gene can be cloned and propagated in *E. coli*. It will also have a eukaryotic origin of replication, such as the SV40 viral origin (so that it will replicate in certain eukaryotic cells), and additional sequences for splicing and polyadenylation that will increase the efficiency of mRNA production (Mulligan and Berg 1980). These vectors can be introduced into cultured cells by DNA-mediated transfection (Graham and Van der Eb 1973; Gorman 1985), a technique that involves the co-precipitation of DNA with calcium phosphate or DEAE–dextran. For higher efficiency transfection, cells can be treated with short, high-voltage electrical pulses that produce small pores in the plasma membrane (electroporation) through which the DNA enters the cell (Potter *et al.* 1984). Once taken up, the DNA is actively but transiently expressed, and can be assayed in a matter of 1–3 days. Co-transfection of the vector with a marker that is selectable in a eukaryotic cell can facilitate the establishment of stable transformants. If these cells are grown in culture for longer periods of time, some of the cells will become permanently transformed by the relatively inefficient integration of the transfected DNA into the chromosomal DNA of the host genome. These stably transformed cells are useful for long-term studies of gene expression. Viral expression vectors, such as bovine papillomavirus (BPV) or certain murine retroviruses, have additional advantages. BPV (Sarver *et al.* 1981; Pavlakis and Hamer 1983; Campo 1985) can reach high copy numbers and be maintained for long periods as episomes (unintegrated). Murine retroviruses can be introduced into cells with high efficiency and can be stably integrated into genomes (Miller *et al.* 1984).

Library construction and screening

There are basically two different kinds of libraries: genomic libraries (Dahl *et al.* 1981), which contain fragments of chromosomal DNA (the genes themselves);

and cDNA libraries (Williams 1981), which contain DNA copies of mRNAs (the expressed gene sequences). Lambda bacteriophage is used frequently for both genomic and cDNA libraries. Cosmids, P1 phage, and yeast artificial chromosomes (YACs) are used for cloning larger genomic DNA fragments, and plasmids may be used for libraries made up of the generally smaller cDNAs.

Genomic libraries can be used: (1) to isolate a gene in order to obtain information about its structure, sequence, or the location and sequence of its regulatory regions; (2) to investigate the molecular basis of a genetic disease (in this case, a genomic library is constructed from the DNA of an individual with an inherited disease); and (3) as a means to locate and identify, by positional cloning, the gene responsible for a particular disease.

In contrast to genomic clones, cDNA clones represent copies of the expressed genes in a particular cell, tissue, or organ. Therefore, cDNA libraries can be used as a means: (1) to identify and isolate cell-specific expressed sequences; (2) cDNA clones can be sequenced to determine the primary amino acid sequence of their encoded proteins, whether normal or mutated; and (3) cDNAs can be expressed as protein products in prokaryotic or eukaryotic cells, to investigate the function of the proteins in cell physiology and metabolism and for production of recombinant eukaryotic proteins.

Genomic libraries

DNA for constructing genomic libraries can be isolated from any cell, tissue, or organ that is convenient to handle. High molecular weight DNA is extracted and purified, partially digested with an appropriate restriction enzyme to generate a range of different size fragments, and size-fractionated by sucrose gradient centrifugation or gel electrophresis. This DNA is then mixed with lambda DNA that has been digested with a compatible restriction enzyme, the fragments are enzymatically ligated together, and the recombinants are packaged into virions using an *in vitro* packaging mixture (Hohn and Murray 1977). A culture of *E. coli* is then infected with the recombinant bacteriophage and the number of infectious units is determined by titrating the library. The number of plaque-forming units indicates how many recombinant viruses were initially made and therefore how representative the library is (Kaiser and Murray 1985). The library is then amplified by carrying out a large-scale infection. The recombinant phage resulting from this process can be stored almost indefinitely and used whenever necessary to grow new preparations for screening.

Genomic libraries should contain enough clones to include all of the DNA sequences in the genome (Maniatis *et al.* 1987; Lawn *et al.* 1978). Genomic DNA is randomly cleaved with restriction enzymes to generate a variety of overlapping fragments of different sizes. Optimally sized fragments are then packaged into enough phage particles so that statistically every sequence is represented in the library. Partial digestion with restriction enzymes that are 4-base cutters provides the best opportunity to obtain fragments that are both optimal in size and representative, given the fact that 4-base cutters have sites every 256 bp on average (in a random sequence) and that the optimal size clone is more than 50 times this size. In fact, many genes are much larger than the 15–20 kb that can be packaged into lambda phage, and it is usually no problem to isolate a family of overlapping clones that represent the entire gene region, no matter how large the gene (Kaiser and Murray 1985).

The size of the human genome is approximately 33×10^9 bp. If it were possible to divide it up into non-randomly generated fragments of 15–20 kb in size, a complete human library would need only 150,000–200,000 of these ideal clones. In practice, a human library (constructed of randomly generated fragments) would actually require about 700,000–900,000 clones to ensure a 99 per cent probability that any particular gene is represented at least once (Clarke and Carbon 1976).

cDNA libraries

The mRNA for constructing cDNA libraries can be purified from any cell, tissue, or organ of interest. Since mRNA usually comprises less than 5 per cent of the total RNA of a cell (much of the rest being ribosomal RNA and transfer RNA), it is usually advantageous to enrich for poly(A)$^+$ mRNA by one or two rounds of oligo(dT)-cellulose chromatography (Jacobson 1987). This is carried out by applying the RNA to a column containing cellulose to which short (15–18 bases) oligo(dT), nucleotides are covalently attached. mRNA containing poly(A) tails (most mRNAs) will anneal to the oligo(dT) by A–T base-pairing in a high salt buffer, allowing poly(A) negative RNAs to pass through. The mRNA is then removed with a low salt elution. The integrity of the purified mRNA can be evaluated by gel electrophoresis, Northern hybridization, or *in vitro* translation to determine whether the preparation is sufficiently intact to yield successful results.

Double-stranded (ds) cDNA is generated from mRNA in two steps (Fig. 1.3). The first cDNA strand is synthesized (using mRNA as a template) by reverse transcriptase, an enzyme that is purified from avian myeloblastosis virus or Moloney murine leukaemia virus. This enzyme is normally found packaged in the retrovirus particle, and is used to replicate the single-stranded viral RNA genome into ds DNA for integration into the host chromosome. Oligo (dT), to be used as a primer for first-strand synthesis, is hybridized to the poly(A) tail of the purified mRNA, and a cDNA strand is synthesized from this primer using reverse transcriptase (Krug and Berger 1987). Completion of the first strand results in an mRNA/cDNA hybrid (cDNA for complementary DNA). A number of different procedures exist for second-strand synthesis. In one procedure that is now used frequently (Gubler 1987), the mRNA strand of this mRNA/cDNA hybrid is nicked at numerous sites by the enzyme RNase H(H for hybrid), which is specific for the RNA strand of an RNA/DNA hybrid. The resulting 3′ ends of these RNA fragments are then used as primers for second-strand synthesis, using DNA polymerase I. This enzyme synthesizes DNA from the 3′ end of the primer in a 5′ to 3′ direction (with respect to the new strand

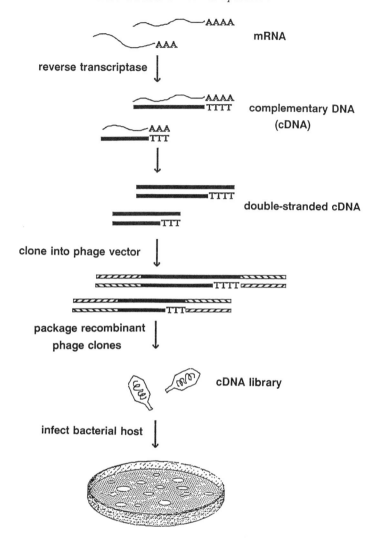

Fig. 1.3 *cDNA library construction in a bacteriophage vector.* mRNA is reverse transcribed to produce the first cDNA strand and is then made double-stranded. The double-stranded (ds) cDNAs are cloned into a region of a phage vector (hatched). The recombinant molecules are packaged into phage particles, which are then used to infect bacteria.

being synthesized). At the same time a 5′ to 3′ exonuclease activity associated with the enzyme removes the RNA (or DNA) strand lying downstream in its path (see nick-translation, below). The ds cDNA products are prepared for cloning by first making the ends compatible with those of the vector. Ragged ends are made blunt, either by enzymatic trimming or filling reactions, and synthetic restriction enzyme sites are ligated onto the blunt ends using the enzyme

DNA ligase. Addition of these so-called linkers (e.g. for EcoRI) makes it possible to anneal the cDNAs to a suitably cut cloning vector.

The lambda vectors, λgt10 and λgt11 (Jendrisak *et al.* 1987), are used for screening with hybridization probes (λgt10) or with antibody probes (λgt11). Both of these vectors have unique EcoRI sites (for cDNAs with EcoRI linkers) and are capable of accepting inserts of up to 7 kb, a size sufficient to handle most mRNAs (as cDNAs). As an alternative strategy, the ds cDNAs can be cloned into plasmid vectors. In addition, cloning can be made directional with respect to the vector by the sequential ligation of different linkers, or by the use of an adaptor–primer containing an oligo (dT) tract attached to a restriction site to prime first-strand synthesis. Construction of cDNA libraries in phagemid-containing bacteriophage vectors, such as Lambda ZAP, provides additional convenience. These vectors are hybrids between a lambda vector and a plasmid, such as pBluescript, the latter containning an M13 phage origin of replication within the plasmid sequence (hence, it is a phagemid). This construct allows the cloning of the cDNA (in the multiple cloning site of the plasmid) and utilizes the advantages of phage for increased infectivity and ease of handling. Once a clone has been identified, the plasmid (phagemid) can be excised by utilizing a helper phage which supplies proteins that recognize the begining and the end of the phagemid sequences, thus allowing the phagemids plus cDNA inserts to be replicated and packaged as a single-stranded (ss) M13-like phage (Short and Sorge 1992). These ss phagemids are extruded into the culture medium from which they can be isolated and used to re-infect bacteria, where they grow as ds plasmids. The pBluescript phagemid vectors have a multiple cloning region containing convenient restriction sites, T3 and T7RNA polymerase transcription start sites that provide a means of synthesizing sense or antisense RNA from the cDNA insert or a sequencing primer (Wu 1994) hybridization site for dideoxy chain-termination DNA sequencing, along with blue/white colour selection and β-galactosidase fusion protein expression (Alting-Mees *et al.* 1992). The primary advantage of these vectors is that they eliminate the need to subclone the cDNA insert. A newer phagemid–bacteriophage vector called ZAP Express (Stratagene) has recently been developed, in which the phagemid vector contains sequences allowing expression of cDNA sequences in both eukaryotic and prokaryotic cells.

Successful library construction depends on the quality and the quantity of clones (Hagen *et al.* 1988). If full-length cDNA clones are necessary, it is important to start with intact mRNA, and to utilize procedures that will maximize full-length cDNA synthesis. The number of clones required for success depends on the purpose of constructing the library (Williams 1981; Jendrisak *et al.* 1987). For example, if one wants to isolate a clone for an mRNA that makes up 10 per cent of the mRNA population of a cell, a library containing only a few hundred clones would be adequate. On the other hand, if one wants to isolate a clone for a rare mRNA, or if one wants a more representative library, many more clones would be necessary. Of the several hundred thousand mRNAs in a typical cell, the vast majority are relatively rare to moderately abundant and are present at about 10–100 copies per cell. The cDNA libraries for these mRNAs would have to contain 10,000 to 100,000 clones to be fully representative. Libraries for the rarest mRNAs would require up to 10^6 clones.

Screening

After constructing a library (genomic or cDNA), what is next required is that the clone of interest be identified and recovered (Kimmel 1987). In practice, the two most common ways to screen a library are by hybridization (with a nucleic acid probe) and by immunological methods (with an antibody probe). Of the two, hybridization is the more general approach (Wahl *et al.* 1987) since immunological techniques can only be used when screening cDNA expression libraries.

Hybridization

Double-stranded DNA consists of perfectly complementary, base-paired strands. If these are separated (denatured or melted) into their constituent single strands by high pH or high temperature and then incubated under conditions that favour the re-formation of duplexes, there will be a trial-and-error process of DNA strands interacting with each other and finding complementary sequences. If these interacting DNA strands are sufficiently complementary to form stably base-paired duplexes under the incubation conditions, they will remain associated with each other. Such duplexes are said to be renatured or reassociated (Hames and Higgins 1985; Marmur 1994). RNA strands can also base-pair with single-stranded DNA (or with other RNA strands), and if so, are said to be hybridized. Generally speaking, the term 'hybridization' applies to the formation of any duplex of nucleic acid strands (DNA/DNA, DNA/RNA, or RNA/RNA) that was not originally base-paired.

Hybridization conditions are important in the design of an experiment. The factors that influence the formation and stability of hybrids are incubation temperature and salt concentration. In general, the optimum temperature is approximately 25 °C below the temperature required to denature the hybrids (T_m). This melting temperature is dependent on the G+C content and can be easily calculated. If the reaction is carried out in an aqueous buffer, the hybridization temperature is usually around 60–65 °C. If the reaction is carried out in a buffer containing formamide (which lowers the melting temperature), the optimum may be around 40–45 °C. Increasing salt concentration (usually NaCl) increases the stability of hybrids. Since the melting temperature and the rate of hybridization are both affected by salt concentration, both salt and temperature can be adjusted to suit the needs of the experiment.

Together, the conditions of salt and temperature are termed the stringency of the reaction. Increased stringency is achieved by increasing the hybridization temperature and decreasing the salt concentration; decreased stringency is obtained by decreasing the temperature and increasing the salt. For perfectly matched DNA or RNA strands there is a set of standard criteria of salt and temperature that provides an optimal rate of hybridization. In practice, however, there is almost always the potential for cross-hybridization between similar (but not identical) sequences in the genome and in mRNA populations. If cross-hybridization is a problem, the stringency can be increased to reduce non-specific interactions.

Some experimental strategies require a certain amount of cross-hybridization. If, for example, one wants to isolate a gene for a human kidney-specific protein using a rat cDNA clone, conditions would have to be found that would allow cross-hybridization between the evolutionarily divergent sequences. This can usually be accomplished by decreasing the stringency. In these cases, one must often strike a balance (usually arrived at empirically) that will tolerate a degree of relatively specific cross-hybridization, but will discourage unwanted, non-specific interactions.

Probes

Hybridization probes are usually labelled with ^{32}P (phosphorus), by one of a variety of methods. A purified DNA fragment can be labelled by the process of nick-translation (Rigby *et al.* 1977; Meinkoth and Wahl 1987). This is a technique by which probe-specific DNA is actually synthesized *in vitro* in the presence of all four deoxynucleoside triphosphates (dNTPs), one labelled with ^{32}P (where the ^{32}P atom is in the α-position of the triphosphate, adjacent to the 5' carbon). As these are incorporated into the newly synthesized DNA chain, the ^{32}P becomes a part of the phosphodiester backbone. The procedure makes use of a DNA clone for a specific gene (or gene segment) or cDNA. First, single-stranded breaks (or nicks) are generated at random locations in the DNA molecule with DNase I. Secondly, DNA polymerase I is used to repair the nicks (in the presence of the labelled dNTPs). However, in doing so, the DNA polymerase (using an endogenous 5' to 3' exonuclease activity) nibbles along the DNA ahead of it while simultaneously filling in the gap that it leaves behind. This synthetic process takes place at every nick on both DNA strands, making use of the existing, opposite strands as the templates for new DNA synthesis. As such, most of the original DNA is replaced with a copy of newly synthesized, labelled DNA.

Several other ways exist to label probes. One technique now in general use is the random primer approach (Feinberg and Vogelstein 1983), which makes use of a collection of short (hexanucleatide) DNAs that represent all of the possible combinations of six nucleotide sequences. These oligonucleotides are hybridized to denatured DNA being used to make the probe, and thus are used as primers for DNA synthesis in the presence of labelled dNTPs and DNA polymerase I. A related method is to utilize Taq DNA polymerase (see discussion of PCR, below) and a thermal cycler to carry out multiple rounds of hybridization and labelling. A disadvantage of double-stranded probes is that they can self-hybridize and are taken out of the reaction. This problem can be overcome by using single-stranded (or asymmetric) probes.

The most frequently employed procedure for making single-stranded probes is to utilize one of the transcription vectors to make a labelled, single-stranded RNA (Melton *et al.* 1984). The DNA sequence that is used as the template for probe construction is cloned adjacent to an SP6, T3, or T7 bacteriophage promoter and RNA is made *in vitro* in the presence of α-^{32}P labelled nucleoside triphosphates (NTPs). These probes have the advantage that unhybridized, single-stranded probe can be removed by ribonuclease treatment to reduce background radioactivity. Another approach for making single-stranded probes is to carry out asymmetric PCR with Taq polymerase and only a single primer, thus making labelled product from only one of the two DNA strands (PCR is discussed below).

Single-stranded, synthetic oligonucleotides (oligos) can also be used as probes (Wallace and Miyada 1987). They can be labelled by the enzymatic addition of ^{32}P to their 5' ends using ^{32}P-labelled ATP and polynucleotide kinase, which transfers the ^{32}P at the gamma (end) position of ATP to the available 5'-hydroxyl group on the DNA. Specific hybrids can usually be expected for oligos that are at least 15–20 nucleotides in length, although longer probes can be easily made. Hybridization probes can be made based on amino acid sequence information for a protein, that will detect the gene or cDNA clone specific to that protein. In these cases, it is usually best to find a region of the protein that has an amino acid sequence specified by a relatively unambiguous set of codons. While some amino acids are specified by up to six different codons, others have only one or two codons. The oligo probe is synthesized as a mixture of DNAs comprising all possible nucleotide sequences that could generate that peptide. This so-called 'degenerate probe' is then labelled and hybridized to the library as a mixture, with the expectation that one of the labelled sequences will match the gene exactly and hybridize specifically.

Plaque hybridization/colony hybridization

Phage libraries are screened by plaque hybridization and plasmid libraries are screened by colony hybridization (Wahl and Berger 1987). A genomic library that has been cloned in one of the phage vectors, for example, can be screened by hybridizing a labelled probe to the bacteriophage plaques, which represent the different recombinant clones. A portion of the library (which may consist of hundreds of thousands of different recombinants) is plated out by mixing the purified phage with a vast excess of bacteria to initiate an infection. The infected (and uninfected) bacteria are then spread on to a number of agar plates. Plating is carried out at a dilution that will allow individual plaques (each representing a clone) to be resolved from one another as they appear on the otherwise uniform lawn of bacteria. A replica of the phage plate is then made by transferring some of the bacteriophage from each plaque onto a nitrocellulose or nylon membrane (Benton and Davis 1977). This is accomplished by laying the membrane filter on to the agar plate and allowing some of the phage to adsorb to it. The phage are then lysed in place to release their DNA. During this process the DNA is denatured into single strands, which adhere to the membrane filter. In effect, therefore, a replica is made that mirrors the pattern of the phage plaques on the original plate, with a small spot of DNA on the membrane corresponding to each clone.

The phage plaques are hybridized in a solution containing the probe in a sealed plastic bag, shallow pan, or covered petri dish, incubated (usually overnight) at the appropriate temperature. After hybridization, the membrane filter is removed and washed in buffers of increasing stringency to remove nonspecifically bound probe. The membrane is then covered with Xray film to reveal the plaques containing complementary DNA sequences, as spots on the X-ray film. To recover phage clones identified by the hybridization procedure, the X-ray film is aligned with the original phage plate. Plaques lying under the autoradiographic spots are removed, and the phage are amplified on plates or in suspension culture. Usually, the phage are re-screened through several rounds of plaque hybridization, in order to isolate pure phage clones. Colony hybridization is similar to plaque hybridization. However, instead of probing for DNA sequences in plaques, the recombinant clones are grown up as isolated bacterial colonies on agar plates. These are then transferred to membrances, lysed in place, and hybridized in the same way that plaques are hybridized (Grunstein and Hogness 1975; Hanahan and Meselson 1980).

Tools for studying gene expression

mRNA levels

To evaluate gene expression, it is often necessary to measure the steady-state levels of specific mRNAs. If a change in steady-state mRNA is observed in development or following induction by a physiological stimulus, the rate of gene transcription can then be examined by nuclear run-on analysis to determine whether the change in the amount of mRNA is caused by transcriptional or post-transcriptional mechanisms.

The most common technique for measuring mRNA levels is Northern blot hybridization (Alwine *et al.* 1977; Wahl *et al.* 1987) (Fig. 1.4). This involves the isolation of unlabelled RNA from the cell or tissue of interest, followed by gel electrophoresis, immobilization of the RNAs on nitrocellulose or nylon membranes, and the subsequent hybridization of this RNA with a labelled probe. The Northern blotting procedure starts with the electrophoresis of RNA on an agarose gel to resolve mRNAs by molecular weight. The RNA is then transferred to the membrane by capillary action, and the blot is hybridized in a sealed plastic bag or in any suitable apparatus with a [^{32}P]-labelled (e.g. antisense RNA) probe. Many abundant and moderately abundant mRNAs can be detected with high specific-activity probes in samples of total cellular RNA, while detection of the less abundant mRNAs may require the purification of poly(A)$^+$ mRNA. Messenger RNA usually comprises less than 5 per cent of the RNA of the cell. (The 18S and 28S ribosomal RNAs are by far the most prominent

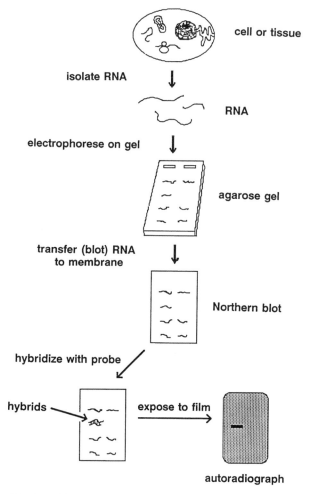

cell or tissue

isolate RNA

RNA

electrophorese on gel

agarose gel

transfer (blot) RNA
to membrane

Northern blot

hybridize with probe

hybrids

expose to film

autoradiograph

Fig. 1.4 *Northern blot hybridization.* mRNA is isolated and fractionated by agarose gel electrophoresis. It is then blotted on to a nitrocellulose or nylon membrane and hybridized with a radioactive probe (specific for an mRNA present in the sample in the left lane but absent in the right lane). The hybridized mRNA is detected by autoradiography.

RNA species resolved on agarose gels, and usually the only discrete RNA species observed by staining these gels for RNA. In contrast, the mRNA population is very heterogeneous in size and would appear as a faint smear through the gel lane, if it were visible at all after staining.) One round of oligo(dT)-cellulose chromatography can enrich for poly(A)$^+$ sequences approximately 10-fold (two or three rounds can provide further enrichment), and thus can allow a corresponding increase in the amount of mRNA that can be loaded on to a gel lane. Although there is a practical limit to the amount of RNA that can be applied to these gels (which places a limit on the sensitivy of the technique), Northern blotting should be able to detect mRNAs that are in the range of only a few copies per cell.

Northern hybridization can be used as a semi-quantitative approach for the comparison of one sample to another, if equal amounts or RNA are applied to each gel lane. Hybridization with the labelled probes is carried out in probe excess (with respect to the mRNA sequences being analysed) in order to saturate the complementary RNA sites on the nitrocellulose. After autoradiography, the hybridization signals can be quantitated by densitometry and compared to one another and to standards. The standards ensure that equal amounts of RNA were electrophoresed and transferred. The blots can be hybridized with an oligo probe specific for 18S ribosomal RNA if total RNA is analysed, or an antisense ribo-probe for a housekeeping enzyme such as GAPDH if poly(A)$^+$ RNA is analsyed.

Rates of RNA synthesis

Nuclear run-on transcription is a technique that involves the labelling of RNA transcripts to high specific activity in isolated nuclei, permitting the subsequent analysis of these labelled transcripts by nucleic acid hybridization with gene-specific probes (McKnight and Palmiter 1979; Lamers *et al.* 1982; Berger *et al.* 1986). Isolated nuclei are permeable to nucleoside triphosphates (NTPs) (the immediate precursors of RNA). Therefore, it is possible to get the incorporation of high specific-activity α-^{32}P-labelled NTPs directly into newly synthesizing RNA transcripts, without encountering the problems of getting a biosynthetic precursor specific to RNA into intact cells. At the time of isolation, nuclei are engaged in transcription, and thus have a number of active RNA polymerase molecules associated with certain genes. After isolation, the nuclei are incubated under conditions that support transcription. The RNA polymerases that were involved in transcription prior to isolation resume transcription and continue it (run-on) until they reach the ends of their respective genes. Thus, the nascent RNA molecules that were already initiated will get radioactively labelled, and the amount of label in any one RNA species will reflect the number or RNA polymerase molecules associated with gene at the time of nuclear isolation.

The transcriptional activities of the genes being studied by nuclear run-on transcription are analysed by blot hybridization. Blots are made on which cloned DNAs are affixed on nitrocellulose or nylon membranes. (The blots are usually made with a dot- or slot-forming manifold.) These blots are hybridized with labelled RNA from the run-on transcription step, and the amount of specifically hybridizing, labelled RNA is determined by autoradiography. The hybridization reaction is carried out with an excess of nucleic acid (cloned DNA) on the blot, so that hybridization of the labelled RNA goes to completion. As such, the intensity of the signal on each dot or slot reflects the number of transcripts on each of the active genes, and thus, their relative rates of transcription. The autoradiographs are quantitated by scanning densitometry of the X-ray films, or alternatively the blots can be directly quantitated by radioanalytic phospho-imaging systems.

Localization of gene expression

Most cells, tissues, and organs are amenable to analysis by the techniques of molecular biology, in large part by having highly specific nucleic acid and antibody probes. The techniques for the isolation and purification of intact RNA are now fairly standard and can be applied to a variety of tissues. These RNA preparations can be used to construct cDNA libraries, which can be screened in a number of ways to isolate tissue-specific clones. Once the clones are isolated, sequence information can be obtained for the preparation of antibodies. The clones can also be used to investigate gene expression in the tissue of origin, and in other cell types, tissues, and organs.

If cDNA clones and antibodies are utilized in conjunction with histological approaches (*in situ* hybridization and immunohistochemical localization), almost any cell can be studied. *In situ* hybridization can be used to assess steady-state mRNA levels in individual cells (Lawrence and Singer 1986) or in tissue sections (Angerer *et al.* 1987). Although there are a variety of approaches, it is now standard to use antisense RNA probes labelled with ^{35}S (Sulphur) NTPs, for sensitivity of detection and for microscopic resolution. Tissue sections are fixed and prepared for hybridization, incubated with the labelled probe, washed and treated with ribonuclease to remove unhybridized probe (hybridized probe is resistant to the RNase), and dipped in liquid autoradiographic emulsion. After exposure, the slides are developed, stained, and examined for silver grains over the tissue. The probe hybridizes directly to mRNA sequences, which can be present in individual cells at an abundance of only a few hundred copies up to thousands of copies (and higher) per cell.

Differential cDNA analysis

Analysis of gene expression by transcriptional run-on, Northern blotting, or *in situ* hybridization depends on having cloned DNA sequences to use as specific hybridization probes. This may require having some prior knowledge about what is expected to happen in the cell and the right clones. If it is believed that differences in gene expression exist between different cell types or in the same cell under different conditions, but it is not known what genes are differentially expressed, it should be possible to find these differences by differential cDNA screening, subtractive cloning, or mRNA differential display.

Differential cDNA screening

The principle behind differential screening (Sargent 1987; Lemke *et al.* 1993; Luo *et al.* 1994) is to compare mRNA populations (e.g. in cells that are induced and uninduced by a hormone or mitogen) utilizing a cDNA library specific to one population that is then differentially screened with labelled cDNA probes representing the two mRNA populations. Most of the mRNAs in the two populations will be the same. The objective is to find the ones that are different. A cDNA library constructed with the mRNA from the induced cells, for example, will contain clones for the mRNAs that are differentially expressed upon induction, as well as a large number of clones that are not unique to induced cells. If this library is screened with a population of labelled cDNAs that is made to the same mRNA population used to make the library, every clone, in theory, should hybridize. If, on the other hand, the library is screened with labelled cDNAs that are made to the mRNAs in the uninduced cell, the clones representing induced mRNAs will not hybridize. These are the clones being sought.

The cDNA library is plated out for screening, and duplicate nitrocellulose or nylon replicas of each plate are prepared for hybridization (Fig. 1.5). The cDNA probes are made by synthesizing first-strand cDNA copies of the mRNAs in the two populations in the presence of α-^{32}P dNTPs to label the cDNAs. Each of the duplicate membrane replicas is then hybridized with a different cDNA probe population, and the hybridization is analysed by autoradiography. The autoradiographs should line up with each other and with the original plate. If a hybridization signal is found on one film (hybridized with the induced cell cDNA) but not the other, it would be a candidate for a cDNA clone representing an induced mRNA. Differential screening can also be sensitive to quantitative changes in mRNA levels, and not simply to their presence or absence. Once positive clones are identified, they can be isolated and analysed in a

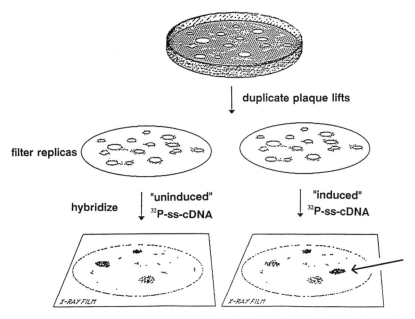

Fig. 1.5 *Differential cDNA library screening.* Duplicate plaque lifts are hybridized with labelled single-stranded (ss) cDNA probes made to the mRNAs in uninduced and induced cells. Plaques representing mRNAs present in both cell populations hybridize with both probes. A plaque representing an mRNA in the induced cells only is shown by the arrow.

number of ways to identify the proteins they encode and the roles these proteins have in cell function.

Subtractive cloning

Subtractive cloning provides a means to enrich a cDNA library for differentially expressed sequences, during the process of constructing it (Sargent 1987). To isolate clones representing genes that are specifically expressed in induced cells, for example, single-stranded cDNAs are synthesized using the induced cell mRNA population. These cDNAs are then hybridized in solution to an excess of mRNA (driver RNA) from uninduced cells. The cDNA sequences representing mRNAs expressed in common will hybridize, while those that are unique to the induced cells will remain single-stranded. The hybrids can then be removed using any number of methods. One method makes use of photobiotin-labelled driver RNA. Following hybridization, streptavidin is bound to the cDNA-biotinylated RNA hybrids, and the hybrid–protein complexes are subsequently removed by phenol–chloroform extraction, leaving the single-stranded cDNAs in the aqueous phase (Sive and St.John 1988; Rubenstein *et al.* 1990). These cDNAs are recovered, hybridized back to mRNA and made into double-stranded cDNA using the RNase H technique, and cloned.

A variation of the subtraction method makes use of phagemid vectors to produce cloned single-stranded, complementary inserts representing the two mRNA populations being subtracted (Duguid *et al.* 1988; Rubenstein *et al.* 1990). Phagemids have the capacity to generate single-stranded recombinant phage-insert sequences specific for one or the other strand. The cDNA libraries are directionally cloned into the phagemids, with the inserts for one mRNA population in the opposite orientation to those for the other mRNA population. Single-stranded, complementary DNAs are generated from the two libraries. If induced cell cDNAs are being sought, these sequences would be hybridized to an excess of a biotin-labelled complementary-strand cDNA preparation representing the uninduced cell. Hybrids would then be removed by streptavidin–biotin affinity column or streptavidin–phenol extraction, leaving the single-stranded induced cell cDNA.

mRNA differential display

Another technique for the rapid identification and isolation of differentially expressed sequences is mRNA differential display (Liang and Pardee 1992; Liang *et al.* 1993) or arbitrarily primed PCR (Welsh *et al.* 1992; Ralph *et al.* 1993). This method makes use of the sensitivity and specificity of the polymerase chain reaction (PCR) (Arnheim and Erlich 1992) and does not require the construction of cDNA libraries. PCR makes use of two priming oligonucleotides that flank a sequence region by hybridizing to sites on the complementary strands. The primers are annealed to the DNA strands and extended by DNA synthesis. Repeated cycles of denaturation, annealing, and synthesis are carried out in a chain reaction, such that the newly synthesized strands are used as templates for further DNA synthesis, exponentially increasing the number of DNA copies of the target region. The process makes use of a heat-stable DNA polymerase, for example from *Thermus aquaticus* (Taq polymerase), which does not require the addition of new enzyme after each round of denaturation (Kogan *et al.* 1987; Orkin 1987; Saiki *et al.* 1988), and permits a 200,000-fold or greater amplification of very small amounts of DNA.

Differentially expressed mRNAs are identified by carrying out cDNA synthesis and subsequent PCR with sets of short oligonucleotide primers of aribitrary sequence (Fig. 1.6). PCR products generated from different populations of mRNA are then compared in a side-by-side fashion following electrophoresis in adjacent lanes of a DNA sequencing gel. PCR bands containing different amounts of DNA indicate levels of a particular sequence in the two mRNA

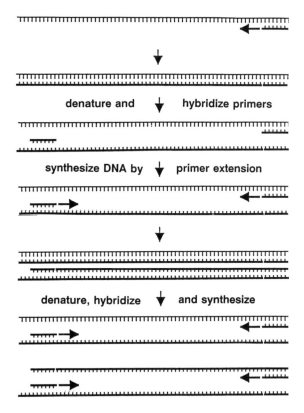

Fig. 1.6 *Reverse transcriptase PCR.* mRNA (thin line) is reverse transcribed using a downstream primer (right). The mRNA–DNA hybrid is then denatured and downstream and upstream (left) primers are hybridized. DNA (thick lines) is then synthesized in both directions by primer extension (arrows) giving rise to another mRNA–DNA hybrid and a double-stranded DNA product. The cycle is then repeated by denaturation, primer hybridization, synthesis, etc., giving rise ultimately to amplified double-stranded copies of the original mRNA.

populations. mRNA preparations from the sources being compared are used as templates for the synthesis of cDNA in a reverse transcriptase-catalysed reaction (RT-PCR or reverse-transcriptase PCR). However, instead of using oligo(dT) for the downstream primer, a set of four anchored primers is used. These primers have the degenerate sequence $5'$-d(T)$_{12}$(A,G,C)N-$3'$ (where N is either A,C,G, or T), and thus should recognize all of the mRNAs in the population. The d(T)$_{12}$ region of the oligos will guide the primers to the poly(A) tail of the mRNAs, and the two $3'$-most nucleotides will ensure that cDNA synthesis starts at exactly the same point adjacent to the poly(A) tail on each mRNA (and PCR product) at each round of synthesis. Each of the anchored primers is then paired with a specific (but arbitrary) upstream 10-mer for PCR (Welsh *et al.* 1992). The amplified DNA is labelled with ^{35}S for optimal resolution on a sequencing gel.

Since only a finite number of PCR products can be displayed on a DNA sequencing gel, a survey of all the mRNAs in a population might require in the order of 20 different upstream primers, each paired with one of the four anchored primers, for a total of about 80 reactions. While the primers are expected to hybridize with considerable mismatching, this interaction (if sufficiently stable) is also specific enough to reproducibly generate discrete-sized PCR products. Analysis of differentially displayed sequences requires isolation of the PCR-generated DNA by cutting out the band from the gel, eluting the DNA, re-amplifying, and re-gel purifying. This DNA is then cloned, so that it can be sequenced and to make probes for Northern blot analysis. One of the advantages of differential display is that comparisons can easily be made between more than two RNA sources, since separate reactions are displayed on adjacent lanes of a sequencing gel (Liang *et al.* 1993).

Partially sequencing the cDNAs is usually sufficient to permit them to be tentatively identified. It is convenient to sequence a short region of about 100–200 nucleotides at each end of the cDNA clone and to then carry out a sequence homology analysis by sending the sequences to the GenBank nucleic acid acid database. If a match is obtained, the clone has been identified, and if no match is found, the clone may represent a new gene that might warrant further sequence analysis.

Gene expression *in vitro*

Studies of gene expression in higher organisms have made use of a wide variety of methods, including a large number of *in vitro* systems for the experimental analysis of gene function. All *in vitro* systems suffer the disadvantage that they are only close (and not identical) to the *in vivo* state. However, their convenience far outweighs this drawback. It is well recognized that cells take on new characteristics almost immediately upon being placed in culture (Jefferson *et al.* 1984), and that they can easily adapt to culture conditions to the extent, in some cases, that they hardly resemble their parent cell. Whether this is a manifestation of changes imposed on the cells by the culture conditions, or the selection of cells that become mutated and gain an advantage, is not clear. However, it is known that these changes in phenotype are a reflection of changes that occur in the expression of their genes. Despite this, cells in culture also retain many of their original characteristics and often express differentiated cell functions, such as regulated transport, hormone responsiveness (Taub 1985), or morphogenetic differentiation (Montesano *et al.* 1991*a*,*b*). Cells in culture utilize established biochemical pathways, and thus, it is presumed that what is learned about molecular control mechanisms *in vitro*, should be relevant to mechanisms at work *in vivo*.

Cells *in vitro* can be manipulated by induction of growth or differentiation (Adamson 1987). In many cases, the response to mitogens or differentiating agents can be analysed at the gene level by quantitating the amounts of certain mRNAs by Northern blot hybridization, by carrying out transcription studies, or by identifying induced genes by differential cDNA cloning. Once genes have been identified by this type of analysis, their functions can be tested *in vitro* in the same cells, or *in vivo* by looking for their expression (and action) in the original cell type.

Gene function can be studied by the manipulation of the gene of interest, followed by its introduction into cells where its expression can be monitored (Rosenthal 1987). There are three basic objectives to these types of studies: (1) to mutate putative control regions to test their function; (2) to mutate translated regions to analyse the functions of amino acid sequence domains; and (3) to express (mutated or unmutated) genes to determine their functions in the cell. Genes are introduced into cells by a variety of means. Among the simplest and most reliable techniques are calcium phosphate and DEAE–dextran-mediated transfection and electroporation. DNA (also mRNA and protein) can also be introduced into cells by microinjection. This is fairly simple with oocytes, because of their large size. Amphibian oocytes will support the functions of the foreign DNA by transcribing it, translating its mRNA, and processing the protein product (Dawid and Sargent 1988). Alternatively, mRNA can be injected directly into the egg cytoplasm where it will be translated into a protein product that can be assayed immunologically or by monitoring its function (Melton 1987).

Studies of gene expression frequently lead to questions of how a particular gene is regulated. One approach to this question is to analyse the promoter of the gene for *cis*-acting regulatory elements and to determine the transcription factors that may be regulating that promoter. If the analysis started with the isolation of a cDNA, it will be necessary to use that cDNA to screen for the gene itself. In this case, a fragment representing the 5′ end of the cDNA is used as a probe to screen for genomic clones. This will ensure that clones containing the upstream region containing the promoter will be isolated.

Deletion studies can then be carried out with the isolated promoter by making use of a promoter–reporter construct that is active in transfected cells. This construct would consist of the promoter region placed adjacent to a reporter gene whose product can be easily assayed. Frequently used reporter genes include bacterial chloramphenicol acetyltransferase (CAT) (Prost and Moore 1986) and firefly luciferase (Williams *et al.* 1989). Deletions that remove small regions of the promoter (Poncz *et al.* 1982; Henikoff 1987) are then tested in transient transfection assays to localize sites that significantly effect the expression of the reporter gene. If the promoter is thought to be under the regulation of a particular external stimulus, it is also possible to determine at what promoter site a deletion confers loss of responsiveness to the inducer. It is frequently possible to find important promoter regions by deletion analysis and to then sequence those regions and identify conserved DNA motifs specific for known transcription factors.

To further establish the identity of a site, or in cases where a site cannot be identified by its sequence alone, protein-mapping and DNA-binding experiments can be carried out. One approach is DNase I footprinting (Brenowitz *et al.* 1986). With this technique, the promoter DNA (labelled at one end) is mixed with a nuclear extract (or purified protein) to allow the transcription factors to bind their sites. The DNA–protein complex is then digested with DNase I such that on average only one cut per molecule is made. The randomly cut fragments are then resolved on a DNA sequencing gel, which will reveal regions of DNA-binding as protected sites along the sequence. Gel-shift or gel-retardation (also called EMSA for electrophoretic mobility shift assay) can then be used to confirm the binding of factors to the sequence region (Chodosh *et al.* 1986). In this case, a short oligonucleotide is labelled and mixed with the nuclear extract or purified factors being tested. Following binding, the mixture is electrophoresed in a non-denaturing polyacrylamide gel to resolve the DNA–protein complexes from the unbound DNA. The higher molecular weight of the DNA–protein complex causes a retarded mobility in the gel which shifts the position of the autoradiographic band. The identity of the bound transcription factors is then confirmed by antibody supershift in which an oligo is first incubated with the nuclear extract and subsequently with an antibody to the transcription factor. The increased molecular weight of the DNA–protein complex results in further retardation in the gel and hence a supershift.

Acknowledgements

The author thanks Robin Maser for help with the figures.

References

Adamson, E. D. (1987). Trends in teratotocarcinoma research. In *Control of animal cell proliferation*, (ed. A. L. Boynton and H. L. Leffert), Vol. 2, pp. 37–72. Academic Press, Orlando, FL.

Angerer, L. M., Cox, K. H., and Angerer, R. C. (1987). Demonstration of tissue-specific gene expression by in situ hybridization. *Methods in Enzymology*, **152**, 649–61.

Alt. F. W., *et al.* (1980). Synthesis of secreted and membrane-bound immunoglobulin μ heavy chains is directed by mRNAs that differ at their 3′ ends. *Cell*, **20**, 293–301.

Alting-Mees, M., Sorge, J. A., and Short, J. M. (1992). pBluescriptII: multifunctional cloning and mapping vectors. *Methods in Enzymology*, **216**, 483–95.

Alwine, J. C., Kemp, D. J., and Stark, G. R. (1977). Method for detection of specific RNAs in agarose gels by transfer to diazobenzyloxymethyl-paper and hybridization with DNA probes. *Proceedings of the National Academy of Sciences USA*, **74**, 5350–4.

Andreadis, A., Gallego, M. E., and Nadal-Ginard, B. (1987). Generation of protein isoform diversity by alternative splicing: Mechanistic and biological implications. *Annual Review of Cell Biology*, **3**, 207–42.

Angel, P., *et al.* (1987). Phorbol ester-inducible genes contain a common cis element recognized by a TPA-modulated trans-acting factor. *Cell*, **49**, 729–39.

Arber, W. (1979). Promotion and limitation of genetic exchange. *Science*, **205**, 361–5.

Arnheim, N. and Erlich, H. (1992). Polymerase chain reaction strategy. *Annual Review of Biochemistry*, **61**, 131–56.

Atchison, M. L. (1988). Enhancers: mechanisms of action and cell specificity. *Annual Review of Cell Biology*, **4**, 127–53.

Ausubel, F. M., *et al.* (ed.) (1994). *Current protocols in molecular biology*, Vols 1 and 2. Wiley, New York.

Benton, W. D. and Davis, R. W. (1977). Screening λgt recombinant clones by hybridization to single plaques in situ. *Science*, **196**, 180–2.

Berger, F. G., Loose, D., Meisner, H., and Watson, G. (1986). Androgen induction of messenger RNA concentrations in mouse kidney is posttranscriptional. *Biochemistry*, **25**, 1170–5.

Berger, S. L. and Kimmel, A. R. (ed.) (1987). *Guide to molecular cloning techniques. Methods in enzymology*, Vol. 152. Academic Press, Orlando, FL.

Brawerman, G. (1987). Determinants of mRNA stability. *Cell*, **48**, 5–6.

Breitbart, R. E., Andreadis, A., and Nadal-Ginard, B. (1987). Alternative splicing: A ubiquitous mechanism for the generation of multiple protein isoforms from single genes. *Annual Review of Biochemistry*, **56**, 467–95.

Brenowitz, M, Senear, D. F., Shea, M. A., and Ackers, G. K. (1986). Quantitative DNase I footprint titration: A method for studying protein-DNA interactions. *Methods in Enzymology*, **130**, 132–81.

Brock, M. L. and Shapiro, D. J. (1983). Estrogen stabilizes vitellogenin mRNA against cytoplasmic degradation. *Cell*, **34**, 207–14.

Brooks, J. E. (1987). Properties and uses of restriction endonucleases. *Methods in Enzymology*, **152**, 113–29.

Calvet, J. P. (1990). Molecular biology, gene expression, and medicine. In *Inheritance of kidney and urinary tract diseases*, (ed. A. Spitzer and E. D. Avner), pp. 3–51. Kluwer, Boston.

Campo, M. S. (1985). Bovine papillomavirus DNA: A eukaryotic cloning vector. In *DNA cloning: A practical approach*, (ed. D. M. Glover), Vol. 2, pp. 213–38. IRL Press, Oxford.

Chodosh, L. A., Carthew R. W., and Sharp, P. A. (1986). A single polypeptide possesses the binding and activities of the adenovirus major late transcription factor. *Molecular and Cellular Biology*, **6**, 4723–33.

Clarke, L. and Carbon, J. (1976). A colony bank containing synthetic Col El hybrid plasmids representative of the entire *E. coli* genome. *Cell*, **9**, 91–9.

Clemens, M. J. (1987). A potential role for RNA transcribed from B2 repeats in the regulation of mRNA stability. *Cell*, **49**, 157–8.

Collins, J. and Hohn, B. (1979). Cosmids: A type of plasmid gene-cloning vector that is packageable in vitro in bacteriophage λ heads. *Proceedings of the National Academy of Sciences USA*, **75**, 4242–6.

Conaway, J. W. and Conaway, R. C. (1991). Initiation of eukaryotic mRNA synthesis. *Journal of Biological Chemistry*, **266**, 17721–4.

Conaway, R. C. and Conaway, J. W. (1993). General initiation factors for RNA polymerase II. *Annual Review of Biochemistry*, **62**, 161–90.

Cullen, B. R. (1987). Use of eukaryotic expression technology in the functional analysis of cloned genes. *Methods in Enzymology*, **152**, 684–704.

Dahl, H. H., Flavell, R. A., and Grosveld, F. G. (1981). The use of genomic libraries for the isolation and study of eukaryotic genes. In *Genetic engineering*, (ed. R. Williamson), Vol. 2, pp. 49–127. Academic Press, New York.

Daum, G., Eisenmann-Tappe, I., Fries, H. W., Troppmair, J., and Rapp, U. R. (1994). The ins and outs of Raf kinases. *Trends in Biochemical Sciences*, **19**, 474–80.

Davis, R. J. (1994). MAPKs: new JNK expands the group. *Trends in Biochemical Sciences*, **19**, 470–3.

Dawid, I. B. and Sargent, T. D. (1988). *Xenopus laevis* in developmental and molecular biology. *Science*, **240**, 1443–8.

Decker, C. J. and Parker, R. (1994). Mechanisms of mRNA degradation in eukaryotes. *Trends in Biochemical Sciences*, **19**, 336–40.

Duguid, J. R., Rohwer, R. G., and Seed, B. (1988). Isolation of cDNAs of scrapie-modulated RNAs by subtractive hybridization of a cDNA library. *Proceedings of the National Academy of Sciences USA*, **85**, 5738–42.

Dynan, W. S. and Tijan, R. (1985). Control of eukaryotic messenger RNA synthesis by sequence-specific DNA-binding proteins. *Nature*, **316**, 774–8.

Early, P., *et al.* (1980). Two mRNAs can be produced from a single immunoglobulin m gene by alternative RNA processing pathways. *Cell*, **20**, 313–19.

Feinberg, A. P. and Vogelstein, B. (1983). A technique for radiolabeling DNA restriction endonuclease fragments to high specific activity. *Analytical Biochemistry*, **132**, 6–13.

Fields, C., Adams, M. D., White, O., and Venter, J. C. (1994). How many genes in the human genome? *Nature Genetics*, **7**, 345–6.

Glover, D. M. (ed.) (1985). *DNA cloning: A practical approach*, Vols 1 and 2. IRL Press, Oxford.

Gorman, C. (1985). High efficiency gene transfer into mammalian cells. In *DNA cloning: A practical approach*, (ed. D. M. Glover) Vol. 2, pp. 143–90. IRL Press, Oxford.

Graham, F. and Van der Eb, L. (1973). A new technique for the assay of infectivity of human adenovirus 5 DNA. *Virology*, **52**, 1156–67.

Grunstein, M. and Hogness, D. S. (1975). Colony hybridization: A method for the isolation of cloned DNAs that contain a specific gene. *Proceedings of the National Academy of Sciences USA*, **72**, 3961–5.

Gubler, U. (1987). Second-strand cDNA synthesis: mRNA fragments as primers. *Methods in Enzymology*, **152**, 330–5.

Hagen, F. S., Gray, C. L., and Kuijper, J. L. (1988). Assaying the quality of cDNA libraries. *BioTechniques*, **6**, 340–5.

Hames, B. D. and Higgins, S. J. (ed.) (1985). *Nucleic acid hybridisation: A practical approach*. IRL Press, Oxford.

Hanahan, D. and Meselson, M. (1980). Plasmid screening at high density. *Gene*, **10**, 63–7.

Helfman, D. M., Fiddes, J. C., and Hanahan, D. (1987). Directional cDNA cloning in plasmid vectors by sequential addition of oligonucleotide linkers. *Methods in Enzymology*, **152**, 349–59.

Henikoff, S. (1987). Unidirectional digestion with exonuclease III in DNA sequence analysis. *Methods in Enzymology*, 155, 156–65.

Hod, Y. and Hanson, R. W. (1988). Cyclic AMP stabilizes the mRNA for phospho-enolpyruvate carboxykinase (GTP) against degradation. *Journal of Biological Chemistry*, 263, 7747–52.

Hohn, B. and Murray, K. (1977). Packaging recombinant DNA molecules into bacteriophage particles in vitro. *Proceedings of the National Academy of Sciences USA*, 74, 3259–63.

Hudson, B. G., Reeders, S. T., and Tryggvason, K. (1993). Type IV collagen: Structure, gene organization, and role in human diseases. *Journal of Biological Chemistry*, 268, 26033–6.

Jacobson, A. (1987). Purification and fractionation of poly(A)⁺ RNA. *Methods in Enzymology*, 152, 254–61.

Jefferson, D. M., Clayton, D. F., Darnell, J. E. Jr, and Reid, L. M. (1984). Post-transcriptional modulation of gene expression in cultured rat hepatocytes. *Molecular and Cellular Biology*, 4, 1929–34.

Jendrisak, J., Young, R. A., and Engel, J. D. (1987). Cloning cDNA into λgt10 and λgt11. *Methods in Enzymology*, 152, 359–71.

Jinno, Y., Merlino, G. T., and Pastan, I. (1988). A novel effect of EGF on mRNA stability. *Nucleic Acids Research*, 16, 4957–66.

Johnson, P. F. and McKnight, S. L. (1989). Eukaryotic transcriptional regulatory proteins. *Annual Review of Biochemistry*, 58, 799–839.

Jones, K. A., Kadonaga, J. T., Rosenfeld, P. J., Kelley, T. J., and Tjian, R. (1987). A cellular DNA-binding protein that activates eukaryotic transcription and DNA replication. *Cell*, 48, 79–89.

Kadonaga, J. T., Jones, K. A., and Tijan, R. (1986). Promoter-specific activation of RNA polymerase II transcription by Sp1. *Trends in Biochemical Sciences*, 11, 20–3.

Kaiser, K. and Murray, N. E. (1985). The use of phage lambda replacement vectors in the construction of representative genomic DNA libraries. In *DNA cloning: A practical approach*, (ed. D. M. Glover), Vol. 1, pp. 1–47. IRL Press, Oxford.

Khoury, G. and Gruss, P. (1983). Enhancer elements. *Cell*, 33, 313–14.

Kimmel, A. R. (1987). Selection of clones from libraries: Overview. *Methods in Enzymology*, 152, 393–99.

King, C. R. and Piatigorski, J. (1984). Alternative splicing of αA-crystallin RNA: Structural and quantitative analyses of the mRNAs for the αA2- and αAins-crystallin polypeptides. *Journal of Biological Chemistry*, 259, 1822–6.

Kogan, S. C., Doherty, M., and Gitschier, J. (1987). An improved method for prenatal diagnosis of genetic disease by analysis of amplified DNA sequences: Application to hemophilia A. *New England Journal of Medicine*, 317, 985–90.

Kozak, M. (1991a). An analysis of vertebrate mRNA sequences: intimations of transla-tional control. *Journal of Cell Biology*, 115, 887–903.

Kozak, M. (1991b). Structural features in eukaryotic mRNAS that modulate the initiation of translation. *Journal of Biological Chemistry*, 266, 19867–70.

Kozak, M. (1994). Features in the 5′ non-coding sequences of rabbit alpha and beta-globin mRNAs that affect translational efficiency. *Journal of Molecular Biology*, 235, 95–110.

Krieg, P. A. and Melton, D. A. (1984). Functional messenger RNAs are produced by SP6 in vitro transcription of cloned cDNAs. *Nucleic Acids Research*, 12, 7057–70.

Krug, M. S. and Berger, S. L. (1987). First-strand cDNA synthesis primed with oligo(dT). *Methods in Enzymology*, **152**, 316–25.

Lamers, W. H., Hanson, R. W., and Meisner, H. M. (1982). cAMP stimulates transcription of the gene for cytosolic phosphoenolpyruvate carboxykinase in rat liver nuclei. *Proceedings of the National Academy of Sciences USA*, **79**, 5137–41.

Lau, Y.-F. and Kan, Y. W. (1983). Versatile cosmid vectors for the isolation, expression, and rescue of gene sequences: Studies with the human α-globin gene cluster. *Proceedings of the National Academy of Sciences USA*, **80**, 5225–9.

Lawn, R. M., Fritsch, E. F., Parker, R. C., Blake, G., and Maniatis, T. (1978). The isolation and characterization of linked δ- and β-globin genes from a cloned library of human DNA. *Cell*, **15**, 1157–74.

Lawrence, J. B. and Singer, R. H. (1986). Intracellular localization of messenger RNAs for cytoskeletal proteins. *Cell*, **45**, 407–15.

Lee, W., Mitchell, P., and Tjian, R. (1987). Purified transcription factor AP-1 interacts with TPA-inducible enhance elements. *Cell*, **49**, 741–52.

Leff, S. E., Rosenfeld, M. G., and Evans, R. M. (1986). Complex transcriptional units: Diversity in gene expression by alternative RNA processing. *Annual Review of Biochemistry*, **55**, 1091–117.

Lemke, S. J., *et al.* (1993). SPOT: An improved differential screening protocol that allows the detection of marginally induced mRNAs. *BioTechniques*, **14**, 415–19.

Liang, P. and Pardee, A. B. (1992). Differential display of eukaryotic messenger RNA by means of the polymerase chain reaction. *Science*, **257**, 967–71.

Liang, P., Averboukh, L., and Pardee, A. B. (1993). Distribution and cloning of eukaryotic mRNAs by means of differential display: Refinements and optimization. *Nucleic Acids Research*, **21**, 3269–75.

Lucas, P. C. and Granner, D. K. (1992). Hormone response domains in gene transcription. *Annual Review of Biochemistry*, **61**, 1131–73.

Luo, G., An, G., and Wu, R. (1994). A PCR differential screening method for rapid isolation of clones from a cDNA library. *BioTechniques*, **16**, 670–75.

Maniatis T., *et al.*, (1978). The isolation of structural genes from libraries of eukaryotic DNA. *Cell*, **15**, 687–701.

Maniatis, T., Goodbourn, S., and Fischer, J. A. (1987). Regulation of inducible and tissue-specific gene expression. *Science*, **236**, 1237–45.

Marmur, J. (1994). DNA strand separation, renaturation and hybridization. *Trends in Biochemical Sciences*, **19**, 343–6.

McKnight, G. S. and Palmiter, R. D. (1979). Transcriptional regulation of the ovalbumin and conalbumin genes by steroid hormones in chick oviduct. *Journal of Biological Chemistry*, 9050–8.

Meinkoth, J. and Wahl, G. M. (1987). Nick translation. *Methods in Enzymology*, **152**, 91–4.

Melton, D. A. (1987). Translation of messenger RNA in injected frog oocytes. *Methods in Enzymology*, **152**, 288–96.

Melton, D. A., Krieg, P. A., Rebagliati, M. R., Maniatis, T., Zinn, K., and Green, M. R. (1984). Efficient in vitro synthesis of biologically active RNA and RNA hybridization probes from plasmids containing a bacteriophage SP6 promoter. *Nucleic Acids Research*, **12**, 7035–56.

Miller, L. K. (1988). Baculoviruses as gene expression vectors. *Annual Review of Microbiology*, **42**, 177–99.

Miller, A. D., Ong, E. S., Rosenfeld, M. G. Verma, I. M., and Evans, R. M. (1984). Infectious and selectable retrovirus containing an inducible rat growth hormone minigene. *Science*, **225**, 993–8.

Montesano, R., Schaller, G., and Orci, L. (1991*a*). Induction of epithelial tubular morphogenesis in vitro by fibroblast-derived soluble factors. *Cell*, **66**, 697–711.

Montesano, R., Matsumoto, K., Nakamura, T., and Orci, L. (1991*b*). Identification of a fibroblast-derived epithelial morphogen as hepatocyte growth factor. *Cell*, **67**, 901–8.

Mulligan, R. C. and Berg, P. (1980). Expression of a bacterial gene in mammalian cells. *Science*, **209**, 1422–7.

Nathans, D. (1979). Restriction endonucleases, simian virus 40 and the new genetics. *Science*, **206**, 903–9.

Orkin, S. H. (1987). Genetic diagnosis by DNA analysis. *New England Journal of Medicine*, **317**, 1023–25.

Orkin, S. H. and Kazazian, H. H. Jr (1984). Mutation and polymorphism of the human β-globin gene and its surrounding DNA. *Annual Review of Genetics*, **18**, 131–71.

Pabo, C. O. and Sauer, R. T. (1992). Transcription factors: Structural families and principles of DNA recognition. *Annual Review of Biochemistry*, **61**, 1053–95.

Pavlakis, G. N. and Hamer, D. H. (1983). Regulation of a metallothionein-growth hormone hybrid gene in bovine papilloma virus. *Proceedings of the National Academy of Sciences USA*, **80**, 397–401.

Poncz, M., Solowiejczyk, D., Ballantine, M., Swartz, E., and Surrey, S. (1982). 'Nonrandom' DNA sequence analysis in bacteriophage M13 by the dideoxy chain-termination method. *Proceedings of the National Academy of Sciences USA*, **79**, 4298–302.

Potter, H., Weir, L., and Leder, P. (1984). Enhancer-dependent expression of human κ immunoglobulin genes introduced into mouse pre-B lymphocytes by electroporation. *Proceedings of the National Academy of Sciences USA*, **81**, 7161–5.

Prost, E. and Moore, D. D. (1986). CAT vectors for analysis of eukaryotic promoters and enhancers. *Gene*, **45**, 107–11.

Ptashne, M. (1988). How eukaryotic transcriptional activators work. *Nature*, **335**, 683–9.

Raghow, R. (1987). Regulation of messenger RNA turnover in eukaryotes. *Trends in Biochemical Sciences*, **12**, 358–60.

Raghow, R., Postlethwaite, A. E., Keski-Oja, J., Moses, H. L., and Kang, A. H. (1987). Transforming growth factor-b increases steady state levels of type I procollagen and fibronectin messenger RNAs posttranscriptionally in cultured human dermal fibroblasts. *Journal of Clinical Investigation*, **79**, 1285–8.

Ralph, D., McClelland, M., and Welsh, J. (1993). RNA fingerprinting using arbitrarily primed PCR identifies differentially regulated RNAs in mink lung (MvlLu) cells growth arrested by transforming growth factor beta 1. *Proceedings of the National Academy of Sciences USA*, **90**, 10710–14.

Rigby, P. W. J., Dieckmann, M., Rhodes, C., and Berg, P. (1977). Labelling deoxyribonucleic acid to high specific activity in vitro by nick translation with DNA polymerase I. *Journal of Molecular Biology*, **113**, 237–51.

Roberts, R. J. (1988). Restriction enzymes and their isoschizomers. *Nucleic Acids Research*, **16**, r271–313.

Roberts, R. G., Coffey, A. J., Bobrow, M., and Bentley, D. R. (1993). Exon structure of the human dystrophin gene. *Genomics*, **16**, 536–8.

Rogers, J., Early, P., Carter, C., Calame, K., Bond, M., Hood, L., and Wall, R. (1980). Two mRNAs with different 3′ ends encode membrane-bound and secreted forms of immunoglobulin m chain. *Cell*, **20**, 303–12.

Rosenthal, N. (1987). Identification of regulatory elements of cloned genes with functional assays. *Methods in Enzymology*, **152**, 704–20.

Rubenstein, J. L. R., Brice, A. E. J., Ciaranello, R. D., Denney, D., Porteus, M. H., and Usdin, T. B. (1990). Subtractive hybridization system using single-stranded phagemids with directional inserts. *Nucleic Acids Research*, **18**, 4833–42.

Sachs, A. and Wahle, E. (1993). Poly(A) metabolism and function in eukaryotes. *Journal of Biological Chemistry*, **268**, 22955–8.

Saiki, R. K., *et al.* (1988). Primer-directed enzymatic amplification of DNA with a thermostable DNA polymerase. *Science*, **239**, 487–91.

Sambrook, J., Fritsch, E. F., and Maniatis, T. (1989). *Molecular cloning: A laboratory manual*. Cold Spring Harbor Laboratory Press.

Sargent, T. D. (1987). Isolation of differentially expressed genes. *Methods in Enzymology*, **152**, 423–32.

Sarver, N., Gruss, P., Law, M.-F., Khoury, G., and Howley, P. M. (1981). Bovine papilloma virus deoxyribonucleic acid: A novel eukaryotic cloning vector. *Molecular and Cellular Biology*. **1**, 486–96.

Sawadogo, M. and Roeder, R. G. (1985). Interaction of a gene-specific transcription factor with the adenovirus major late promoter upstream of the TATA box region. *Cell*, **43**, 165–75.

Schleif, R. (1988). DNA binding by proteins. *Science*, **241**, 1182–7.

Schwarzbauer, J. E., Tamkun, J. W., Lemischka, I. R., and Hynes, R. O. (1983). Three different fibronectin mRNAs arise by alternative splicing within the coding region. *Cell*, **35**, 421–31.

Sharp, P. (1994). Split genes and RNA splicing. *Cell*, **77**, 805–15.

Shatzman, A. R. and Rosenberg, M. (1987). Expression, identification, and characterization of recombinant gene products in Escherichia coli. *Methods in Enzymology*, **152**, 661–73.

Shaw, G. and Kamen, R. (1986). A conserved AU sequence from the 3′ untranslated region of GM-CSF mRNA mediates selective mRNA degradation. *Cell*, 46, 659–67.

Short, J. M. and Sorge, J. A. (1992). In vivo excision properties of bacteriophage λ ZAP expression vectors. *Methods in Enzymology*, **216**, 495–508.

Sive, H. L. and St. John, T. (1988). A simple subtractive hybridization technique employing photoactivatable biotin and phenol extraction. *Nucleic Acids Research*, **16**, 10937.

Smith, H. O. (1979). Nucleotide sequence specificity of restriction endonucleases. *Science*, **205**, 455–62.

Taub, M. (ed.) (1985). *Tissue culture of epithelial cells*. Plenum, New York.

Tsai, M. J. and O'Malley, B. W. (1994). Molecular mechanisms of action of steroid/thyroid receptor superfamily members. *Annual Review of Biochemistry*, **63**, 451–86.

Takami, H., Burbelo, P. D., Fukuda, K., Chang, H. S., Phillips, S. L., and Yamada, Y. (1994). Molecular organization and gene regulation of type IV collagen. *Contributions in Nephrology*, **107**, 36–46.

Wahl, G. M. and Berger, S. L. (1987). Screening colonies or plaques with radioactive nucleic acid probes. *Methods in Enzymology*, **152**, 415–23.

Wahl, G. M., Berger, S. L., and Kimmel, A. R. (1987). Molecular hybridization of immobilized nucleic acids: Theoretical concepts and practical considerations. *Methods in Enzymology*, **152**, 399–407.

Wahle, E. and Keller, W. (1992). The biochemistry of 3′-end cleavage and polyadenylation of messenger RNA precursors. *Annual Review of Biochemistry*, **61**, 419–40.

Wallace, R. B. and Miyada, C. G. (1987). Oligonucleotide probes for the screening of recombinant DNA libraries. *Methods in Enzymology*, **152**, 432–42.

Wassarman, D. A. and Steitz, J. A. (1992). Interactions of small nuclear RNA's with precursor messenger RNA during in vitro splicing. *Science*, **257**, 1918–25.

Welsh, J., *et al.* (1992). Arbitrarily primed PCR fingerprinting of RNA. *Nucleic Acids Research*, **20**, 4965–70.

Williams, J. G. (1981). The preparation and screening of a cDNA clone bank. In *Genetic engineering*, (ed. R. Williamson), Vol. 1, pp. 1–59. Academic Press, New York.

Williams, B. G. and Blattner, F. R. (1979). Construction and characterization of the hybrid bacteriophage lambda Charon vectors for DNA cloning. *Journal of Virology*, **29**, 555–75.

Williams, T. M., Buerlein J. E., Ogden, S., Kricka, L. J., and Kant, J. A. (1989). Advantages of the firefly luciferase as a reporter gene: Application to the interleukin-2 gene promoter. *Analytical Biochemistry*, **176**, 28–32.

Wormington, M. (1993). Poly(A) and translation: development control. *Current Opinion in Cell Biology*, **5**, 950–4.

Wu, R. (1994). Development of the primer-extension approach: A key role in DNA sequencing. *Trends in Biochemical Sciences*, **19**, 429–33.

Wu, R., Wu, T., and Ray, A. (1987). Adaptors, linkers, and methylation. *Methods in Enzymology*, **152**, 343–9.

Young, R. A., Hagenbuchle, O., and Schibler, U. (1981). A single mouse α-amylase gene specifies two different tissue specific mRNAs. *Cell*, **23**, 451–8.

2

In vitro models in the study of renal cystogenesis

Roberto Mangoo-Karim, Lawrence P. Sullivan, Min Ye, and Jared J. Grantham

Introduction

Epithelial cyst configuration is a physiological design in the function of certain organs such as ovarian follicles, thyroid follicles, and blastocysts. Similarly, the cylindrical design of nephrons and collecting ducts and the juxtaposition of renal tubules and microvessels are essential for proper renal function. In the kidney, however, the cyst phenotype deriving from tubules is distinctly abnormal. These pathological structures distort the functional, vascular, and structural integrity of the kidney, and are associated in many instances with the progressive deterioration of renal function. Polycystic kidney disease encompasses a spectrum of clinical conditions that have renal enlargement secondary to cyst expansion as a common feature.

The autosomal dominant pattern of inheritance (ADPKD) is the most prevalent genetic form of the disease, accounting for approximately 6–10 per cent of patients with end-stage renal disease. A rarer but more aggressive form of hereditary cystic disease is seen in infants. Autosomal recessive polycystic kidney disease (ARPKD) is characterized by collecting duct cyst development, hepatic fibrosis, and death early in life. However, an heritable predisposition is not a requirement for cyst formation since an acquired form of the disease occurs in chronically scarred kidneys with an apparent normal genome (Grantham 1991). Therefore, hypotheses of renal cystic disease pathophysiology should be consistent with the fact that all renal epithelial cells have the potential to form cysts. In addition, other organs are affected in ADPKD, and in these, the central elements of epithelial cystogenesis are probably similar to those operating in the kidneys.

Experimental models are used to investigate the aetiology of cyst formation and to study the individual elements participating in the generation of cysts: epithelial cellular proliferation, cavity fluid accumulation, and extracellular matrix remodelling (Grantham 1992, 1993). This chapter considers some of the *in vitro* models that have been used to study epithelial cystogenesis in the context of the pathogenesis of polycystic kidney disease (PKD).

Cell culture systems

The creation of cysts *in vitro* requires cells that aggregate or actively proliferate within a supportive matrix to form a confluent epithelium that accumulates intracavitary fluid.

Madin–Darby canine kidney cells

The Madin–Darby canine kidney (MDCK) is an established cell line of renal origin (Madin and Darby 1975). MDCK cells express in culture many of the differentiated characteristics of cells from the distal portion of the nephron and collecting duct (Rindler *et al.* 1979). The exponential clonal growth of MDCK cells suspended within hydrated collagen matrices create polarized epithelial cysts (Fig. 2.1). The MDCK cysts are composed of a single layer of epithelium that secretes solutes to form a fluid-filled cavity (McAteer *et al.* 1987). The basolateral surface of these cysts is in contact with the collagen matrix and the apical membrane faces the cyst lumen mimicking the orientation of human renal tubules and cysts. The development of a hormone-supplemented culture medium to promote the growth of MDCK cells enhanced the study of specific factors that influence cell proliferation and solute transport (Taub *et al.* 1979; McAteer *et al.* 1987; Grantham *et al.* 1989*b*).

The wild-type MDCK stock obtained from ATCC is composed of at least two cell phenotypes. One of these proliferates in collagen gel and secretes fluid, leading to cyst formation (McAteer *et al.* 1987; Grantham *et al.* 1989*b*). This strain of MDCK cells (termed C5A by Grantham *et al.* 1989*b*) does not form

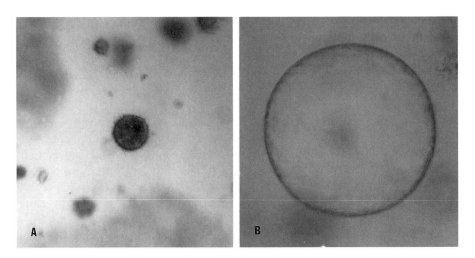

Fig. 2.1 Photomicrographs (×100) of MDCK cells grown in hydrated collagen gel and fed with DMEM/F12, insulin, transferrin, selenium, hydrocortisone, and triiodothyronine. (A) Control. (B) PGE_1. The presence of AMP agonists change the growth pattern of MDCK cells from 'tumour' to cystic configuration.

domes when grown on plastic surfaces. The other phenotype absorbs fluid and forms domes when grown on plastic dishes (Table 2.1). This strain of cells will not form cysts when cultured in type I collagen matrix, but in polymerized agarose, cells will aggregate with apical surface facing the matrix. In this state the absorptive cells will form cyst-like structures (McAteer *et al.* 1985*a*). Comparable behaviour has been described by Wang *et al.* (1990*a,b*), which they attribute to a single type of MDCK cell that adapts polarity in response to alterations in extracellular composition.

LLC-PK$_1$ cells

LLC-PK$_1$ cells express characteristics of mammalian proximal tubules (Hull *et al.* 1976). A subpopulation of these cells form spherical cysts when embedded in collagen gel (Wohlwend *et al.* 1985), similar to that observed with the C5A subculture of MDCK cells. In contrast, wild-type LLC-PK$_1$ cells primarily absorb fluid and form clusters of cells in hydrated collagen gel rather than cysts (Mangoo-Karim *et al.* 1989*b*; Grantham *et al.* 1989*a*). LLC-PK$_1$ cells grown as polarized monolayers do not secrete fluid when stimulated with cyclic AMP (Grantham *et al.* 1989*a*).

Human kidney cortex cells

Cells obtained from superficial nephrons of normal human kidney cortex (HKC) grow well in primary cultures (Mangoo-Karim *et al.* 1989*b*; Neufeld and Grantham 1990; Neufeld *et al.* 1990, 1992). When subcultured in type I collagen matrix, HKC cells form spherical microcysts, but only if critical growth factors epidermal growth factor/transforming growth factor-alpha (EGF/TGFα) are included in the medium (Neufeld and Grantham 1990; Neufeld *et al.* 1992). This experiment proved that a genetic defect is not an essential requirement for the development of the cyst phenotype *in vitro*, a conclusion supported by the fact that cysts develop in advanced renal disease (acquired PKD) in patients without hereditary predisposition (Grantham 1991) and in conditions associated with low body potassium (Torres *et al.* 1990). Thus, ostensibly normal nephrons have the intrinsic components required for cyst development.

Autosomal dominant polycystic kidney cells

Primary cultures of epithelial cell outgrowths of ADPKD cyst walls proliferate (Wilson *et al.* 1986; McAteer *et al.* 1988). Epithelial outgrowths obtained in this manner appear to retain the morphological features found in the progenitor kidney tissue (McAteer *et al.* 1988). Epithelial cells derived from primary cultures of cyst walls by enzymatic digestion of extracellular matrix also form microcysts in type I collagen matrix (Mangoo-Karim *et al.* 1989*b*). These methods to grow human cyst-derived cells *in vitro* are powerful tools for investigating the mechanism of renal cyst biogenesis.

Autosomal recessive polycystic kidney cells

Cells derived from the cysts of infants with ARPKD propagate *in vitro* (Hjelle *et al.* 1990). These cells retain ultrastructural features and lectin staining characteristics compatible with a collecting tubule origin. ARPKD cells in culture contain large electron-dense cytoplasmic glycogen granules which decrease upon administration of a cyclic AMP (cAMP) analogue.

C57BL/6J cpk/cpk cell culture

The cpk rodent model of hereditary kidney disease develops collecting duct cysts and dies of uraemia at 3 weeks of age (Gattone and Grantham 1991). The course of the renal disease resembles that seen in infants with ARPKD (Gattone and Grantham 1991). Primary cultures of cpk kidney cysts proliferate at approximately the same rate as kidney cells obtained from normal animals (Rankin *et al.* 1992). Cells from affected mice exhibit a twofold increase above normal in the synthesis of the extracellular matrix proteins collagen IV and laminin (Taub *et al.* 1990*a*). This report identified an *in vitro* phenotypic difference between normal renal epithelial cells and polycystic cells.

Polarized renal epithelial cell monolayers in culture

An additional tool for the study of vectorial fluid transport utilizes confluent monolayers of renal cells grown on permeable membranes (Mangoo-Karim 1989; Mangoo-Karim *et al.* 1989*b*, Grantham *et al.* 1989*a*; Neufeld *et al.* 1991). This technique allows the study of bidirectional transepithelial solute and fluid movement (i.e. absorption and secretion). By adjusting hydrostatic pressure gradients between the apical and basolateral compartments (Fig. 2.2), net fluid movement (absorption and secretion) has been unequivocally demonstrated in

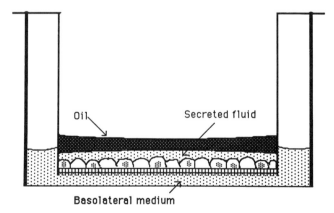

Fig. 2.2 Method of determining fluid transport across cell monolayers grown on permeable support. The apical surface faces the oil which collects the fluid secreted.

MDCK (Mangoo-Karim *et al.* 1989*b*; Grantham *et al.* 1989*a*; Grant *et al.* 1991; Ye *et al.* 1992; Grantham 1993), HKC (Mangoo-Karim *et al.* 1989*b*; Ye *et al.* 1992; Neufeld *et al.* 1992; Grantham 1993), and ADPKD (Mangoo-Karim *et al.* 1989*b*; Grantham *et al.* 1989*a*; Ye *et al.* 1992; Grantham 1993) monolayers. This methodology has recently been adapted to study fluid transport in tracheal epithelial cells from normal individuals and patients with cystic fibrosis (Smith *et al.* 1994).

Monolayers of renal epithelial cells have been studied in Ussing chambers to determine the transepithelial electrical potential difference, the short circuit current and transepithelial resistance as an indication of the species of solute actively transported by the cells (Simmons 1993; Grantham *et al.* 1994; Mangoo-Karim *et al.* 1994).

Renal tubulogenesis

In collagen matrices, renal epithelial cells may form spherical cysts or tubule-like structures. MDCK cells form cysts ordinarily, but addition of hepatocyte growth factor (HGF) causes the cysts to develop branching structures with the characteristics of renal tubules (Montesano *et al.* 1991*a,b*). Primary culture of baby mouse kidney cells in a matrix of type IV collagen (matrigel) form tubule-like structures in response to epidermal growth factor (EGF) or transforming growth factor-alpha (TGFα) (Taub *et al.* 1990*b*). In contrast, TGF-beta (TGFβ) inhibits tubule formation by baby mouse kidneys (Taub *et al.* 1990*b*). In collagen matrix, ADPKD and HKC cells form polarized cysts in response to EGF, TGFα and human cyst fluid (Neufeld *et al.* 1992; Mangoo-Karim *et al.*, 1989*b*). *In vitro* cyst formation that is initiated by EGF or TGFα can be accelerated by agonists of cAMP formation (forskolin, PGE_1, PGE_2, AVP, PTH, isomethylbutylxanthine) and inhibited by TGFβ (Neufeld *et al.* 1992). As opposed to HKC cells, ADPKD cells do not form tubular structures in collagen matrix in response to HGF suggesting that impaired tubulogenesis may lead to cystogenesis (Carone *et al.* 1993).

Isolated intact ADPKD cysts

Intact cysts dissected from kidneys of ADPKD subjects have been maintained *in vitro* for several days (Ye and Grantham 1993). The composition of the intracavitary fluid and the surrounding medium can be manipulated to stimulate or inhibit fluid transport. ADPKD cysts secrete fluid if the native fluid is kept inside the cyst or cAMP agonists (e.g. forskolin) are added to the external culture medium.

Extracellular matrix components in cystic disorders

Cysts initiate as small dilations in renal tubules and collecting ducts which progressively enlarge and reach several centimetres in diameter. Extracellular matrix and interstitial remodelling is obviously envolved in cyst enlargement as these structures take on some of the features of locally invasive neoplasms. Evidence for a pathogenetic role for abnormalities of ECM in PKD is supported by the abnormal development of cysts in liver, pancreas, spleen, and brain, as well as vascular aneurysms, heart valve defects, and colonic diverticuli (Gabow 1991).

Viscoelastic properties of renal cyst basement membrane

To determine if increased basement membrane compliance was a factor in the abnormal distention of renal tubules to form cysts, the deformability of renal cysts was compared to that of normal renal tubules. A micropipet aspiration method demonstrated that the cyst membrane deformability values were not different from normal tubule membranes. Furthermore, estimations of the intratubular hydrostatic pressures required to cause tubular stretching and cyst formation were beyond those physiologically achievable. These studies established that the tensile strength of the cyst wall can be attributed to the collagenous domain of basement membranes since elasticity was lost when tubules or cysts were treated with collagenase (Grantham *et al.* 1987*a*). These findings demonstrated that increased basement membrane compliance was not sufficient to account for the massive distention of renal tubules to form cysts.

ADPKD basement membrane

Surface receptors, enzymes, channels, and structural proteins located in the renal cell membrane are in close association with the basement membrane (BM). Common histopathological findings in ADPKD include duplication of the glomerular BM (Milutinovic *et al.* 1980), thickening of the tubular BM (Cuppage *et al.* 1980), and highly variable appearance and thickness of the cystic BM (Cuppage *et al.* 1980). Basement membrane abnormalities are also seen in hereditary murine models of PKD (Gattone *et al.* 1988) and xenobiotic-induced PKD (Kanwar and Carone 1984; Carone *et al.* 1989*a*). However, thickening of the BM does not lead to cyst formation since it is seen in many non-cystic causes of renal dysfunction (Calvet 1993).

   The composition of the basement membrane and extracellular matrix of cystic cells has been investigated. Primary cultures of murine cpk kidneys have demonstrated increased incorporation of [^{35}S] methionine into type IV collagen and laminin (Taub *et al.* 1990*a*). Normal and polycystic porcine (Beavan *et al.* 1991) and human (Jin *et al.* 1992) renal cells have similar proteoglycan synthesis. The abnormal production of extracellular matrix proteins seen in cystic cells may arise from altered synthesis, defective post-translational modification or abnormal cellular transport of sulphated proteoglycans (Jin *et al.* 1992; Kovacs *et al.* 1994).

   Preliminary data have shown the presence of mesenchymal proteins in ADPKD cystic cells in culture (Bacallao *et al.* 1993*a,b*) which supports the hypothesis that abnormal cellular differentiation may lead to cyst formation in PKD (Calvet 1993; Grantham 1993). Alterations in the composition of the base-

ment membrane may affect cell–matrix interactions causing abnormal cell proliferation, adhesion, differentiation, morphogenesis, and gene expression leading to
cyst formation (Calvet 1993). However, a unique abnormality in the extracellular
matrix to account for cystogenesis has not been identified. It remains to be
determined if extracellular matrix changes represent a primary lesion or a
compensatory response to the cystic transformation.

Cell proliferation in cystic disorders

MDCK cells

The cell doubling time of cyst-forming MDCK cells in hydrated-collagen gel is
approximately two days during the initial phases of growth when serum is added
to the culture medium (McAteer *et al.* 1985*b*; Grantham *et al.* 1989*b*). The
proliferation of subconfluent monolayers of MDCK cells grown in hormonally
defined medium including insulin, transferrin, selenium, hydrocortisone, and
triiodothyronine is enhanced by the addition of cAMP agonists (Mangoo-Karim
et al. 1989*a*). In addition, MDCK cells produce epithelial cysts in serum-free
medium when intracellular cAMP is stimulated with PGE_1 arginine vaso-
pression, forskolin, cholera toxin, or permeable cAMP analogue. Culture
medium not supplemented with fetal bovine serum or adenylate cyclase agonists
leads to the stratification of cells in clusters (Fig. 2.1) resembling epithelial
adenomas (Mangoo-Karim *et al.* 1989*a*).

When MDCK cells are embedded in collagen gel and co-cultivated with
mouse embryo-derived or adult fibroblasts, paracrine factors change their growth
phenotype into branching colonies with apical microvilli and junctional complexes resembling tubular structures (Montesano *et al.* 1991*a*). The effect of
fibroblast-conditioned medium can be duplicated by the addition of exogenous
hepatocyte growth factor (HGF) and blocked by antibodies to HFG, suggesting
that this polypeptide is responsible for epithelial tubulogenesis (Montesano *et al.*
1991*b*). HGF also induces an immortalized inner medullary collecting duct cell
line to grow into branching tubular structures (Barros *et al.* 1993). The differential phenotype expressed by MDCK cells in hydrated collagen gel has also been
attributed to the presence of cell subpopulations within the MDCK cell line.
Wild-type MDCK cells produce both cysts and tubular structures upon
stimulation with hepatocyte growth factor or cAMP agonists suggesting that the
morphological product of MDCK cell proliferation depends on cell heterogeneity as well as on the effect of mitogenic agents (Orellana *et al.* 1993).

Normal and cystic human renal cells

Studies that compare HKC and ADPKD cells grown *in vitro* have demonstrated
different functional, structural, and growth properties among these renal cells.
Controversial data on the growth rate of cystic and non-cystic epithelia in

culture have been obtained. Initial observations showed that ADPKD cells exhibited faster growth rates compared to HKC cells (Wilson *et al.* 1986). Furthermore, cyst-derived cells demonstrated increased [³H] thymidine incorporation in culture compared to normal kidney cortex and medulla, supporting an hyperproliferative behaviour of ADPKD cells *in vitro* (Torres *et al.* 1992). In contrast, others have found a similar growth rate and cell-doubling time between epithelial cells from autosomal dominant polycystic kidneys and HKC cells grown *in vitro* (Carone *et al.* 1989*b*).

The response of ADPKD cells to cyclic nucleotide agonists has also been inconsistent among different laboratories. Adenylate cyclase activity was not impressively stimulated in response to PTH, AVP, and forskolin in the landmark study of Wilson *et al.* (1986). In contrast, cAMP stimulation of cystic cells has been shown to promote transepithelial fluid secretion in monolayer cultures and excised intact ADPKD cysts indicating responsiveness of ADPKD cells to stimulation with the cyclic nucleotide (Mangoo-Karim *et al.* 1989*b*; Grantham 1993; Ye and Grantham 1993). The different culture results may be due to the use of tissue explants in one laboratory (Wilson *et al.* 1986), and the use of primary cultures prepared with collagenase in the other (Mangoo-Karim *et al.* 1989*b*; Grantham 1993).

Epidermal growth factor (EGF, 0.25–25 ng/ml) is a critical factor in the initiation of cyst formation by normal human kidney cortex cells dispersed in a collagen matrix (Neufeld and Grantham 1990; Neufeld *et al.* 1992; Carone *et al.* 1993). The effect of EGF can be mimicked by TGFα (Neufeld *et al.* 1992) or cyst fluid from human ADPKD cysts (Ye *et al.* 1992). Cyclic AMP agonists do not initiate cystogenesis in the absence of EGF or TGFα, but potentiate the effect of such mitogens suggesting a co-ordinated interplay between cell proliferation and fluid secretion (Neufeld and Grantham 1990; Neufeld *et al.* 1992). Abundant levels of EGF receptor and one ligand (TGFα) have been found in human cyst and renal cell carcinoma cells, further suggesting a role for tyrosine kinase activation in renal cell proliferation (Klingel *et al.* 1992). Insulin and dexamethasone also stimulate mitogenesis in ADPKD epithelia *in vitro* (Wilson 1991; Wilson *et al.* 1993).

TGFβ1- and 2-chloroadenosine inhibit HKC cell cyst formation *in vitro* (Neufeld and Grantham 1990; Neufeld *et al.* 1992; Wilson 1991; Wilson *et al.* 1993). Platelet-derived growth factor has no effects on epithelial cell proliferation, but stimulates the growth of ADPKD-derived fibroblasts (Wilson 1991).

Epithelial polarity in cyst biogenesis

Differences in the composition and properties of the apical and basolateral membranes are fundamental features of epithelial cells that support transcellular solute and fluid transport. The establishment of membrane polarity is made possible by the development of junctions between neighbouring cells.

MDCK cell polarity

MDCK cell cyst polarity depends on culture conditions. The apical surface faces the cyst cavity in MDCK cysts embedded in type I collagen, but cysts grown in agarose display an opposite polarity (McAteer *et al.* 1985*a*). Similarly, MDCK cell cysts in suspension culture polarize with the basolateral membrane facing the central lumen and the apical surface toward the outside medium (Wang *et al.* 1990*a*). Furthermore when MDCK cysts grown in suspension culture are transferred to a collagen gel, cell polarity is reversed and the basolateral membrane orients to face the collagen matrix. The reversal of polarity follows the sequential internalization of plasma membrane proteins into cytoplasmic vesicles and subsequent degradation, followed by the protein assembly into the new domains (Wang *et al.* 1990*b*).

The formation of apical junctions is an important factor in the development of cyst polarity. Increasing the calcium concentration from <5 μM to 1.8 μM in media bathing MDCK cells leads to the development of lateral cell-to-cell contact via tight junctions and desmosomes. The development of polarity is associated with a >10-fold increase in intracellular calcium without a change in intracellular pH (Nigam *et al.* 1992). H7, an inhibitor of protein kinase A, C, and G, blocks the development of transepithelial electrical resistance, a reflection of permeable junctional complexes, presumably by blocking the phosphorylation of junctional proteins (Nigam *et al.* 1991).

Reversal of polarity in cystic disorders

Some experimental data implicate changes in cellular polarity as a factor in the conversion of a reabsorptive epithelium into one that predominantly secretes fluid. It has been suggested that localization of the Na^+-K^+ ATPase to the apical surface of renal cysts will cause transepithelial sodium secretion with concomitant water transport. Initial observations using metanephric organ culture made cystic with hydrocortisone or triiodothyronine correlated cyst development with increases in the Na^+-K^+ ATPase activity and inhibition with ouabain (Avner *et al.* 1985, 1987*b*). However, non-cystic control explants after 120 hours of incubation have similar rates of Na^+-K^+ ATPase activity as cystic explants at 84 hours of incubation but do not become cystic, implicating additional factors involved in cyst formation (Avner *et al.* 1985, 1987*b*). These studies demonstrated the role of epithelial fluid transport and the permissive role of active Na^+-K^+ ATPase in the genesis of renal cysts.

The association between Na^+-K^+ ATPase activity and the development of ADPKD was supported by the finding of an abnormal Na^+ pump distribution from the basolateral domain to the apical plasma membranes (Wilson *et al.* 1991). Immunocytochemical localization of the Na^+-K^+ ATPase using a polyclonal antibody against the alpha subunit of guinea-pig and dog kidney Na^+-K^+ ATPase showed that the Na^+ pump was restricted primarily to the apical membrane in ADPKD cysts and cultured epithelium. The abnormal immunolocalization was selective for the Na^+-K^+ ATPase since other basolateral and apical membrane proteins were normally distributed. Transport of ^{22}Na in confluent monolayers of ADPKD cells grown on permeable supports demonstrated movement of sodium in the secretory direction and inhibition of sodium transport by ouabain in medium bathing the apical surface of the cells.

Although the effect of ouabain to inhibit a secretory Na^+ flux is consistent with a role for active Na^+ transport in the secretion of fluid, several corroborative pieces of information were not included in the initial study by Wilson and co-workers (1991). The electrical polarity and short circuit current of the tissue under study was not examined and the net movement of liquid coupled to the Na^+ flux was not measured. Recently, Grantham *et al.* (1995) and Mangoo-Karim *et al.* (1994) have studied intact excised human ADPKD cysts and polarized monolayers of ADPKD cyst epithelia cells *in vitro*. Preliminary results indicate that cultured ADPKD epithelia have lumen negative electrical voltages and positive short circuit currents, neither of which is consistent with active Na^+ secretion. Moreover, the application of ouabain, an inhibitor of Na-K ATPase, to the applical surface of the cells had no effect on fluid transport, whereas basolateral application inhibited net fluid secretion. Bumetanide, which inhibits the Na-K-2Cl co-transport mechanism and diphenylamine-2-carboxylate (DPC), which inhibits chloride channels, also diminished short circuit current and net fluid secretion by cultured ADPKD epithelial. The response of these intact and cultured epithelia to ouabain, bumetanide, and diphenylamine-2-carboxylate are consistent with chloride transport as the motive force behind net fluid secretion (Grantham *et al.* 1995; Mangoo-Karim *et al.* 1994).

Carone and collaborators have been unable to confirm a predominant apical display of immunoreactive Na^+-K^+ ATPase in ADPKD cysts (Carone *et al.* 1994). In spontaneous and transgenic murine models of PKD, the polarity of the Na^+ pump protein was basolateral (Barisoni *et al.* 1993; Kawa *et al.* 1994). Although the Na^+ pump is located in the apical membranes of cyst cells in cpk mice (Avner *et al.* 1992), the enzyme is located in basolateral membranes of humans with ARPKD (Avner and Sweeney, 1992). The weight of current evidence would seem to indicate that the location of the functional Na^+-K^+ ATPase is primarily basolateral in cyst epithelium, and that net secretory movement of solute and water is driven by the transport of solutes other than sodium.

Fluid transport in cystic disorders

Everson *et al.* (1990) provided an important clue to the mechanism of fluid secretion in human cysts. Catheters were inserted into several liver and renal cysts of patients with ADPKD. Using an indicator dilution technique, these investigators found that secretin, a cAMP agonist, stimulated net secretion of fluid into the cysts. The cyst fluid had a higher chloride concentration than plasma, suggesting that anion transport may have had a primary role in the process of fluid secretion.

Fluid secretion has not received much attention in kidney research since it has been overshadowed by robust reabsorption of NaCl and water along the nephron. Grantham and colleagues (1973, 1974) demonstrated that the proximal straight tubule of rabbit kidney was capable of fluid secretion. Lumen formation in isolated tubules was induced by uraemic human serum and *p*-aminohippurate (PAH). Fluid secretion was inhibited by probenecid and ouabain (Grantham *et al.* 1974; Grantham 1993). Using *in vitro* microperfusion of renal tubules, Beyenbach observed fluid secretion in the proximal tubule of the winter flounder *Pseudopleuronectes americanus*. The secreted fluid in this teleost was hyperosmolal and apparently driven by NaCl secretion that could be stimulated by cAMP (Beyenbach 1982). Later observations in isolated vertebrate (shark) proximal tubules showed that net transepithelial fluid secretion was driven by chloride transport (Sawyer *et al.* 1985). Isolated rabbit proximal tubules and collecting ducts *in vitro* embedded in hydrated collagen gel and incubated in chemically defined culture medium develop lumens after treatment with cAMP (Figs 2.3 and 2.4) (Mangoo-Karim 1989). Chronic stimulation caused progressive tubular dilation.

In view of the fact that most renal cysts are isolated sacs that reaccumulate fluid shortly after percutaneous drainage (Saini *et al.* 1983; Everson *et al.* 1990) there is little doubt that they must fill with fluid by the transepithelial secretion of solute and fluid (Grantham *et al.* 1987*b*). Renal tubule epithelial cells also have the capacity to secrete solutes and fluid. Thus, renal epithelial solute and fluid secretion does not appear to be a unique function of renal cysts, but rather an exaggerated property that is normally present in these cells but ordinarily overshadowed by the forces of solute and fluid absorption.

Chloride transport in MDCK cell cysts

MDCK cells, which secrete chloride in response to cAMP, provide an *in vitro* model for the systematic examination of epithelial fluid secretion mechanisms (Simmons 1993). The original MDCK cell line is composed of at least two different cell subpopulations based on functional phenotypes. Cultures of wild-type MDCK cells (ATTC stock) can absorb and secrete fluid. The high resistance (HR) strain of MDCK cells available to some investigators absorb fluid and form domes when grown on plastic surfaces, but do not form cysts when they are suspended in collagen matrix. In contrast, when wild-type MDCK cells are suspended in collagen matrix some of them are able to form cysts by clonal growth (McAteer *et al.* 1987). These microcysts obviously must secrete liquid. A subculture of cells (C5A) derived from an individual MDCK microcyst grown in collagen matrix does not form domes when cultured on plastic surfaces but predominantly secretes fluid in polarized cultures (Table 2.1). In the absence of cAMP agonists, wild-type and HR monolayers exhibit a small degree of fluid absorption, consistent with their capacity to form domes when cultured on plastic surfaces. In contrast, C5A cells ordinarily secrete fluid to a small degree in the absence of cAMP stimulation. Addition of forskolin, a potent agonist of adenylate cyclase in MDCK cells, stimulates net fluid secretion in C5A cells,

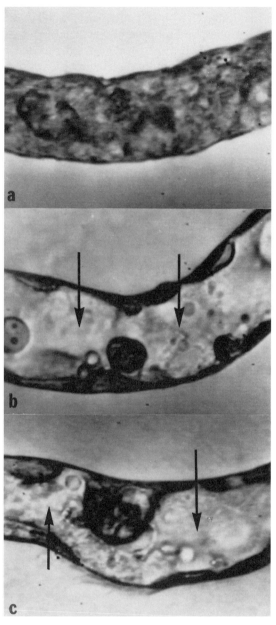

Fig. 2.3 Photomicrographs (×100) of living rabbit straight proximal tubule suspended placed within collagen matrix. (a) Control medium (DMEM/F12, insulin, transferrin, selenium, and triiodothyronine). (b) Addition of 8-Br-cAMP 1 mM and IBMX 0.1 mM for 2 days. (c) Addition of cholera toxin 1 µg/ml and IBMX 0.1 mM to another tubule for 2 days.

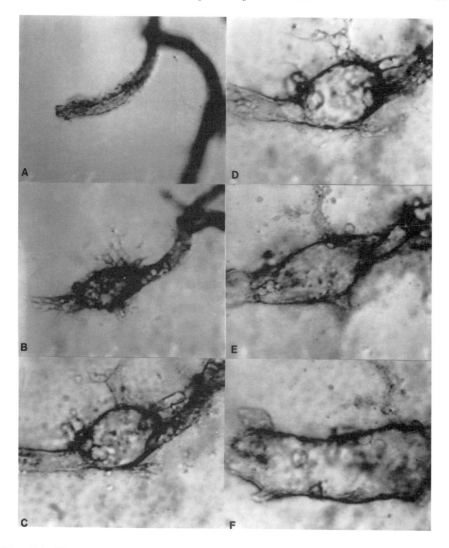

Fig. 2.4 Photomicrographs (×40) of living rabbit cortical collecting duct suspended within collagen matrix. Culture media contained DMEM/F12, insulin, transferrin, selenium, and triiodothyronine, cholera toxin 1 μg/ml and IBMX 0.1 mM. (A) Day 0. (B) Day 6. (C) Day 11. (D) Day 13. (E) Day 29. (F) Day 32.

and to a lesser extent in the wild-type cells composed of heterogenous elements. On the other hand, forskolin has no discernible effect on fluid transport in the HR strain of MDCK. Thus, subcultures of the original MDCK cell line respond quite differently when stimulated with cAMP agonists, further emphasizing that, to determine the mechanisms of fluid secretion in renal epithelia, it is necessary to link the vectorial movement of liquid to the net movements of Na and Cl.

Table 2.1 Comparison of the secretory/absorptive activities in polarized monolayers of wild-type MDCK cells, MDCK C5A, and 'high resistance' HR-type MDCK cells cultured on collagen-coated filters sealed with oil on the apical surface in the presence and absence of forskolin (Fsk) 10 μM in the basolateral medium. One-half of each pair was treated with Fsk on Day 2 and Day 3

MDCK	Day 1		Day 2		Day 3	
	Control	Control	Control	+ Fsk	Control	+ Fsk
Wild-type	0.05	0.04	−0.08	**0.28**	−0.08	**0.13**
C5A	0.13	0.12	0.12	**0.92**	0.37	**0.85**
HR	0.04	0.04	−0.14	−0.04	−0.06	−0.07

Units: μl/cm^2/h. Negative numbers indicate fluid absorption. **Bold** numbers indicate forskolin significantly increased fluid secretion. (Ye and Grantham, unpublished observations.)

The intracavitary hydrostatic pressure of MDCK cysts suspended in collagen matrix is greater than that of the external bath (Mangoo-Karim *et al.* 1989*b*). Ouabain and vanadate (Na$^+$-K$^+$ ATPase inhibitors), L-645,695 (Na$^+$-dependent Cl/HCO$_3$ and K$^+$/Cl transport inhibitor) and amiloride analogues (primarily via Na$^+$- and Ca^{2+}-dependent transport inhibition) slow the expansion of MDCK cysts derived from the C5A cell subculture. These findings suggest that fluid accumulation into the cyst cavity is secondary to solute transport (Grantham *et. al.* 1989*b*).

The stimulation of cAMP production is a crucial factor in the promotion of fluid secretion by C5A MDCK cells. In the absence of a cAMP agonist, C5A MDCK cells grow into solid colonies composed of stratified cells in hydrated collagen gel (Fig. 2.1). The addition of PGE$_1$, arginine vasopressin, cholera toxin, forskolin, or 8-Br-cAMP to chemically defined culture medium promotes cyst formation. The effect of these drugs is potentiated by isobutylmethylxanthine, a phosphodiesterase inhibitor. Cyclic AMP stimulation increases both cell proliferation and fluid transport.

Fluid collected from MDCK cyst contains Na and Cl in nearly isomolal proportions to the culture medium (Mangoo-Karim *et al.* 1989*a*). The osmolality, sodium, potassium, and chloride levels of fluid secreted by MDCK monolayers were slightly greater than those of the culture medium. Macias *et al.* (1990, 1992*b*) demonstrated that MDCK cysts derived from ATTC stock utilized the potential energy of the trans-basolateral concentration gradient of Na to develop an electrochemical gradient for intracellular chloride that favours the net movement of this anion from culture medium to cyst cavity. Thus, in MDCK microcyst the net driving force for net solute transport that originates in the sodium pump is transduced to secondary active anion transport by favourable electrochemical gradients and membrane proteins that selectively increase cell chloride concentrations.

Stimulation of vasopressin-2 receptors in MDCK cells causes sustained cAMP-mediated fluid secretion. The effects of vasopressin are blocked by ouabain, bumetanide, and a sodium-dependent Cl/HCO$_3$ exchange inhibitor (Grant *et al.* 1991). MDCK cyst enlargement in collegen matrix is weakly inhibited by basolateral diphenylamine-2-carboxylate (DPC), a low-affinity chloride channel blocker, without affecting the rate of cellular proliferation (McAteer *et al.* 1990). However, MDCK cells organized in cyst configuration may prevent drugs, such as DPC, from gaining access to the apical surface of the cells. MDCK cells grown on permeable supports and mounted in Ussing chambers have an apex negative potential and apical to basolateral positive short circuit current. Stimulation with forskolin is followed by fluid secretion, cell hyperpolarization, and increased short circuit current compatible with anion secretion (Mangoo-Karim *et al.* 1994). The application of DPC to the apical surface caused a reduction of electrical potential that occured within seconds. Longer incubation of polarized MDCK monolayers with DPC in the apical medium also decreased net fluid secretion. These preliminary data indicate that anion secretion, and more specifically chloride secretion, is the motive element in the net transepithelial secretion of fluid (Mangoo-Karim *et al.* 1994).

Microelectrode studies of electrical potential profiles of resting MDCK microcysts in basal medium in response to 4-acetamido-4′ isothiocyanatostilbene-2, 2′-disulphonic acid (SITS), and furosemide suggested that chloride transport across the basolateral plasma occurs via an Na$^+$-dependent Cl-HCO$_3$ exchange mechanism (Macias *et al.* 1992*a*). The basolateral sodium conductance was low, suggesting that sodium moved through a paracellular pathway. The effects of cAMP agonists were not examined in these studies.

Analysis of the rate of fluid transport, cell volume, and membrane potential changes of isolated MDCK cell cysts following stimulation with arginine vasopressin (AVP) and isobutylmethylxanthine (IBMX) showed a change in the direction of fluid transport from absorption to net secretion (Sullivan *et al.* 1994). During the transition, cell volume decreased and stabilized at 92.6 per cent of control. Fluid secretion was not affected by DIDS and cell pH did not change suggesting that cAMP-driven secretion was not dependent on Cl-HCO$_3$ exchange. Bumetanide blocked secretion, reduced cell volume, and caused cell hyperpolarization. However, the drug had no effect on any of these parameters in the absence of secretagogues. This suggests that the Na-K-2Cl co-transporter is quiescent until cAMP production is stimulated. The effects of AVP and IBMX were also blocked by ouabain and barium. The studies by Macias *et al.* and Sullivan *et al.* suggest that the basolateral Cl-HCO$_3$ exchanger may mediate chloride entry into 'resting' MDCK cells and that activation of the basolateral Na-K-2Cl co-transporter by cAMP may govern the net secretion of chloride and fluid. There is extensive evidence to support a role for a basolateral Na-K-2Cl co-transporter in different strains of MDCK cells (Simmons 1993).

Chloride channels have been identified in the apical membranes of proximal convoluted tubule primary cultures, A6 cells, M-1 mouse and rabbit cortical collecting duct cells, and inner medullary collecting ducts (Anagnostopoulos *et al.* 1984: Darvish *et al.* 1990; Chalfant *et al.* 1992; Korbmacher *et al.* 1992; Ling and Kokko 1992; Vandorpe *et al.* 1993; Rocha and Kudo 1990; Wang *et al.* 1993). The transepithelial electrical polarity, positive short circuit current, and the response of these elements to the apical application of DPC are consistent with chloride movement through the apical plasma membranes of cultured ADPKD epithelial cells. Cystic fibrosis transmembrane conductance regulator (CFTR) protein has been localized to the apical membranes of ADPKD epithelial cells (Caplan and Grantham, unpublished observations), a strong indication that cAMP-activated chloride channels have a role in the movement of chloride and fluid across cyst epithelial cells.

Hydraulic conductivity of renal epithelia

The capacity to generate osmotic gradients by MDCK cysts and monolayers is possible, given the low rates of transport, only if the hydraulic conductivity of the epithelium is low. The hydraulic conductivity of MDCK cysts and mono-layers was estimated from the osmotic flow of water. (Mangoo-Karim 1989; Mangoo-Karim and Grantham 1990; Grant *et al.* 1991). The value of 6.8 μm/s approximates the water permeability of the thick ascending limb of Henle, a tubule segment in which transepithelial osmotic gradients are generated. Although vasopressin stimulates NaCl and liquid transport, there was no effect of the hormone on hydraulic conductivity in MDCK cells. Thus, it appears that net fluid secretion is regulated by changes in net solute transport and not by changes in water permeability or reflection coefficients.

Organic acid transport in renal cells

Although organic anion secretion can promote fluid secretion in normal proximal tubules, the potential impact of organic anion transport by cyst epithelia has received little attention. Antibiotics transported by the renal organic anion system do not appear to be concentrated within renal cysts and renal cyst fluids do not have unusual concentrations of naturally occurring organic acids (unpublished observations). Nonetheless, Avner *et al.* (1987*a*) reported that probenecid inhibited the formation of cysts in hydrocortisone-induced murine metanephric cultures and Neufeld *et al.* (1990) observed that probenecid blocked the formation of cysts in collagen matrix by renal cells. Transepithelial fluid secretion by polarized mono-layers of MDCK and HKC cells was also inhibited by probenecid but not by hippuric acid. Proximal tubule cyst formation in murine metanephric organ cultures was inhibited by bumetanide (Sliman *et al.* 1993). These findings indicate that the transport of organic acids, acting either as osmotic solutes or as secretagogues, may play a role in the development of renal cysts.

Fluid transport by human normal and cyst cells

Transepithelial fluid secretion across human kidney epithelia was first demonstrated in primary cell cultures grown on permeable supports (Mangoo-Karim *et al.* 1989*b*). Stimulation of cells derived from ADPKD cysts, normal human renal cortex, and established cell lines with cAMP agonists cause 'uphill' fluid movement in monolayer cultures and cyst formation in hydrated collagen gel (Grantham *et al.* 1989*a*; Neufeld *et al.* 1992; Ye *et al.* 1992). Excised, intact, ADPKD cysts incubated *in vitro* and containing natural cyst fluid gained weight as a reflection of net transepithelial fluid secretion. Excised cysts did not secrete liquid when natural fluid was replaced with a mixture of Dulbecco's modified Eagle's medium and Ham's F12 medium (DMEM-F 12). The addition of forskolin to the culture medium restored fluid secretion. This suggests that cyclic AMP-mediated transport may play a role in the pathogenesis of cyst enlargement in ADPKD (Ye and Grantham 1993).

Fluid secretion caused by cAMP has also been shown in non-renal epithelia. Human rectal adenocarcinoma cells (HRA-19) form polarized monolayers on plastic and develop large intercellular spaces as a consequence of fluid absorption (the equivalent of 'dome' formation). Stimulation of transepithelial chloride secretion with cAMP agonists cause disappearance of the intercellular spaces.Vasopressin-stimulated sodium reabsorption of HRA-19 cells and increased the width of intercellular spaces. HRA-19 cells embedded in hydrated collagen gel grow in cyst configuration when stimulated with cAMP agonists, or when co-cultivated with 3T3 cells. 3T3 cells appear to participate in the paracrine regulation of HRA-19 cyst formation through their capacity to produce prostaglandins, since their stimulatory effect is blocked by indomethacin (Kirkland 1990).

Cyclic AMP and PKD

Chloride transport mediated by cAMP and organic anion transport are the only known solute-driven mechanisms of fluid secretion by renal cells. Evidence of fluid secretion has been demonstrated in primary cell cultures derived from ADPKD and HKC. Cyclic AMP appears to have a dual function since the nucleotide also stimulates the proliferation of renal cells in culture (Mangoo-Karim 1989). The cAMP cascade is ubiquitous and could play a role in the development of cysts in different organs. Most organs affected by ADPKD are probably subject to hormonal regulation of cAMP levels including; kidney (PTH, calcitonin, AVP, vasoactive intestinal peptide, eicosanoids, secretin); liver (secretin); thyroid (TSH, long-acting thyroid stimulator); testis (LH); ovaries (FSH,LH); parathyroid (PTH); adrenals (ACTH); and pancreas (secretin). In addition, receptors for neurotransmitters are prevalent in all of these tissues, and their activation could lead to cAMP production. The wide distribution of this signal transduction and its role in cellular proliferation and fluid secretion make it an attractive candidate for a central role in PKD pathogenesis.

Endogenous cystogens

Natural cyst fluid has been examined to determine if endogenous mitogens or secretagogues are sequestered there.

ADPKD cyst fluid

Excised human ADPKD cysts secrete fluid *in vitro* at higher rates when natural cyst fluid, rather than culture medium, is placed in the cavity (Ye and Grantham 1993). ADPKD cyst fluid stimulates fluid secretion in polarized monolayers of ADPKD, HKC, and MDCK cells (Ye *et al.* 1992; Grantham, unpublished). Forskolin mimics the effect of cyst fluid on solute and water secretion. Since cyst fluid stimulates cAMP production (Ye *et al.* 1992) there is reason to think that the nucleotide mediates the action of the cyst fluid secretagogue. Preliminary evidence suggests that the secretagogue is a neutral lipid (Sharma and Grantham 1993).

Human ADPKD cyst fluid also stimulated the formation and enlargment of HKC and MDCK cysts derived from solitary cells suspended in collagen matrix (Ye *et al.* 1992). In unpublished work from this laboratory, ADPKD cells have also been shown to form cysts in collagen matrix in response to human cyst fluid. The capacity of cyst fluid to stimulate cyst formation and growth is attributed to 'cystogenic' activity. Since HKC cells only form cysts in collagen matrix when EGF or its homologue TGFα is present in the medium, the cystogen in cyst fluid was presumed to be from that family of mitogens. However, cystogenic activity was not removed by treatment with antiserum to EGF, and gel filtration experiments indicate that the cystogenic activity travels in a fraction with a molecular weight approximating that of albumin, too high to be EGF or TGFα.

Thus, ADPKD cyst fluid contains a lipophilic secretagogue and a peptidic mitogen that may stimulate cyst growth.

Murine renal cyst fluid

Cyst fluid, obtained from DBA-2FG PCY mice with recessively inherited renal cystic disease, stimulates transepithelial fluid secretion and cAMP production in MDCK cells (Yamaguchi *et al.* 1993).

Conclusions

The phenotypic features of renal cysts can be reproduced *in vitro* with primary and immortalized renal epithelial cell cultures. Thus, solitary cells of normal and abnormal genetic background have the biological components required for the formation of epithelial cysts *in vitro*. Orderly proliferation and net transepithelial fluid secretion appear to be minimal requirements for cyst formation in a three-dimensional collagen matrix.

The rate of cyst growth *in vitro* depends on the presence of mitogens and secretagogues in the culture medium. The cAMP signal transduction system appears to have a prominent role in promoting cell proliferation and fluid secretion in MDCK, normal human cortex, and ADPKD cyst cells, although the human cells require an additional initiating factor (EGF, TGFα or cyst fluid) to form cysts in collagen matricies. *In vitro* fluid secretion by intact human cysts, and microcysts composed of HKC, ADPKD, or MDCK cells, depend on a functioning Na$^+$-K$^+$ ATPase in the basolateral membrane. The extent to which mislocation of functioning Na$^+$-K$^+$ ATPase to the apical membrane contributes to the secretion of fluid by cyst epithelial cells is unclear. Evidence from studies of rodent, rabbit, dog, and human renal epithelial cells *in vitro* indicate that chloride secretion, mediated by cAMP, is a strong candidate for the primary mechanism that drives net fluid secretion in renal cysts.

References

Anagnostopoulos, T., Edelman, A., Planelles, G., Teulon, J., and Thomas, R. (1984). Chloride transport in proximal tubule. Its effect on water and electrolyte absorption. *Journal of Physiology*, **70**, 132–8.

Avner, E. D. and Sweeney, W. E. (1992). Epidermal growth factor receptor (EGFR), but not NaKATPase, is mislocated to apical cell surfaces of collecting tubule cysts in human autosomal recessive polycystic kidney disease (ARPKD) (Abstract). *Journal of the American Society of Nephrology*, **3**, 292.

Avner, E. D., Sweeney, W. E., Finegold, D. N., Piesco, N. P., and Ellis, D. (1985). Sodium-potassium ATPase activity mediates cyst formation in metanephric organ culture. *Kidney International*, **28**, 447–55.

Avner, E. D., Sweeney, W. E., and Ellis, D. (1987*a*) Increased organic anion uptake mediates proximal tubular cyst formation in metanephric organ culture (Abstract). *Kidney International*, **31**, 159.

Avner, E. D., Sweeney, W. E., Piesco, N. P., and Ellis, D. (1987*b*). Triiodothyronine-induced cyst formation in metanephric organ culture: the role of increased Na-K-adenosine triphosphatase activity. *Journal of Laboratory and Clinical Medicine*, **109**, 441–53.

Avner, E. D., Sweeney, W. E., and Nelson, W. J. (1992). Abnormal sodium pump distribution during renal tubulogenesis in congenital murine polycystic kidney disease. *Proceedings of the National Academy of Sciences USA*, **89**, 7447–51.

Bacallao, R., Nakamura, S., and Carone, F. A. (1993*a*). ADPKD epithelial cells express fibroblast surface protein and the fibronectin receptor (Abstract). *Journal of the American Society of Nephrology*, **4**, 811.

Bacallao, R., Nakamura, S., and Carone, F. A. (1993*b*). Intermediate filament expression suggests a block in the differentiation pathway of ADPKD epithelial cells (Abstract). *Journal of the American Society of Nephrology*, **4**, 811.

Barisoni, L., Trudel, M., Chretien, N., Ward, L., and D'Agati, V. (1993). Membrane polarity in the SBM transgenic (TG) mouse model of polycystic kidney disease (PKD) (Abstract). *Journal of the American Society of Nephrology*, **4**, 811.

Barros, E. J. G., Cantley, L. G., Santos, O. F. P., Rauchman, M. I., and Nigam, S. K. (1993). HGF induces the formation of branching tubular structures in an immortalized inner medullary collecting duct cell line (Abstract). *Journal of the American Society of Nephrology*, **4**, 461.

Beavan, L. A., Carone, F. A., Nakamura, S., Jones, J. K., Reindel, J. F., and Price, R. G. (1991). Comparison of proteoglycans synthesized by porcine normal and polycystic renal tubular epithelial cells *in vitro*. *Archives of Biochemistry and Biophysics*, **284**, 392–9.

Beyenbach, K. W. (1982). Direct demonstration of fluid secretion by glomerular renal tubules in a marine teleost. *Nature*, 299, 54–6.

Calvet, J. P. (1993). Polycystic kidney disease: Primary extracellular matrix abnormality or defective cellular differentiation. *Kidney International*, 43, 101–8.

Carone, F. A., Hollenberg, P. F., Nakamura, S., Punyarit, P., Glogowski, W., and Flouret, G. (1989a). Tubular basement membrane change occurs *pari passu* with the development of cyst formation. *Kidney International*, 35, 1034–40.

Carone, F. A., Nakamura, S., Schumacher, B. S., Punyarit, P., and Bauer, K. D. (1989b). Cyst-derived cells do not exhibit accelerated growth or features of transformed cells *in vitro*. *Kidney International*, 35, 1351–7.

Carone, F. A., Nakamura, S., Caputo, M., Bacallao, R., Nelson, W. J., and Kanwar, Y. S. (1994). Cell polarity in human renal cystic disease. *Laboratory Investigation*, 70, 648–55.

Carone, F. A., Nakamura, S., Bacallao, R., and Kanwar, Y. S. (1993). Impaired tubulogenesis of human renal cyst-derived cells in collagen gel (Abstract). *Journal of the American Society of Nephrology*, 4, 463.

Chalfant, L., Coupaye-Gerard, B., Civan, M., and Kleyman, T. R. (1992). Rapid activation of Cl secretion by arginine vasopressin in the epithelial cell line A6 (Abstract). *Journal of the American Society of Nephrology*, 3, 805.

Cuppage, F. E., Huseman, R. A., Chapman, A., and Grantham, J. J. (1980). Ultrastructure and function of cysts from human adult polycystic kidneys. *Kidney International*, 17, 372–81.

Darvish, N., Marom, S., Winaver, J., and Dagan, D. (1990). cAMP-dependent chloride channels in apical membranes of cultured proximal convoluted tubule cells (Abstract). *Journal of the American Society of Nephrology*, 1, 715.

Everson, G. T., Emmett, M., Brown, W. R., Redmond, P., and Thickman, D. (1990). Functional similarities of hepatic cystic and biliary epithelium: studies of fluid constituents and *in vivo* secretion in response to secretin. *Hepatology*, 11, 557–65.

Gabow, P. A. (1991). Polycystic kidney disease: Clues to pathogenesis. *Kidney International*, 40, 989–96.

Gattone, V. H. II and Grantham, J. J. (1991). Understanding human cystic disease through experimental models. *Seminars in Nephrology*, 11, 617–31.

Gattone, V. H. II, *et al.* (1988). Autosomal recessive polycystic kidney disease in a murine model. *Laboratory Investigation*, 59, 231–8.

Grant, M. E., Neufeld, T. K., Cragoe, E. J., Welling, L. W., and Grantham, J. J. (1991). Arginine vasopressin stimulates net fluid secretion in a polarized subculture of cyst-forming MDCK cells. *Journals of the American Society of Nephrology*, 2, 219–27.

Grantham, J. J. (1991). Acquired cystic kidney disease. *Kidney International*, 40, 143–52.

Grantham, J. J. (1992). Regulation of cell proliferation and fluid secretion in the progressive enlargement of renal cysts. In *Polycystic kidney disease*, (ed. M. H. Breuning, M. Devoto, and G. Romeo), pp. 15–22. Karger, Basel.

Grantham, J. J. (1993). Fluid secretion, cellular proliferation, and the pathogenesis of renal epithelial cysts. *Journal of the American Society of Nephrology*, 3, 1843–57.

Grantham, J. J., Irwin, R. L., Qualizza, P. B., Tucker, D. R., and Whittier, F. C. (1973). Fluid secretion in isolated proximal straight renal tubules: Effect of human uremic serum. *Journal of Clinical Investigation*, 52, 2441–50.

Grantham, J. J., Qualizza, P. B., and Irwin, R. L. (1974). Net fluid secretion in proximal straight renal tubules *in vitro*: Role of PAH. *American Journal of Physiology*, 226, 191–7.

Grantham, J. J., Donoso, V. S., Evan, A. P., Carone, F. A., and Gardner, K. D. (1987*a*). Viscoelastic properties of tubule basement membranes in experimental renal cystic disease. *Kidney International*, **32**, 187–97.

Grantham, J. J., Geiser, J. L., and Evan, A. P. (1987*b*). Cyst formation and growth in autosomal dominant polycystic kidney disease. *Kidney International*, **31**, 1145–52.

Grantham, J. J., *et al.* (1989*a*). Net fluid secretion by mammalian renal epithelial cells: stimulation by cAMP in polarized cultures derived from established renal cells and from normal and polycystic kidneys. *Transactions of the Association of American Physicians*, **102**, 158–162.

Grantham, J. J., *et al.* (1989*b*). Chemical modification of cell proliferation and fluid secretion in renal cysts. *Kidney International*, **35**, 1379–89.

Grantham, J. J., Ye, M., and Sullivan, L. P. (1995). *In vitro* fluid secretion by epithelium from polycystic kidneys. *Journal of Clinical Investigation*, **95**, 195–202.

Hjelle, J. T., *et al.* (1990). Autosomal recessive polycystic kidney disease: characterization of human peritoneal and cystic kidney cells *in vitro*. *American Journal Kidney of Diseases*, **15**, 123–36.

Jin, H., Carone, F. A., Nakamura, S., Liu, Z. Z., and Kanwar, Y. S. (1992). Altered synthesis and intracellular transport of proteoglycans by cyst-derived cells from human polycystic kidneys. *Journal of the American Society of Nephrology*, **2**, 1726–33.

Kanwar, Y. S. and Carone, F. A. (1984). Reversible changes of tubular cell and basement membrane in drug-induced renal cystic disease. *Kidney International*, **26**, 35–43.

Kawa, G., *et al.* (1994). Sodium pump distribution is not reversed in the DBA/2FG-pcy polycystic kidney disease model mouse. *Journal of the American Society of Nephrology*, **4**, 2040–9.

Kirkland, S. C. (1990). Control of fluid transport in human rectal adenocarcinoma cells (HRA-19) in monolayer and collagen gel cultures. *Journal of Cell Science*, **95**, 167–74.

Klingel, R., Dippold, W., Störkel, S., Meyer, K. H., and Köhler, H. (1992). Expression of differentiation antigens and growth-related genes in normal kidney, autosomal dominant polycystic kidney disease, and renal cell carcinoma. *American Journal of Kidney Diseases*, **19**, 22–30.

Korbmacher, C., Segal, A. S., Boulpaep, E. L., Schröder, U. H., and Frömter, E. (1992). Forskolin stimulates a chloride conductance in M-1 mouse cortical collecting duct cells (Abstract). *Journal of the American Society of Nephrology*, **3**, 812.

Kovacs, J., Carone, F. A., Liu, Z. Z., Nakumara S., Kumar, A., and Kanwar Y. S. (1994). Differential growth factor-induced modulation of proteoglycans synthesized by normal human renal versus cyst-derived cells. *Journal of the American Society of Nephrology*, **5** 44–54.

Ling, B. N. and Kokko, K. E. (1992). PGE_2 activates apical chloride channels in rabbit cortical collecting tubule (RCCT) principal cells via a cAMP-dependent pathway (Abstract) *Journal of the American Society of Nephrology*, **3**, 813.

Macias, W. L., Carrigan, A. L., Graber, S. D., McAteer, J. A., and Armstrong, W. M. (1990). Chloride uptake in MDCK cells (Abstract). *Journal of the American Society of Nephrology*, **1**, 724.

Macias, W. L., McAteer, J. A., Tanner, G. A., Fritz, A. L., and Armstrong, W. M. (1992*a*). NaCl transport in Madin Darby canine kidney cyst epithelial cells. *Kidney International*, **42**, 308–19.

Macias, W. L., McAteer, J. A., Tanner, G. A., and Armstrong, W. M. (1992*b*). Electrogenic chloride secretion by Madin-Darby canine kidney (MDCK)-cyst epithelial cells (Abstract). *Journal of the American Society of Nephrology*, 3, 298.

Madin, S. H. and Darby, N. B. (1975). *American type culture collection catalogue of strains*, 2, 47. American Type Culture Collection, Rockville, MD.

Mangoo-Karim, R. (1989). The biogenesis of renal cysts *in vitro*. Dependence on cyclic AMP.D.Phil.thesis. University of Kansas.

Mangoo-Karim, R. and Grantham, J. J. (1990). Transepithelial water permeability in an *in vitro* model of renal cysts. *Journal of the American Society of Nephrology*, 1, 278–85.

Mangoo-Karim, R., Uchic, M., Lechene, C., and Grantham, J. J. (1989*a*). Renal epithelial cyst formation and enlargement *in vitro*: Dependence on cAMP. *Proceedings of the National Academy of Sciences USA*, 86, 6007–11.

Mangoo-Karim, R., *et al.* (1989*b*). Renal epithelial fluid secretion and cyst growth: the role of cyclic AMP. *Federation of American Societies for Experimental Biology Journal*, 3, 2629–32.

Mangoo-Karim, R., Ye M., Grantham, J. J., and Sullivan, L. P. (1994). Anion secretion drives fluid secretion by monolayers of cultured autosomal dominant polycystic kidney (ADPKD) cells (Abstract). *Journal of the American Society of Nephrology*, 5, 630.

McAteer, J. A., Vance, E. E., Gardner, K. D., and Evan, A. P. (1985*a*). Polarity reversal by MDCK cells *in vitro* (Abstract). *In Vitro*, 21, 12A.

McAteer, J. A., Welling, D. J., Evan, A. P., Connors, B. A. and Welling, L. W. (1985*b*). Determination of growth rate for MDCK-cysts cultured within collagen gel. *Federation Proceedings*, 44, 1039.

McAteer, J. A., Evan, A. P., and Gardner, K. D. (1987). Morphogenetic clonal growth of kidney epithelial cell line MDCK. *Anatomical Record*, 217, 229–39.

McAteer, J. A., Carone, F. A., Grantham, J. J., Kempson, S. A., Gardner, K. D., and Evan, A. P. (1988). Explant culture of human polycystic kidney. *Laboratory Investigation*, 59, 126–36.

McAteer, J. A., Cusick, D. A., Macias, W. L., Evan, A. P., and Armstrong, W. M. (1990). Inhibition of MDCK-cyst growth by DPC (Abstract). *Journal of the American Society of Nephrology*, 1, 725.

Milutinovic, J., Agodoa, L. C. Y., Cutler, R. E., and Striker, G. E. (1980). Autosomal dominant polycystic kidney disease. Early diagnosis and consideration of pathogenesis. *American Journal of Clinical Pathology*, 73, 740–7.

Montesano, R., Schaller, G., and Orci, L. (1991*a*). Induction of epithelial tubular morphogenesis *in vitro* by fibroblast-derived soluble factors. *Cell*, 66, 697–711.

Montesano, R., Matsumoto, K., Nakamura, T., and Orci, L. (1991*b*). Identification of a fibroblast-derived epithelial morphogen as hepatocyte growth factor. *Cell*, 67, 901–8.

Neufeld, T. K. and Grantham, J. J. (1990). Epidermal growth factor promotes cyst formation by human renal epithelial cells *in vitro*. *Transactions of the Association of American Physicians*, 103, 48–52.

Neufeld, T. K., Ye, M., Kornhaus, J., and Grantham, J. J. (1990). Probenecid inhibits cyst formation and net fluid secretion of renal epithelial cells *in vitro* (Abstract). *Journal of the American Society of Nephrology*, 1, 726.

Neufeld, T. K., Grant, M. E., and Grantham, J. J. (1991). A method to measure the rate of net fluid secretion by monolayers of cultured renal epithelial cells. *Journal of Tissue Culture Methods*, 13, 229–34.

Neufeld, T. K., *et al.* (1992). *In vitro* formation and expansion of cysts derived from human renal cortex epithelial cells. *Kidney International*, 41, 1222–36.

Nigam, S. K., Denisenko, N., Rodriguez-Boulan, E., and Citi, S. (1991). The role of phosphorylation in development of tight junctions in cultured renal epithelial (MDCK) cells. *Biochemical and Biophysical Research Communications*, 181, 548–53.

Nigam, S. K., Rodriguez-Boulan, E., and Silver, R. B. (1992). Changes in intracellular calcium during the development of epithelial polarity and junctions. *Proceedings of the National Academy of Sciences USA*, 89, 6162–6.

Orellana, S. A., Sweeney, W. E., and Avner, E. D. (1993). Spontaneous tubule formation by Madin Darby canine kidney cells is independent of exogenous hepatocyte growth factor (Abstract). *Journal of the American Society of Nephrology*, 4, 473.

Rankin, C. A., Grantham, J. J., and Calvet, J. P. (1992). C-fos expression is hypersensitive to serum-stimulation in cultured cystic kidney cells from the C57Bl/6J-cpk mouse. *Journal of Cellular Physiology*, 152, 578–86.

Rindler, M., Chuman, L. M., Shaffer, L., and Saier, M. H. (1979). Retention of differentiated properties in an established dog kidney epithelial cell line (MDCK). *J. Cell. Biol*, 81, 635–48.

Rocha, A. S. and Kudo, L. H. (1990). Factors governing sodium and chloride transport across the inner medullary collecting duct. *Kidney International*, 38, 654–67.

Saini, S., Mueller, P. R., Ferrucci, J. T., Simeone, J. F., Wittenberg, J., and Butch, R. J. (1983). Percutaneous aspiration of hepatic cysts does not provide definitive therapy. *American Journal of Radiology*, 141, 559–60.

Sawyer, D. B., Cliff, W. H., Wilhelm, M. M., Frömter, R. O., and Beyenbach, K. W. (1985). Mechanism of fluid secretion by proximal tubules in the glomerular kidney of the shark (Abstract). *Kidney International*, 27, 319.

Sharma, M., Ye, M., and Grantham, J. J. (1993). Partial purification of a secretagogue isolated from cyst fluid in autosomal dominant polycystic kidney disease (Abstract). *Journal of the American Society of Nephrology*, 4, 824.

Simmons, N. L. (1993). Renal epithelial Cl secretion. *Experimental Physiology*, 78, 117–37.

Sliman, G. A., Sweeney, W. E., and Avner, E. D. (1993). Organic anion (OA) uptake and chloride (Cl) secretion mediate tubular cyst formation (TCF) in murine metanephric organ culture (MOC) (Abstract). *Journal of the American Society of Nephrology*, 4, 824.

Smith, J. J., Karp, P. H., and Welsh, M. J. (1994). Defective fluid transport by cystic fibrosis airway epithelia. *Journal of Clinical Investigation*, 93, 1307–11.

Sullivan, L. P., Wallace, D. P., and Grantham, J. J. (1994). Coupling of cell volume and membrane potential changes to fluid secretion in a model of renal cysts. *Kidney International*, 45, 1369–80.

Taub, M., Chuman, L., Saier, M. H., and Sato, G. (1979). Growth of Madin-Darby canine kidney epithelial cell (MDCK) line in hormone-supplemented, serum-free medium. *Proceedings of the National Academy of Sciences USA*, 76, 3338–42.

Taub, M., Laurie, G. W., Martin, G. R., and Kleinman, H. K. (1990a). Altered basement membrane protein biosynthesis by primary cultures of cpk/cpk mouse kidney. *Kidney International*, 37, 1090–7.

Taub, M., Wang, Y., Szczesny, T. M., and Kleinman, H. K. (1990b). Epidermal growth factor or transforming growth factor alpha is required for kidney tubulogenesis in matrigel cultures in serum-free medium. *Proceedings of the National Academy of Sciences USA*, 87, 4002–6.

Torres, V. E., Young, W. F., Offord, K. P., and Hattery, R. R. (1990). Association of hypokalemia, aldosteronism and renal cysts. *New England Journal of Medicine*, **322**, 345–51.

Torres, V. E., Mujwid, D. K., and Johnson, C. M. (1992). Proliferative potential of cyst-derived epithelial cells in ADPKD (Abstract). *Journal of the American Society of Nephrology*, **3**, 303.

Vandorpe, D., Kizer, N., Ciampolillo, F., Memoli, V. A., Guggino, W. B., and Stanton, B. (1993). cAMP stimulates CFTR (cystic fibrosis transmembrane conductance regulator) chloride channels in inner medullary collecting duct (Abstract). *Journal of the American Society of Nephrology*, **4**, 882.

Wang, A. Z., Ojakian, G. K., and Nelson, W. J. (1990*a*). Steps in the morphogenesis of a polarized epithelium. I. Uncoupling the roles of cell-cell and cell-substratum contact in establishing plasma membrane polarity in multicellular epithelial (MDCK) cysts. *Journal of Cell Science*, **95**, 137–51.

Wang, A. Z., Ojakian, G. K., and Nelson, W. J. (1990*b*). Steps in the morphogenesis of a polarized epithelium. II. Disassembly and assembly of plasma membrane domains during reversal of epithelial cell polarity in multicellular epithelial (MDCK) cysts. *Journal of Cell Science*, **95**, 153–65.

Wang, T., Segal, A., Giebisch, G., and Aronson, P. S. (1993). Stimulation of chloride transport by cAMP in the rat proximal tubule (Abstract). *Journal of the American Society of Nephrology*, **4**, 883.

Wilson, P. D. (1991). Aberrant epithelial cell growth in autosomal dominant polycystic kidney disease. *American Journal of Kidney Diseases*, **17**, 634–7.

Wilson, P. D., Schrier, R. W., Breckon, R. D., and Gabow, P. A. (1986). A new method for studying human polycystic kidney disease epithelia in culture. *Kidney International*, **30**, 371–8.

Wilson, P. D., Sherwood, A. C., Palla, K., Du, J., Watson, R., and Norman, J. T. (1991). Reversed polarity of Na^+-K^+-ATPase: mislocation to apical plasma membranes in polycystic kidney disease epithelia. *American Journal of Physiology*, **260**, F420–30.

Wilson, P. D., Du, J., and Norman, J. T. (1993). Autocrine, endocrine and paracrine regulation of growth abnormalities in autosomal dominant polycystic kidney disease. *European Journal of Cell Biology*, **61**, 131–8.

Wohlwend, A., Montesano, R., Vassalli, J. D., and Orci, L. (1985). LLC-PK1 cysts: a model for the study of epithelial polarity. *Journal of Cellular Physiology*, **125**, 533–9.

Yamaguchi, T., Nagao, S., Takahashi, H., Ye, M., and Grantham, J. J. (1993). Cyst fluid from DBA-2FG PCY mice stimulates fluid secretion and cyclic AMP accumulation by MDCK cells (Abstract). *Journal of the American Society of Nephrology*, **4**, 827.

Ye, M. and Grantham, J. J. (1993). The secretion of fluid by renal cysts from patients with autosomal dominant polycystic kidney disease. *New England Journal of Medicine*, **329**, 310–3.

Ye, M., *et al.* (1992). Cyst fluid from human autosomal dominant polycystic kidney promotes cyst formation and expansion by renal epithelial cells *in vitro*. Journal of the American Society of Nephrology, **3**, 984–94.

3

Mouse models of polycystic kidney disease

Ruth A. McDonald and Ellis D. Avner

Introduction

Experimental studies in a variety of model systems have identified three major factors of potential pathophysiological significance in tubular cyst formation and enlargement: (1) tubular epithelial hyperplasia in response to a variety of physical or chemical stimuli, or cell cycle control abnormalities; (2) altered tubular epithelial cell metabolism and transport leading to intratubular fluid accumulation; and (3) extracellular matrix abnormalities leading to increased tubular wall compliance or alteration of the tubular microenvironment (Avner 1993; Avner *et al.* 1990). The relative importance of each of these factors and their complex interaction in mediating naturally occurring cystic abnormalities remains unknown, but are beginning to be delineated in experimental murine models. In this chapter we will review these models, focusing on their roles in the pathogenesis of renal cystic disease.

Chemically induced renal cystic disease: glucocorticoids

The renal cystogenic effects of glucocorticoids have been studied in mice as well as other species (Avner *et al.* 1990). Despite interspecies differences, several conclusions can be drawn. For the most part, the initial cystic lesions produced by glucocorticoids are localized to developing cortical collecting tubules. Following initial localization to cortical collecting tubules, cystic lesions produced by glucocorticoids extended to glomeruli and proximal tubules (Oikarien *et al.* 1986; Ojeda and Garcia-Porrero 1982; Ojeda *et al.* 1972; Ros *et al.* 1987; Whitehouse *et al.* 1980). It has become apparent that all of the corticosteroid-induced cystic models are highly influenced, if not directly mediated, by hypokalaemia and electrolyte imbalance (Avner *et al.* 1990).

The induction of polycystic kidney disease (PKD) by glucocorticoids in newborn mice behaves as a 'threshold' trait, with prevalence of PKD varying in different inbred strains after exposure to an inducing steroid (McDonald *et al.* 1990). Ogborn and Crocker (1991), showed that kidneys of C3H mice (low threshold for PKD) demonstrated greater specific dexamethasone binding than kidneys of DBA mice (high threshold for PKD) on the second day of life and treatment with methylprednisolone down-regulated dexamethasone binding in the C3H strain. C3H mice demonstrated greater whole kidney homogenate Na-K ATPase activity than DBA mice within 24 hours of methylprednisolone injection. The investigators concluded that specific renal glucocorticoid binding may regulate the species-specific threshold for induction of PKD through a variety of Na-K ATPase-mediated transport processes (Avner *et al.* 1990; Ogborn *et al* 1993). Their findings are supported by *in vitro* evidence that glucocorticoids induce Na-K ATPase activity in parallel with cystic tubulogenesis during critical periods of nephron development (Avner *et al.* 1985).

Although the precise mechanisms of cyst formation and progressive enlargement in the corticosteroid models are unknown, the regular production of cystic lesions at different sites along the nephron makes these models potentially useful for studying the differential susceptibility of specific nephron segments to cyst formation. The reproducibility of cyst formation following corticosteroid administration permits study of environmental factors that might modulate cyst formation or enlargement. The corticosteroid models may also be of value in the study of renal epithelial differentiation and the assembly of the glomerular filtration surface (Ojeda *et al.* 1972; Reeves *et al.* 1980; Ros *et al.* 1987). A major drawback to the corticosteroid-induced whole animal models is the well-known multiple effects of corticosteroids on renal and cellular physiology, growth, differentiation, the inflammatory response, and the metabolism of extracellular matrix (Beauwens and Crabbe 1985; Ojeda *et al.* 1986; Slater *et al.* 1986). Such effects make delineation and study of precise pathophysiological processes difficult in these models.

Genetically transmitted renal cystic disease: spontaneous mutations

The study of cyst formation and enlargement in genetically transmitted animal models has the potential of identifying both specific cystogenic gene products and biological and environmental factors that modulate cyst formation. The spontaneous mutations that result in genetically transmitted murine renal cystic diseases are listed in Table 3.1.

The CFWwd mouse

In 1984, Werder *et al.* described a new mutation in the CFW strain of inbred AKR mice, which developed a form of autosomal dominant renal cystic disease (CFWwd). Affected animals developed progressive bilateral renal enlargement and died with progressive uraemia by 16 to 24 months of age. The renal cystic lesions occurred in the glomerulus as well as the distal and cortical collecting tubules. Approximately 15 per cent of the affected mice that died with cystic kidneys also had hepatic cysts, and an unspecified proportion developed thoracic aortic aneurysms. Only 4 per cent of CFWwd animals that lived their entire lives in a germ-free environment develop cystic kidneys whereas almost 100 per cent of the affected mice raised in a clean conventional environment died from

Table 3.1   Genetically transmitted murine polycystic kidney disease: spontaneous mutations

Mouse model	Inheritance	Mouse chromosome	Human chromosome
CFWwd	AD	–	–
CPK	AR	12	2
JCK	AR	Not allelic to CPK, JCK	–
PCY	AR	9	3
BPK	AR	Not allelic to CPK or TGN737	–
nm1633	?AR	8	–
CBA/Ca-KD	AR	–	–
CBA/N	XR	X	–

AD, autosomal dominant; AR, autosomal recessive; XR, X-linked recessive.

cystic disease 24 months of age. The CFWwd model provides dramatic evidence of environmental modulation of a cystic disease.

The CPK mouse

In 1977, a spontaneous mutation in C57BL/6J mice at Jackson Laboratories, Bar Harbor, Maine produced an autosomal recessive polycystic kidney disease (Russell and McFarland 1977). The C57BL/6J cpk/cpk (CPK) strain has subsequently been maintained through controlled breeding of obligatory heterozygotes. CPK animals, which appeared normal at birth, developed progressive lethargy and abdominal protuberance and died in renal failure at 3 to 4 weeks of post-natal age with massively enlarged kidneys (Gattone *et al.* 1988; Mandell *et al.* 1983; Preminger *et al.* 1982). Although abnormalities are limited to the kidneys in affected CPK mice (Preminger *et al.* 1982), hepatic cysts have been reported in aged heterozygous breeders (Crocker *et al.* 1987). Injection of plastic into the biliary tree of these animals as well as histological and electron microscopic studies revealed that the hepatic cysts arise from focal dilations of the epithelial lining that may enlarge to the point that they obstruct the bile ducts (Grimm *et al.* 1990). The cystic gene has produced pancreatic and hepatic fibrosis and ductal dilatation when crossbred into the basic DBA/2J strain (Fry *et al.* 1985). Therefore, the CPK mouse has been suggested as an animal model of human autosomal recessive polycystic kidney disease (Avner *et al.* 1987*a*; Crocker *et al.* 1987; Mandell *et al.* 1983; Preminger *et al.* 1982). By positional cloning, the cpk gene has been localized to a site near D12Nyu2, approximately 7 cM from the centromere of chromosome 12 (Davisson *et al.* 1991). Guay-Woodford *et al.* (1993), have shown that the syntenic linkage for the human cpk homologue is chromosome 2p23-p25.

The morphology and ontogeny of tubular cyst formation in the CPK mouse were studied by light and transmission electron microscopy and intact nephron microdissection (Avner *et al.* 1987*a*, Fry *et al.* 1985; Gattone *et al.* 1988; Nidess

reports that immunohistological expression of basement membrane components was normal in tubular cyst walls at one week (Avner *et al.* 1988*b*), focal decreases in basement membrane antigen expression were later demonstrated in enlarged cysts (Ebihara *et al.* 1988). The immunohistological findings were inversely correlated with whole kidney mRNA levels for type IV collagen and laminin. Thus, while decreased message levels were associated with immunohistologically normal antigen expression, increased message levels were associated with focal decreases in immunohistological expression of these components. Despite these alterations, the viscoelasticity (a measure of deformability) of tubular basement membranes from CPK kidneys does not differ from those of controls (Grantham *et al.* 1987). Thus matrix abnormalities may contribute to cystogenesis in this model by altering the cystic cellular microenvironment rather than altering tubular wall compliance.

Cowley *et al.* (1987), described elevated c-myc proto-oncogene expression in CPK kidneys during the later stages of cystogenesis. It was subsequently shown that there was also marked overexpression of the proto-oncogenes c-fos and c-Ki-ras consistent with an increased rate of cell proliferation and an altered state of differentiation (Cowley *et al.* 1991). Harding *et al.* (1992), has demonstrated increased c-fos and c-myc transcription by nuclear run-on transcription in cystic kidneys and localized c-myc mRNA by *in situ* hybridization in nephron anlagen and elongating tubules of normal and cystic kidneys during late fetal and early neonatal kidney development. They suggest that increased c-myc expression in CPK kidneys is linked to the proliferation of cystic epithelium.

Sulphated glycoprotein-2 (SGP-2) is a secreted, dimeric, glycosylated protein synthesized by a number of different epithelial cell types. SGP-2 has been hypothesized to be involved in the promotion of cell-cell interaction and programmed cell death and has been shown to developmentally regulated in the mouse kidney (Harding *et al.* 1991). Abnormally high levels of SGP-2 mRNA were found in the cyst wall epithelium of CPK kidneys (Harding *et al.* 1991). This suggests that PKD may, in part, be a defective developmental process in which there is delay in terminal differentiation. This is supported by additional data demonstrating that the expression of epithelial cell adhesion molecules N-CAM and E-cadherin, believed to be involved in guiding the sequential differentiation and polarization of normal renal epithelium, is decreased in CPK cystic kidneys (Rocco *et al.* 1992) as well as the persistence of apical/lateral EGFR expression in cystic collecting tubules (Avner *et al.* 1992) as previously noted.

Additional abnormalities reported in CPK kidneys include increased expression of endothelin (ET-1) and its receptor, proliferating cell nuclear antigen (PCNA), transforming growth factor-beta (TGF-β), and tumour necrosis factor-alpha (TNFα) (Nakamura *et al.* 1993*a*) and decreased expression of Ke 6 (Aziz *et al.* 1993). Further studies will be required to clearly link these findings to specific cystogenic processes.

Woo *et al.* (1994), studied the effect of weekly Taxol on the progression of cystic kidney disease in 10-day-old CPK mice. Although the treatment was lethal in some animals, Taxol prolonged the life span and slowed the progression of kidney disease in other affected animals. This report demonstrates the promise of pharmacotherapy in decreasing cyst enlargement and suggests that the microtubular network may have a particular role in mediating PKD. Additional studies are required to determine the specific mechanisms of microtubular inhibitors in modulating cystogenesis, and to determine their potential role as treatment options in human PKD.

The JCK mouse

A new recessive mutation called juvenile cystic kidneys (JCK) arose in a transgenic line of mice, but appears unrelated to the MMTV/c-myc transgene since it segregates freely from it (Atala *et al.* 1993). Affected mice had palpably enlarged kidneys from 4 to 7 weeks of age, and survived 5 to 6 months. No histological abnormalities were found in any other organs. Although the jck gene has not yet been completely mapped, complementation analysis demonstrated that it is not allelic to either cpk or pcy (Atala *et al.* 1993).

Focal cysts were evident in affected animals as early as 3 days of life. By 15 days, cysts were evident in about 15 per cent of the kidney cortex. Progressive cystic changes were found with increasing age, shifting from cortical disease, to outer medullary involvement (Atala *et al.* 1993).

The relatively late onset and longer life span in this model of recessive PKD offers a unique opportunity to study the pathophysiology of cystic renal disease. Further study is needed to identify the nephron segments involved and the location of the candidate gene to determine whether this model is suitable for the study of human autosomal recessive PKD (ARPKD).

The PCY mouse

In 1973, a spontaneous mutation in the KK mouse strain transmitted a form of PKD in an autosomal recessive fashion (Takahashi *et al.* 1986). The cystic gene was originally designated cy but currently is designated pcy. The pcy locus has been mapped to a region of mouse chromosome 9 homologous to human chromosome 3 (Takahashi *et al.* 1991). Due to poor reproduction of the original KK-pcy strain, a congenic pcy strain was developed in DBA/2 mice, DBA/2FG-pcy/pcy (Takahashi *et al.* 1991).

DBA/2FG-pcy/pcy mice inherited a slowly progressive PKD in an autosomal recessive fashion which was similar in many clinical and morphological respects to human ADPKD (Takahashi *et al.* 1991). Affected homozygotes developed enlarged kidneys after 8 weeks of age and became azotaemic after 18 weeks of age. Renal cysts developed in all segments of the nephron and progressively enlarged with age. Individual cysts were lined by a single layer of epithelial cells. Focal polyps and mounds of cells were found principally in collecting ducts. The early stage of cyst formation was characterized by slight, non-specific, tubular and glomerular basal lamina abnormalities and associated with accelerated eruption of incisors. Azotaemia and chronic interstitial inflammation characterized later stages of cyst development in all affected animals and 10 per cent developed cerebral vascular aneurysms. On another genetic background, C57FB/6, macroscopic renal cysts did not develop until 30 weeks of age and overall the disease progression was slower (Nago *et al.* 1991). This suggests that phenotypic expression of the pcy gene in the mouse depends on genetic background and that variations in the severity of human PKD may be explained in part by individual genetic differences.

Although Na-K ATPase mislocates to apical plasma membrane of renal epithelia in some, but not all studies of ADPKD (Wilson *et al.* 1991; Carone *et al.* 1994) and CPK mouse (Avner *et al.* 1992), only normal basolateral location was identified in PCY renal tubular epithelia (Kawa *et al.* 1994). This suggests, as noted earlier, that abnormal Na pump polarity is not a consistent feature of PKD.

Nakamura *et al.* (1993*b*), examined mRNA expression of growth-related proteins in the PCY model. The mRNA levels encoding for PCNA, TGFβ, platelet-derived growth factor-A and -B (PDGF-A, PDGF-B), insulin-like growth factor-I (IGF-I), and basic fibroblast growth factor (bFGF) were increased with the progression of cystic lesions in the kidneys of PCY mice from 8 to 30 weeks of age when compared to controls. Consistent with other models (Gattone *et al.* 1990), EGF mRNA levels decreased with age in the PCY kidney. Aukema *et al.* (1992*c*), found abnormal ratios of various membrane lipid components in 4-month-old PCY kidneys. This indicates a possible abnormality in polyunsaturated fatty acid metabolism in this model of PKD. These lipid abnormalities may influence membrane-mediated events such as receptor activation, signal transduction, ion transport, and enzyme activities.

Polyphosphoinositidol-phosphate (PIP) isomers have been demonstrated to be important mediators of cell proliferation *in vitro* (Whitman *et al.* 1988). Recently it has been demonstrated that activated cells possess a PIP metabolic pathway involving the D-3 phosphorylation of PIP by 3-kinase enzymes. Various oncogenes, hormones, and growth factors have been associated with the activity of the 3-kinase enzymes (Aukema *et al.* 1992*a*) and the elevation of 3-kinase products has been found in transformed cells (Serunian *et al.* 1990). Aukema *et al.* (1992*a*), demonstrated the *in vivo* formation of a 3-kinase product, phosphatidylinositol(3)phosphate(PI3P), in the kidney and liver of PCY mice, after intraperitoneal injection of [^{3}H] myoinositol. The formation of renal [^{3}H] PI3P relative to [^{3}H] PIP was positively correlated with cyst proliferation and renal enlargement.

Based on the data suggesting a role for abnormal lipid metabolism in PCY cystogenesis, Aukema *et al.* (1992*b*) studied the effects of dietary protein restriction and fatty acid composition (oils high in omega-3 fatty acids vs. oils high in omega-6 fatty acids) on the early progression of PKD in PCY mice. Although dietary lipids had no effect on disease progression, early dietary protein restriction resulted in decreased total cyst area per kidney. These results indicate that early dietary protein restriction in PKD prior to clinical manifestation of the disease may have a significant impact on disease progression. However, a recent clinical trial including humans with ADPKD found that protein restriction had little or no benefit on slowing the progression of renal disease (Klahr *et al.* 1994).

The BPK mouse

We have recently characterized a new murine model of PKD. A spontaneous mutation in an inbred colony of Balb/c mice transmitted a form of PKD in an autosomal recessive fashion was designated Balb/c bpk/bpk (BPK) (*Balb/cPolycysticKidney*) (Nauta *et al.* 1993). The animals developed massively enlarged kidneys and died of renal failure in the first month of post-natal life. The chromosomal location of the bpk mutation has not yet been mapped.

Similar to the CPK strain, initial cystic lesions occurred in the proximal tubules with a subsequent shift in the site of cystic lesions to collecting ducts by day 21 as determined by segment-specific lectin binding (Nauta *et al.* 1993). The immunocytochemical composition of basement membranes of cystic tubular walls during post-natal development was normal during the earliest stage of cyst formation. However, with disease progression, cystic tubular basement membranes demonstrated decreased immunoreactivity to antilaminin and antientactin antibodies. This suggests that basement membrane abnormalities are not a primary feature of early cyst formation but may be secondary to progressive cystic enlargement in this model (Ozawa *et al.* 1993). Animals homozygous for the BPK gene also demonstrated liver abnormalities consisting of proliferative intrahepatic biliary tract ectasia and nonobstructive dilation of the common bile duct (Nauta *et al.* 1993). Like the renal tubular epithelial hyperplasia demonstrated in the CPK model (see above), biliary epithelial hyperplasia in the BPK model appears to be mediated by a mitogenic cycle driven by the TGFα/EGF/EGFR axis (Nauta *et al.* 1995). The hyperplastic abnormalities in both renal and biliary epithelium make this mouse strain a good model for the study of the dual organ cellular pathophysiology of ARPKD.

The NM1633 mouse

Recently, a new mutant mouse, with heritable PKD, was identified in the C57BL/6J mouse line at the Jackson Laboratory (Janaswami and Berkenmeier 1995). Affected mice are small, with short limbs and tail, and have a peculiar facial dysmorphism. Approximately half die before 21 days of age and the survivors die between 6 to 12 months with massively enlarged cystic kidneys. Other organs are affected including the liver with abnormal proliferation of portal bile ducts. The severe form of the disease appears to be inherited as autosomal recessive. The nm1633 mutation has been linked to markers on chromosome 8. The morphology and pathophysiology of cyst formation in this new model have yet to be characterized.

The CBA/Ca-KD mouse

In 1971, Lyon and Hulse described a new autosomal recessive medullary cystic kidney disease that arose in an inbred strain of CBA/Ca mice and called the affected mice 'kdkd' for kidney disease. The kidneys of the mice were normal at birth but at 10 weeks of age they developed a focal peritubular mononuclear cell infiltrate. Over the next several weeks of life tubular dilation occurred in the medulla and cortex, primarily in areas of inflammatory infiltrate. By 4 months of age, the tubulo-interstitium became fibrotic and the glomeruli became sclerotic. During this period, the animals developed a concentrating defect followed by progressive renal failure. Lyon and Hulse (1971), proposed that the kdkd mice were a model of human nephronophthisis.

It is now known that the kdkd mice inherit a T cell-mediated autoimmune disease which has histological features of interstitial nephritis and microcyst formation (Kelly and Neilson 1990). CD8$^+$T cells recognize a tubulo-interstitial antigen in association with class I major histocompatibility complex antigens (Kelly *et al.* 1986). This is potentially useful model to study the mechanisms by which immune cells and their cytokine products contribute to cystogenesis.

CBA/N immunodeficient mouse

Rahilly *et al.* (1992), described a polycystic lesion of the kidney in the CBA/N mouse with an X-linked recessive immunodeficient syndrome. This mouse carries an X chromosome-linked recessive mutation (xid) which specifically affects B lymphocyte differentiation. The xid mutation leads to an inability to generate antibodies to thymus-independent type 2 antigens and to poor proliferative response to B cell mitogens. All CBA/N mice of greater that 3 months of age exhibited PKD.

The kidneys appeared normal at birth but progressively enlarged with hyperplastic cysts up to 1 mm in diameter throughout the renal parenchyma. Light microscopy localized cystic dilation to glomeruli, proximal tubules, loops of Henle, and distal tubules. The collecting ducts and the remainder of the collecting system were normal and there was no evidence of luminal obstruction. The cystically dilated tubules showed markedly thickened PAS-positive basement membranes with positive reactivity for laminin and type IV collagen. In older animals, interstitial fibrosis, mixed mononuclear cell infiltrates, and glomerulosclerosis were seen. The liver was morphologically normal. The finding of a polycystic kidney lesion in these mice as well as the CBA/Ca-KD model discussed above, offers an opportunity to investigate the relationship between the immune system and renal cyst formation.

Genetically transmitted renal cystic disease: transgenic models

One approach to defining disease-specific genes is to create models in which the genetic background of the animal is modified in a specific manner. The recently

Table 3.2 Genetically transmitted murine polycystic kidney disease: transgenic models

Mouse model	Expression	Chromosome		Defect
		Mouse	Human	
TgN7373Rpw	Recessive	14	13	Disruption of a possible cell cycle control gene
SBM	Dominant	–	–	C-myc overexpression
Bcl–2 'knockout'	Recessive	1	18	Abnormal regulation of apoptosis
SV40 early region	Dominant	–	–	Expression of large T antigen
SR2–3 chimeric	Dominant	–	–	v-src integration

acquired ability to produce specific alterations in the genetic background of mice affords a unique opportunity to asses the effect of the increased or decreased expression of a specific gene on the structure and function of an organ of interest. Such modifications have been carried out in the creation of the transgenic mice described in this section and summarized in Table 3.2.

TgN737Rpw

A line of transgenic mice has been generated at the Oak Ridge National Laboratory which demonstrate a phenotype similar to ARPKD. This line was developed as part of a large-scale insertional mutagenesis programme and is designated TgN(lmorpk)-737Rpw, abbreviated as TgN737Rpw (Moyer *et al.* 1994).The transgenic line was generated on the FVB/N inbred genetic background by pronuclear microinjection of a construct which contains the bacterial chloramphenicol acetyltransferase gene under the control of a mutated version of the polyoma early region promoter (Bohnlein *et al.* 1985). In the FVB/N inbred genetic background, homozygous mutant animals had scruffy fur, pre-axial poly-dactyly on all limbs, PKD, abnormalities of the intrahepatic biliary tract, and were severely growth-retarded. Most of the TgN737Rpw mutant mice on the FVB/N background died during the first week of life, although a few animals lived for several months. In contrast, on the C3H inbred genetic background, TgN737Rpw mice had a less severe phenotype. These animals lived longer, had polydactyly that was more variable, developed renal cysts at a slower rate, and had a less aggressive liver lesion. The significant difference in the lesions when the mutation is expressed on a different genetic background suggests the presence of important modifier genes. This may also be the case in human ARPKD, in which the severity of the phenotype and the nature of the liver lesion can be quite variable (Bernstein 1986). The mutant locus in the TgN737Rpw line has been mapped to mouse chromosome 14. This chromo-somal assignment rules out allelism of TgN737Rpw with pcy and cpk, which map to chromosomes 9 and 12 respectively (Takahashi *et al.* 1991; Guay-Woodford *et al.* 1993). Moreover, complementation testing with the BPK mouse has ruled out allelism between TgN737Rpw and bpk (Moyer *et al.* 1994).

Therefore, it appears likely that the TgN737Rpw mutation represents a novel murine PKD mutation.

Histologically, the lesions in the kidneys and livers of TgN737Rpw mutant mice were remarkably similar to those seen in the BPK mouse (Nauta *et al.* 1993) and human ARPKD (Moyer *et al.* 1994). Both renal collecting tubule ectasia and the biliary ectasia and/or portal hepatic fibrosis were a constant finding of the disease in the mutant animals. In the kidneys, an initial mild, microscopic dilation of the proximal tubules was followed by marked dilation and cyst formation of the collecting tubules. This pattern of early proximal tubule dilation followed by a shift to predominant dilation of the collecting tubule is similar to that seen in the CPK and BPK murine models (Avner *et al.* 1988*b*; Nauta *et al.* 1993) as well as human ARPKD (Bernstein 1986). The liver lesion was characterized by the proliferation of epithelial cells that arise from the portal triads and form primitive, dysplastic, tortuous structures that expand the portal and periportal areas. On the C3H genetic background, the kidney lesions were morphologically similar with all cysts being localized to collecting tubules by post-natal day 70, and the liver lesions were characterized by biliary hyperplasia, dysplasia, and portal fibrosis.

The mutant locus was cloned and characterized through use of the transgene as a molecular marker. Northern blot analysis revealed that the primary wild-type transcript of 3.2 kb was normally expressed in a number of tissues including kidney and liver and was absent in all mutant tissues examined including the adult kidney and liver from TgN737Rpw homozygotes. The predicted protein is unique and the primary amino acid sequence revealed that the protein contains 10 copies of an internally repeated 34 amino acid sequence referred to as the tetratricopeptide repeat (TPR) (Sikorski *et al.* 1990). The TPR was first described in lower eukaryotes as a motif associated with several genes involved in cell cycle control (Sikorski *et al.* 1990). More recently, TPR containing proteins in yeast and Drosophila have been discovered that function in various cellular processes including protein import, transcription, and neurogenesis (Goebl and Uanagida 1993; Van der Leij *et al.* 1993). The finding that the interrupted gene at the mutant locus in the TgN737Rpw line contains a motif common to several cell cycle control genes suggests that this gene normally functions to regulate the cell cycle in the epithelial component of the kidney. Inactivation of the gene in the mutant animals may cause epithelial hyperplasia by a pertubation in the cell cycle progression that results either in activation of the cellular proliferative response, or in the alteration of the normal pattern of apoptosis in the developing kidney.

Utilizing the mouse cDNA as a probe, most of the corresponding human gene has been cloned and mapped to human chromosome 13 (Moyer *et al.* 1994). Though probably not identical to the gene mutated in ARPKD that has been linked to human chromosome 6 (Zerres *et al.* 1994), the identification and characterization of this unique cystic gene and its protein product will likely add new and important insight into the molecular and cell biology of PKD.

SBM transgenic mouse

The c-myc proto-oncogene is believed to be involved in the regulation of cell proliferation (Luscher and Eisenman 1990) and is transiently expressed in the uninduced mesenchyme and developing tubular epithelium during normal mouse renal embryogenesis (Zimmerman *et al.* 1986; Mugrauer and Ekblom 1991; Schmid *et al.* 1989). Trudel *et al.* (1991), described a transgenic mouse with continued renal expression of c-myc post-natally which develops dominantly transmitted PKD. The transgenic mice carried a fusion gene including the *s*imian virus 40 (SV40) enhancer, the β-globin promoter, and the c-*myc* coding region (SBM) which was expressed at high levels in the renal tubular epithelium with weak or absent expression in other organs. The SBM transgene was completely penetrant and the affected mice developed markedly enlarged kidneys, muscular atrophy, and runting. The mice died a 1 to 5 months of age due to renal failure (D'Agati and Trudel 1992). Recently Trudel *et al.* (1994), reported the disappearance of PKD in revertant SBM mice in which a spontaneous mutation results in loss of the c-myc transgene expression.

On histological examination of the kidneys, there were multiple cortical and medullary cysts. A spectrum of cystic hyperplasia and papillary hyperplasia was present in most mice and a few contained renal epithelial microadenomas. Lectin, immunohistochemical, and electron microscopic studies showed that the cysts were present at birth and increased in number and diameter with age (D'Agati and Trudel 1992). Cysts predominantly involved the collecting tubules of young transgenic mice but progressively affected the proximal tubules. With advanced disease, focal segmental and global glomerulosclerosis and interstitial fibrosis were also observed. In 80 per cent of the adult SBM transgenic mice examined, the kidneys also contained focal interstitial aggregates of atypical plasma cells. In a small percentage of mice more generalized involvement of lymphoid organs by these atypical plasma cell infiltrates was also observed. No hepatic or pancreatic cysts were detected, nor were cerebral aneurysms observed.

The overexpression of c-myc in the renal tubular epithelium of the SBM mouse appears to trigger cyst formation. While c-myc is best known for its oncogenic potential as a promoter of cell proliferation, this work demonstrates that the proto-oncogene may also play an important role in certain non-neoplastic genetic diseases. The specific localization of c-myc expression to the renal tubular cyst epithelia associated with hyperplasia in SBM transgenic mice as well as elevated c-myc expression in renal cysts of CPK mice (Harding *et al.* 1992) again suggest that cyst formation can arise through the deregulation of tubular epithelial cell proliferation.

The Bcl-2 -/- 'Knockout' mouse

Bcl-2 is a proto-oncogene that plays a key role in protecting cells against apoptosis or programmed cell death. Coles *et al.* (1993), has shown that apoptosis is found in both the nephrogenic and medullary regions of the developing rat kidney and follows a distinct developmental time course. The Bcl-2 protein is expressed in the developing human (Lu *et al.* 1993) and murine kidney (Veis *et al.* 1993). Veis *et al.* (1993), reported that bcl-2 -/- 'knockout' mice developed polycystic kidneys soon after birth. The bcl-2 -/- mice appeared normal at birth but by approximately one week of age, they could be identified by their decreased size, small external ears, and immature facial features. The mice turned gray with the second hair follicle cycle implicating a defect in redox-regulated melanin synthesis. Haematopoiesis including lymphocyte differentiation was initially normal but the thymus and spleen underwent massive apoptotic involution. Renal failure was associated with PKD characterized by hyperplastic, dilated proximal and distal tubular segments associated with interstitial proliferation. Histological examination showed various degrees of cystic disease from small or moderate cysts in small kidneys to extremely dilated cysts in grossly enlarged kidneys. Many glomeruli were encapsulated within an abnormal cuboidal epithelium and some glomeruli were surrounded by multilayered immature epithelial crescents. Most other organs, including the liver, appeared normal.

Abnormal regulation of apoptosis may prove to be an important link between the various models of PKD. Programmed cell death is one suggested mechanism for the B cell depletion in CBA/N polycystic *xid* mice (Rahilly *et al.* 1992). Comparison of the SBM model (Trudel *et al.* 1991) to the bcl-2 -/- mice is of interest given the interplay between c-myc and Bcl-2 in oncogenesis (Vaux *et al.* 1988; McDonnell and Korsmeyer 1991) and the ability of Bcl-2 to counter c-myc induced apoptosis (Bissonnette *et al.* 1992; Fanidi *et al.* 1992). C-myc expression is also increased in the hyperplastic epithelium lining the cyst walls in CPK mice. Perhaps the elimination of Bcl-2 in -/- mice leads to unregulated c-myc resulting in proliferation and cell death. The observation that Bcl-2 regulates an antioxidant pathway (Hockenbery *et al.* 1993) suggests a link between the PKD induced by antioxidant drugs in rodent models (Avner *et al.* 1990) and that seen in bcl-2 -/- mice. Whether abnormalities of bcl-2 gene family expression occur in other mouse models of PKD or human polycystic disease remains to be determined.

The SV40 early region transgenic mouse

Mackay *et al.* (1987), have examined the kidneys of transgenic mice which express the transformation antigen called large-T antigen, encoded by the early region of simian virus 40 (SV40). Numerous functions have been attributed to SV40 large-T antigen including initiation of viral DNA replication (Tegtmeyer 1972), regulation of early and late region gene expression (Alwine *et al.* 1977), and immortalization and transformation of tissue culture cells (Tegtmeyer 1975). The mice appeared normal until 3 to 4 months of age when they developed choroid plexus tumours followed by death. In addition to these tumours, renal abnormalities were found in the majority of animals associated with thymic hyperplasia, thymomas, and rarely, liver tumours. Immunoprecipitation with antibody against large-T antigen revealed expression in affected tissues but not normal organs (Brinster *et al.* 1984). Kelley *et al.* (1991), produced another

SV40 early region transgenic line which consistently developed polycystic kidneys, with significant kidney enlargement and death in the most severely affected animals between 1 and 2 months of age.

The MacKay *et al.* (1987) transgenic line showed heterogeneity in the type and severity of renal lesions but the majority of the older mice displayed glomerulosclerosis and/or proliferative tubular lesions which in some were associated with multiple, large tubular cysts. In the animals described by Kelley *et al.* (1991), found marked proliferation of tubular epithelial cells with focal neoplastic areas and occasional replacement of normal renal parenchyma by invading tumour was characteristic. Glomerulosclerosis was not a significant feature but overall the numbers of glomeruli were decreased.

The appearance of proliferative cystic lesions in mice transgenic for a transforming gene suggests a clear link between expression of a gene which controls cell proliferation and the development of renal cysts. It is interesting to note that renal cysts are a prominent feature of tuberous sclerosis and Von Hippel–Lindau syndrome, two disorders characterized by the presence of tumours in many organs. Tumours and cysts may represent different degrees of the same pathological process differing only in the degree of escape from cell cycle control.

SR2-3 chimeric mouse model

Embryonic stem (ES) cells are developmentally pluripotent cells which, on successful introduction into the mouse embryo, contribute to all cell lineages of the fetus (Bradley *et al.* 1984).The SR2-3 ES cell line which has a single integrated copy of the v-src retroviral vector SR2 reproducibly gives rise to chimeric mice with cystic kidney disease (Boulter *et al.* 1992). The severity of the disease ranged from the presence of a few small cysts in otherwise normal renal tissue to greatly enlarged cystic kidneys. The dominant transmission and variable severity of kidney involvement were similar to human ADPKD. However, no extrarenal manifestations were present even though other tissues were found to be chimeric. On histological examination, numerous epithelial macroscopic and microscopic cysts were present in the cortex and medullary involvement was seen in severely affected animals.

The cause of kidney disease in the chimeric mice is unclear. The v-src oncogene might be responsible for the hyperplasia in this disorder as seen in the SV40 large-T antigen and c-myc SBM models. However, the v-src activity in the kidneys of the chimeric mice is low. Alternatively, the disease may result from a dominant mutation at a cystic locus. This could have arisen either spontaneously in the SR2-3 cell line, or may have been caused by insertion of the retroviral vector leading to disruption of a critical gene resulting in cystogenesis.

In vitro murine models: renal organ culture

Because of the uncontrolled variables inherent in the study of *in vivo* cysts formation, several investigators have recently turned to the *in vitro* study of cystic renal tubular epithelium. *In vitro* studies, which include cyst-induction in renal organ culture and cell culture of cyst-derived tubular epithelia and established epithelial cell lines, permit highly controlled experimental conditions. *In vitro* models thereby allow precise study of abnormalities of cellular metabolism and function that promote cyst development.

Organ culture methodology is particularly suited to controlled studies of renal cystogenesis because cyst formation can be induced in a tissue undergoing advanced organotypic differentiation (Avner *et al.* 1988*a*). Tubular cysts can be experimentally produced in renal explants incubated in chemically defined, serum-free medium in the absence of vascularization, perfusion, or urine production (Avner *et al.* 1983, 1984*a,b*, 1985, 1986, 1987*a,b,c*, 1988*a,b*, 1989*b*). Thus, the processes of cyst formation and progressive enlargement can be experimentally isolated from the influences of glomerular filtration and flow-related phenomena, endothelial-mesangial cell interaction, and the effects of growth factors and transport substrates present in mammalian serum or urine.

Following initial studies demonstrating the potential of organ culture methodology (Crocker 1973; Crocker and Vernier 1970; Resnick *et al.* 1973), Avner *et al.* subsequently reported that proximal tubular cyst formation could be induced in developing metanephric organ culture tissue under completely defined conditions by *cis*-dichlorodiamine II platinum (1983), glucocorticoids (1984*a,b*), and triiodothyronine (1987*c*). Proximal tubular cyst formation was induced in the metanephric culture system amid a background of normal organotypic epithelial differentiation. Cyst induction in the glucocorticoid and triiodothyronine models was directly linked to increases in Na-K ATPase activity and was completely inhibited by specific Na-K ATPase blockade with ouabain (Avner *et al.* 1985, 1987*c*). Subsequent studies suggested that the mechanism of cyst formation in these models involved increases in metanephric organic anion uptake driven by sodium gradients, with intratubular sequestration of osmotically active substances obligating net intratubular fluid accumulations. Abnormal transtubular transport under these experimental conditions led to net fluid secretion in discrete nephron segments, playing a significant role in cyst formation and enlargement. Additional studies (Avner and Sweeney 1990; Pugh *et al.* 1995) demonstrated that EGF and transforming growth factor-alpha (TGFα) acted as cystogens during nephrogenesis in fetal metanephric explants. Blockade of ligand-EGFR interaction or inhibition of the EGFR tyrosine kinase activity by tyrophostin S25, tyrophostin B42, or genistein abolished all growth factor effects and blocked tubular cyst formation (Pugh *et al.* 1995). Avner *et al.* (1986), showed that cystic lesions of CPK renal explants undergo complete regression when cultured under defined environmental conditions in serum-free organ culture medium. *In vitro* tubular cyst regression in CPK explants was directly correlated with increases in explant Na-K ATPase activity and could be directly modulated by experimental stimulation of Na-K ATPase activity with triiodothyronine or by blockade of Na-K ATPase activity with ouabain (Avner *et al.* 1989*a*). Experimental modulation of tubular cyst regression and formation in this model was effected without alterations in tubular epithelial hyperplasia or tubular basal lamina composition. As in the organ culture studies of normal fetal murine tissue, preliminary studies have demonstrated that sodium pump dependent alterations in transtubular organic anion transport promote proximal tubular cyst enlargements. Thus, organ culture studies have delineated precise mechanisms by which cysts may be produced in normal developing tubules as well as a genetically determined renal cystic disease, and suggested specific targets (i.e. Na-K transporter, EGFR) for possible pharmacotherapy to decrease progressive cystic enlargement in PKD.

The relationship of experimental models to human cystic disease states

It should be obvious that the theories of renal cyst formation generated in experimental murine models are not mutually exclusive, and that they are largely complementary. On the basis of mathematical models it has been suggested that if tubular epithelial hyperplasia is present any additional factor or combination of factors such as obstruction, abnormal tubular basement membrane compliance, or fluid secretion, is sufficient to explain the observed kinetics of cyst growth in ADPKD (Welling 1990). Thus, a hypothesis has been generated to interrelate such factors in experimental renal cyst formation and to provide a theoretical framework for future investigations (Fig. 3.1). In this hypothesis, a mutant gene or certain environmental factors can directly lead to alterations in tubular epithelial metabolism. Further, environmental factors can modulate the expression of a mutant gene or directly lead to tubular cell death. An induced alteration in tubular cell metabolism may subsequently lead directly to abnormal sorting of transport proteins, growth factor receptors, or cell adhesion molecules; abnormal extracellular matrix production; or to the production of growth factors mediating tubular hyperplasia. Induced changes in transtubular transport energetics may lead to hyperplasia secondary to increased transmembrane sodium flux, while programmed cell death may lead to further hyperplasia secondary to tubular regeneration. Alterations in sodium pump polarity or sodium pump-mediated transtubular transport could lead to net intratubular fluid accumulation. Subsequent increases in tubular wall tension may further increase stimulation of epithelial proliferation, leading to tubular hyperplasia. The presence of a particular pattern of tubular hyperplasia and necrotic debris from cell death could lead to partial tubular obstruction and further increases in tubular wall tension. Finally, abnormal extracellular matrix production could alter the epithelial microenvironment further increasing hyperplasia and transtubular transport, thereby contributing to cyst formation and progressive cyst enlargement. Such a hypothesis of renal cyst formation appropriately focuses future investigations on the molecular mechanisms by which tubular epithelial hyperplasia is controlled and tubular metabolism is altered in both experimental and human cystic diseases.

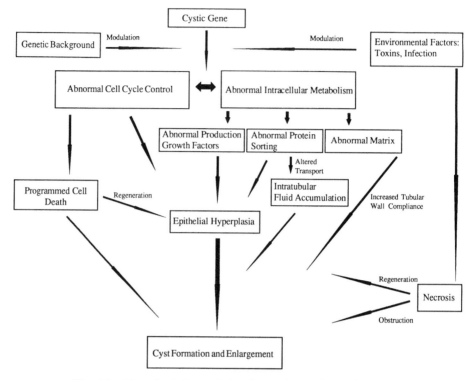

Fig. 3.1   Hypothesis interrelating factors in renal cyst formation.

References

Alwine, J. C., Reed, S. I., and Stark, G. S. (1977). Characterization of the autoregulation of simian virus 40 gene *American Journal of Virology*, **4**, 22–7.

Atala, A., Freeman, M. R., Mandell, J., and Beier, D. R. (1993). Juvenile cystic kidneys (jck): A new mouse mutation which causes polycystic kidneys. *Kidney International*, **43**, 1081–5.

Aukema, H. M., Chapkin, R. S., Tomobe, K., Takahashi, H., and Holub, B. J. (1992*a*). In vivo formation of polyphosphoinositide isomers and association with progression of murine polycystic kidney disease. *Experimental and Molecular Pathology*, **57**, 39–46.

Aukema, H. M., Ogborn, M. R., Tomobe, K., Takahashi, H., Hibino, T., and Holub, B. J. (1992*b*). Effects of dietary protein restriction and oil type on the early progression of murine polycystic kidney disease. *Kidney International*, **42**, 837–42.

Aukema, H. M., Yamaguchi, T., Takahashi, H., Celi, B., and Holub, B. J. (1992*c*). Abnormal lipid and fatty acid compositions of kidneys from mice with polycystic kidney disease. *Lipids*, **27**, 429–35.

Avner, E. D. (1988). Renal cystic disease: insights from recent experimental investigations. *Nephron*, **48**, 89–93.

Avner, E. D. (1993). Renal developmental diseases. *Seminars in Nephrology*, **13**, 427–35.

Avner, E. D. and Sweeney, W. E. (1990). Polypeptide growth factors in metanephric growth and segmental nephron differentiation. *Pediatric Nephrology*, **4**, 372–7.

Avner, E. D., Sweeney, W. E., and Ellis, D. (1983). Cyst formation in metanephric organ culture induced by cis-dichlorodiammine platinum (II). *Experientia*, **39**, 74–6.

Avner, E. D., Piesco, N. P., Sweeney, W. E., Studnick, F. M., Fetterman, G. H., and Ellis, D. (1984*a*). Hydrocortisone-induced cystic metanephric maldevelopment in serum-free organ culture. *Laboratory Investigation*, **50**, 208–18.

Avner, E. D., Sweeney, W. E., Piesco, N. P., and Ellis, D. (1984*b*). A new model of glucocorticoid-induced cystic metanephric maldevelopment. *Experientia*, **40** 489–90.

Avner, E. D., Sweeney, W. E., Finegold, D. N., Piesco, N. P., and Ellis, D. (1985). Sodium-potassium ATPase activity mediates cyst formation in metanephric organ culture. *Kidney International*, **28**, 447–55.

Avner, E. D., Sweeney, W. E., Piesco, N. P., and Ellis, D. (1986). Regression of genetically-determined polycystic kidney disease in murine organ culture. *Experientia*, **42**, 77–80.

Avner, E. D., *et al.* (1987*a*). Congenital murine polycystic kidney disease. I. The ontogeny of tubular cyst formation. *Pediatric Nephrology*, **1**, 587–96.

Avner, E. D., Sweeney, W. E. and Ellis, D. (1987*b*). Increased organic anion uptake mediates proximal tubular cyst formation in metanephric organ culture. *Kidney International*, **31**, 159.

Avner, E. D., Sweeney, W. E., Piesco, N. P., and Ellis, D. (1987*c*). Triiodothyronine-induced cyst formationin metanephric organ culture: the role of increased Na-K ATPase activity. *Journal of Laboratory and Clinical Medicine*, **109**, 441–54.

Avner, E. D., Sweeney, W. E., and Ellis, D. (1988*a*). Transtubular organic anion transport mediates congenital murine renal tubular cyst formation *in vitro*. *Clinical Research*, **36**, 782a.

Avner, E. D., Sweeney, W. E., Young, M. C., and Ellis, D. (1988*b*). Congenital murine polycystic kidney disease. II. Pathogenesis of tubular cyst formation. *Pediatric Nephrology*, **2**, 210–18.

Avner, E. D., Sweeney, W. E., and Ellis, D. (1989*a*). Isolated proximal tubules and proximal tubular cyst of CPK mice have increased Na-K ATPase activity. *Kidney International*, **35**, 423.

Avner, E. D., Sweeney, W. E., and Ellis, D. (1989*b*). In vitro modulation of tubular cyst regression in murine polycystic kidney disease. *Kidney International*, **36**, 960–8.

Avner, E. D., McAteer, J. A., and Evan, A. P. (1990). Models of cysts and cystic kidneys. In *The cystic kidney*, (ed. K. D. Gardner and J. Bernstein), pp. 55–98. Kluwer, Boston.

Avner, E. D., Sweeney, W. E. and Nelson, W. J. (1992). Abnormal sodium pump distribution during renal tubulogenesis in congenital murine polycystic kidney disease. *Proceedings of the National Academy of Sciences USA*, **89**, 7447–51.

Aziz, N., Maxwell, M. M., St.-Jacques, B., and Brenner, B. M. (1993). Downregulation of Ke 6, a novel gene encoded within the major histocompatibility complex, in murine polycystic kidney disease. *Molecular and Cellular Biology*, **13**, 1847–53.

Beauwens, R, and Crabbe, J. (1985). Biochemistry of hormone action. In *Renal biochemistry*, (ed. R. K. H. Kinne), pp. 273–335. Elsevier, Amsterdam.

Bernstein, J. (1986). Hepatic and renal involvement in malformation syndromes. *Mount Sinai Journal of Medicine*, **53**, 421–8.

Bissonnette, R. P., Echeverri, F., Mahboubi, A., and Green, D. R. (1992). Apoptotic cell death induced by c-myc is inhibited by bcl-2. *Nature*, **359**, 552–4.

Bohnlein, E., Chowdhury, K., and Gruss, P. (1985). Functional analysis of the regulatory region of polyoma mutant F9-1 DNA. *Nucleic Acids Research*, **13**, 4789–809.

Boutler, C. A., Aguzzi, A., Evans, M. J., and Affara, N. (1992). A chimaeric mouse model for autosomal-dominant polycystic kidney disease. *Contributions to Nephrology*, **97**, 60–70.

Bradley, A., Evans, M. J., Kaufman, M. H., and Robertson, H. J. (1984). Formation of germline chimaeras from embryo-derived teratocarcinoma cell lines. *Nature*, **309**, 255–6.

Breyer, M. D., Jacobson, H. R., and Breyer, J. (1988). Epidermal growth factor inhibits the hydroosmotic effect of vasopressin in the isolated perfused rabbit cortical collecting tubule. *Journal of Clinical Investigation*, **82**, 1313–20.

Brinster, R. L., Chen, H. Y., Messing, A., VanDyke, T., Levine, A. J., and Palmiter, R. D. (1984). Transgenic mice harboring SV40 T-antigen genes develop characteristic brain tumors. *Cell*, **37**, 367–79.

Carone, F. A., Nakamura, S., Caputo, M., Bacallao, R., Nelson, W. J., and Kanwar, Y. S. (1994). Cell polarity in human renal cystic disease. *Laboratory Investigation*, **70**, 648–55.

Coles, H. S. R., Burne, J. F., and Raff, M. C. (1993). Large-scale normal cell death in the developing rat kidney and its reduction by epidermal growth factor. *Development*, **118**, 777–84.

Crowley, B. D., Smardo, F. L., Grantham, J. J., and Calvet, J. P. (1987). Elevated c-myc protooncogene expression in autosomal recessive polycystic kidney disease. *Proceedings of the National Academy of Sciences USA*, **84**, 8394–8.

Cowley, B. D., Chadwick, L. J., Grantham, J. J., and Calvet, J. P. (1991). Elevated proto-oncogene expression in polycystic kidneys of the C57BL/6J (cpk) mouse. *Journal of the American Society of Nephrology*, **1**, 1048–53.

Crocker, J. F. S. (1973). Human embryonic kidneys in organ culture: abnormalities of development induced by decreased potassium. *Science*, **181**, 1178–9.

Crocker, J. F. S. and Vernier, R. L. (1970). Fetal kidney in organ culture: abnormalities of development induced by decreased amounts of potassium. *Science*, **169**, 485–7.

Crocker, J. F. S., Blecher, S. R., Givner, M. L., and McCarthy, S. C. (1987). Polycystic kidney and liver disease and corticosterone changes in the CPK mouse. *Kidney International*, **31**, 1088–91.

D'Agati, V. and Trudel, M. (1992). Lectin characterization of cystogenesis in the SBM transgenic model of ploycystic kidney disease. *Journal of the American Society of Nephrology*, **3**, 975–83.

Davison, M. T., Guay-Woodford, L. M., Harris, H. W., and D'Eustachio, P. (1991). The mouse polycystic kidney disease mutation (cpk) is located on proximal chromosome 12. *Genetics*, **9**, 778–81.

Ebihara, I., *et al.* (1988). Altered mRNA expression of basement membrane components in a murine model of polycystic kidney disease. *Laboratory Investigation*, **58**, 262–9.

Fanidi, A., Harrington, E. A., and Evan, G. I. (1992). Cooperative interaction between c-myc and bcl-2 proto-oncogenes. *Nature*, **359**, 554–6.

Freiberg, J. M., Kinsella, J., and Sacktor, B. (1982). Glucocorticoids increased the Na^+-H^+ exchange and decrease the Na^+ gradient-dependent phosphate-uptake systems in renal brush border membrane vesicles. *Proceedings of the National Academy of Sciences, USA*, **79**, 4932–6.

Fry, J. L., Koch, W. E., Jennette, J. C., McFarland, E., Fried, F. A., and Mandel, J. (1985). A genetically determined murine model of infantile polycystic kidney disease. *Journal of Urology*, **134**, 828–33.

Garg, L. C., Narang, N., and Wingo, C. S. (1985). Glucocorticoid effects on Na-K ATPase in rabbit nephron segements. *American Journal of Physiology*, **248**, F487–91.

Gattone, V. H., II, *et al.* (1988). Autosomal recessive polycsytic kidney disease in a murine model: a gross and microscopic description. *Laboratory Investigation*, **59**, 231–8.

Gattone, V. H. II. Andrews, G. K., Nie, F. W., Chadwich, L. J., Klein, R. M., and Calvet, J. P. (1990). Defective epidermal growth factor gene expression in mice with polycsytic kidney disease. *Developmental Biology*, **138**, 225–30.

Goebl, M. and Yanagida, M. (1991). The TPR snap helix: a novel protein repeat motif from mitosis to transcription. *Trends in Biochemical Sciences*, **16**, 173–7.

Grantham, J. J., Donoso, V. S., Evan, A. P., Carone, F. A., and Gardner, K. D. Jr (1987). Viscoelastic properties of tubule basement membranes in experimental renal cystic disease. *Kidney International*, **32**, 187–97.

Grimm, P. C., Crocker, J. F., Malatjalian, D. A., and Ogborn, M. R. (1990). The microanatomy of the intrahepatic bile duct in polycystic disease: comparison of the cpk mouse and human. *Journal of Experimental Pathology*, **71**, 119–31.

Guay-Woodford, L. M., D'Eustachio, P., and Bruns, G. A. P. (1993). Identification of the syntenic human linkage for the mouse congenital polycystic kidney (cpk) locus. *Journal of the American Society of Nephrology*, **4**, 814.

Harding, M. A., Chadwich, L. J., Gattone, V. H. II, and Calvet, J. P. (1991). The SGP-2 gene is developmentally regulated in the mouse kidney and abnormally expressed in collecting duct cysts in polycystic kidney disease. *Developmental Biology*, **146**, 483–90.

Harding, M. A., Gattone, V. H., Grantham, J. J. and Calvet, J. P. (1992). Localization of overexpressed c-myc mRNA in polycystic kidneys of the cpk mouse. *Kidney International*, **41**, 317–15.

Hockenberry, D. M., Oltvai, Z. N., Yin, X-M., Milliman, C. L., and Korsmeyer, S. J. (1993). Bcl-2 functions in an antioxidant pathway to prevent apoptosis. *Cell*, **75**, 241–51.

Horikoshi, S., Kubota, S., Martin, G. R., Yamada, Y., and Klotman, P. E. (1991). Epidermal growth factor (EGF) expression in the congenital polycystic mouse kidney. *Kidney International*, **39**, 57–62.

Igarashi, Y., Aperia, A., Larsson, L., and Zetterstrom, R. (1983). Effect of beta-methasone on Na-K ATPase activity and basal and lateral cell membranes in proximal tubular cells during early development. *American Journal of Physiology*, **245**, F232–7.

Janaswami, P. and Berkenmeier, E. H. (1995). Role of modifier genes in polycystic kidney disease *Kidney International*, **47**, 731–2.

Kawa, G., *et al.* (1994). Sodium pump distribution is not reversed in the DBA/2FG-pcy, polycystic kidney disease model mouse. *Journal of the American Society of Nephrology*, **4**, 2040–9.

Kelley, K. A., Agarwal, N., Reeders, S., and Herrup, K. (1991). Renal cyst formation and multifocal neoplasia in transgenic mice carrying the simian virus 40 early region. *Journal of the American Society of Nephrology*, **2**, 84–97.

Kelly, C. J. and Neilson, E. G. (1990). The interstitium of the cystic kidney. In *The cystic kidney*, (ed. K. D. Gardner and J. Bernstein), pp. 43–53. Kluwer, Boston.

Kelly, C. J., Korngold, R., Mann, R., Clayman, M., Haverty, T., and Neilson, E. G. (1986). Spontaneous interstitial nephritis in kdkd mice. II. Characterization of tubular antigen-specific H-2K-restricted Lyt-2+ effector T cell that mediates destructive tubulointerstitial injury. *Journal of Immunology*, **136**, 526–31.

Klahr, S., *et al.* (1994). The effects of dietary protein restriction and blood-pressure control on the progression of chronic renal disease. *New England Journal of Medicine*, **330**, 877–84.

Lakshmanan, J. and Fisher, D. A. (1993). An inborn error in epidermal growth factor prohormone metabolism in a mouse model of autisomal recessive polycystic kidney disease. *Biochemical and Biophysical Research Communications*, **196**, 892–901.

Lu, Q. L., Poulsom, R., Wong, L., and Hanby, A. M. (1993). Bcl-2 expression in adult and embryonic non-haematopoietic tissues. *Journal of Pathology*, **169**, 431–7.

Luscher, B. and Eisenman, R. N. (1990). New light on Myc and Myb. Part I. Myc. *Genes and Development*, **4**, 2025–35.

Lyon, M. F. and Hulse, E. V. (1971). An inherited kidney disease of mice resembling human nephronophthisis. *Journal of Medical Genetics*, **8**, 41–8.

MacKay, K., Striker, L. J., Pinkert, C. A., Brinster, R. L., and Striker, G. E. (1987). Glomerulosclerosis and renal cysts in mice transgenic for the early region of SV40. *Kidney Internationl*, **32**, 827–37.

Mandell, J., Koch, W. K., Nidess, R., Premlinger, G. M., and McFarland, E. (1983). Congenital polycystic kidney disease. *American Journal of Pathology*, **113**, 112–4.

McDonlad, A. T. J., Crocker, J. F. S., Digout, S. C., McCarthy, S. C., Blecher, S. R. and Cole, D. E. (1990). Glucocorticoid-induced polycystic kidney disease-a-threshold trait. *Kidney International*, **37**, 901–8.

McDonnell, T. J. and Korsmeyer, S. J. (1991). Progression from lymphoid hyperplasia to high grade malignant lymphoma in mice transgenic for the t(14;18). *Nature*, **349**, 254–6.

Moyer, J. H., *et al.* (1994). Candidate gene associated with a mutation causing recessive polycystic kidney disease in mice. *Science*, **264**, 1329–33.

Mugrauer, G. and Ekblom, P. (1991). Contrasting expression patterns of three members of the myc family of protooncogenes in the developing and adult mouse kidney. *Journal of Cell Biology*, **112**, 13–25.

Nagao, S., Hibino, T., Koyama, Y., Marunouchi, T., Konishi, H., and Takahashi, H. (1991). Strain difference in expression of the adult-type polycystic kidney disease gene, pcy, in the mouse. *Jikken-Dobutsu Experimental Animals*, **40**, 45–53.

Nakamura, T., *et al.* (1993*a*). Increased endothelin and endothelin receptor mRNA expression in polycystic kidneys of cpk mice. *Journal of the American Society of Nephrology*, **4**, 1064–72.

Nakamura, T., *et al.* (1993*b*). Growth factor gene expression in kidney of murine polycystic kidney disease. *Journal of the American Society of Nephrology*, **3**, 1378–86.

Nauta, J., Ozawa, Y., Sweeney, W. E., Rutledge, J. C., and Avner, E. D. (1993). Renal and biliary abnormalities in a new murine model of autosomal recessive polycystic kidney disease. *Pediatric Nephrology*, **7**, 163–72.

Nauta, J., Sweeney, W. E., Rutledge, J. C., and Avner, E. D. (1995). Biliary epithelial cells from mice with congential polycystic kidney disease are hyperresponsive to epidermal growth factor. *Pediatric Research*, **37**, 55–63.

Nidess, R., Koch, W. E., Fried, F. A., McFarland, E., and Mandell, J. (1984). Development of the embryonic murine kidney in normal and congenital polycystic kidney disease: characterization of a proximal tubular degenerative process as the first observable light microscopic defect. *Journal of Urology*, **131**, 156–62.

Ogborn, M. R. and Crocker, J.F. (1991). Ontogeny of dexamethasone binding and sodium potassium ATPase activity in experimental murine polycystic kidney disease. *Journal of Steroid Biochemistry and Molecular Biology*, **39**, 181–4.

Ogborn, M. R., Crocker, J. F. S., and McCarthy, S. C. (1987). RU 38486 prolongs survival in murine congenital polycystic kidney disease. *Journal of Steroid Biochemistry*, **28**, 783–4.

Ogborn, M. R., Sareen, S., and Grimm, P. C. (1993). Renal tubule Na, K-ATPase polarity in glucocorticoid-induced polycystic kidney disease. *Journal of Histochemistry and Cytochemistry*, **41**, 555–8.

Oikarinen, A. I., Uitto, J., and Oikarinen, J. (1986). Glucocorticoid action on connective tissue. *Medical Biology*, **64**, 221–30.

Ojeda, J. L. and Garcia-Porrero, J. A. (1982). Structure and development of parietal podocytes in renal glomerular cysts induced in rabbits with methylprednisole acetate. *Laboratory Investigation*, **47**, 167–76.

Ojeda, J. L., Barbosa, E., and Gomez-Bosque, P. (1972). Morphological analysis of renal polycystosis induced by corticoids. *Journal of Anatomy*, **111**, 399–413.

Ojeda, J. L., Ros, M. A. and Garcia-Porrero, J. A. (1986). Polycystic kidney disease induced by corticoids. *Nephron*, **42**, 240–8.

Orellana, S. A., Sweeney, W. E., Neff, C. D., and Avner, E. D. (1995). Epidermal growth factor receptor expression is abnormal in murine polycystic kidney. *Kidney International*, **47**, 490–9.

Ozawa, Y., Nauta, J., Sweeney, W. E. and Avner, E. D. (1993). A new murine model of autosomal recessive polycystic kidney disease. *Nippon-Jino-Gakkai-shi*, **35**, 349–54.

Pouyssegur, J., Franchi, A., L'Allemain, G., Magnaido, I., Paris, S., and Sardet, C. (1987). Genetic approach to structure function, and regulation of the Na$^+$/H$^+$ antiporter. *Kidney International*, **32**, S144–9.

Preminger, G. M., Koch, W. E., Fried, F. A., McFarland, E., Murphy, E. D., and Mandell, J. (1982). Murine congenital polycystic kidney disease: a model for studying development of cystic disease. *Journal of Urology*, **127**, 556–60.

Pugh, J. L., Sweeney, W. E., and Avner, E. D. (1995). The tyrosine kinase activity of the EGF receptor in murine metanephric organ culture. *Kidney International*, **47**, 774–81

Rahilly, M. A., Samuel, K., Ansell, J. D., Michelem, H. S., and Fleming, S. (1992). Polycystic kidney disease in the CBA/N immunodeficient mouse. *Journal of Pathology*, **168** 335–42.

Reeves, W. H., Kanwar, Y. S., and Farquhar, M. G. (1980). Assembly of the glomerular filtration surface. *Journal of Cell Biology*, **85**, 735–53.

Resnick, J. S., Brown, D. M., and Vernier, R. L. (1973). Oxygen toxicity in fetal organ culture. *Laboratory Investigation*, **28**, 437–45.

Rocco, M. V., Neilson, E. G., Hoyer, J. R., and Ziyadeh, F. N. (1992). Attenuated expression of epithelial cell adhesion molecules in murine polycystic kidney disease. *American Journal of Physiology*, **262**, F679–86.

Ros, M. A., Garcia-Porrero, J. A., and Ojeda, J. L. (1987). Duplication of slit diaphragms in the cystic glomeruli of rabbits treated with methylprednisolone acetate. *Acta Anatomica*, **130**, 362–5.

Russell, E. S. and McFarland, E. C. (1977). Cystic kidneys. *Mouse Newsletter*, **56**, 40–3.

Schmid, P., Schultz, W. A. and Hameister, H. (1989). Dynamic expression pattern of the myc protooncogene in midgestation mouse embryos. *Science*, **24**, 225–9.

Serunian, L. A., Auger, K. R., Roberts, T. M., and Cantley, L. C. (1990). Production of novel polyphosphoinositides in vivo is linked to cell transformation by polyomavirus middle T antigen. *Journal of Virology*, **64**, 4718–25.

Slater, E. P., *et al.* (1986). Mechanisms of glucocorticoid hormone action. *Advances in Experimental Medical Biology*, **196**, 67–80.

Sikorshi, R. S., Boguski, M. S., Goebl, M., and Hieter, P. (1990). A repeating amino acid motif in CDC23 defines a family of proteins and a new relationship among genes required for mitosis and RNA synthesis. *Cell*, **60**, 307–17.

Takahashi, H., *et al.* (1986). A new mouse model of genetically transmitted kidney disease. *Journal of Urology*, **135**, 1280–3.

Takahashi, H., Calvet, J. P., Dittemore-Hoover, D., Yoshida, K., Grantham, J. J., and Gattone V. H. (1991). A hereditary model of slowly progressive polycystic kidney disease in the mouse. *Journal of the American Society of Nephrology*, **1**, 980–9.

Tegtmeyer, P. (1972). Simian virus 40 deoxyribonucleic acid synthesis: The viral replicon. *Journal of Virology*, **10**, 591–8.

Tegtmeyer, P. (1975). Function of simian virus 40 gene A in transforming infection. *Journal of Virology*, **15**, 613–18.

Trudel, M., D'Agati, V., and Costantini, F. (1991). C-myc as an inducer of polycystic kidney disease in transgenic mice. *Kidney International*, **39**, 665–71.

Trudel, M., D'Agati, V. (1994). Disappearence of polycystic kidney disease in transgenic mice. *Mammalian Genome*, **5**, 149–52.

Uchida, S., Tsutsumi, O., Hise, M. K., and Oka, T. (1988). Role of epidermal growth factor in compensatory renal hypertrophy in mice. *Kidney International*, **33**, 387.

Van der Leij, I., Franse, M. M., Elgersma, Y., Distel, B., and Tabak, H. F. (1993). PAS10 is a tetratricopeptide-repeate protein that is essential for the import of most matrix proteins into peroxisomes of saccharomyes cerevisiae. *Proceedings of the National Academy of Sciences USA*, **90**, 11782–6.

Vaux, D. L., Cory, S., and Adams, J. M. (1988). Bcl-2 gene promotes haemopoietic cell survival and cooperates with c-myc to immortalize pre-B cells. *Nature*, **335**, 440–2.

Veis, D. J., Sorenson, C. M., Shutter, J. R., and Korsmeyer, S. J. (1993). Bcl-2-deficient mice demonstrate fulminant lymphoid apoptosis, polycystic kidneys, and hypo-pigmented hair. *Cell*, **75**, 229–40.

Welling, L. W. (1990). Pathogenesis of cysts and cystic kidneys. In *The cystic kidney*, (ed. K. D. Gardner and J. Bernstein), pp. 99–116. Kluwer, Boston.

Werder, A. A., Amos, M. A., Nielsen, A. H., and Wolfe, G. H. (1984). Comparative effects of germ-free and ambient environments on the development of cystic kidney disease in CFM_{wd} mice. *Journal of Laboratory and Clinical Medicine*, **103**, 399–407.

Whitehouse, R. W., Lendon, R. C., and Lendon, M. (1980). Renal polycytosis in the rat induced by prednisolone tertiary butylacetate. *Experientia*, **36**, 244–5.

Whitman, M., Downes, C. P., Keller, M., Keller, T., and Cantley, L. (1988). Type 1 phosphatidylinositol kinase makes a novel inositol phospholipid, phosphatidyl-inositol-3-phosphate. *Nature*, **332**, 644–6.

Wilson, P. D., Dillingham, M. A., Breckon, R., and Anderson, R. J. (1985). Defined human renal tubular epithelia in culture: growth characterization, and hormonal response. *American Journal of Physiology*, **248**, F436–43.

Wilson, P. D., Sherwood, A. C., Palla, K., Du, J., Watson, R., and Norman, J. T. (1991). Reversed polarity of $Na(^+)$-$K(^+)$-ATPase: mislocation to apical plasma membranes in polycystic kidney disease epithelia. *American Journal of Physiology*, **260**, F420–30.

Woo, D. D., Miao, S. Y., Pelayo, J. C., and Woolf, A. S. (1994). Taxol inhibits progression of congenital polycystic kidney disease. *Nature*, **368**, 750–3.

Zerres, K., *et al.* (1994). Mapping of the gene for autosomal recessive polycystic kidney disease (ARPKD) to chromosome 6p21-cen. *Nature Genetics*, **7**, 429–32.

Zimmerman, K. A., *et al.* (1986). Differential expression of myc family genes during murine development. *Nature, London*, **319**, 780–3.

4

In vivo models of PKD in non-murine species

Benjamin D. Cowley Jr and Vincent H. Gattone II

Introduction

Cystic kidney disease has been reported in numerous animal species (Table 4.1) and murine models of this disease are reviewed in another chapter. Many of the reports listed in Table 4.1 described isolated or limited numbers of cases, and therefore the characteristics of cystic disease in these animals are not well defined. In this review, we will concentrate on non-murine models of cystic kidney disease that have been used or continue to be used in attempts to understand pathogenetic mechanisms of polycystic kidney disease (PKD).

In humans, there are two inherited forms of PKD, autosomal dominant (ADPKD) and autosomal recessive (ARPKD), and there is an acquired form of PKD found in patients with end-stage renal disease (each reviewed in other chapters). Human ADPKD and acquired PKD take many years to develop and involve many different tubule segments, whereas ARPKD tends to be a rapidly progressive disease affecting, principally, collecting ducts (Welling and Grantham 1994). In view of these differences, the non-murine models of PKD are considered under the following three headings: (1) inherited, rapidly progressive (mainly involving collecting ducts); (2) inherited, slowly progressive (involving multiple tubule segments); and (3) chemically induced forms.

Inherited, rapidly progressive polycystic kidney disease

Rapidly progressive forms of PKD are typically equated with infantile PKD which, in humans, is inherited as an autosomal recessive trait. This condition is characterized by the development of numerous collecting duct cysts which replace the normal parenchyma (Welling and Grantham 1994). In addition, humans afflicted by ARPKD also exhibit liver pathology in the form of biliary duct cysts and hepatic fibrosis (see other chapter in this monograph). A number of inherited models of rapidly progressive or collecting duct PKD have been described (Table 4.1). Of those listed in Table 4.1, all but the rat model appear to have been lost. However, cells derived from the porcine model have recently been used in a culture study (Beavan *et al.* 1991) and may still be available. While hepatic pathology has not been described in the rat model (Ohno and Kondo 1989; Inage *et al.* 1991, 1993), hepatic pathology (biliary cysts and

Table 4.1   Polycystic kidney disease in non-human, non-murine animals

Inherited rapidly progressive (primarily collecting duct cysts)
Cat (AR)	Crowell *et al.* (1979)
Coyote	Roher and Nielsen (1983)
Dog (AR)	McKenna and Carpenter (1980)
Mink	Henriksen (1988)
Monkey	Baskin *et al.* (1981)
Pig (AR)	Beavan *et al.* (1991)
Rat (AR)*	Ohno and Kondo 1989; Minato *et al.* 1990; Inage *et al.* 1991, (1993)
Springbok (AR)	Iverson *et al.* (1982)

Inherited slowly progressive (multiple nephron site cysts)
Cat	Stebbins (1989)
Cat (AD)*	Biller *et al.* 1990; DiBartola *et al.* (1994)
Cat (AD)	Podell *et al.* (1992)
Ferret	Dillberger (1985)
Horse	Scott and Vasey (1986)
Monkey	Kessler *et al.* (1984)
Pig (AR)	Wijeratne and Wells (1980); Wells *et al.* (1980)
Rat (AR)*	(Kaspareit-Rittinghausen *et al.* (1989, 1990*a,b*, 1991); Cowley *et al.* (1993*b*); Schafer *et al.* (1994)
Rat	Solomon (1973)
Sheep (AD)	Jones *et al.* (1990)
Rabbit (AR)	Fox *et al.* (1971)

Inherited, unknown progression
Cat	Silvestro (1967)
Cat	Battershell and Garcia (1969)
Cat	Rendano and Parker (1976)
Cat	Northington and Juliana (1977)
Dog	McQueen *et al.* (1975)
Dog	Robertson (1986)
Horse	Ramsay *et al.* (1987)
Monkey	Miyoshi *et al.* (1984)
Pigeon	Van Alstine and Trampel (1984)
Sheep	Pazameta (1970)
Sheep	Dennis (1979)
Woodchuck	Young and Webster (1985)

Drug-induced
Biphenyl	Rat	Sondergaard and Blom (1979)
cis-Platin	Rat	Dobyan *et al.* (1981)
Corticosteroid	Rat	Crocker *et al.* (1976); Whitehouse *et al.* (1980); Crocker and McDonald (1988)
	Rabbit	Perey *et al.* (1967); Garcia Porrero *et al.* (1978); Ojeda and Garcia Porrero (1981, 1982); Ros *et al.* (1985, 1987); Ojeda *et al.* (1989, 1993)
	Hamster	Filmer *et al.* (1973)

Table 4.1   *Continued*

DPA	Chicken	Sorrentino *et al.* (1978)
	Guinea-pig	Sorrentino *et al.* (1978)
	Rat	Thomas *et al.* (1957); Crocker *et al.* (1972); Eknoyan *et al.* (1976); Evan and Gardner (1976); Gardner *et al.* (1976); Clegg *et al.* (1981); Alvarez *et al.* (1987)
DPT/phenol II	Rat	Filmer *et al.* (1973); Carone *et al.* (1974); Gardner and Evan (1983); Kanwar and Carone (1984); Butkowski *et al.* (1985); Hjelle *et al.* (1987); Lelongt *et al.* (1988); Torres *et al.* (1988); Carone (1988); Carone *et al.* (1988*a,b*; 1989, 1992); Hjelle *et al.* (1990); Ehara *et al.* (1994)
NDGA	Rat	Goodman *et al.* (1970); Gardner *et al.* (1986, *et al.* 1987); Hjelle *et al.* (1990)
5,6,7,8-Tetrahydrocarbozole-3-acetic acid	Rat	Mcgeoch *et al.* (1972); Mcgeoch and Darmady (1976)

*Inherited model still available; AR, autosomal recessive; AD, autosomal dominant.

fibrosis) similar to that seen in humans was described in the springbok (Iverson *et al.* 1982), cat (Crowell *et al.* 1979), and dog (McKenna and Carpenter 1980). All of these later models had a neonatal presentation of PKD but are no longer available.

Rat ARPKD

The remaining inherited model of autosomal recessive, collecting duct PKD still in use is a rat model of ARPKD originally described by Ohno and Kondo (1989). This rat develops skeletal abnormalities (small torso, broad skull, shortened limbs, flattened thorax, lordosis of thoracic vertebrae) and collecting duct cysts within the polycystic kidneys. The degree of renal enlargement secondary to cyst progression appears to be minimal based on published pictures of the normal and cystic kidneys. Unlike the other inherited forms of collecting duct PKD, which are very rapidly progressive, in this rat, cysts take many months to develop, leading to renal death at 6–11 months of age. There is no evidence of other visceral organ pathology. With the pattern and time frame of PKD development and the associated basement membrane alterations (Inage *et al.* 1993), this inherited PKD appears very similar to the form of PKD induced by diphenylthiazole (see below and Chapter 5). The defective gene (*chi*) in this rat model has not been assigned to a chromosome, however, no linkage was identified with fur colour (Ohno and Kondo 1989).

Inherited, slowly progressive polycystic kidney disease

Slowly progressive forms of polycystic kidney disease are typically equated with the 'adult' form of PKD which, in humans, is inherited as an autosomal dominant trait. This condition is characterized by the development of numerous cysts arising from all nephron segments (Welling and Grantham 1994). Human ADPKD usually develops over a period of decades, although childhood cases have been reported. Renal failure occurs in approximately 50 per cent of cases and typically does not occur until the fourth or fifth decade of life. Extrarenal manifestations of human ADPKD are common and include colonic diverticula, hepatic cysts, pancreatic cysts, cardiac valvular abnormalities, intracranial aneurysms, and arachnoid cysts (Welling and Grantham 1994) (see also other chapters in this book).

Han:SPRD rat

In 1989, Kaspareit-Rittinghausen and co-workers described a model of hereditary polycystic kidney disease, the Han-SPRD, which arose spontaneously in Sprague–Dawley rats (Kaspareit-Rittinghausen *et al.* 1989). Analysis of these rats showed an autosomal dominant inheritance pattern.

Homozygous Cy/Cy disease

PKD in the Han:SPRD rat has been described as an autosomal dominant trait. However the Han:SPRD mutation may not be dominant in the strict definition, since the phenotypic expression of dominant acting mutations is not altered by gene dose, and in the Han:SPRD rat there is a gene dose effect. This may not represent a difference between the Han:SPRD rat and human ADPKD. Human ADPKD is a common disease (Welling and Grantham 1994), and the lack of reported homozygous cases has led to speculation that homozygosity results in more severe disease and intrauterine death. Homozygous Han:SPRD rats develop a rapidly progressive form of PKD typified by massively enlarged cystic kidneys (Fig. 4.1), profound azotaemia, and death near 3 weeks of age, while heterozygotes develop a more slowly progressive form of PKD (Kaspareit-Rittinghausen *et al.* 1989; Cowley *et al.* 1993*b*; Schafer *et al.* 1994). In homozygotes, cysts involve all regions of the kidney, although cyst development in the inner medulla may be less pronounced (Cowley *et al.* 1993*b*; Schafer *et al.* 1994). Kidney weights and serum urea nitrogen levels are dramatically increased in homozygotes compared to normals (Kaspareit-Rittinghausen *et al.* 1989; Cowley *et al.* 1993*b*; Schafer *et al.* 1994).

Heterozygous Cy/+ disease

Kidneys from heterozygotes are clearly enlarged compared to normals (Fig. 4.2), and cysts continue to enlarge over a period of months. Kidney size decreases between 8 and 24 weeks of age due to regression of cysts and development of interstitial inflammation and fibrosis. In the young adult heterozygote, cysts affect primarily the cortex, particularly the juxtamedullary region, whereas, as in

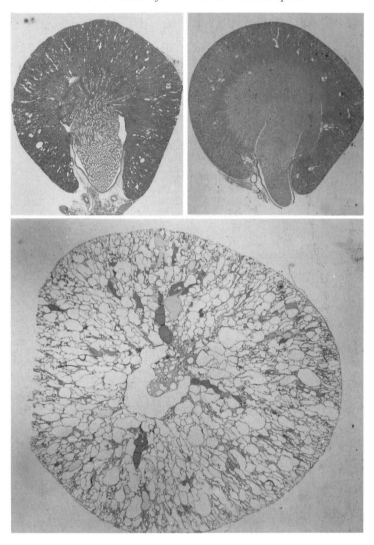

Fig. 4.1 Light micrographs of kidneys from 3-week-old normal +/+ (top right), heterozygous Cy/+ (top left), and homozygous Cy/Cy cystic (bottom) Han:SPRD rats. The heterozygous Cy/+ kidney exhibits several inner cortical, proximal tubular cysts. The kidney of the homozygous Cy/Cy cystic rat is massively enlarged by innumerable renal cysts throughout the cortex and outer medulla. All photographs are at the same magnification (×7). Reprinted from Cowley *et al.* (1993*b*) with permission.

homozygotes, the medulla is less severely involved (Cowley *et al.* 1993*b*; Schafer *et al.* 1994). Approximately 75 per cent of cysts appear to be derived from proximal tubules (Schafer *et al.* 1994). To date, extrarenal manifestations in heterozygous Han:SPRD males are those associated with uraemia and may not be specific to the Han:SPRD gene (Kaspareit-Rittinghausen *et al.* 1989, 1991).

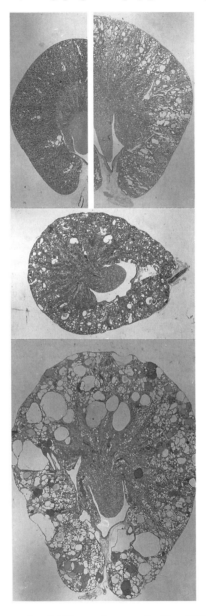

Fig. 4.2 Light micrograph of kidneys from male Han:SPRD rats: normal +/+ 10-week-old (top left), heterozygous Cy/+ 10-week-old (top right), heterozygous Cy/+ 24-week-old (middle), heterozygous Cy/+ 44-week-old (bottom). The numerous small inner cortical cysts in the 10-week-old Cy/+ largely regress by 24 weeks, however, numerous very large cysts, as well as small cysts, develop by 44 weeks. All photographs are at the same magnification (×5). Reprinted from Cowley *et al.* (1993*b*) with permission.

Cystic disease differs in severity in male and female heterozygotes (Kaspareit-Rittinghausen *et al.* 1989; Cowley *et al.* 1993*b*).The heterozygous disease is more aggressive in males, as manifest by a more rapid increase in renal size and cystic change in young adults and by the occurrence of progressive interstitial fibrosis in older male heterozygotes. Female heterozygotes show less pronounced renal enlargement in young adults. Prominence of cysts diminishes in older females, and little interstitial fibrosis is evident even in 24-week-old female heterozygotes (Cowley *et al.* 1993*b*).

The anatomical manifestations of the heterozygous disease are reflected in renal function. Heterozygous males have significantly elevated serum urea nitrogen levels at 8 weeks of age, before development of obvious interstitial fibrosis by light microscopy. Serum urea nitrogen levels become progressively elevated in older males, coincident with advancing interstitial fibrosis (Cowley *et al.* 1993*b*). Early reports indicated that male heterozygotes die near 6 months of age (Kaspareit-Rittinghausen *et al.* 1989; Cowley *et al.* 1993*b*). However, in our inbred colony and another inbred colony in Germany (N. Gretz, personal communication), male heterozygotes are now living into the second year of life. In contrast, female heterozygotes, which have less renal enlargement and interstitial fibrosis than males, have minimal elevations in serum urea nitrogen levels and appear to have a normal life span (Kaspareit-Rittinghausen *et al.* 1989; Cowley *et al.* 1993*b*). This gender difference in the development of renal failure is analogous to that seen in several studies of human ADPKD (Gretz *et al.* 1989; Gabow *et al.* 1992; Hannedouche *et al.* 1993*a,b*), although more pronounced.

Heterozygotes show patchy thickening of tubular basement membrane surrounding both cysts and normal appearing tubules. Frequently, cells overlying thickened basement membrane appear immature, as manifest by an increased nuclear to cytoplasmic ratio and an increased cell-packing density, consistent with an interaction between cells and the underlying basement membrane. Immunohistochemical studies indicate that thickened basement membrane contains type IV collagen, laminin, and fibronectin, but not type I collagen (Cowley *et al.* 1993*b*; Schafer *et al.* 1994). A reversal of epithelial basolateral Na^+-K^+ ATPase polarity, as reported in other forms of PKD (Wilson *et al.* 1991), is not seen in Han:SPRD heterozygotes (Schafer *et al.* 1994).

Pathophysiology of PKD in Han:SPRD

Hormonal abnormalities have been documented in Han:SPRD rats. Evidence of hyperparathyroidism has been seen, but is likely a manifestation of renal failure and may not be specific to the Han:SPRD gene (Kaspareit-Rittinghausen *et al.* 1991). Immunoreactive renin and renin mRNA are decreased in both homozygotes and heterozygotes. Mild anaemia has been noted with decreased renal erythropoietin mRNA, however, serum erythropoietin levels are not significantly decreased (Schafer *et al.* 1994).

Evaluation of whole kidney mRNA levels by Northern hybridization (Fig. 4.3) reveals elevated c-myc mRNA levels in homozygous cystic animals at 2 and more prominently at 3 weeks of age (Cowley *et al.* 1993*b*). Heterozygotes show

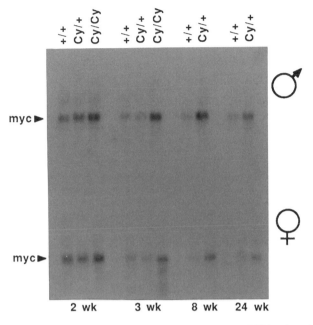

Fig. 4.3 Northern blot hybridization showing c-*myc* mRNA abundance in whole kidneys from normal +/+, heterozygous Cy/+, and homozygous Cy/Cy Han:SPRD rats. Each lane contains 5 μmg of total cellular RNA. Reprinted from Cowley *et al.* (1993*b*) with permission.

elevated c-myc mRNA levels at later ages. Elevated levels of c-fos mRNA have also been seen (Cowley *et al.* 1993*b*). These findings, earlier studies showing elevations of cell cycle-associated mRNAs in the *cpk* mouse model of autosomal recessive PKD (Cowley *et al.* 1987, 1991), and the histological evidence of cellular proliferation noted in several of the other models of PKD described in this chapter are consistent with the concept that abnormal regulation of proliferation is a component common to several forms of PKD.

A recent study (Lakshmanan and Eysselein 1993) reported abnormal expression of epidermal growth factor (EGF) in Han:SPRD rats. Using immunoblotting, these authors noted decreased expression of a 165 kDa EGF prohormone isoform in homozygotes and heterozygous males and detected a 66 kDa immunoreactive product in cyst fluid of these same animals. They suggested that the smaller protein, suggested to be a proteolytic EGF breakdown product, may act to promote cyst formation or growth.

We envision the development of renal failure in PKD as a cascade of events with several steps that may potentially be altered by many, as yet, undefined mediators (Fig. 4.4). The gender difference in the development of renal failure in heterozygous Han:SPRD rats indicates that factors other than the primary genetic defect are important in causing renal failure in this model of PKD. Recent studies have sought to advance the understanding of the development

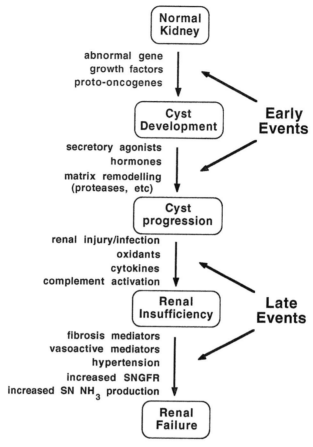

Fig. 4.4 Theoretical scheme for the progression of PKD to renal failure. Progression may stop or proceed through any stage due to endogenous or exogenous factors. The indicated mediators represent plausible, but not exhaustive, examples.

and progression of both cystic changes and renal insufficiency in Han:SPRD rats by attempts to alter the disease with exogenous interventions.

Hormonal differences due to gender

The difference in the expression of PKD in male and female Han:SPRD rats has led to speculation that gonadal hormones may affect the expression of PKD in this model. In a preliminary study from age 4 to 10 weeks of age, ovariectomy of female heterozygotes had no effect on renal size or renal function. Castration of male heterozygotes reduced the renal enlargement and the degree of cystic change without affecting renal function. In females, testosterone was a renotropic factor and worsened renal function. Thus there appeared to be a complex inter-action of gender and hormonal status in these animals (Cowley *et al.* 1994). In a similar study of Han:SPRD heterozygotes from 9 to 23 weeks of age, castration also did not affect renal function (Zeier *et al.* 1992).

Agents targeted to interstitial abnormalities

Methylprednisolone ameliorates both renal enlargement and renal failure in the Han:SPRD rat and in the *pcy*mouse, a model of slowly progressive, inherited PKD (Barash *et al.* 1993). The mechanism of this amelioration has not been defined, but may be related to anti-inflammatory effects, antifibrogenic effects, and/or other effects of the glucocorticoid.

Renal growth-promoting agents

Torres *et al.* (1990) demonstrated an association between hypokalemia and renal cysts in patients without inherited PKD. In preliminary studies, dietary potassium restriction (Cowley *et al.* 1993*a*) in Han:SPRD heterozygotes exacerbated cystic disease in both males and females as manifest by greater kidney enlargement in males and females, more severe azotaemia in males, and azotaemia in females, which normally develop PKD but not azotaemia. In complementary studies, dietary potassium bicarbonate supplementation ameliorated both cystic disease and renal failure in heterozygous Han:SPRD males (Torres *et al.* 1993); dietary sodium bicarbonate supplementation has a similar effect, but results in less body growth retardation (V. Torres, personal communication). The mechanism underlying exacerbation of cystic disease and renal failure in rats fed a potassium-depleted diet has not been determined, but may involve changes in renal ammonia production, hormones (e.g. renin, aldosterone, angiotensin), or another effect of potassium depletion. In similar experiments, ammonium chloride loading (Cowley *et al.* 1993*a*; Torres *et al.* 1993) in Han:SPRD heterozygotes exacerbated cystic disease in heterozygous Han:SPRD males and females. The mechanism whereby ammonium chloride exacerbated cystic disease and renal failure in Han:SPRD rats has also not been described. Ammonium chloride is a known cause of renal hypertrophy, and thus may act as a growth stimulus that is superimposed on the intrinsic tendency for growth seen in PKD. The observation that both sodium bicarbonate and potassium bicarbonate have a similar protective effect in male Han:SPRD heterozygotes may indicate that ammonium chloride loading, potassium depletion (which increases renal ammonia production), and potassium bicarbonate supplementation act by altering renal ammonia and/or acid handling. Ammonia has also been suggested to have a role in the progression of tubulo-interstitial diseases (Clark *et al.* 1991; Nath *et al.* 1985) and other causes of chronic renal insufficiency associated with increased renal ammonia production per unit nephron (Nath *et al.* 1994). Specifically, ammonia may be involved in complement activation in the kidney (Nath *et al.* 1985) and may also react with reactive oxygen species to from long-lived oxidants (Nath *et al.* 1994).

Chemically induced polycystic kidney disease

Several chemicals, frequently termed 'cystogens', will cause renal cystic disease when administered to laboratory animals (Table 4.1; see also (Avner *et al.* 1990; Gretz *et al.* 1992)). In addition, ureteral ligation in fetuses (Thomasson *et al.* 1970; Beck 1971; Tanagho 1972; Fetterman *et al.* 1974) and 5/6 nephrectomy (Kenner *et al.* 1985) in adults have both been reported to cause renal cystic disease, but will not be reviewed here. Characteristics of cystogen-induced PKD have been well described for only selected agents in selected species. Only these models will be reviewed here.

Corticosteroid-induced PKD

There is an extensive literature on the use of glucocorticoids to induce PKD in neonatal mammals. While the mouse seems to be the most commonly used mammal for studying glucocorticoid-induced PKD, several other animal species have been used (see Table 4.1). In all species, the glucocorticoid exposure needs to occur in the neonate, thus implicating an action as a modulator of renal cell differentiation. In mouse and rabbit, the cysts develop primarily in collecting ducts, however, in hamster, glucocorticoid-induced cysts develop mainly in the proximal and distal convoluted tubules (Filmer *et al.* 1973). *In vitro*, glucocorticoid treatment of murine metanephric cultures induces proximal tubule cysts (Avner *et al.* 1984) possibly through the induction of Na^+-K^+ ATPase (Avner *et al.* 1985). It is presently unclear what mechanism underlies glucocorticoid cystogenesis since it induces cysts in so many different tubule segments. Hypokalaemia has been proposed as one explanation based on an amelioration of glucocorticoid-induced PKD by co-administration of potassium chloride in rabbits (Perey *et al.* 1967). However, Crocker *et al.* (1976) found that potassium bicarbonate did not similarly ameliorate PKD in rats, thus implicating chloride rather than potassium in this effect. Recent evidence suggests cyst formation may be due to delayed maturation of the collecting duct. However, in rabbits, Ojeda *et al.* (1986) showed that intercalated cell development is not impaired in glucocorticoid-induced PKD. As yet, it is unclear what underlies the cystogenic action of glucocorticoids in any animal species.

Diphenylamine-induced PKD

Diphenylamine (DPA) is an antioxidant and has been used as a plastic stabilizer. Thomas *et al.* (1957) first reported the development of renal cystic disease caused by long term feeding of DPA to rats. Early studies indicated that DPA feeding in adult rats resulted in primarily collecting ducts cysts (Safour *et al.* 1970), but that DPA feeding of pregnant female rats caused proximal tubular cysts in offspring (Crocker *et al.* 1972). Later studies suggested that DPA-induced cysts occurred in all nephron segments in a pattern similar to human ADPKD (Evan and Gardner 1976). Several authors (Kime *et al.* 1962; Safour *et al.* 1970) have emphasized apparent functional, as well as structural, similarities between DPA-induced cystic disease and human ADPKD. Particular attention has been given to defects in urinary concentration, present even in early human ADPKD and seen in DPA-treated animals before the onset of severe structural abnormalities (Eknoyan *et al.* 1976).

Signs of tubular injury are prominent in DPA-induced cystic disease (Crocker *et al.* 1972; Evan and Gardner 1976; Gardner *et al.* 1976). Additionally, basement membranes surrounding cysts and tubules are thickened, and interstitial inflammation and fibrosis occur. Evidence of cellular repair with areas of hyperplasia has also been seen. One study of DPA-induced cystic disease (Gardner *et al.* 1976) suggested that tubular hyperplasia could lead to partial obstruction, elevated intratubular pressure, and subsequent cyst formation. However, the finding that many cysts in human ADPKD lose their tubular connections altogether (Grantham *et al.* 1987*b*) has led others to suggest that tubular obstruction may not be of primary importance in cyst progression in human ADPKD and that transepithelial secretion has an important role in this process. In a detailed ultrastructural examination of human ADPKD and DPA-induced cystic disease (Evan and Gardner 1976), the authors highlighted the hyperplasia seen in DPA-induced cystic disease and suggested that epithelial hyperplasia itself may have an important role in the development of renal cysts.

DPA is only one of several compounds that have been shown to cause renal cystic disease (see below and Table 4.1). Although there appear to be several similarities between DPA-induced cystic disease and human ADPKD, interest in this model has diminished, perhaps due in part to the finding that the active moiety is not DPA itself but rather an oxidative by-product present in varying abundance in commercial preparations of DPA (Crocker *et al.* 1972; Safe *et al.* 1977; Clegg *et al.* 1981).

Diphenylthiazole-induced PKD

Another antioxidant 2-amino-4,5-diphenylthiazole (DPT), has also been shown to cause renal cystic disease. Carone *et al.* (1974) reported that rats fed DPT for several weeks developed diffuse, progressive renal cystic disease that began in the medullary collecting ducts and then extended into cortical collecting ducts, distal tubules, and Henle's loops. Micropuncture studies revealed no evidence of tubular obstruction or increased intratubular pressures in DPT-induced cystic disease. Proximal tubules are relatively unaffected, and glomerular filtration and tubular transport functions remain normal. As with human ADPKD and DPA-induced cystic-disease, a defect in urinary concentration is an early event (Carone *et al.* 1974) and is in part mediated by decreased responsiveness of the collecting duct to vasopressin (Dousa *et al.* 1973; Carone *et al.* 1974). With longer periods of treatment, rats develop a decrease in glomerular filtration and moderate proteinuria (Carone *et al.* 1988*b*).

It was originally suggested that an abnormality of tubular basement membrane (BM) elasticity, caused by a DPT-induced alteration in BM structural protein, might account for cyst development in this model (Carone *et al.* 1974). Subsequent analysis of BM deformability in this and other models of PKD demonstrated normal deformability and elasticity (Grantham *et al.* 1987*a*). Additional studies (Gardner and Evan 1983) demonstrated hyperplasia prior to cyst development and papillary micropolyps, sometimes near branch points for coalescing collecting ducts. Microperfusion analysis in these same studies showed normal basal intratubular pressures in DPT-treated animals but a more rapid increase when tubules were challenged with increasing rates of tubular fluid flow. Thus, these authors suggested that partial tubular obstruction was a more likely explanation for cyst development in this model. The relevance of possible tubular obstruction to human ADPKD remains in doubt as described above for DPA.

More recent studies using this model have focused on the nature of the BM alterations seen. Abnormal BM thickening and lamination have been noted, and abnormal staining of these same structures is consistent with altered sulphated proteoglycans or anionic glycoproteins. Structural alterations in cells lining cysts occur before BM changes are are consistent with the notion that DPT affects cellular metabolism. Early biochemical studies of BMs in DPT-induced cystic kidneys noted an increase in the concentration of high molecular weight components and a decrease in the concentration of low molecular weight components (Butkowski *et al.* 1985). Altered activity of several enzymes including catalase, UDP-glucuronosyltransferase, galactosyltransferase, and sulphatase B occurs early after DPT feeding and correlates with cellular ultrastructural changes (Hjelle *et al.* 1987). Subsequent studies demonstrated inhibition of catalase and the related epoxide hydrolase by DPT, phenol II (a more potent cystogenic metabolite of DPT, see below), and the known cystogen nordihydroguaiaretic acid (Hjelle *et al.* 1990), although the pathophysiological significance of this finding remains unclear. Immunohistochemical analysis of human ADPKD and DPT-induced cystic kidneys revealed similar results, indicating a marked decrease of heparan sulphate proteoglycan, little change in type IV collagen and laminin, and an increase in peritubular and interstitial fibronectin (Carone *et al.* 1988*a*).

In spite of the above analyses, the mechanism(s) responsible for renal cyst development in DPT-fed rats remains unclear. Torres *et al.* (1988) demonstrated alterations in cyst development in response to manipulations that altered the renin–angiotensin system and suggested that angiotensin II might be an important modulator of cyst development in DPT-induced cystic disease. A hydroxy-metabolite of DPT, 2-amino-4-hydroxyphenyl-5-phenyl thiazole (designated phenol II), is a much more potent inducer of cystic disease (Carone *et al.* 1989). Studies in phenol II-fed rats showed rapid development of renal cysts which was reversible upon discontinuation of phenol II (Fig. 4.5) Additional findings included BM thickening, decreased staining for heparan sulphate proteoglycan, and increased staining for fibronectin (Carone *et al.* 1992). Analysis of several specific basement membrane components shortly after phenol II feeding revealed a rapid decrease in chondroitin sulphate proteoglycan (Ehara *et al.* 1994). Basement membrane changes coincide with cyst development and precede evidence of cellular proliferation or abnormal cellular localization of Na^+-K^+ ATPase (Carone *et al.* 1992), leading to the suggestion that BM alterations occur

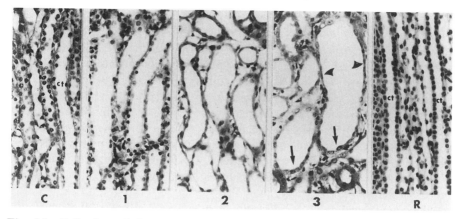

Fig. 4.5 Collecting tubules (ct) in renal outer medulla in control (C), phenol II-treated for 1, 2, and 3 days, and recovery (R) (7 days after 5 days of phenol II) kidneys. Cysts are lined by plump cells with prominent nuclei (arrows) or flattened cells (arrowheads) (Panel 3), (×200). Reprinted from Carone *et al.* (1992) with permission.

early in the cascade of events leading to cyst development and that studies of extracellular matrix–cell interactions may be of value in attempting to understand this process.

In a recent preliminary study, clusterin mRNA and immunoreactive protein were induced in tubular epithelium early after initiation of phenol II treatment in rats (Rosenberg *et al.* 1993). Clusterin, which is known by several names but was first identified as the sulphated glycoprotein SGP-2, has been associated with cell adhesion and tissue remodelling, and the authors of this recent study in phenol II-treated rats suggested that SGP-2 normally functions in cell–cell and cell–substrate interactions that are disrupted during the process of cyst formation (Rosenberg *et al.* 1993). SGP-2 is expressed at high levels in fetal and neonatal animals and its expression is down-regulated during normal development (Harding *et al.* 1991; French *et al.* 1993). SGP-2 is also abnormally expressed in the *cpk* mouse model of ARPKD, a finding that has been suggested to reflect developmental immaturity of epithelium in PKD (Harding *et al.* 1991). DPT-treated rat kidneys show evidence of epithelial injury, which in other circumstances results in dedifferentiation of epithelial cells, and may have role in the abnormal induction of this protein. SGP-2 is induced by other causes of renal injury (Rosenberg and Paller 1991; Aulitzky *et al.* 1992; Correa Rotter *et al.* 1992; Eti *et al.* 1993).

Nordihydroguaiaretic acid

Nordihydroguaiaretic acid (NDGA) is another antioxidant and has been shown to inhibit numerous enzyme systems (Goodman *et al.* 1970). Adult rats fed a diet containing 2 per cent NDGA for 6 weeks or longer develop renal cystic disease (Goodman *et al.* 1970). Cyst development is preceded by evidence of tubular injury, including necrotic and desquamated cells, particularly in proximal tubules, which have been hypothesized to accumulate an NDGA metabolite. Evidence of tubule cell degeneration is accompanied by evidence consistent with attempted tubule cell regeneration. The authors of these early studies suggested that necrotic debris and foreign material cause tubular obstruction, and in the face of continued glomerular filtration, result in increased intratubular pressure and ultimately cyst formation. Cysts initially develop in proximal tubules, but subsequently appear to involve all nephron segments. Degenerating (atrophic) tubules are seen surrounding cystic tubules. Cyst development is accompanied by interstitial inflammatory cell, fibroblast, and histiocyte infiltration and interstitial fibrosis.

Subsequent studies supported the concept that tubular obstruction is important in the development of renal cysts in NDGA-treated animals (Evan and Gardner 1979). In microperfusion studies of kidneys from NDGA-treated rats, microperfusion of dilated tubules resulted in greater increases in intratubular pressure than did microperfusion of non-dilated tubules or tubules from normal kidneys. Additionally, when [3H] inulin was instilled into tubules, the rate of excretion was lower from non-dilated tubules in NDGA-treated rats than from normal tubules in untreated rats and was even lower from dilated (cystic) tubules. Additionally, ^{3}[H] thymidine-labelling studies indicated maximal collecting tubule hyperplasia after 2 to 3 weeks of NDGA exposure, before structural evidence of cellular degeneration/regeneration or cyst formation was apparent. Furthermore, in a few cases it was possible to follow dilated tubules to the points where tubular diameters became normal, and micropolyps were consistently found at these locations. Based on this information, it was suggested that partial nephron obstruction was a likely contributor to cyst formation in NDGA-induced renal cystic disease. Once again, the relevance of tubular obstruction to human ADPKD remains in doubt as described above.

More recent studies in NDGA-treated rats have emphasized the importance of environmental factors and renal inflammation in the development of cystic disease caused by NDGA treatment. Germ-free rats treated with NDGA for 6 weeks in germ-free conditions show no evidence of renal cystic disease. In contrast, germ-free rats treated for 6 weeks with NDGA, but moved to a non-germ-free environment after 3 weeks, develop even more severe cystic disease than conventional rats treated for the same period (Fig. 4.6) (Gardner *et al.* 1986). Subsequent studies have shown that germ-free animals fed NDGA for three weeks in germ-free conditions develop cystic disease if exposed for the final week to endotoxin, either by oral feeding of endotoxin-containing bacteria or by alternate day injections of endotoxin. The severity of cystic disease correlates with the number of circulating lymphocytes and polymorphonuclear leucocytes, and cystic kidneys have a greater degree of leucocyte infiltration. The authors of these studies suggested an important role for leucocytes and possibly leucocyte-mediated injury in the pathophysiology of renal cystic disease in

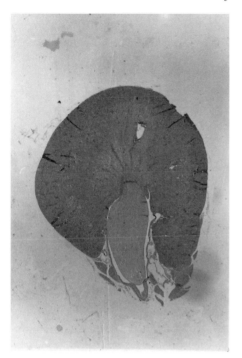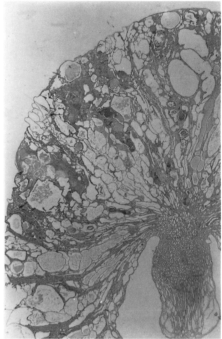

Fig. 4.6 Photomicrographs of kidneys from germ-free rats fed NDGA for 6 weeks. Animals represented in (left) remained in germ-free conditions for the entire 6 weeks, while those represented in (right) were removed from the germ-free environment after 3 weeks. Similar photomicrographs were presented in Gardner *et al.* (1986).

NDGA-treated animals (Gardner *et al.* 1987). The subsequent demonstration of several different cytokines in renal cyst fluid from patients with ADPKD gives these studies added relevance (Gardner *et al.* 1991).

Acknowledgements

The authors thank Dr Frank Carone and Dr Kenneth Gardner for providing figures used in this chapter and Dr Stephen DiBartola for providing a preprint describing ADPKD in the cat.

References

Alvarez, F., Diaz Alferez, F. J., Perez Munoz, P. J., Arteaga Serrano, F., and Martin Rodriguez, A. (1987). Cystic kidney disease induced by diphenylamine in rats [In Spanish]. *Actas Urologicas Espanolas*, **11**, 656–9.
Aulitzky, W. K., *et al.* (1992). Measurement of urinary clusterin as an index of nephrotoxicity. *Proceedings of the Society for Experimental Biology and Medicine*, **199**, 93–6.

Avner, E. D., Piesco, N. P., Sweeney, W. E., Studnick, F. M., Fetterman, G. H., and Ellis, D. (1984). Hydrocortisone-induced cystic metanephric maldevelopment in serum-free organ culture. *Laboratory Investigation*, **50**, 208–18.

Avner, E. D., Sweeney, W. E. J., Finegold, D. N., Piesco, N. P., and Ellis, D. (1985). Sodium-potassium ATPase activity mediates cyst formation in metanephric organ culture. *Kidney International*, **28**, 447–55.

Avner, E.D., McAteer, J. A., and Evan, A. P. (1990). Models of cysts and cystic kidneys. In *The Cystic Kidney*, (ed. K. D. Gardner, Jr and J. Bernstein), pp. 55–97. Kluwer, Dordrecht.

Barash, B. D., Cowley, B. D. Jr, Takahashi, H., Yamaguchi, T., Grantham, J. J., and Gattone, V. H. II (1993). Glucocorticoid inhibition of renal cystic disease in two rodent models of inherited polycystic kidney disease. *Journal of the American Society of Nephrology*, **3**, 292.

Baskin, G. B., Roberts, J. A., and McAfee, R. D. (1981). Infantile polycystic renal disease in a rhesus monkey *(Macaca mulatta)*. *Laboratory Animal Science*, **31**, 181–3.

Battershell, D. and Garcia, J. P. (1969). Polycystic kidney in a cat. *Journal of the American Veterinary Medical Association*, **154**, 665–6.

Beavan, L. A., Carone, F. A., Nakamura, S., Jones, J. K., Reindel, J. F., and Price, R. G. (1991). Comparison of proteoglycans synthesized by porcine normal and polycystic renal tubular epithelial cells *in vitro*. *Archives of Biochemistry and Biophysics*, **284**, 392–9.

Beck, A. D. (1971). The effect of intrauterine urinary obstruction upon the development of the fetal kidney. *Journal of Urology*, **105**, 784–9.

Biller, D. S., Chew, D. J., and DiBartola, S. P. (1990). Polycystic kidney disease in a family of Persian cats. *Journal of the American Veterinary Medical Association*, **196**, 1288–90.

Butkowski, R. J., Carone, F. A., Grantham, J. J., and Hudson, B. G. (1985). Tubular basement membrane changes in 2-amino-4,5-diphenylthiazole-induced polycystic disease. *Kidney International*, **28**, 744–51.

Carone, F. A. (1988). Functional changes in polycystic kidney disease are tubulo-interstitial in origin. *Seminars in Nephrology*, **8**, 89–93.

Carone, F. A., Rowland, R. G., Perlman, S. G., and Ganote, C. E. (1974). The pathogenesis of drug-induced renal cystic disease. *Kidney International*, **5**, 411–21.

Carone, F. A., Makino, H., and Kanwar, Y. S. (1988a). Basement membrane antigens in renal polycystic disease. *American Journal of Pathology*, **130**, 466–71.

Carone, F. A., Ozono, S., Samma, S., Kanwar, Y. S., and Oyasu, R. (1988b). Renal functional changes in experimental cystic disease are tubular in origin. *Kidney International*, **33**, 8–13.

Carone, F. A., Hollenberg, P. F., Nakamura, S., Punyarit, P., Glogowski, W., and Flouret, G. (1989). Tubular basement membrane change occurs pari passu with the development of cyst formation. *Kidney International*, **35**, 1034–40.

Carone, F. A., Nakamura, S., Punyarit, P., Kanwar, Y. S., and Nelson, W. J. (1992). Sequential tubular cell and basement membrane changes in polycystic kidney disease. *Journal of the American Society of Nephrology*, **3**, 244–53.

Clark, E. G., Nath, K. A., Hostetter, M. K., and Hostetter, T. H. (1991). Role of ammonia in progressive interstitial nephritis. *American Journal of Kidney Diseases*, **17**, 15–19.

Clegg, S., Safe, S., and Crocker, J. F. (1981). Identification of a toxic impurity in commercial diphenylamine. *Journal of Environmental Science and Health. Part B*, **16**, 125–30.

Correa Rotter, R., Hostetter, T. H., Nath, K. A., Manivel, J. C., and Rosenberg, M. E. (1992). Interaction of complement and clusterin in renal injury. *Journal of the American Society of Nephrology*, **3**, 1172–9.

Cowley, B. D. Jr., Smardo, F. L. Jr, Grantham, J. J., and Calvet, J. P. (1987). Elevated c-myc protooncogene expression in autosomal recessive polycystic kidney disease. *Proceedings of the National Academy of Sciences USA*, **84**, 8394–8.

Cowley, B. D. Jr, Chadwick, L. J., Grantham, J. J., and Calvet, J. P. (1991). Elevated proto-oncogene expression in polycystic kidneys of the C57BL/6J (*cpk*) mouse. *Journal of the American Society of Nephrology*, **1**, 1048–53.

Cowley, B. D. Jr, Grantham, J. J., Muessel, M. J., and Gattone, V. H. ii (1993*a*). Accelerated progression of inherited polycystic kidney disease (PKD) caused by non-genetic interventions. *Journal of the American Society of Nephrology*, **4**, 261.

Cowley, B. D. Jr, *et al.* (1993*b*). Autosomal dominant polycystic kidney disease in the rat. *Kidney International*, **43**, 522–34.

Cowley, B. D. Jr, Muessel, M. J., Rupp, J. C., and Gattone, V. H. ii (1994). Effect of gonadal hormones on progression of inherited polycystic kidney disease in Han:SPRD rats. *Journal of the American Society of Nephrology*, 619.

Crocker, J. F. and McDonald, A. T. (1988). Effects of lithium chloride and ethacrynic acid on experimental polycystic kidney disease. *Clinical and Investigative Medicine*, **11**, 16–21.

Crocker, J. F., Brown, D. M., Borch, R. F., and Vernier, R. L. (1972). Renal cystic disease induced in newborn rats by diphenylamine derivatives. *American Journal of Pathology*, **66**, 343–50.

Crocker, J. F., Steward, A. G., Sparling, J. M., and Bruneau, M. E. (1976). Steroid-induced polycystic kidneys in the newborn rat. *American Journal of Pathology*, **82**, 373–80.

Crowell, W. A., Hubbell, J. J., and Riley, J. C. (1979). Polycystic renal disease in related cats. *Journal of the American Veterinary Medical Association*, **175**, 286–8.

Dennis, S. M. (1979). Urogenital defects in sheep. *Veterinary Record*, **105**, 344–7.

DiBartola, S., Biller, D., Eaton, K., Wellman, M., and Radin, M. J. (1994). Animal model: Autosomal dominant polycystic kidney disease in Persian cats. *Journal of Heredity*.

Dillberger, J. E. (1985). Polycystic kidneys in a ferret. *Journal of the American Veterinary Medical Association*, **186**, 74–5.

Dobyan, D. C., Hill, D., Lewis, T., and Bulger, R. E. (1981). Cysts formation in rat kidney induced by cis-platinum administration. *Laboratory Investigation*, **45**, 260–8.

Dousa, T. P., Rowland, R. G., and Carone, F. A. (1973). Renal medullary adenylate cyclase in drug-induced nephrogenic diabetes insipidus. *Proceedings of the Society for Experimental Biology and Medicine*, **142**, 720–2.

Ehara, T., Carone, F. A., McCarthy, K. J., and Couchman, J. R. (1994). Basement membrane chondroitin sulfate proteoglycan alterations in a rat model of polycystic kidney disease. *American Journal of Pathology*, **144**, 612–21.

Eknoyan, G., *et al.* (1976). Renal function in experimental cystic disease of the rat. *Journal of Laboratory and Clinical Medicine*, **88**, 402–11.

Eti, S., Cheng, C. Y., Marshall, A., and Reidenberg, M. M. (1993). Urinary clusterin in chronic nephrotoxicity in the rat. *Proceedings of the Society for Experimental Biology and Medicine*, **202**, 487–90.

Evan, A. P. and Gardner, K. D. Jr (1976). Comparison of human polycystic and medullary cystic kidney disease with diphenylamine-induced cystic disease. *Laboratory Investigation*, **35**, 93–101.

Evan, A. P. and Gardner, K. D. Jr (1979). Nephron obstruction in nordihydroguaiaretic acid-induced renal cystic disease. *Kidney International*, 15, 7–19.

Fetterman, G. H., Ravitch, M. M. and Sherman, F. E. (1974). Cystic changes in fetal kidneys following ureteral ligation: studies by microdissection. *Kidney International*, 5, 111–21.

Filmer, R. B., Carone, F. A., Rowland, R. G., and Babcock, J. R. (1973). Adrenal corticosteroid-induced renal cystic disease in the newborn hamster. *American Journal of Pathology*, 72, 461–72.

Fox, R. R., Krinsky, W. L., and Crary, D. D. (1971). Hereditary cortical renal cysts in the rabbit. *Journal of Heredity*, 62, 105–9.

French, L. E., *et al.* (1993). Murine clusterin: molecular cloning and mRNA localization of a gene associated with epithelial differentiation processes during embryogenesis. *Journal of Cell Biology*, 122, 1119–30.

Gabow, P. A., *et al.* (1992). Factors affecting the progression of renal disease in autosomal-dominant polycystic kidney disease. *Kidney International*, 41, 1311–19.

Garcia Porrero, J. A., Ojeda, J. L., and Hurle, J. M. (1978). Cell death during the post-natal morphogenesis of the normal rabbit kidney and in experimental renal polycy-stosis. *Journal of Anatomy*, 126, 303–18.

Gardner, K. D. Jr and Evan, A. P. (1983). Renal cystic disease induced by diphenylthia-zole. *Kidney International*, 24, 43–52.

Gardner, K. D. Jr, Solomon, S., Fitzgerrel, W. W., and Evan, A. P. (1976). Function and structure in the diphenylamine-exposed kidney. *Journal of Clinical Investigation*, 57, 796–806.

Gardner, K. D. Jr, Evan, A. P., and Reed, W. P. (1986). Accelerated renal cyst development in deconditioned germ-free rats. *Kidney International*, 29, 1116–23.

Gardner, K. D. Jr, Reed, W. P., Evan, A. P., Zedalis, J., Hylarides, M. D., and Leon, A. A. (1987). Endotoxin provocation of experimental renal cystic disease. *Kidney International*, 32, 329–34.

Gardner, K. D. Jr, Burnside, J. S., Elzinga, L. W., and Locksley, R. M. (1991). Cytokines in fluids from polycystic kidneys. *Kidney International*, 39, 718–24.

Goodman, T., Grice, H. C., Becking, G. C., and Salem, F. A. (1970). A cystic nephropathy induced by nordihydroguaiaretic acid in the rat. Light and electron microscopic investigations. *Laboratory Investigation*, 23, 93–107.

Grantham, J. J., Donoso, V. S., Evan, A. P., Carone, F. A., and Gardner, K. D. Jr (1987a). Viscoelastic properties of tubule basement membranes in experimental renal cystic disease. *Kidney International*, 32, 187–97.

Grantham, J. J., Geiser, J. L., and Evan, A. P. (1987b). Cyst formation and growth in autosomal dominant polycystic kidney disease. *Kidney International*, 31, 1145–52.

Gretz, N., Zeier, M., Geberth, S., Strauch, M., and Ritz, E. (1989). Is gender a deter-minant for evolution of renal failure? A study in autosomal dominant polycystic kidney disease. *American Journal of Kidney Disease*, 14, 178–83.

Gretz, N., *et al.* (1992). Rat models of polycystic kidney disease. *Contributions to Nephrology*, 97, 35–46.

Hannedouche, T., Albouze, G., Chauveau, P., Lacour, B., and Jungers, P. (1993a). Effects of blood pressure and antihypertensive treatment on progression of advanced chronic renal failure. *American Journal of Kidney Diseases*, 21, 131–7.

Hannedouche, T., Chauveau, P., Kalou, F., Albouze, G., Lacour, B., and Jungers, P. (1993b). Factors affecting progression in advanced chronic renal failure. *Clinical Nephrology*, 39, 312–20.

Harding, M. A., Chadwick, L. J., Gattone, V. H. ii, and Calvet, J. P. (1991). The SGP-2 gene is developmentally regulated in the mouse kidney and abnormally expressed in collecting duct cysts in polycystic kidney disease. *Developmental Biology*, **146**, 483–90.

Henriksen, P. (1988). Polycystic disease of the kidney in related mink. *Journal of Comparative Pathology*, **99**, 101–4.

Hjelle, J. T., Hjelle, J. J., Maziasz, T. J., and Carone, F. A. (1987). Diphenylthiazole-induced changes in renal ultrastructure and enzymology: toxicologic mechanisms in polycystic kidney disease? *Journal of Pharmacology and Experimental Therapeutics*, **243,**, 758–66.

Hjelle, J. T., Guenthner, T. M., Bell, K., Whalen, R., Flouret, G., and Carone, F. A. (1990). Inhibition of catalase and epoxide hydrolase by the renal cystogen 2-amino-4,5-diphenylthiazole and its metabolites. *Toxicology*, **60**, 211–22.

Inage, Z., *et al.* (1991). Autosomal recessive polycystic kidney in rats. *Nephron*, **59**, 637–40.

Inage, Z., *et al.* (1993). Cystic basement membrane with increased negative charge in rat autosomal recessive polycystic kidney (Letter). *Nephron*, **63**, 107–8.

Iverson, W. O., Fetterman, G. H., Jacobson, E. R., Olsen, J. H., Senior, D. F., and Schobert, E. E. (1982). Polycystic kidney and liver disease in Springbok: I. Morphology of the lesions. *Kidney International*, **22**, 146–55.

Jones, T. O., Clegg, F. G., Morgan, G., and Wijeratne, W. V. (1990). A vertically transmitted cystic renal dysplasia of lambs. *Veterinary Record*, **127**, 421–4.

Kanwar, Y. S. and Carone, F. A. (1984). Reversible changes of tubular cell and basement membrane in drug-induced renal cystic disease. *Kidney International*, **26**, 35–43.

Kaspareit-Rittinghausen, J., Rapp, K., Deerberg, F., Wcislo, A., and Messow, C. (1989). Hereditary polycystic kidney disease associated with osteorenal syndrome in rats. *Veterinary Pathology*, **26**, 195–201.

Kaspareit-Rittinghausen, J., Deerberg, F., Rapp, K. G., and Wcislo, A. (1990*a*). Renal hypertension in rats with hereditary polycystic kidney disease. *Zeitschrift für Versuchstierkunde*, **33**, 201–4.

Kaspareit-Rittinghausen, J., Deerberg, F., Rapp, K. G., and Wcislo, A. (1990*b*). A new rat model for polycystic kidney disease of humans. *Transplantation Proceedings*, **22**, 2582–3.

Kaspareit-Rittinghausen, J., Deerberg, F., and Wcislo, A. (1991). Hereditary polycystic kidney disease: Adult polycystic kidney disease associated with renal hypertension, renal osteodystrophy, and uremic enteritis in SPRD rats. *American Journal of Pathology*, **139**, 693–6.

Kenner, C. H., Evan, A. P., Blomberg, P., Aronoff, G. R., and Luft, F. C. (1985). Effect of protein intake on renal function and structure in partially nephrectomized rats. *Kidney International*, **27**, 739–50.

Kessler, M. J., Roberts, J. A., and London, W. T. (1984). Adult polycystic kidney disease in a rhesus monkey (*Macaca mulatta*). *Journal of Medical Primatology*, **13**, 147–52.

Kime, S. W., McNamara, J. J., Luse, S., Farmer, S., Silberg, C., and Bricker, N. S. (1962). Experimental polycystic renal disease in rats: Electron microscopy, function, and susceptibility to pyelonephritis. *Journal of Laboratory and Clinical Medicine*, **60**, 64–78.

Lakshmanan, J. and Eysselein, V. (1993). Hereditary error in epidermal growth factor prohormone metabolism in a rat model of autosomal dominant polycystic kidney disease. *Biochemical and Biophysical Research Communications*, **197**, 1083–93.

Lelongt, B., Carone, F. A., and Kanwar, Y. S. (1988). Decreased de novo synthesis of proteoglycans in drug-induced renal cystic disease. *Proceedings of the National Academy of Sciences USA*, **85**, 9047–51.

Mcgeoch, J. E., Woodhouse, M. A., and Darmady, E. M. (1972). Experimental infantile polycystic kidney in rats. The influence of age and sex. *British Journal of Experimental Pathology*, **53**, 322–40.

Mcgeoch, J. E. and Darmady, E. M. (1976). Polycystic disease of kidney, liver and pancreas; a possible pathogenesis. *Journal of Pathology*, **119**, 221–8.

McKenna, S. C. and Carpenter, J. L. (1980). Polycystic disease of the kidney and liver in the Cairn Terrier. *Veterinary Pathology*, **17**, 436–42.

McQueen, S. D., Directo, A. C., and Llorico, B. F. (1975). Bilateral congenital polycystic kidneys with vague symptomatology in a dog (a case report). *Veterinary Medicine — Small Animal Clinician*, **70**, 1167–71.

Minato, M., Inage, Z., Ohwada, M., and Ohno, K. (1990). A study of an autosomal recessive polycystic kidney disease with facial and skeletal abnormalities in rat [In Japanese]. *Nippon Jinzo Gakkai Shi*, **32**, 1211–20.

Miyoshi, M., Ogawa, K., Shingu, K., and Omagari, N. (1984). Scanning and transmission electron microscopy of cysts in the renal cortex of the macaque monkey. *Archivum Histologicum Japonicum*, **47**, 259–69.

Nath, K. A., Hostetter, M. K., and Hostetter, T. H. (1985). Pathophysiology of chronic tubulinterstitial disease in rats: Interaction of dietary acid load, ammonia, and complement component C3. *Journal of Clinical Investigation*, **76**, 667–75.

Nath, K. A., Fischereder, M., and Hostetter, T. H. (1994). The role of oxidants in progressive renal injury. *Kidney International*, **45**, S111–15.

Northington, J. W. and Juliana, M. M. (1977). Polycystic kidney disease in a cat. *Journal of Small Animal Practice*, **18**, 663–6.

Ohno, K. and Kondo, K. (1989). A mutant rat with congenital skeletal abnormalities and polycystic kidneys. *Jikken Dobutsu*, **38**, 139–46.

Ojeda, J. L. and Garcia Porrero, J. A. (1981). Proximal tubule changes in the polycystic kidney induced by methylprednisolone acetate in the newborn rabbit. A microdissection-SEM study. *Experentia*, **37**, 894–96.

Ojeda, J. L. and Garcia Porrero, J. A. (1982). Structure and development of parietal podocytes in renal glomerular cysts induced in rabbits with methylprednisolone acetate. *Laboratory Investigation*, **47**, 167–76.

Ojeda, J. L., Ros, M. A., and Garcia Porrero, J. A. (1986). Polycystic kidney disease induced by corticoids. A quantitative and qualitative analysis of cell populations in the tubular cysts. *Nephron*, **42**, 240–8.

Ojeda, J. L., Ros, M. A., and Garcia Porrero, J. A. (1989). Structural and morphometric characteristics of the basement membrane of rabbit parietal podocytes induced by corticoids. *Acta Anatomica (Basel)*, **135**, 307–17.

Ojeda, J. L., Ros, M. A., and Icardo, J. M. (1993). Lectin-binding sites during postnatal differentiation of normal and cystic rabbit renal corpuscles. *Anatomy and Embryology (Berlin)*, **187**, 539–47.

Pazameta, Z. (1970). An unusual case of congenital cystic kidney in a lamb. *New Zealand Veterinary Journal*, **18**, 225.

Perey, D. Y., Herdman, R. C., and Good, R. A. (1967). Polycystic renal disease: a new experimental model. *Science*, **158**, 494–6.

Podell, M., DiBartola, S. P., and Rosol, T. J. (1992). Polycystic kidney disease and renal lymphoma in a cat. *Journal of the American Veterinary Medical Association*, **201**, 906–9.

Ramsay, G., Rothwell, T. L., Gibson, K. T., Moore, J. D., and Rose, R. J. (1987). Polycystic kidneys in an adult horse. *Equine Veterinary Journal*, **19**, 243–4.

Rendano, V. T. and Parker, R. B. (1976). Polycystic kidneys and peritoneopericardial diaphragmatic hernia in the cat: a case report. *Journal of Small Animal Practice*, **17**, 479–85.

Robertson, J. L. (1986). Spontaneous renal disease in dogs. *Toxicologic Pathology*, **14**, 101–8.

Roher, D. P. and Nielsen, S. W. (1983). Polycystic kidneys in a western coyote. *Journal of the American Veterinary Medical Association*, **183**, 1276–7.

Ros, M. A., Ojeda, J. L., and Garcia Porrero, J. A. (1985). Vascular architecture modifications in the steroid-induced polycystic kidney. *Nephron*, **40**, 332–40.

Ros, M. A., Garcia Porrero, J. A., and Ojeda, J. L. (1987). Duplication of slit diaphragms in the cystic glomeruli of rabbits treated with methylprednisolone acetate. *Acta Anatomica (Basel)*, **130**, 362–5.

Rosenberg, M. E. and Paller, M. S. (1991). Differential gene expression in the recovery from ischaemic renal injury. *Kidney International*, **39**, 1156–61.

Rosenberg, M. E., Manivel, J. M., Carone, F. A., and Kanwar, Y. S. (1993). Genesis of renal cysts is associated with clusterin induction. *Journal of the American Society of Nephrology*, **4**, 822.

Safe, S., Hutzinger, O., Crocker, J. F., and Digout, S. C. (1977). Identification of toxic impurities in commercial diphenylamine. *Bulletin of Environmental Contamination and Toxicology*, **17**, 204–7.

Safour, M., Crocker, J. F. S., and Vernier, R. L. (1970). Experimental cystic disease of the kidney–sequential, functional, and morphological studies. *Laboratory Investigation*, **23**, 392–400.

Schafer, K., *et al.* (1994). Characterization of the Han:SPRD rat model for hereditary polycystic kidney disease. *Kidney International*, **46**, 134–52.

Scott, P. C. and Vasey, J. (1986). Progressive polycystic renal disease in an aged horse. *Australian Veterinary Journal*, **63**, 92, xv.

Silvestro, D. (1967). On a case of bilateral polycystic kidney in a cat [In Italian]. *Acta Medica Veterinaria (Napoli)*, **13**, 349–61.

Solomon, S. (1973). Inherited renal cysts in rats. *Science*, **181**, 451–2.

Sondergaard, D. and Blom, L. (1979). Polycystic changes in rat kidney induced by biphenyl fed in different diets. *Archives of Toxicology Supplement*, 499–502.

Sorrentino, F., Fella, A., and Pota, A. (1978). Diphenylamine-induced renal lesions in the chicken. *Urological Research*, **6**, 71–5.

Stebbins, K. E. (1989). Polycystic disease of the kidney and liver in an adult Persian cat. *Journal of Comparative Pathology*, **100**, 327–330.

Tanagho, E. A. (1972). Surgically induced partial obstruction in the fetal lamb: III. Ureteral obstruction. *Investigative Urology*, **10**, 35–52.

Thomas, J. O., Cox, A. J., and DeEds, F. (1957). Kidney cysts produced by diphenylamine. *Stanford Medical Bulletin*, **15**, 90–3.

Thomasson, B. H., Esterly, J. R., and Ravitch, M. M. (1970). Morphologic changes in the fetal rabbit kidney after intrauterine ligation. *Investigative Urology*, **8**, 261–72.

Torres, V. E., *et al.* (1988). Mechanisms affecting the development of renal cystic disease induced by diphenylthiazole. *Kidney International*, **33**, 1130–9.

Torres, V. E., Young, W. F. J., Offord, K. P., and Hattery, R. R. (1990). Association of hypokalemia, aldosteronism, and renal cysts. *New England Journal of Medicine*, **322**, 345–51.

Torres, V. E., Mujwid, D. K., Keith, D. S., Wilson, D. M., and Holley, K. H. (1993). Effect of ammonium chloride and potassium bicarbonate on the development of polycystic kidney disease (PKD) in Han:SPRD rats. *Journal of the American Society of Nephrology*, **4**, 825.

Van Alstine, W. G. and Trampel, D. W. (1984). Polycystic kidneys in a pigeon. *Avian Diseases*, **28**, 758–64.

Welling, L. W. and Grantham, J. J. (1994). Cystic diseases of the kidney. In *Renal pathology with clinical and functional correlations*, (2nd edn), (ed. C. C. Tisher and B. M. Brenner), pp. 1312–54. Lippincott, Philadelphia, PA.

Wells, G. A., Hebert, C. N., and Robins, B. C. (1980). Renal cysts in pigs: prevalence and pathology in slaughtered pigs from a single herd. *Veterinary Record*, **106**, 532–5.

Whitehouse, R. W., Lendon, R. G., and Lendon, M. (1980). Renal polycystosis in the rat induced by prednisolone tertiary butyl acetate. *Experientia*, **36**, 244–5.

Wijeratne, W. V. and Wells, G. A. (1980). Inherited renal cysts in pigs: results of breeding experiments. *Veterinary Record*, **107**, 484–8.

Wilson, P. D., Sherwood, A. C., Palla, K., Du, J., Watson, R., and Norman, J. T. (1991). Reversed polarity of $Na(^+)$-$K(^+)$-ATPase: mislocation to apical plasma membranes in polycystic kidney disease epithelia. *American Journal of Physiology*, **260**, F420–30.

Young, R. A. and Webster, W. S. (1985). Tumors and polycystic renal disease in two captive woodchucks (*Marmota monax*). *Laboratory Animal Science*, **35**, 493–6.

Zeier, M., Pohlmeyer, G., Deerberg, F., Fehrenbach, P., Waldherr, R., and Ritz, E. (1992). Progression of renal failure in a rat model of dominant cystic kidney disease. *Journal of the American Society of Nephrology*, **3**, 306.

5

Pathogenesis of polycystic kidney disease: basement membrane and extracellular matrix

Frank A. Carone, Robert Bacallao, and Yashpal S. Kanwar

Introduction

Polycystic kidney disease (PKD) is a genetic or acquired disorder with progressive dilatation of multiple tubular segments and/or enlargement of glomerular capsules, accompanied by fluid accumulation, growth of non-neoplastic epithelial cells, and deranged remodelling of the extracellular matrices. This results ultimately in a certain degree of renal functional impairment, which potentially can regress to normal after removal of the inductive agent(s) in experimental animal models (Carone *et al.* 1994; Kanwar and Carone 1984). These localized events with segmental dysmorphogenetic lesions are conceivably related to an aberration of one or more factors which maintain normal tubular and glomerular morphological features.

The evolution of epithelial-lined cystic spaces may be the result of normal or abnormal developmental processes prevalent during embryonic or adult life. Normally, during embryogenesis, the cells divide and form cellular condensates. At the morula stage, cell–cell contacts generate a polarized transporting epithelium, the trophoectoderm, leading ultimately to the formation of a cystic structure, the blastocyst (Rodriguez-Boulan and Nelson 1989). Conceivably, in an similar manner, although accompanied with certain aberrational morphogenetic steps, the formation of cysts, often multiple, occur in many benign and malignant neoplasms and in other disorders (Cotran *et al.* 1994). With reference to PKD, one can summarize by stating that the tissue expression of cystogenesis is a unique process that is dynamic, progressive, and possesses the features as defined above.

The three phenotypic features, in respect to intra- and extracellular compartments, in autosomal dominant polycystic kidney disease (ADPKD) are: (1) impaired structure and function of the Golgi complex; (2) an altered extracellular matrix (ECM); and consequentially (3) an arrest in epithelial cell maturation (dedifferentiation). These changes seem to be closely interrelated and are thus central to the pathogenesis of PKD.

Altered structure and function of the Golgi complex

To generate and maintain polarity, epithelial cells transport newly synthesized proteins from the endoplasmic reticulum (ER) through the Golgi complex to intracellular and extracellular target sites (Griffiths and Simons 1986; Simons and Zerial 1993). Movement of proteins occurs via the vesicular transport, and release from these compartments is modulated by proteins coating the intra-cellular vesicles. Movement along this pathway is facilitated by cytoplasmic microtubules or actin cables, thus propelling the vesicle cargo to the defined docking site. Docking is tightly regulated by specific proteins on the membranes of both the transport and acceptor compartments, the interactions of which leads to the release of transported proteins. Thus, it appears that the Golgi complex plays an important role in protein maturation pathways. The Golgi complex consists of a series of compartments with distinct biochemical and spatial polar-ity. Via vesicular transport, secretory proteins move from the ER to the inter-mediate compartment and thence to the *cis*-face of the Golgi complex. Post-translational modifications of proteins in the Golgi complex are numerous and diverse. However, most of the covalent additions can be classified as: (1) ad-dition of charged groups (e.g. sulphation); (2) modification of charged amino acids by addition of uncharged groups (e.g. carboxymethylation); (3) addition of hydrophilic groups (e.g. *O*-linked *N*-glycosylation); or (4) addition of hydro-phobic groups (e.g. fatty acid acylation).

Our studies in ADPKD cells indicate abnormalities in post-translational modifications during the processing of glycoproteins, principally of proteoglycans exported to the matrix and glycolipids (Carone *et al.* 1994). The major covalent protein modifications involved appear to include glycosylation, fatty acylation, and sulphation.

Proteoglycans (PGs) are complex glycoconjugates containing one or more glycosaminoglycan (GAG) chains and often *N*- and *O*-linked oligosaccharides covalently bound to a protein core via xylose–serine linkages (Hascall and Hascall 1983). The great diversity of PGs is due to the large number of different core proteins and to the polydispersity produced by a great variety of post-translational modifications involved in their biosynthesis. These modifications are relevant in the interactions of PGs with other glycoproteins (i.e. type IV col-lagen and laminin, and in their final assemblage into a mature defined matrix).

Similar to a previous study in a drug-induced model of PKD in rats (LeLongt *et al.* 1988), a decrease was seen in the *in vitro* synthesis of PGs by cyst-derived cells from autosomal dominant PKD kidneys compared to normal renal cortical epithelial (NK) cells from human kidneys (Liu *et al.* 1992). *In vitro*, the *de novo* synthesis and ECM incorporation of sulphated PGs by NK and ADPKD cells was investigated by pulse–chase experiments. The *de novo* synthesis of PGs by ADPKD vs. NK cells was significantly reduced. The charge density characteristics revealed decreased sulphation, suggestive of alteration in the post-translational modification of PGs. In addition, a delayed release of PGs to the cell exterior suggested an altered Golgi function. Furthermore, ADPKD cells synthesized PGs of higher molecular weight with an increased proportion of chondroitin sulfate PG vs. heparan sulphate PG similar to PGs synthesized during renal development, suggesting a dedifferentiated embryonic state of the

ADPKD cells. Collectively, these data indicate defect(s) in the synthesis, post-translational modification, and cellular transport of PGs by ADPKD cells. Additional pulse–chase experiments revealed that ADPKD vs. NK cells had a marked prolongation of the exit time for cellular sulphated glycoproteins into the exterior milieu (Carone *et al.* 1993). Transport kinetics revealed a substantial delay in processing and release of these macromolecules by the Golgi apparatus in ADPKD cells (Fig. 5.1). During the chase period, the kinetics for the cellular transport of sulphated glycoproteins by secretory vesicles and their incorporation into the ECM were comparable in ADPKD and NK cells. However, the percentage of total sulphated glycoproteins incorporated into the ECM of ADPKD vs. NK cell monolayers was notably diminished. These findings indicate that in ADPKD vs. NK cell monolayers, synthesis of sulphated glycoproteins in impaired, processing of sulphated glycoproteins by the Golgi apparatus is prolonged and assembly of these macromolecules into the ECM is reduced. In addition, recent studies suggest a delay in the exit of lipid from the Golgi complex in ADPKD (Bacallao *et al.* 1994).

Altered extracellular matrix

Several studies on human and experimental forms of PKD have demonstrated a number of extracellular matrix (ECM) abnormalities, suggesting that an abnormal matrix may be responsible for the development of tubular cysts (Carone *et al.* 1994). In cell–matrix interactions, there is a reciprocal dependency between the cell and its ECM (Hay 1984). The tubular epithelial cells may be primarily responsible for the synthesis/degradation of ECM components, and the composition of the ECM, in turn, plays a regulatory role in cell mobility, shape, differentiation, growth, and gene expression. The major well-characterized components of basement membranes (BM) are type IV collagen, laminin, PGs, nidogen, and entactin. In addition, several other less well-characterized BM components have also been isolated. The basic 3-dimensional structure of the BM is apparently a network of type IV collagen to which other BM components are attached by lateral or end-to-end associations. Assembly of type IV collagen monomers into large molecular aggregates provides a supporting structure for the BM. This collagen network is complex and variable and may include interactions between 7S and NC1 cross-linking domains, lateral associations along the triple helix and binding of NC1 domains into triple helical segments. BMs are heterogenous and their architecture and the concentrations of individual components may be determined by their synthesis, degradation, and remodelling. These ECM macromolecules interact with cell membrane adhesion receptors (integrins) to maintain proper cell–matrix relationships (Horwitz 1987).

The integrins are transmembrane macromolecules that link the cell cytoskeleton with ECM via interactions with talin and vinculin. Recent studies indicate that a majority of the ECM glycoproteins have peptide sequences, such as the tripeptide Arg-Gly-Asp (RGD), which are recognized by the extracellular domains of the integrins (Ruoslahti and Pierschbacher 1987). Binding affinities

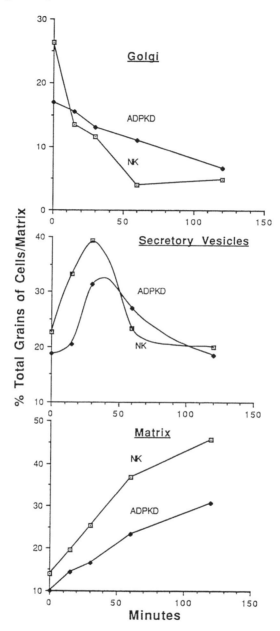

Fig. 5.1 Percentage of total grains of combined cell–matrix, determined by electron micrograph autoradiography, in Golgi complexes, secretory vesicles, and extracellular matrix of NK and ADPKD cells at 0, 15, 30, 60, and 120 min after a 150-min pulse with [^{35}S]sulphate to label sulphated glycoproteins *in vitro*.

between ECM proteins and integrins vary widely and may account for rapid dissolution and re-formation of glycoprotein–glycoprotein complexes in one situation or tissue stability in another, where these macromolecules display strong binding characteristics.

Altered cell–basement membrane interactions may be central to the pathogenesis in some forms of PKD. In a number of human and experimental models of PKD, the ECM of the various segments of the tubule is abnormal. 2-amino-4,5-diphenulthiazole (DPT)-induced PKD in rats involves collecting ducts, while the glomerular morphology, tubular functions, and the intratubular pressure are normal, suggesting that cystic transformation is due to an inherent alteration in the ECM of the tubule (Carone *et al.* 1974). The BMs lining cystic tubules are thickened, and have a loss of staining with ruthenium red, a cationic dye characteristically binding to the PGs (Fig. 5.2) (Kanwar and Carone 1984). Analysis of isolated, purified tubular basement membrane (TBM), revealed an increased content of low molecular weight glycoproteins, fibronectin, and type I collagen, but a normal content of laminin, entactin, and type IV collagen (Butkowski *et al.* 1985). Thus, DPT-induced PKD cyst formation may be due to a change in TBM compliance. However, the deformability and visco-elastic properties of BM lining cysts are not significantly different from normal TBMs (Grantham *et al.* 1987). By immunohistochemisty, compared with controls, ECM of cysts showed uneven staining for type IV collagen and laminin, weak or absent staining for heparan sulphate proteoglycans, and intense staining for fibronectin (Carone *et al.* 1988). DPT induced a marked reduction in the *de novo* synthesis of PGs, an increase in chondroitin sulphate PGs compared with heparan sulphate PGs, and an apparent reduction in their sulphation in the Golgi saccules (Lelongt 1988). The major urinary metabolite of DPT, 4-hydroxyphenyl-5-phenylthiazole (phenol II) induces PKD rapidly so that sequential tubular cell and BM changes can be correlated with the development of cysts (Carone *et al.* 1989). In this model, BM change and cyst formation developed in tandem and preceded the onset of tubular cell proliferation (Fig. 5.3).

In an autosomal recessive murine model (cpk/cpk) of PKD, mRNA expression of BM components was found to be altered (Ebihara *et al.* 1988). At an early stage, expression was reduced, while at a later stage, the mRNA transcript messages were abnormally high, which may be related to the compensatory synthesis of BM components due to rapid cyst enlargement. These alterations, presumably, were related to the changes in the mRNA expression of the interstitial cells, as elucidated in *in situ* hybridization studies with cRNA probes generated from the nucleotide sequences of the alpha-1 chain of type IV collagen. Similar altered BM protein biosynthesis was found in the primary cultures of cpk/cpk mouse kidney, suggesting that there is an intrinsic cellular defect that is not related to systemic factors (Taub *et al.* 1990). Also, the findings of reduced mRNA levels of specific cell adhesion molecules in this model, reinforces the concept that the aberrant cell–matrix interactions may ultimately be responsible for nephro-cystogenesis (Rocco *et al.* 1992).

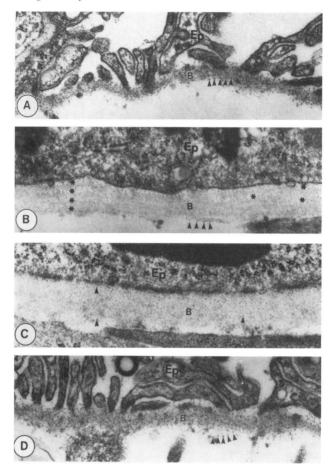

Fig. 5.2 Electron micrographs of basement membranes of collecting tubules stained with ruthenium red (RR). A, Control; (B) and (C), rats treated with DPT for 4 and 8 weeks, respectively; and (D) rats treated with DPT for 8 weeks followed by a normal diet for 8 weeks (recovery). In A, there is a normal lattice-like network of RR-stainable granules (arrows) consisting of heparan sulphate PGs. In B (DPT 4 weeks), the basement membrane (B) is thickened and laminated (*). The RR granules stain less intensely and have lost their normal lattice-like network. In C, (DPT 8 weeks), the basement membrane (B) is extremely thick, and particles only reminiscent of RR-stainable granules (arrows) are present. In D (recovery), the basement membrane (B) regains its normal thickness and RR-stained granules with a normal lattice arrangement. Ep, epithelium. (×30 000).

In PKD induced by methylprednisone in rabbits, there was a definitive correlation between the BM alterations and the development and regression of tubular cysts (Ojeda and Ros 1990). During cyst regression, an increase in the number of interstitial cells was observed, and it closely related to the changes in

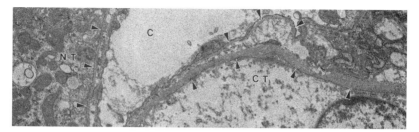

Fig. 5.3 Three-day phenol II-treated rat kidney. Basement membrane (arrowheads) of a cystic tubule (CT) is several fold thickened compared to basement membranes of a normal tubule (NT) or a peritubular capillary (C). (×24 000).

BM components. Most recently, such BM alterations have been reported in a hereditary model of slowly progressive PKD in mice resembling ADPKD.

In human ADPKD, basement membrane lining cysts are markedly thickened and laminated (Fig. 5.4), and immunohistochemical studies reveal a loss of reactivity to antiheparan sulphate PGs in the basal lamina, and an enhanced interstitial reactivity to antifibronectin (Carone *et al.* 1988). *In vitro*, post-confluent normal human renal epithelial cells (NK) and cyst-derived cells elab-

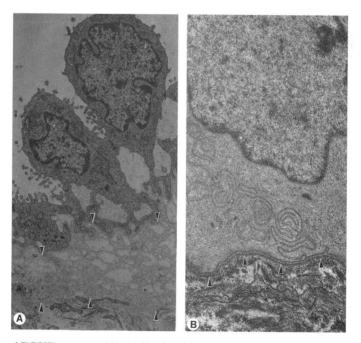

Fig. 5.4 ADPKD: a cyst (A) is lined with cuboidal cells adherent to a basement membrane (arrowheads) which is extremely thick and reticulated compared to the thin basement membrane (arrowheads) of a non-cystic tubule (B). (A, ×24 000; B, ×48 000.)

orate BMs (Carone and Kanwar 1991). The ECMs of NK cells are dense and display uniform intense reactivity to antifibronectin, antilaminin, antitype IV collagen, and antiheparan sulphate PG core peptide, whereas the ECMs of ADPKD cells are thicker, less distinct, and show diminished reactivity to anti-heparan sulphate PG and increased reactivity to antifibronectin. Furthermore, [^{35}S] sulphate-labelling studies revealed decreased synthesis and altered processing of sulphated glycoproteins by the Golgi complex by ADPKD cells (Liu *et al.* 1992; Carone *et al.* 1993). Altered biosynthesis of several of the other BM and matrix macromolecules was also observed in the cyst-derived cells of human ADPKD kidneys (Granot *et al.* 1990). Recent studies suggest a role for degradative events involving the ECM in PKD. Degradation of specific basement membrane components by metalloproteinases by processes closely regulated by tissue inhibitors of these enzymes may permit restructuring of the ECM associated with cyst development and growth (Rankin *et al.* 1994). Alterations in the expression of metalloproteinases and their inhibitors have been described in human and experimental forms of PKD (Norman *et al.* 1993; Schaefer *et al.* 1994), suggesting that degradation as well as biosynthesis of ECM are operative in PKD. Taken together, the above observations suggest that the alterations in the cell–matrix interactions may contribute to the development of PKD. In support of evidence for the concept that PKD is a primary disorder of ECM, are the findings of connective tissue anomalies affecting heart valves, cerebral arteries, and other organs, such as liver (Gabow 1990).

Impaired cell differentiation

It has been proposed that the gene defect in ADPKD causes a block in the differentiation of renal epithelial cells. During nephrogenesis, a number of growth factors have been shown to influence the various differentiation events and biosynthesis of sulphated PGs (Liu *et al.* 1990) in the development of the kidney. In cpk/cpk mice, there is a marked reduction in expression of epidermal growth factor (EGF) in the kidney (Gattone *et al.* 1990; Horikoshi 1991). There is some ancillary evidence that EGF has a regulatory role in the differentiation of renal cells, so that the loss of EGF expression may contribute to an arrest in the differentiation of cells lining the cystic collecting ducts. Compatible with this, are studies on the gene expression of the sulphated glycoprotein-2 in mice. The sulphated glycoprotein-2 (SGP-2, also known as clusterin) is expressed early in the course of nephrogenesis, and is down-regulated in normal collecting ducts but is persistently expressed at all stages in the epithelium lining cyst in cpk/cpk mice (Harding *et al.* 1991). It is known that certain proteins are transiently expressed in epithelial cells during nephrogenesis. One group of well-characterized markers of differentiation are the intermediate filament proteins. The expression of the intermediate filament proteins, vimentin and cytokeratin have been used to characterize the differentiation state of malignancies and to identify the cell lineage of carcinomas (Cotran *et al.* 1994). During nephrogenesis in the mouse embryo it has been shown that metanephric mesenchyme expresses vimentin (Ekblom 1991*a*). On induction, the metanephric mesenchyme begins to differentiate and leads to the formation of a polarized epithelium. Cytokeratin rather than vimentin becomes the intermediate filament expressed in these epithelial cells. To assess the pattern of intermediate filament expression, ADPKD and normal kidney tissue sections were fixed and stained using antibodies to vimentin and cytokeratin and the expression of cytokeratin and vimentin in cells grown in culture was also assessed (Bacallao *et al.* 1993). Cytokeratin was noted in both normal kidney and ADPKD epithelial cells. Vimentin staining was observed exclusively in the interstitium in normal kidney. However, vimentin was also expressed in the epithelial cells lining the cysts in ADPKD kidneys. About 70 per cent of the cysts examined stained positive for vimentin. The expression of vimentin and cytokeratin in primary cultures of confluent ADPKD and NK epithelial cells was examined. Cytokeratin staining was observed in 98 per cent of the NK and ADPKD cells 1 day after plating. This percentage remained relatively constant for both cell lines even after 7 days in culture. One day after plating, 98 per cent of the NK and ADPKD cells displayed reactivity to vimentin. On day 7, the percentage of NK cells that were vimentin-positive decreased to less than 10 per cent. In contrast, 45 per cent of the ADPKD cells remained vimentin-positive, consistent with a maturational arrest in these cells. Intermediate filaments are cytoskeletal proteins whose function is still unknown (Green and Stappenbeck 1994). These filaments do form stable attachments with specialized cellular junctions called desmosomes and hemidesmosomes. The junctions help mediate cell–cell and cell–matrix interactions. Given the alteration in intermediate filament expression in ADPKD, we examined the distribution of desmosomal proteins (Carone and Bacallao 1994). Kidney sections from ADPKD and NK were stained with antibodies that recognize desmoplakin I/II. In NK tubules, the staining is exclusively basolateral and is punctuate in nature. Apical desmoplakin staining was noted in ADPKD cells lining the cysts. Basolateral staining was also observed in the ADPKD cells. In order to determine whether the apical desmoplakin was due to a protein sorting defect or a differentiation block, we examined the distribution of desmoplakin in a human embryonic kidney. Apical desmoplakin was observed in immature nephron segments of 13–21-week embryonic kidneys. This suggests that the apical desmoplakin staining observed in ADPKD renal cells is another manifestation of the block in differentiation. In cultured NK epithelial cells, punctate desmoplakin staining was noted at the sites of cell–cell contact. ADPKD cells had large aggregates of desmoplakin at the cell borders and in a cytoplasmic location.

These results are consistent with the hypothesis that the genetic defect in ADPKD may be responsible for a block in the differentiation pathway of renal epithelial cells. Other findings indicate that ADPKD renal epithelial cells express a number of additional markers that are consistent with the idea that the cells are immature or dedifferentiated. For example, SGP-2, a cell adhesion molecule associated with apoptosis and transiently expressed developmentally, is expressed in ADPKD cells (Dvergsten *et al.* 1994). In addition to SGP-2, other developmentally regulated genes, PAX-2 and the proto-oncogene N-myc, are expressed in ADPKD renal epithelial cells and in embryonic kidneys (Harding *et al.* 1991). Taken together the data indicate that in ADPKD there is a block in renal epithelial differentiation pathways.

Cell–matrix interactions in normal and cystic tubular morphogenesis

Under normal conditions, cell–matrix interactions are essential for the maintenance of normal morphology and polarity of tubular epithelium (Rodriguez-Boulan and Nelson 1989; Molitoris and Nelson 1990). Disturbance of these biological processes would be expected to result in tubular dysmorphogenesis. In tubulogenesis, the induction of mesenchymal cells by the ureteric bud (Saxen *et al.* 1968; Ekblom and Willer 1991*b*; Ekblom 1992) leads to the expression of distinct cell adhesion molecules, which are specific for cell–cell (CAM, uvomorulin) communication and cell–matrix (integrins) interaction. After induction and aggregation of mesenchymal cells, the cells polarize and acquire vectorial transport properties (Rodriguez-Boulan and Nelson 1989; Wang *et al.* 1990). The development of cell polarity requires the expression of specialized structures such as tight junctions and glycoproteins at the apical and basolateral membrane domains. To achieve successful vectorial transport by the polarized cells, the membrane proteins are segregated to specific plasmalemmal domains in line with specialized functions (e.g. the restriction of Na-K ATPase to basolateral membranes). The conversion of mesenchymal cells to polarized epithelium may require an external signal (soluble factors?) for mitogenesis and differentiation (Klein *et al.* 1988; Ekblom and Weller 1991*b*). Growth factors stimulate the expression of matrix proteins that probably provide orientation signals for the cell. Interaction of matrix proteins with cell surface receptors induces organization of the cytoskeletal actin network, the major scaffolding for modulating further differentiation and development of cell membrane domains. The formation of cell–cell contacts and expression of adhesion molecules integrate the cells into a polarized monolayer and maintains the separation of the cell membrane domains. Microtubules and microfilaments appear essential for the spatial organization of intracellular organelles and aid in the delivery of transport vesicles to specific membrane domains.

Thus, the cell polarity and tubular structural organization are dependent upon tightly regulated cell–cell and cell–matrix interactions. Cell-matrix interactions are interdependent: the cell has a major role in matrix synthesis and degradation, whereas the composition of the matrix and its signals affect cell division, differentiation and gene expression (Fig. 5.5). Tubular cells and matrix components are in a state of dynamic turnover, and these processes must be closely regulated to maintain normal tubular morphology. One or more defects in this intricate process could lead to tubular dysmorphogeneis, particularly cystic disease. In ADPKD, the tubular dysmorphogenesis is associated with an altered Golgi complex, an altered matrix, and an impairment of cell differentiation (Fig. 5.5). These alterations may be interrelated: defective biosynthesis of matrix com-

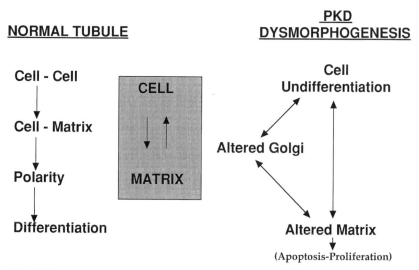

Fig. 5.5 Cell–matrix interactions are reciprocal: the cell has a major role in matrix synthesis and degradation, whereas matrix composition and signalling affect cell division, motility, shape, differentiation, and gene expression. Normal cell–cell and cell–matrix interaction(s); along with cell polarity and concomitant vectorial structure and function (cell differentiation) are required to establish and maintain normal tubular morphology. Under normal conditions, the dynamic turnover of tubular epithelia and matrices are tightly regulated to maintain tubular morphology. The basic defect in PKD is tubular dysmorphogenesis. The principal phenotypic features of ADPKD are altered structure and function of the Golgi complex, altered structure and composition of the matrix, and cell undifferentiation. These changes are probably interrelated (see text). If the gene defect in PKD results in a defective matrix, the abnormal Golgi function and cell differentiation could be due to perturbed matrix–cell communication.

ponents in the Golgi complex could result in a defective matrix which, in turn, could impair cell maturation. On the other hand, if the primary gene defect in ADPKD is an arrest in cell differentiation, this could secondarily alter Golgi complex function and ECM structure. Similarly, a primary ECM defect could block cell maturation and alter the Golgi complex functions.

Apoptosis, a regulated process of programmed cell death, has been reported in human and animal forms of PKD (Woo 1993; Veis *et al.* 1993). It has also been shown that altered matrices can induce apoptosis of attached cells (Frisch and Francis 1994). Thus, in PKD, an abnormal matrix may induce apoptosis which may account for increased oncogene expression and cell proliferation.

Certain phenotypic features of ADPKD cells may be manifestations of altered matrix–cell interaction. Mislocalization of membrane proteins (Na-K ATPase, desmoplakin, etc.) or inappropriate expression of cytoplasmic (intermediate filaments) or secreted proteins (SGP-2) are reminiscent of tubules in their embryonic forms and, therefore, are probably features of an arrest in cell differentiation.

It has recently been shown that the *PKD1* gene which accounts for about 85 per cent of ADPKD encodes a 14 kb transcript (Harris *et al.* 1994). Partial sequence analysis of this transcript reveals that it encodes a novel protein whose function is unknown at present. The large size of the transcript indicates that it encodes a high molecular weight protein of about 500 kDa. The large size of the ADPKD1 gene product and the occurrence of structural defect in tissues not lined by epithelia (heart valve, cerebral artery, etc.) suggests a defect in a matrix protein (Gabow 1990). If this proves to be the case, then ADPKD could be due to altered synthesis, assembly, or degradation of one or more matrix components. In conclusion, altered Golgi function and impaired cell differentiation could be due to aberrant signals of defective matrix–cell interactions.

Acknowledgements

This research was supported by NIH grants DK42304, DK28492, and a grant from the Polycystic Kidney Disease Research Foundation.

References

Bacallao, R., Nakamura, S., Carone, F. A. (1993). Intermediate filament expression suggests a block in the differentiation pathway of ADPKD epithelial cells. *J. Am. Soc. Nephrol.* **4**, 811.

Bacallao, R, Carone, F. A., Nakamura, S., and Wandinger-Ness, A. (1994). Evidence for a Golgi complex defect in autosomal dominant polycystic kidney disease. *J. Am. Soc. Nephrol.*, **5**, 618.

Butkowski, R. J., Carone, F. A., Grantham, J. J., and Hudosn, G. F. (1985). Tubular basement membrane changes in 2-amino-4,5-diphenylthiazole-induced polycystic disease. *Kidney Int.*, **28**, 744–51.

Carone, F. A. and Kanwar, Y. S. (1991). Pathology of tubular basement membranes in renal cystic disease. In *Proceedings of the XIth International Congress of Nephrology*, (ed. H. Hatano), pp. 876–84. Springer-Verlag, Tokyo.

Carone, F. A., and Bacallao, R. (1994). Epithelial apical localization of desmosome proteins in human fetal kidney and autosomal dominant polycystic kidneys. *J. Am. Soc. Nephrol.*, **5**, 619.

Carone, F. A., Rowland, R. G., Perlman, S. G., and Ganote, C. E. (1974). The pathogenesis of drug-induced renal cystic disease. *Kidney Int.*, **5**, 411–21.

Carone, F. A., Makino, H., and Kanwar, Y. S. (1988). Basement membrane antigens in renal polycystic disease. *Am. J. Pathol.*, **130**, 466–71.

Carone, F. A., Hollenberg, P. F., Nakamura, S., Punyarit, P., Glogowski, W., and Flouret, G. (1989). Tubular basement membrane changes occur pari passu with the development of cyst formation. *Kidney Int.*, **35**, 1034–40.

Carone, F. A., Jin, H., Nakamura, S., and Kanwar, Y. S. (1993). Decreased synthesis and delayed processing of sulfated glycoproteins by cells from human polycystic kidneys. *Lab. Invest.*, **68**, 413–18.

Carone, F. A., Bacallao, R., and Kanwar, Y. S. (1994). Biology of polycystic kidney disease. *Lab. Invest.*, **70**, 437–48.

Cotran, K. S., Kumar, V., and Robbins, S. L. (1994). *Pathologic basis of disease*, (5th edn). Saunders, Philadelphia PA.

Dversten, J., Maivel, J. C., Correa-Rotter, R., and Rosenberg, M. E. (1994). Expression of clusterin in human renal diseases. *Kidney Int.*, **45**, 828–35.

Ebihara, I., *et al.* (1988). Altered mRNA expression of basement membrane components, in a murine model of polycystic kidney disease. *Lab. Invest.*, **58**, 262–9.

Ekblom, P. (1991*a*). Developmentally regulation conversion of mesenchyme to epithelium. *FASEB J.*, **10**, 2141–50.

Ekblom, P. (1992). Renal development. In *The kidney*, (ed. D. W. Seldin, and G. Giebisch), pp. 475–501. Raven, New York.

Ekblom, P. and Weller, A. (1991*b*). Ontogeny of tubulointerstitial cells. *Kidney Int.*, **39**, 394–400.

Frisch, S. M. and Francis, H. (1994). Disruption of epithelial cell-matrix interactions induces apoptosis. *J. Cell. Biol.*, **124**, 619–26.

Gabow, P. A. (1990). Autosomal dominant polycystic kidney disease — more than renal disease. *Am. J. Kidney Dis.*, **16**, 403–13.

Gattone, V. H. II Andrews, G. K., Niu, F. W., Chadwick, L. J., Klein, R. M., and Calvet, J. P. (1990). Defective epidermal growth factor gene expression in mice with polycystic kidney disease. *Dev. Biol.*, **138**, 225–30.

Granot, Y., Van Putten, V., Przekwas, J., Gabow, P. A., and Schrier, R. W. (1990). Intra- and extracellular proteins in human normal and polycystic kidney epithelial cells. *Kidney Int.*, **37**, 1301–9.

Grantham, J. J., Danos, V. S., Evan, A. P., Carone, F. A., and Gardner, K. D. (1987). Viscoelastic properties of the tubular basement membranes in experimental renal cystic disease. *Kidney Int.*, **32**, 187–97.

Green, K. J. and Stappenbeck, T. S. (1994). The desmosomal plaque: Role in attachment of intermediate filaments to the cell surface. In *Molecular mechanisms of epithelial cell junctions: From development to disease*, (ed. S. Citi and R. G. Landes), pp. 157–71. CRC Press, Boca Raton, Fl.

Griffiths, G. and Simons, K. (1986). The trans Golgi network: Sorting at the exit site of the Golgi complex. *Science*, **234**, 438–43.

Harding, M. A., Chadwick, L. J., Gattone, V. H., and Calvet, J. P. (1991). The SGP-2 gene is developmentally regulated in the mouse kidney and is abnormally expressed in collecting duct cysts in polycystic kidney disease. *Dev. Biol.*, **146**, 483–90.

Harris, P. C., *et al.* (1994). The polycystic kidney disease 1 gene encodes a 14 kb transcript and lies within a duplicated region on chromosome 16. *Cell*, **17**, 881–94.

Hascall, V. and Hascall, G. K. (1983). Proteoglycans In *Cell biology of extracellular matrix*, (ed. E. H. Hay), pp. 39–63. Plenum, New York.

Hay, E. D. (1984). Cell-matrix interaction in the embryo: Cell shape, cell surface, cell skeletons and their role in differentiation. In *The role of the extracellular matrix in development* (ed. R. L. Trelstad), pp. 1–31. Liss, New York.

Horikoshi, S., Kubota, S., Martin, G. R., Yanada, Y., and Klotman, P. E. (1991). Epidermal growth factor (EGF) expression in the congenital polycystic mouse kidney. *Kidney Int.*, **39**, 57–62.

Horwitz, A. F. (1987). Cell surface receptors for extracellular matrix molecules. *Ann. Rev. Cell. Biol.*, **3**, 179–205.

Kanwar, Y. S. and Carone, F. A. (1984). Reversible tubular cell and basement membrane changes in drug-induced renal cystic disease. *Kidney Int.*, **26**, 35–43.

Klein, G., Hanegger, M., Timple, R., and Ekblom, R. (1988). Role of laminin A chain in the development of epithelial cell polarity. *Cell*, **55**, 331–41.

Lelongt, B., Carone, F. A., and Kanwar, Y. S. (1988). Decreased de novo synthesis of proteoglycans in drug-induced renal cystic disease. *PNAS*, **85**, 9047–51.

Liu, Z. Z., Dalecki, T., Kashohara, N., Watanabe, Y., and Kanwar, Y. S. (1990). Promoted metanephric development by insulin-like growth factor-I. *J. Am. Soc. Nephrol.*, **1**, 458.

Liu, Z. Z., Carone, F. A., Nakamura, S., and Kanwar, Y. S. (1992). Altered de novo synthesis of proteoglycans by cyst-derived cells from patients with autosomal dominant polycystic kidneys. *Am. J. Physiol.*, **263**, F697–704.

Molitoris, B. A. and Nelson, W. J. (1990). Alterations in the establishment and maintenance of epithelial cell polarity as a basis for disease processes. *J. Clin. Invest.*, **85**, 3–9.

Norman, J. T. K., Gatti, L., and Wilson, P. D. (1993). Abnormal matrix metalloproteinase (MMP) regulation in human autosomal dominant polycystic disease (ADPKD). *J. Am. Soc. Nephrol.*, **3**, 819.

Ojeda, J. L. and Ros, M. A. (1990). Basement membrane alterations during development and regression of tubular cysts. *Kidney Int.*, **37**, 1270–80.

Rankin, C. A., Suzuki, K., Ziemer, D. M., Calvet, J. P., and Nagase, H. (1994). Abnormally high levels of MMPs and TIMPs are synthesized by kidney cells from c57BL/6J mice. *J. Am. Soc. Nephrol.*, **5**, 634.

Rocco, M. V., Nielson, E. G., Hoyer, J. R., and Ziyadeh, F. N. (1992). Attenuated expression of epithelial cell adhesion molecules in congenital murine polycystic kidney disease. *Am. J. Physiol.*, **262**, F679–86.

Rodriguez-Boulan, E. and Nelson, W. J. (1989). Morphogenesis of the polarized epithelial cell phenotype. *Science*, **245**, 718–25.

Ruoslahti, E. and Pierschbacher, M. D. (1987). New perspectives in cell adhesion: RGD and integrins. *Science*, **238**, 491–3.

Saxen, L., Koskimies, O., Lahti, A., Miettinen, H., Rapola, J., and Wartiovaara, J. (1968). Differentiation of kidney mesenchyme in an experimental model system. *Adv. Morphol.*, **7**, 251–93.

Schaefer, L., Gretz, N., Bachmann, S., Xiao, H., and Schaefer, R. M. (1994). Deficit of tubular proteinases in polycystic kidney disease: the role of aberrant secretion. *J. Am. Soc. Nephrol.*, **5**, 635.

Simons, K. and Zerial, M. (1993). Rab proteins and the road maps for intracellular transport. *Neuron*, **11**, 789–99.

Taub, M., Laurie, G. M., Martin, G. R., and Cleinman, H. K. (1990). Altered basement membrane protein biosynthesis in cpk/cpk mouse kidney. *Kidney Int.*, **37**, 1090–7.

Veis, D., Sorenson, C. M., Shutter, J. R., and Korsmeyer, S. J. (1993). Bcl-2-deficient mice demonstrate fulminant lymphoid apoptosis, polycystic kidneys and hypopigmented hair. *Cell*, **75**, 229–40.

Wang, A. Z., Ojakian, G. K., Nelson, W. J. (1990). Steps in the morphogenesis of a polarized epithelium. I. Uncoupling the role of cell–cell and cell substratum contact in establishing plasma membrane polarity in multicellular epithelial (MDCK) cysts. *J. Cell. Sci.*, **95**, 137–51.

Woo, D. (1993). Loss of renal function in polycystic kidneys is a result of apoptosis. *J. Am. Soc. Nephrol.*, **4**, 268.

6

Pathogenesis of polycystic kidney disease: altered cellular function

Patricia D. Wilson

Introduction

There may be several different mechanisms leading to the formation of cysts in kidneys, which can be broadly divided into those of genetic and non-genetic in origin. Within the genetic group, to date, no exact animal model has been shown to reflect a human genetic polycystic kidney disease (PKD) as judged by chromosome assignment, inheritance trait or rate of disease progression. Nevertheless, animal models have been of value in analysing cellular mechanisms involved in renal cyst formation (Table 6.1), and are particularly useful when viewed in comparison to findings in human tissues (Table 6.2). For instance, there are common themes of identified abnormalities with regard to proliferation, secretion, polarity, and extracellular matrix regulation. The few genes identified within the groups of cystic disease in humans and adults so far include transcription factors, cell cycle-related motifs, and GTPase-activating proteins. Unfortunately, although the ADPKD-1 gene has recently been identified, to date there is no known homology of sequence to any known motif, protein, or family of proteins, and has not yet increased our knowledge concerning the biology and underlying mechanisms of the pathogenesis of cyst expansion in autosomal dominant PKD.

The aim of this chapter is to provide an overview of findings related to the pathogenesis of cyst expansion in human PKD. The majority of information has been derived from studies on autosomal dominant PKD tissues and rather less from autosomal recessive PKD tissues, both of which have been studied *in vivo* and *in vitro*. Medullary cystic diseases, have been little studied and our knowledge is at present limited to pathological findings. Results from non-human *in vivo* and *in vitro* experimental model systems will not be reviewed in depth here, but conclusions will be drawn where relevant and pertinent to findings in the human disease.

Pathology of human polycystic kidney disease

Renal cysts in human ADPKD and ARPKD arise throughout the kidney and result in dramatic bilateral enlargement of the organs. Lectin profiling, micro-

Table 6.1 Properties of animal models of polycystic kidney disease

Segments	Mouse								Rat			
	Spontaneous				Manipulated				Spontaneous	Drug-induced		
	cpk	pcy	bpk	CBA/N	SV40	c-myc	pax-2	Insertional	Han	DPT	Cort.	MPA
	PT CT	All	PT CT	All		CT PT						CT
Proliferation												
Hyperplasia	+	+	+		+	+						
Neoplasia					+	+						
Biliary tract	–		+					+				
PCNA	+	+										
c-myc	+	+				+			+			
c-fos	+	+										
c-Ki-ras	+											
T antigen					+							
Pax-2							+					
Growth factors												
TGFβ	0,+	+										
PDGF		+										
IGF-I		+										
FGFb		+										
EGF	–	–										
TNFα	+											
Growth factor receptors												
EGFR	+											

Table 6.1 *Continued*

| | Mouse | | | | | | | | Rat | | | |
| | Spontaneous | | | | Manipulated | | | | Spontaneous | Drug-induced | | |
	cpk	pcy	bpk	CBA/N	SV40	c-myc	pax-2	Insertional	Han	DPT	Cort.	MPA
Matrix												
BM change	–								+	+		
Collagen IV	0,+								+	0		
Laminin	0,+								+	–		
Nidogen	0								+			
Fibronectin	0								+			
Proteoglycans										C–H+		
Adhesion												
N–Cam	–											
E–cadherin	–											
Cytoskeleton												
Actin	0											
Transport												
Na–KATPase	+*	0,*							0	+,0*	+*	+*
Enzymes												
Alk. Pase	–											
KE–6	–											
Apoptosis												
SGP–2	+											

+, increase; 0, no change; –, decrease; C, chondroitin sulphate; H, heparan sulphate; PT, proximal tube; CT, collecting tubule.

Table 6.2 Characteristics of human ADPKD and ARPKD

	ADPKD	ARPKD
Kidney		
Segment origin of cyst	All	PT then CT
Hyperplasia	+	+
Neoplasia	–	–
Fibrosis	+	–
Liver		
Cysts	+	–
Fibrosis	–	+
Proliferation		
PCNA	+	+
N-myc	+	+
Transcription factors		
Pax-2	+	+
WT-1	+	+
Growth Factors		
EGF	+ protein in epithelia	
TGFα	+ mRNA	
TGFβ	+ protein, some epithelia, mRNA *in vitro*	
FGF-acidic	+ protein, some epithelia	
PDGF	+ protein	
Growth factor receptors		
EGF Receptor	+ mRNA, protein, binding, tyr. phosphorylation	
	+ apical mislocation	+ apical mislocation
c-met: HGF receptor	+ in epithelia, apical and basal localization	
		+ apical and basal
FGF-acidic	Fibroblasts hypersensitive, novel cross-linked sp.	
IGF-I	Fibroblast hypersensitive	
IGF-II	Fibroblasts hypersensitive	
Signal transduction		
Phosphotyrosine	+	+
EGFR	Hyperphosphorylated	
FGF-acidic	More rapid and sustained phosphorylation	
ERK	+	+
AKT, RAC (ser.thr PTK)	+ in hyperplastic cyst epithelia	

Table 6.2 *Continued*

	ADPKD	ARPKD
Matrix proteins		
Collagen IV	+ mRNA, protein	
Collagen I, III, VI	+	
Laminin	+, protein	
Fibronection	+, protein	
Proteoglycans	−, +, HSPG, CSPG, sulphation, abnormal forms	
Tenascin	−, focal +	
Matrix receptors		
Integrin		
alpha-2	+distal cysts	
alpha-3		+
alpha-6	+, all basal	+, all basal
beta-1	+	
beta-4	+	
Adhesion		
E-cadherin	Some apical	
ZO-1	No change	
Cytoskeleton		
Actin	+, protein, microfilaments	+, epithelia
α-Actinin	+, some cysts	
Vinculin	+, some cysts	
Calpactins I and II	+ protein, intracellular to apical localization	
Cytokeratin	no change: epithelial	No change, epithelia
Vimentin	+, some cysts	epithelia
Transporters, enzymes		
Na-K-ATPase	+, mRNA, protein, activity +, apical mislocalization, beta-2 isoform	+, beta-2 isoform, mRNA, protein apical, and basolateral localization
Amiloride-sensitive Na transport	No change, apical	
Na/glucose	−	−
Na$^+$K$^+$2Cl$^-$	+, basal	
Cl$^-$ (CFTR)	+, apical	
MDR P-glycoprotein	No change, apical	
AQP-CHIP	+, some cysts apical, some basal	+, some cysts, all apical
AQP-CD	+, some cysts, all apical	+, some cysts, all apical
Phospholipase	+, secretion	

AQP, aquaporin; CT, collecting tubule; EGF, epidermal growth factor; FGF, fibroblast growth factor; HGF, hepatocyte growth factor; IGE, insulin-like growth factor; MDR, multidrug resistance; PDGE, platelet derived growth factor; PT, proximal tubule; TGF, transforming growth factor; TIMP, tissue inhibitor of metallo proteinase; WT, Wilms' tumor.

dissection, and tissue culture studies have shown that in ADPKD kidneys there is expansion and enlargement of tubule segments from every region of the nephron, while in end-stage ARPKD the cysts are of collecting tubule origin (Baert 1978; Faraggiana *et al.* 1985). In medullary cystic diseases, there is no enlargement of the kidney, and cysts are confined to the inner (medullary sponge) or outer medulla. Examination of 15 early stage, pre-azotemic ADPKD kidneys reveal 'microcysts' with clear proximal tubule, distal tubule, or glomerular epithelial phenotypes (Wilson and Falkenstein 1994) and no spatial or temporal preference in sequence of segment expansion has been noted during the early stages of disease. This contrasts with ARPKD where in the early stages, proximal tubule expansion was detected, but as the disease progressed *in utero*, collecting tubule expansion ensued and accounted for the majority of cystic expansion in end-stage kidneys after birth, as determined by lectin profiling. Marker analysis in ADPKD also suggested that in the early stages of disease, distinct cysts were labelled with markers characteristic of proximal tubule, thick ascending limb, thin limb, distal convoluted tubule, or collecting tubule origin (Faraggiana *et al.* 1985; Silva *et al.* 1993; Wilson *et al.* 1991, 1994). As either ADPKD or ARPKD progressed towards end-stage, however, there seems to be further morphological and marker profile modifications, since cysts are detected without distinct morphological features or lectin profiles of any clear tubule segment.

Cysts are typically lined by a single layer of epithelium and filled with fluid. In early ADPKD, epithelial phenotypes range from columnar, to cuboidal to flattened and in some cases, cysts contain light cells with an occasional profile showing a single cilium and dark cells containing several organelles, suggestive of collecting tubule origin (Figs 6.1–6.3). At the electron microscope level, apical brush borders are clearly seen in some cells, and are rudimentary or absent in others. Later, in end-stage ADPKD these clear distinctions are less evident in cyst-lining epithelia. However, several phenotypes are still distinguishable, including tightly apposed, regular cuboidal, or columnar cells and also loosely apposed foamy and flattened cells (Figs 6.2 and 6.3). All epithelial cells at all stages of disease exhibit a range of tight junctions including junctional complexes and desmosomes. In ADPKD and ARPKD, occasional layering of cells into hyperplastic foci is seen, but this is a rare event. This contrasts sharply with the severely hyperplastic and even metaplastic epithelial lesions seen in medullary sponge kidney, tuberous sclerosis, and von Hippel–Lindau disease, and in the c-myc and SV40 transgenic mouse models of PKD (Bernstein *et al.* 1987; Heptinstall 1992; Kelley *et al.* 1991; Trudel *et al.* 1991). This suggests that renal cyst formation is associated with a wide spectrum of hyperproliferative lesions, but that ADPKD and ARPKD represent the least aggressive, untransformed, non-neoplastic end of the spectrum. This is further supported by proliferative studies carried out in tissue culture and the absence of evidence of increased incidence of renal carcinoma in ADPKD or ARPKD patients, but a clear increase in incidence in von Hippel–Lindau disease and acquired cystic disease (Bernstein *et al.* 1987; Hughson *et al.* 1980).

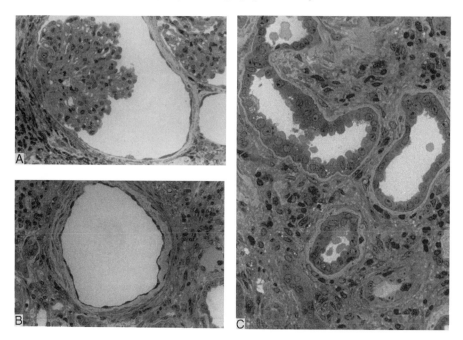

Fig. 6.1 Light micrographs of early-stage ADPKD kidneys, fixed with 2.5 per cent glutaraldehyde, embedded in Araldite resin, sectioned at 1 μmm and stained with toluidine blue. (A) Glomerular cyst with thick basement membrane, thin layer of epithelial cells, and resorbing glomerular tuft. (B) Glomerular cyst with thickened basement membrane and thin layer of cyst epithelial cells. Interstitial cellularity can also be seen. (C) Renal tubule cysts showing epithelial cells with various morphologies ranging from columnar to cuboidal. Light and dark cells can be seen in one cyst (lower right). Fragmentation bodies can be seen in some cyst lumens. Basement membrane thickening, fibroblastic interstitial cellularity, and fibrillar deposition can be seen.

All epithelial cells cysts in ADPKD and ARPKD are polarized and rest on a distinct basement membrane (BM). A characteristic feature of ADPKD cysts is a thickening of the BM (Cuppage *et al.* 1980; Wilson *et al.* 1986), (Figs 6.1–6.3), and can be seen even during the early stages of cyst formation and at the electron microscope level, there is often evidence of layering, lamination, and a loss of homogeneity of protein content (Milutinovic and Agodoa 1983; Milutinovic *et al.* 1980; Wilson *et al.* 1994). In contrast, in ARPKD, thickening of the BM is less common, and it has not been reported in cpk mice. Additional expansion of the extracellular matrix is seen in ADPKD which includes an increase in cellularity and fibroblast content of the interstitium together with an increase in fibrillar collagen deposition (Figs 6.1C and 6.4A). As progression to end-stage renal failure ensues, the contribution of interstitial fibrosis also usually increases, but the degree of fibrosis varies in different individuals in end-stage ADPKD. Although inflammatory infiltrates are sometimes seen, (CD4-positive

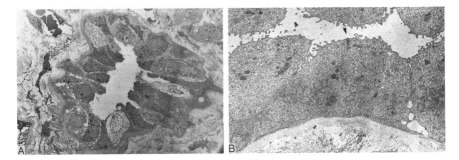

Fig. 6.2 Electron micrographs of distal cysts in ADPKD kidneys. (A) Low power micrograph of an early-stage ADPKD cyst showing light and dark cells which are polarized with apical brush borders and a thickened basement membrane. (B) Higher power electron micrograph of an end-stage ADPKD cyst showing cuboidal epithelia with apical microvilli and intercellular tight junctions. Note the base of a cilium (arrow) consistent with collecting tubule origin.

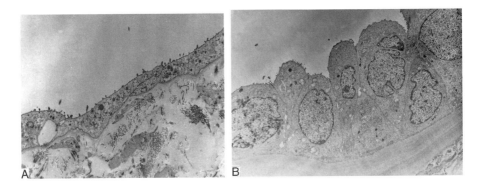

Fig. 6.3 Electron micrographs of end-stage ADPKD cyst walls. (A) Flattened epithelia with apical microvilli, intercellular spaces, and a laminated basement membrane. (B) Columnar and cuboidal epithelia with rudimentary apical microvilli, dense intercellular tight junctions, and tightly apposed lateral cell membranes.

macrophages) these are absent from many ADPKD kidneys, suggesting that they do not exhibit a major causative function (Zeier *et al.* 1992). Although not as extensive, some expansion in the interstitium is also seen in end-stage ARPKD as evidenced by increased cellularity and fibrillar deposition (Fig. 6.4B).

The vascular supply to ADPKD kidneys is modified and arteriolar lesions increase with progression. Thin-walled arterioles in the interstitium adjacent to cysts often contain renin, as do remnant normal and hypertrophied juxtaglomerular apparatus, stromal cells, and cyst epithelial cells (Graham and Lindop 1988; Torres *et al.* 1992; Zeier *et al.* 1992). This correlates with increased plasma renin levels in ADPKD patients with hypertension. In addition, erythropoietin-containing cells are seen in stromal cell surrounding cyst walls (Eckardt *et al.* 1989).

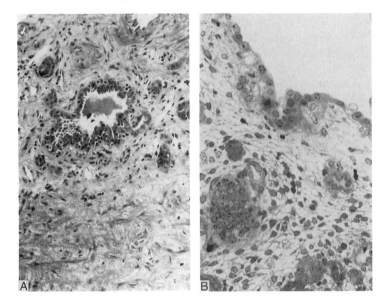

Fig. 6.4 Light micrographs of end-stage ADPKD and ARPKD kidneys fixed with 4 per cent paraformaldehyde, embedded in paraffin wax, sectioned at 6 μmm, and stained with haematoxylin and eosin. (A) End-stage ADPKD kidney showing a hyperplastic cyst and extensive expansion of the extracellular matrix seen in the form of fibroblastic cells and extracellular fibril deposition. (B) End-stage ARPKD kidney showing cellular and fibrillar deposition in the extracellular matrix.

The degree of cyst expansion in ADPKD is widely variable ranging from a few millimetres to several centimetres, and their contents vary from fluid to viscous and from clear to dark brown in colour, reflecting secretion and degree of cystic haemorrhage, which is a highly variable feature from individual to individual. In contrast, ARPKD cysts are more uniform, of small (millimetre) size, and clear contents. Microdissection and electron microscope studies (Baert 1978; Evan and McAteer 1990; Osathanondh and Potter 1964) have demonstrated further differences between ADPKD and ARPKD cysts, in that ADPKD cysts quickly close off from their nephron segment of origin and continue to expand by fluid secretion. In contrast, ARPKD cysts and those of acquired cystic disease induced by dialysis, remain connected to their nephron of origin. These differences may have implications for the relative contribution of secretion and proliferation in cyst expansion in ADPKD and ARPKD.

Cyst fluid contents

The contents of ADPKD cyst fluids has been determined in several studies. Their composition differs from either blood plasma or urine as determined by [¹H]-NMR (Foxall *et al.* 1992) and high levels of amino acids, glucose, organic acids and bases, and presence of epidermal growth factor (EGF), interleukin-1,

TNFα, stromelysin, renin, erythropoietin, and ammonia, are consistent with extensive epithelial secretory activity (Du *et al.* 1991; Eckardt *et al.* 1989; Gardner *et al.* 1991; Torres *et al.* 1992, 1994; Wilson 1991*b*). The inability of antibiotics to reach cyst fluids effectively also suggest that secretion, rather than filtration, is the major mechanism for entry into a cyst cavity (Muther and Bennett 1981). Sodium and chloride contents of cysts vary over a wide range from < 20 mM/l to > 160mM/l, with peaks at low and high NaCl levels suggesting varied capacities for secretion and reabsorption, thought to be related to cyst tubule cell type of origin. It is of interest to note that fluids of breast cysts also show similar profiles of contents including EGF, high NaCl types, low NaCl types, proteases, and a digoxin-like steroid-binding protein (Angeli *et al.* 1990). ADPKD cyst lumens also often contain secretion or fragmentation bodies (Fig. 6.1C) which under electron microscope examination are anuclear portions of cells containing dense cytoplasm, and numerous normal appearing organelles including mitochondria, lysosomes, and also microfilament bundles (Wilson *et al.* 1994). The mechanism of origin of these bodies is unclear since they are clearly different from cell membrane blebs or cellular castes seen after ischaemic damage. Nor do they have the features of apoptotic bodies.

Several conclusions can be drawn from pathological examination of ADPKD and ARPKD kidneys by comparison to normal adult and fetal kidneys. Such analyses have suggested several lines of experimental investigation which might shed light on the cellular mechanisms leading to cyst formation. These include alterations in differentiation, matrix turnover, epithelial and fibroblast proliferation, epithelial secretion, and polarity.

Experimental analysis of ADPKD and ARPKD

In addition to pathological analysis, the contents, activities, and distribution of specific proteins and mRNAs have been examined in ADPKD and to a lesser extent in ARPKD using standard biochemical assays, Western immunoblot, Northern blot and RNAase protection analyses, tissue immunolocalization, and *in situ* hybridization techniques. This has allowed an overall description of differences between tissues of age-matched normal and diseased origins. The derivation of primary cell culture techniques has also allowed for more detailed cellular and mechanistic studies to be carried out.

Cell and tissue culture

Cell culture analysis is a particularly useful approach for studying genetic diseases, since by placing cells in culture, intrinsic, genetically determined properties will be retained through serial passages, whereas non-specific, epigenetic phenomena are not retained. This is particularly important for studies with polycystic kidneys, where, for instance, any non-specific, confounding effects due to ischaemia would be lost in culture where oxygen and substrates are freely available. In addition, as in all cell culture systems, the effects of single manipulations can be readily examined, for example, with regard to growth factor and matrix interactions, allowing for the separation of autocrine, paracrine, and endocrine mechanisms of regulation.

Since 1985, it has been possible to microdissect and grow *in vitro* in defined, growth factor-supplemented, serum-free media, human renal tubule epithelia derived from proximal convoluted tubules (PCT); proximal straight tubules (PST), thick ascending limbs of the loop of Henle (TAL), and cortical and medullary collecting tubules (CCT, MCT) (Wilson 1991*c*; Wilson *et al.* 1985). Tubule epithelia derived and grown in this fashion on collagen-coated Teflon or polycarbonate membranes retain a wide array of normal differentiated characteristics as defined by marker analyses with antibodies and enzymes, tubule segment-specific hormone responsiveness, and physiological polarized transport functions. Similar microdissection techniques, matrix, and growth factor-supplementation of serum-free defined tissue culture media resulted in establishment of primary cultures from ADPKD cyst epithelia which also retained a wide range of the properties of freshly isolated cyst walls (Wilson *et al.* 1986). These techniques have also recently been applied to generate primary cultures of functional ARPKD epithelia (Falkenstein *et al.* 1994; Hjelle *et al.* 1990) Such primary cultures of ADPKD and ARPKD cyst-lining epithelia can be passaged for a finite number (5–15) of passages but eventually die out. Recently, a retroviral transfection system has been used to transduce cells with the temperature-sensitive SV40 T antigen and has resulted in the establishment of immortalized clones of normal fetal and adult proximal tubule, thick ascending limb and collecting tubule, and ADPKD and ARPKD epithelia, some of which show several characteristics of non-transduced epithelia *in vitro* (Eng *et al.* 1994). The advantages of such immortalized cell lines will be the ability to carry out stable transfections with candidate genes and to allow full characterization of the effects through multiple generations. Other techniques for the growth of ADPKD epithelia have been utilized including explant into hydrated collagen gels, which appears to favour the growth of cuboidal cells with small microvilli (McAteer *et al.* 1988). This points to the potential for a 3 dimensional analysis of the effects of various matrix and soluble growth factors on the tubulogenesis vs. cystogenesis of normal and polycystic epithelia, as has successfully been applied in the Madin Darby Canine kidney (MDCK) cell system, where hepatoctye growth factor was found to be a potent morphogen allowing branching tubulogenesis (Montesano *et al.* 1991*a,b*).

Recently, fibroblast cultures have also been generated from ADPKD, ARPKD, and normal human kidneys (Kuo and Wilson 1990). Typically, these cultures can be generated by growth of explants, including the stroma, in media containing 10 per cent serum instead of defined media used for epithelia. Initial epithelial outgrowths soon die out and are overtaken by fibroblast proliferation. These cells are then purified by serial passaging with trypsin until all cells have the morphology and marker patterns of fibroblasts (passage 2–5). These cultured cells have been characterized and shown to retain several properties of interstitial fibroblasts *in vivo* from normal or polcystic kidneys, respectively, and therefore provide a valuable tool for detailed analysis of the reciprocal influence between stroma and epithelia in cyst formation, by co-culture techniques.

The advent of these culture systems has allowed extensive analysis of not only protein and gene expression, but also, kinetic, synthetic and polarized secretion, and transport analyses. Early studies identified several differences in protein synthesis by ADPKD epithelia vs. normal renal tubule epithelia, including alterations in the overall pattern of intracellular protein content and reduced numbers of secreted proteins, including a novel 220 kDa form of heparan sulphate proteoglycan (Granot *et al.* 1990; Wilson 1991*b*; Wilson, *et al.* 1992). More recently, ADPKD epithelia *in vitro* have been shown to synthesize a variety of enzymes including Na-K ATPase, renin, and other proteases and growth factors (Hartz and Wilson 1994; Torres *et al.* 1992; Wilson 1991*a*, Wilson *et al.* 1991). Alterations in biosynthetic activities and secretion are not limited to proteins in ADPKD, since alterations in arachidonic acid secretion have also been seen (Sherwood and Wilson 1990*b*).

Based on pathological studies, it was reasoned that at least two criteria are essential for the formation of a cyst: (1) epithelial cell proliferation, and (2) apical secretion fluid. Both of these features are readily accessible for studying *in vitro* systems. In addition, the roles of matrix, growth factors, mispolarization of critical membrane proteins, and vectorial transport were all implicated by *in vivo* analyses of ADPKD, ARPKD, and some animal model studies (Tables 6.1 and 6.2) and have subsequently led to a more extensive analysis *in vitro*.

Cell proliferation

It was argued from pathological analysis that increased cell proliferation would be a necessary prerequisite to allow for cystic expansion (Welling and Welling 1988). This has been addressed *in vivo* and *in vitro*. *In vivo*, human fetal ADPKD and ARPKD kidneys, show nuclear staining for proliferating cell nuclear antigen (PCNA)-DNA polymerase-delta, indicative of cells that have exited G_0 of the cell cycle, whereas in normal adult kidneys no staining is seen. This suggests that cyst-lining epithelial cells are primed for proliferation and contrasts with normal adult tubules in which cells are terminally differentiated in G_0 having exited the cell cycle. This increased capacity for proliferation was further confirmed *in vitro* since ADPKD epithelia were able to proliferate through significantly more rounds of cell division than adult epithelial cells derived from age-matched, microdissected renal tubule segments (Wilson *et al.* 1992). This suggests that the potential for extended proliferation is intrinsic to the genetically modified ADPKD cells and would be a mechanism for increased cell number production *in vivo*. There were no differences in the rate of cell division *in vitro*, however, and ADPKD cyst epithelial cells did not grow in soft agar, suggesting that these cells do not share an important property of neoplastically transformed cells in culture (Carone *et al.* 1989*b*). Hyperproliferation is also a marked property of human ADPKD fibroblasts *in vitro*, by comparison to age-matched normal adult fibroblasts of cortical or medullary origin *in vitro*

(Kuo 1991). These cells were able to complete up to three fold more doublings (up to 15 passages, 6 months) *in vitro* and, interestingly, did exhibit the capacity for focal growth in soft agar. This suggests that ADPKD fibroblasts do share a property with neoplastically transformed cells *in vitro*, but it should be emphasized that the cells are not immortal. Taken together, these findings suggest that more cells are proliferatively active in ADPKD and ARPKD than in normal kidneys, that this is associated with cyst formation and hyperplasia, but that the proliferative lesion is relatively mild, in that cells are not immortalized and do not undergo neoplastic transformation or tumour formation. This is an important difference from SV40- and c-myc-induced cystic disease in transgenic mice suggesting that caution should be applied in the use of those models to study the proliferative mechanisms in human PKD.

Oncogenes

Aberrant c-myc, c-fos, and c-Ki-ras oncogene expression has been reported in cystic cpk mice (Calvet 1993; Cowley *et al.* 1987). In addition, the overexpression of c-myc as a transgene results in a polycystic phenotype in mice (Trudel *et al.* 1991). We have carried out a wide survey of protein expression by immunostaining analysis of early and end-stage ADPKD and ARPKD kidneys by comparison to normal age-matched controls. N-myc, which is expressed in normal kidneys in medullary collecting tubules only, is strongly expressed in all cysts in end-stage ADPKD and ARPKD. Also, c-myc was detected in a single ADPKD patient (Klingel *et al.* 1992).

Growth factors and their receptors

Growth factor activation is an important mechanism for the induction of cells to enter and traverse through the cell cycle of proliferation. For instance, platelet-derived growth factor (PDGF) and fibroblast growth factor (FGF) act as competence factors, stimulating exit from G_0 into G_1, the quiescent phase of the cell cycle. Epidermal growth factor (EGF) and insulin act as entry factors during early G_1, and insulin-like growth factors I and II (IGF-I, IGF-II) and glucocorticoids act as progression factors later in G_1 (Pardee 1989). Normal, orderly cell division is the product of interactions between cells and one or more of these growth factors via ligand–receptor stimulation and requires strict spatio-temporal control. Virtually all cell proliferation and nephrogenesis is thought to be complete before birth in humans and only a limited capacity for sporadic cell renewal has been demonstrated after renal tubule damage by temporary ischaemia or nephrotoxins. Since proliferation appears to be widespread in cyst epithelia and fibroblasts in ADPKD, it was reasoned that abnormal growth factor content, localization, or receptor-mediated mechanisms may be responsible, at least in part. Immunolocalization studies showed that ADPKD cyst epithelia expressed several growth factor ligands including EGF, PDGF, TGFβ and TGFα (Klingel *et al.* 1991; Wilson 1991*a*; Wilson *et al.* 1993*b*). Also,

ADPKD cyst fluids have been demonstrated to exert strong mitogenic activity, and to contain mitogenic concentrations of EGF, in addition to interleukins and TNFα (Du *et al.* 1991; Du and Wilson 1994; Gardner *et al.* 1991; Ye *et al.* 1992). *In vitro* studies of the proliferative responses of normal and human ADPKD epithelia to several growth factors further showed that ADPKD cyst epithelia were hyper-responsive to EGF and that this was the most potent mitogen of those tested (Wilson *et al.* 1993*b*). A mechanism for this increased responsiveness was suggested by [^{125}I] EGF-binding studies *in vitro*, immuno-staining *in vivo* and *in vitro*, cross-linking, and Western analysis with anti-phosphotyrosine antibodies. Whereas in normal renal tubule epithlia *in vivo* and *in vitro* mitogenic receptors for EGF are restricted to the basolateral membranes, ADPKD epithelia *in vivo* and *in vitro* have significant binding and immuno-reactive receptor staining on the apical, cyst-lining epithelial cell membranes. Ligand binding, mRNA quantitation, and phosphotyrosine activity analyses suggested that total EGF receptor number was increased, partially due to increased synthesis and that these receptors were fully functional with regard to ligand-induced phosphorylation capacity and even show evidence of hyperstimulation in the absence of ligand (Du and Wilson 1994; Wilson 1991*b*; Wilson and Burrow 1992; Wilson *et al.* 1993*b*). Measurement of cyst fluid contents from > 100 cysts from eight ADPKD patients using radioimmunoassay detected EGF in mi-togenic concentrations (> 1 ng/ml), with highest levels in cysts in the maximally proliferative early stages of the disease (2.9 ng/ml). In addition, the application of cyst fluid was highly mitogenic to normal and ADPKD epithelia *in vitro*, as was tissue culture media conditioned by growth of confluent monolayers of ADPKD epithelia. These findings led to the conclusion that EGF was secreted by ADPKD epithelia *in vivo* and *in vitro*. Taken together, these results suggest that EGF is an important mediator of the increased proliferation associated with cyst enlargement in ADPKD. This may be because of an autocrine mechanism of regulation in which EGF is synthesized and/or stored in cyst epithelia, se-creted in mitogenic quantities apically into the cyst lumen where it is trapped due to lack of connections with other nephron elements, and is able to stimulate those same cyst epithelia to proliferate due to the presence of functionally responsive, EGF receptors on the apical cell membranes. It is also of interest that EGF processing is modified, with fully processed 6 kDa forms being less common than higher molecular weight forms (30 kDa, 37 kDa), although these have also been shown to have mitogenic activity. This suggest an abnormality in the proteolytic processing of EGF in ADPKD epithelia, since in normal renal epithelia EGF is synthesized as a 170 kDa pre-pro-form and sequestered at the apical plasma membrane for release by proteolytic degradation, to the 6 kDa form detected in normal urine (Bell *et al.* 1986). It is of interest that similar abnormalities of EGF processing have also been reported in the Han rat and CPK mouse (Lakshmanan and Eysselein 1993; Lakshmanan and Fisher 1993).

In comparison to EGF, the effects of other growth factors tested singly on ADPKD epithelia *in vitro* were unimpressive and showed little difference from effects on normal renal tubule epithelia. Growth factors frequently act in concert, however, and the comparisons of effects of combinations of growth factors on normal and ADPKD epithelia showed that responses to dexamethasone + insulin ± triiodothyronine were significantly increased in ADPKD epithelia. Interestingly, also, the ability of TGFβ to inhibit epithelial proliferation was reduced in ADPKD epithelia where it was ineffective in abrogating the effects of EGF (Wilson *et al.* 1993*b*). It is therefore likely that combined effects of growth factor ligands may be important in ADPKD epithelial cell proliferation.

Much less information is available concerning growth factor alterations in human ARPKD. It is of interest, however, that EGF receptor protein is abundant and localized on the apical membranes of cystic epithelia (Falkenstein *et al.* 1993, 1994) Fig. 6.5. This correlates with findings in the cpk mouse, a model for recessive PKD in which increased EGF receptor synthesis and abnormalities in receptor inhibition profiles using tyrosine kinase inhibitors have also been shown (Avner, personal communication). It can be hypothesized, therefore, that EGF mitogenesis via an autocrine mechanism plays an important role in cyst epithelial proliferation in human ARPKD as well as in ADPKD.

In addition to epithelial proliferation in ADPKD and ARPKD, increases in interstitial fibroblast proliferation are seen, most notably in ADPKD. Together

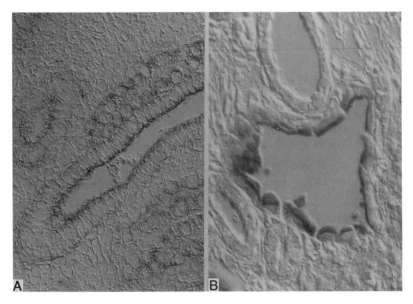

Fig. 6.5 Light micrograph of immunolocalization of EGF receptor on paraformaldehyde fixed 5 μmm sections, stained using an avidin-biotin-peroxidase technique followed by colour development with aminoethylcarbazole as substrate. (A) Human fetal kidney (19 weeks gestation) showing a collecting duct with dark reaction product lining the apical, luminal cell membranes. (B) Early-stage ARPKD kidney showing a cyst with intense apical epithelial cell membrane staining of EGF receptor. An adjacent cyst is unstained.

with extracellular matrix protein accumulation these changes contribute to the fibrosis which can be extensive in end-stage ADPKD, and has been suggested to accelerate decline in renal function. The localization of PDGF in cyst epithelia may suggest a potential role for its release into the interstitium and stimulation of interstitial fibroblast proliferation by a paracrine mechanism (Ritz *et al.* 1993). *In vitro* studies using fibroblasts derived from ADPKD and age-matched normal human kidneys showed that several growth factors were capable of increasing stimulation of ADPKD fibroblast proliferation in excess of normal, including acidic FGF, IGF-I, IGF-II, and PDGF (Kuo *et al.* 1991). The strongest and most increased response was that of acidic FGF which not only induced hyper-stimulation of ADPKD fibroblasts *in vitro*, but was also demonstrated at sub-stantially increased levels in ADPKD fibroblasts *in vitro* and ADPKD kidneys *in vivo*, and to be predominantly localized in the interstitium and in the epithelia of a few cysts. In addition, conditioned media derived from ADPKD fibroblasts contained increased levels of immunoreactive acidic FGF (FGF-a), consistent with increased synthesis and secretion. [^{125}I] FGF-a-binding studies, covalent cross-linking, and phosphotyrosine analysis showed increased affinity for binding, more rapid and sustained receptor stimulation, and the presence of ab-normal receptor species. Taken together, these results suggested that the abnor-mal proliferation of ADPKD fibroblasts is in part due to autocrine and possibly paracrine stimulation by FGF-a. PDGF has also been suggested as a paracrine regulator of ADPKD fibroblast proliferation due to its localization in cyst ep-ithelia and the mitogenic action of PDGF in renal fibroblasts. In addition to growth factors secreted by epithelia having an influence on interstitial fibroblasts, it is also possible that fibroblast-derived secreted growth factors might exert influence on cyst epithelial cells. Recent *in vitro* studies have clearly demon-strated that hepatocyte growth factor (HGF) secreted by fibroblasts was able to promote proliferation and tubule formation in MDCK cells in gels (Montesano *et al.* 1991*a*). This has potential implications in ADPKD since the kidney is a source of HGF and its receptor, the c-*met* oncogene is widely expressed on tubule epithelial cell membranes as well as on the epithelial cell membranes lining ADPKD and ARPKD cysts, both in the apical and basolateral domains.

Signal transduction

Growth factors exert their mitogenic actions via specific membrane receptors, the occupancy of which by the ligand, results in a cascade of events which often includes phosphorylation of tyrosine residues contained at the *C*-terminal intra-cellular domain. Such is the case for EGF, FGF, and PDGF receptor–ligand in-teractions. Cross-linking and Western analysis with antiphosphotyrosine antibodies before and after ligand stimulation have shown that several types of abnormality in signalling may be present in ADPKD kidneys. EGF receptors seem to be in a permanent state of hyperstimulation, even in the absence of ex-ogenous EGF ligand (Du and Wilson 1994). Unique molecular weight species of FGF-a receptor have been detected in ADPKD tissues and in ADPKD fibroblasts and *in vitro* receptor occupancy resulted in a more rapid (1 minute) and sustained tyrosine phosphorylation response than in normal fibroblasts which show a tight peak of stimulation at 15 minutes (Kuo and Wilson 1994; Wilson *et al.* 1993*a*). This increase in tyrosine phosphorylation also correlate with more intense staining with a monoclonal antibody against phosphotyrosine in ADPKD and ARPKD kidneys, with little staining in normal adult kidneys. In addition to tyrosine kinases, serine-threonine kinases also play a role in growth factor–receptor signalling as either as part of membrane receptors, such as TGBβ receptor and extracellular signal-related kinase-1 (ERK-1), or as part of the intracellular phosphorylation cascade which ultimately leads to activation of nuclear transcription factors and controlled gene expression. In this regard, it is of interest that an antibody against the membrane serine-threonine kinase, ERK-1 stains more intensely in ADPKD and ARPKD than in normal kidneys, while expression of the AKT (Bac) gene product, a cytoplasmic serine-threonine protein kinase was particularly associated with the hyperplastic regions of ADPKD cyst expansion (Amsler, personal communication).

Transcription factors

The regulation of gene transcription is controlled by DNA-binding proteins of which there are families with different structures: helix-turn-helix, zinc-finger, homeo box, POU, and paired box. As would be predicted, the spatial and temporal control of expression of genes of this type is critically important in the regulation of development and differentiation since mutations in this class of genes are frequently associated with deregulation of normal development and organ differentiation. In the kidney, for instance, important roles for the expression of the paired box genes, Pax-2 and Pax-8, and the zinc-finger gene, WT-1, during specific stages and at specific sites during development are crucial for normal organogenesis. Aberrant overexpression of Pax-2 results in renal cyst formation (Dressler *et al.* 1993) and WT-1 mutation results in Wilms' tumour (Pelletier *et al.* 1991). In addition, the absence of WT-1 gene expression has been shown to result in the absence of kidneys (Kreidberg *et al.* 1993). We routinely carry out immunostaining analysis to establish patterns of protein expression in human kidneys using a panel of tissue sections including at least 10 fetal, 10 normal adult, 5 early-stage ADPKD, 10 end-stage ADPKD, and 4 ARPKD kidneys. Pax-2 expression is nuclear and restricted to fetal, ADPKD and ARPKD kidney epithelia (Eng *et al.* 1994; Falkenstein *et al.* 1993). In fetal kidneys staining is seen in condensing mesenchyme, S-bodies and collecting ducts, but not in epithelial tubules derived from mesenchyme. No staining was seen in normal adult kidneys, but in ADPKD and ARPKD, the nuclei of several epithelial cells lining cysts were stained. WT-1 antibodies stained fetal kidneys in the mesenchyme and in glomerular podocytes of immature glomeruli. In adult kidneys, some residual staining in glomeruli was also seen while in ADPKD and ARPKD kidneys, staining was seen in cyst-lining epithelia. This aberrant staining for both Pax-2 and WT-1 in cyst epithelia suggests a deregulation of transcription factor expression in ADPKD and ARPKD in comparison to normal adult tissues, and more closely resembles the fetal kidney.

Extracellular matrix

Stromal–epithelial cell interactions are of central importance in renal development and differentiation. The extracellular matrix in the kidney is comprised of the interstitium and the specialized basement membranes which line tubule epithelia and serve to separate epithelial sheets from the interstitial compartments. Components of the interstitium include fibroblasts and extracellular collagenous proteins types I, III, and V, and non-collagenous proteins including tenascin. Basement membranes are specialized regions of the extracellular matrix and typically contain type IV collagen, non-collagenous glycoproteins laminin, entactin, and fibronectin,and sulphated proteoglycans, which together confer tensile strength, elasticity, adhesion, and permselectivity. The glomerular basement membrane is highly specialized and is secreted by both the endothelial and epithelial cell (podocyte) layers. The basement membrane acts as a molecular sieve by virtue of structural pores and heparan sulphate proteoglycan content which select molecules on the basis of size and charge, respectively. The renal tubule basement membrane is more typical of that lining epithelial organs in that it is composed of a lamina lucida and lamina densa and is secreted by the epithelial cells. During renal development the extracellular matrix plays an early and important role where it directs cell migration and spatial organization. In addition, extracellular matrix composition has been shown to influence proliferation, epithelial cell polarization, and differentiation (Ekblom 1992; Ekblom *et al.* 1986). The mechanism of interaction between epithelial and stromal compartments can be effected via direct cell contact via matrix receptor proteins present on cell membranes, such as the intergrins and syndecan, which, in turn, interact with components of the cell cytoskeleton. Also, it has been shown that secretion of soluble growth factors from either the epithelia or stromal fibroblasts can have paracrine effects by activation of specific cell membrane receptors. Therefore, there are clearly complex, reciprocal interactions between stroma and epithelia which are necessary for normal renal morphogenesis and for the retention of the differentiated state in adult tissues. The basement membrane is a dynamic structure, the structure and composition of which is the product of simultaneous synthesis and degradation processes. Increased deposition of basement membrane, therefore, can be the result of increased synthesis and secretion of matrix proteins or decreased matrix metalloproteinase synthesis, secretion, or activity.

Abnormal structure in the form of thickening of the basement membrane is a common pathological feature of renal ageing and diseases including nephronophthisis and ADPKD, and is also seen associated with drug-induced cystic disease in rats (Carone *et al.* 1989*a*). Abnormal basement membrane structure and composition was also seen in the first studies in which human ADPKD epithelia were grown *in vitro* (Wilson *et al.* 1986) suggesting this as a fundamental feature of genetically altered ADPKD cells. Ruthenium red staining and $^{35}SO_4$ incorporation studies demonstrated major changes in the synthesis, intracellular accumulation, turnover, and deposition of sulphated proteoglyans by ADPKD epithelia, resulting in abnormal structure including a loss of integrity of the lamina densa and lamina lucida when cells were grown on plastic and increased fibrillar deposition when cells were grown in a 3-dimensional gel matrix (Matrigel) (Wilson *et al.* 1992). In addition, abnormal molecular weight forms were detected (220 kDa), but no changes in the heparan sulphate proteoglycan core protein were seen, suggesting a post-translational abnormality. Subsequent studies have further confirmed abnormalities in the sulphation and intracellular processing of proteoglycans in ADPKD epithelia and also detected reduced charge density of proteoglycans in ADPKD and an increased proportion of chondroitin sulphate over the normal heparan sulphate proteoglycan species (Kovacs *et al.* 1994; Liu *et al.* 1992). It is also of interest that the growth factors TGFβ and HGF were able to modulate proteoglycan synthesis in ADPKD epithelia: HGF increasing the relative proportion of synthesis of heparan sulphate and TFGβ increasing the relative proportion of chondroitin sulphate proteoglycan. Taken together, with the expression of TGFβ in cyst epithelia, this suggests a role for this growth factor in ADPKD epithelial–stromal interactions.

Although immunostaining analysis is not rigorously quantitative, strong staining likely to be indicative of large amounts of the basement membrane proteins type IV collagen, laminin, and fibronectin, and of interstitial type I, III, and VI collagens have been detected in human ADPKD kidneys (Klingel *et al.* 1993; Wilson *et al.* 1992). Analysis of steady-state levels of mRNA also confirmed substantial increases in type IV collagen synthesis in ADPKD kidneys, particularly in the later stages of the disease (Wilson 1991*d*). Subsequently, *in vitro* studies also suggested substantial increases in collagen synthesis using [^{3}H] proline analysis, particularly of alpha-(III)3 and type IV, together with unidentified forms (Candiano, *et al.* 1992). Further *in vitro* analysis showed that the type of proteins secreted by ADPKD epithelial cells had a significant influence on the proliferative potential of ADPKD cells, since exogenous type I and type IV collagen resulted in hyperproliferation of ADPKD epithelia in comparison to normal human renal tubule epithelia of defined proximal or distal origin. Additional alterations in the interstitial matrix protein tenascin have been detected in the form of focal accumulations adjacent to cysts, which contrasts with the homogeneous localization in the mesenchyme surrounding developing epithelia in normal fetal kidneys (Klingel *et al.* 1993; Norman *et al.* 1994). This is of interest since tenascin C is often associated with active tissue regeneration or tumour formation (Chiquet-Ehrisman *et al.* 1986), that the protein contains EGF-like and fibronectin III domains (Erikcson and Bouirdon 1989) and recent studies have implicated annexin II (Calpactin I) as a high-affinity receptor for an alternatively spliced form of tenascin C (Chung and Erickson 1994).

Matrix receptors

Cell–matrix interactions are mediated through different families of receptors including the integrins, syndecan, and proteoglycans. Integrins are heterodimeric molecules comprised of alpha and beta subunits in several tissue-restricted combinations (Albeda and Buck 1990). For instance, of the laminin receptors: $\alpha_3\beta_1$ is characteristic of the glomerular basement membrane, whereas $\alpha_6\beta_1$ is characteristic of tubule epithelia and its appearance is correlated with polarization of epithelia during renal development (Ekblom 1992; Ruoslahti *et al.* 1994; Sorokin *et al.* 1990). Little information has been collected to date concerning integrin expression in human ADPKD or ARPKD, although studies of the cpk mouse suggest possible alterations in beta-1 expression related to cystic disease (van Adelsberg, personal communication). We have recently carried out immunostaining analysis on human tissue sections with specific monoclonal antibodies and have detected alpha-2 integrin expression in ADPKD cysts and in normal adult distal tubules; strong beta-1 and beta-4 expression in ADPKD cysts and alpha-6 integrin in all fetal, adult, and ADPKD tubules and cysts. It was of interest to note that alpha-6 integrin was also always associated with the basal membrane in all epithelial cells. Alpha-3 integrin was detected in the ureter and collecting tubules of fetal kidneys, also showed strong staining in ARPKD cyst epithelia, which are considered to be of distal origin.

Cell–cell interactions are also mediated via integrins and other families of proteins including the cadherins. In the kidney, N-CAM is expressed during renal development and is associated with the undifferentiated mesenchyme, while E-cadherin (uvomorulin) expression is associated with early events of adhesion and polarization of epithelial tubule structures during development (Ekblom 1992; Rodrigues-Boulan and Nelson 1989). E-cadherin localization is associated with the lateral and basal membranes and is thought to be involved in the early intercellular adhesion events prior to tight junction formation. E-cadherin is first seen in S-Bodies in developing kidneys and in normal renal tubules from adult kidneys where it is basolateral in distribution. Immunostaining and Western analysis of apical and basolateral membrane vesicles from ADPKD kidneys has suggested that there may be some deregulation of polarization of E-cadherin expression since additional immunoreactivity was seen in apical membranes of cyst epithelia (Du and Wilson 1991). This may also have implications for mispolarization of Na-K ATPase with which this protein is reportedly associated in MDCK cells (Nelson *et al.* 1990).

Proteolytic enzymes

Proteolytic enzymes play important roles in cellular and extracellular metabolism and in the turnover of proteins. In the intracellular domain, they may be localized within lysosomes, in the cytoplasm or at the plasma membrane. Lysosomal enzymes include a wide range of proteolytic activities including proteases, hydrolases, and sulphatases, where they play an important role in catabolic processes. Protease activities of the cysteine- and serine-types are also found in the cytoplasm, and at the plasma membrane where they have been implicated in protein processing, for instance of prohormones and growth factors, and also in activation of membrane-bound receptors. In the extracellular domain, proteases of the metalo and serine families are the major enzymes responsible for extracellular matrix turnover by appropriate degradation of proteins (Murphy and Reynolds 1993; Von der Mark *et al.* 1993). They are of particular importance during development when they aid migration and secretion of proteases *in vitro* was associated with tubulogenesis response of MDCK cells in gels to HGF (Montesano *et al.* 1991*b*). It is clear that abnormalities in protease activity, expression or localization could result in deleterious consequences for cellular processes and inappropriate secretion of matrix metalloproteinases (MMP) or of cysteine protease (cathepsin B) have been implicated in tumour cell invasion prior to metastasis. Since abnormalities in the basement membrane and interstitial matrix are common pathological features of ADPKD, matrix metalloproteinases and serine proteinases have been investigated. The first demonstration of abnormality in protease secretion in ADPKD was that plasminogen activator (uPA), a serine protease, which was increased 5- to 10-fold in cultured ADPKD fibroblasts in comparison to normal age-matched renal fibroblasts and this was further stimulated by FGF-a (Kuo 1991; Kuo *et al.* 1995). Zymogram analysis also suggested increased proteolytic enzyme secretion from ADPKD and ARPKD epithelial cells in culture and this was substantiated by immunolocalization of antibodies to MMPs in tubule epithelia *in vivo*. Further *in vitro* and zymogram analysis demonstrated substantial increases in secretion of gelatinases A and B and of stromelysin from both epithelia and fibroblasts derived from ADPKD kidneys during the early stages of disease progression. Later, in end-stage disease these enzymes declined but levels of the secreted inhibitor of tissue metalloproteinases (TIMP) increased, suggesting a mechanism for extracellular matrix accumulation during the fibrosis associated with end-stage ADPKD (Norman *et al.* 1993).

A detailed analysis of lysosomal enzymes has also been carried out in normal, ADPKD and ARPKD cells *in vivo* and *in vitro* (Hartz and Wilson 1995). Decreased proteolytic activity by enzymes in the acidic pH range was shown to be due to reductions in the synthesis of intracellular, predominantly epithelial, cathepsins B, L, and H, beta-galactosidase, and beta-hexosaminidase. No changes in cathepsin D were seen, suggesting specific, enzyme-related modifications. In addition, Western immunoblot and immunoprecipitation analysis showed that abnormal molecular weight species of cathepsin B and beta-galactosidase together with an ADPKD-specific high molecular weight form of cathepsin H, consistent with abnormal molecular processing and post-translational modifications in ADPKD. This is of interest since it correlates with previous findings of abnormal molecular processing of EGF and of post-translational modifications of heparan sulphate proteoglycans in ADPKD and suggests this may reflect some fundamental defect in protein processing in ADPKD cells. Further evidence of a protein-trafficking abnormality was found since in

ADPKD immunolocalization studies detected extralysosomal cathepsin B and H in association with cell membranes in ADPKD cyst epithelia, not seen in normal renal tubules. In addition to intracellular alterations, secretion abnormalities were also detected in conditioned media derived from ADPKD epithelia grown on filter membranes, suspended in tissue culture wells which separate apical from basalmedia compartments. While secretion of these proteolytic enzymes by normal cells was almost exclusively apically directed, that from ADPKD cells showed an increase in basally directed secretion, which in the case of cathepsins B and L resulted in a reversal of polarity from apical to basal. These increases in basal secretion of proteolytic enzymes and decreases in TIMP secretion *in vivo*, might contribute to the abnormal processing and degradation of integrity of the basement membrane and fibrosis of the interstitium.

Cytoskeleton

The cellular cytoskeleton provides structural support and is broadly divisible into microfilaments composed of actin, microtubules composed of tubulin, and intermediate filaments composed of cytokeratin in epithelial cells and vimentin in mesenchymal cells including fibroblasts. A switch from a vimentin to cytokeratin cytoskeletal content is characteristic of the conversion of undifferentiated mesenchyme to differentiated epithelia during renal development (Burrow and Wilson 1993, 1994). Western analysis of Tirton-X-100 insoluble cytoskeletal proteins revealed significant differences characterized by overabundance of actin (42 kDa), calpactin II (lipocortin 1, 36 kDa, 35 kDa), and calpactin I (lipocortin II 11 kDa) (Sherwood and Wilson 1990*a*; Wilson 1991*b*). Increased actin abundance was reflected by increased profiles of intracellular microfilament bundles characteristic of ADPKD cells *in vivo* and *in vitro* as detected by electron microscopy (Falkenstein *et al.* 1993). The calpactins (lipocortins, annexins) are calcium-and phospholipid-dependent actin binding proteins and are of considerable interest in ADPKD since they have been implicated in apical sorting mechanisms and calpactin II is thought to be an intracellular substrate for the EGF receptor. Immunostaining analysis further confirmed their up-regulation in ADPKD cyst epithelia and suggested a shift from intracellular cytoplasmic localization in normal tubule epithelia to the apical membrane of some cysts in ADPKD. Other actin-binding proteins associated with the membrane cytoskeleton also show alterations in polarized distribution in ADPKD kidneys. Ankyrin and fodrin are normally distributed to the basalateral membranes of distal tubules and in the apical and basolateral domains of normal proximal tubules. In ADPKD cysts, staining with antibodies against these proteins are clearly apical membrane-associated (Wilson 1991*b*; Wilson *et al.* 1992) where they co-localize with Na-K ATPase. This is of interest with regard to (mis)polarization mechanisms for Na-K ATPase in these epithelia, since these proteins have been implicated in the control or maintenance of Na-K ATPase polarity in MDCK cells (Nelson and Hammerton1989).

Alpha-actinin and vinculin are cross-linking actin proteins found in adhesion plaques and thought to be involved in cytoskeletal attachment to the cell membrane and matrix via integrins. In normal kidneys these proteins are localized to the medullary collecting ducts and in ADPKD strong staining is seen in some cyst epithelia.

Cytokeratin analysis shows no major changes in that different subtypes of keratin, characteristic of distal vs. proximal tubules are expressed in subsets of cysts in ADPKD and ARPKD epithelia and relect the tubule-type patterns of expression in normal kidneys. It is also of interest that some ADPKD cyst epithelia also show staining for vimentin which may suggest an aberrant differentiation in intermediate filament expression.

Secretion

Several abnormalities in secretion are found in ADPKD and ARPKD epithelia *in vivo* and *in vitro*. The expansion of cysts after early closing of connections with the tubule of origin in ADPKD predicts secretion as a major mechanism of fluid increase in cystic enlargement. This is borne out by cyst fluid analysis where the volume of aspirated fluid can range from milliliters (ARPKD and small cysts of early-stage ADPKD) to tens of centiliters in end-stage ADPKD cysts. In normal kidneys, large amounts of water are reabsorbed and this is via paracellular and transcellular routes as a result of diffusion or through constitutive or regulated water channels. The osmotic gradient driving these fluid movements is generated predominantly by the activity of the Na-K ATPase sodium pump localized on the basolateral membranes of renal tubule epithelia and creating hyperosmotic fluid at the basolateral extracellular domains. Water channels have recently been cloned and detected in the normal kidney. The aquaporin (AQP)-CHIP water channel is constitutive and is expressed at the basolateral and apical membranes of proximal tubules and thin descending limbs of Henle (Nielsen *et al.* 1993; Preston and Agre 1991), while the vasopressin-sensitive AQP-CD is restricted to collecting ducts in rat kidneys (Fushimi *et al.* 1993). A survey study of immunostaining for these proteins in human fetal, adult, early, and end-stage ADPKD and ARPKD kidneys has confirmed these localizations in normal human adult kidneys and demonstrated mutually exclusive staining patterns in ADPKD and ARPKD cyst epithelia. This suggests that although cyst epithelia may become quite extensively modified with regard to structural characteristics, particularly in end-stage ADPKD kidneys, some discriminatory differentiated proteins are well preserved. In addition, although AQP-CD showed a clear apical location in all normal and cystic sites, AQP-CHIP showed alterations in membrane polarity in ADPKD where in early-stage kidneys it was basal in some cysts, apical in others, and in end-stage cysts it was both apical and basal. Of particular interest, in ARPKD kidneys, some cysts showed clear staining in an apical membrane location only (DeVuyst *et al.* 1995). Fluid secretion has also been studied in primary cultures of normal renal cortical cells and ADPKD epithelia *in vitro* where 8-bromocyclic adenosine monophosphate (8-BrcAMP), forskolin, isebutylmethylxanthine (IBMX), PGE_1, and cyst fluid itself have been shown to induce fluid secretion. (Grantham 1993; Mangoo-Karim *et al.* 1989). It was of interest that arginine vasopressin (AVP) was unable to stimulate fluid secretion in ADPKD epithelia, which correlates with the initial findings in these epithelia that AVP failed to stimulate adenylate cyclase activity, despite the ability of normal human collecting tubule epithelia *in vitro* to exhibit a 10-fold response (Wilson *et al.* 1986). Taken together, these findings suggest that cAMP plays a role in fluid secretion and that there may be deficiencies in vasopressin signalling, possibly at the receptor or G protein transducer level in ADPKD epithelia. This may not be restricted to vasopressin, since parathyroid hormone (PTH) response was also very limited in ADPKD but not in normal proximal tubule epithelia (Wilson *et al.* 1986).

Sodium ions are the major osmotic determinant in normal kidneys, Na-K ATPase levels are extremely high and account in large part for the high-energy expenditure and oxygen demand of the kidney. The vectorial transport of sodium ions from the apical (luminal) to the basolateral (blood) side of normal renal tubules is associated with the exclusively basolateral distribution of Na-K ATPase. This polarized distribution is characteristic of absorptive epithelia. More rarely, exclusively apical location of Na-K ATPase is seen in normal tissues, where it is associated with sodium secretion, such as in the choroid plexus and retinal epithelia. Since ADPKD epithelia were thought to be secretory, it was hypothesized that this might be associated with abnormal polarized distribution of the Na-K ATPase in cystic epithelia in ADPKD and ARPKD. Immunostaining analysis of normal human fetal and adult kidneys and of early and end-stage ADPKD and ARPKD confirmed this hypothesis, since in expanding cysts, even from the earliest stages of lumen dilation, clear apical location of Na-K ATPase was seen (Wilson 1991 and Fig. 6.6). Biochemical and enzyme cytochemical studies confirmed that Na-K ATPase was not only fully functional but showed increased activity, in the early stages of ADPKD, the time of maximal cyst expansion. Although some up-regulation was seen in the steady-state mRNA levels of Na-K ATPase subunit levels, the increased activity was predicted to be in part due to post-translational mechanisms. Further confirmation of apical mislocation of functional Na-K ATPase in ADPKD epithelia was obtained by exclusive binding of [^{3}H] ouabain to apical membrane vesicle preparations derived from ADPKD kidneys while all specific binding was to basolateral membrane vesicles from normal adult kidneys (Wilson *et al.* 1991). A similar set of studies confirmed that these properties of increased activity and apical mislocation of Na-K ATPase were retained in primary cultures derived from ADPKD epithelia which were then grown on polarized permeable membrane filters suspended in tissue culture wells. Since the apical and basal media compartments are separated in these preparations, they are ideal for the study of transepithelial ion transport using radiotracers such as ^{22}NaCl. Parallel studies of normal and ADPKD epithelia showed that normal collecting tubule epithelia were capable of transporting ^{22}NaCl Only from the apical to the basal compartment, and that this could be inhibited by the addition of ouabain

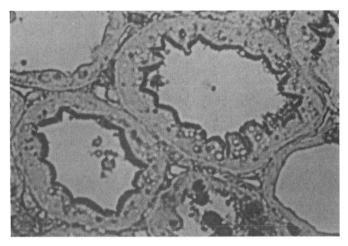

Fig. 6.6 Light micrograph of immunolocalization of Na–K ATPase (alpha-1 subunit) in early-stage ADPKD; 1 μmm sections were stained using an peroxidase-antiperoxidase technique with diamonobenzidine as substrate. Intense staining is seen on the apical, lumenal epithelial cell membranes of columnar and cuboidal morphology. No staining is seen at the basal or lateral cell membranes.

to the basal but not to the apical compartment. In contrast, ADPKD epithelia transported [22]NaCl from the basal to the apical compartment and this vectorial movement was inhibitable by ouabain but only when it was added to the apical medium compartment (Wilson 1991*b*). Therefore this was functional evidence that ADPKD epithelia conducted basal to apical Na transport due to the action of an apically mislocated Na–K ATPase.

Potential mechanisms underlying this mispolarization of Na–K ATPase have been examined. Co-localization with ankyrin and fodrin and to some extent, E-cadherin suggest that these membrane cytoskeletal and adhesion proteins may play a role, possibly in the maintenance of polarity in ADPKD epithelia as they do in MDCK cells (Nelson *et al.* 1990). Na–K ATPase is a heterodimer comprising two alpha and two beta subunits which are transcribed as the products of separate genes and co-translationally inserted into the endoplasmic reticulum where they associate to form a complex prior to post-translational modification in the Golgi apparatus and targeting to the appropriate plasma membrane domain. Since different isoforms of alpha and beta subunits had been cloned and shown to exhibit specific developmental and tissue distribution, it was hypothesized that isoform switching might be of significance in the missorting events in ADPKD and ARPKD. Normal adult kidneys express alpha-1 and beta-1 only, while early and end-stage ADPKD and ARPKD were shown to express alpha-1, beta-1, and beta-2 mRNA and protein as detected by RNAase protection and Western analysis. Distribution analysis using *in situ* hybridization analysis and immunolocalization studies with isoform-specific peptide antibodies showed that all three isoforms were expressed by cyst epithelia (Wilson *et al.*

1993*c*). However, beta-1 expression was seen only in the endoplasmic reticulum and not at the membrane in ADPKD epithelia and by electron microscopy was seen to be retained in the endoplasmic reticulum (Wilson *et al.* 1994). This is consistent with the hypothesis that in ADPKD alpha-1–beta-2 complex formation may be favoured and is able to tranverse the sorting and trafficking machinery of the epithelial cells, albeit to reach the wrong (apical) membrane. Alpha-1–beta-1 heterodimers, however, if they form seem to be unable to exit the endoplasmic reticulum after which they are presumably degraded.

In the studies of ^{22}Na transport in normal and ADPKD epithelium, it was also demonstrated that an apical to basal vectorial transport, albeit of a lower magnitude, was seen in ADPKD epithelium and that this Na uptake was inhibitable by amiloride which implicates an apical sodium channel or Na/H exchanger, and correlates with findings of amiloride sensitivity of some whole cysts isolated from ADPKD kidneys which are similar to normal proximal renal tubule epithelium (Perrone 1985). Bumetamide and furosemide, in contrast, were capable of inhibiting basal uptake of ^{22}Na consistent with the presence of a basally located Na^+K^+2Cl co-transporter in ADPKD epithelia (Wilson *et al.* 1992). Recently, chloride transport has also been studied in ADPKD. In primary cultures of ADPKD epithelium it has been possible to demonstrate a cAMP-activated, voltage-independent chloride conductance which is inhibitable by diphenylamine carboxylic acid (DPC) but not by 4,4′-diisothiocyano stilbene-2, 2′-disulfonic acid (DIDS) (Hanaoka *et al.* 1994). Immunostaining analysis has also demonstrated the presence of intense apical staining of cystic fibrosis transmembrane conductance regulator (CFTR) on ADPKD cyst epithelium (Devuyst *et al.* in prep.). Immunoreactivity against the P-glycoprotein product of the multidrug resistance (MDR) gene is also present in ADPKD and ARPKD cysts where it is located on apical epithelial cell membranes. Other transport-related membrane proteins present in ADPKD cysts include carbonic anhydrase IV and band 3 exchanger, although no Na–glucose transport was detected (Hammel and Wilson 1989).

Polarity

A detailed study of several polarized membrane proteins in normal and ADPKD and ARPKD kidneys has allowed several conclusions to be drawn about this fundamental feature of polycystic epithelia. Properties between ADPKD and ARPKD epithelia are not identical in this regard, nor do they necessarily reflect the findings in animal studies. However, it is clear that several specific and critical mispolarization events take place early in cyst formation in both ADPKD and ARPKD and that some of these have dramatic functional consequences for the pathogenesis of cyst formation. In ADPKD, apical mislocation Na-K ATPase is a primary event and widespread in the majority of cysts and is presumed to be related to the extensive degree of cyst dilation in ADPKD. In ARPKD, there appear to be different subsets of cysts, some of which have purely apical, some with solely basal and some with both apical and basolateral staining. This may be correlated with cpk mouse where apical Na-K ATPase staining is associated with distal cysts and basolateral location is seen proximal cysts (Avner *et al.* 1992) again suggesting a correlation between maximal expansion of cysts and apical Na-K ATPase. Another important membrane protein which undergoes polarity changes in ADPKD and ARPKD and has dramatic functional consequences for cyst expansion is the EGF receptor that is mispolarized to the apical membranes of cysts and allows access to the binding of the mitogen EGF or TGFα, which subsequently leads to aberrant proliferation.

A wide survey of the distribution of polarized membrane proteins has been carried out in our laboratory at the light and electron microscope levels *in vivo* and *in vitro* and demonstrates clearly that specific proteins undergo specific patterns of change. Not all normally basolaterally located proteins are mislocated on the apical surface of cyst epithelia (Table 6.3). For instance, heparan sulphate proteoglycan, type IV collagen, laminin, and alpha-6 integrin remain exclusively basal. Similarly, many normally apically located proteins remain apical such as glycosyl-phopshatidyl inositol (GPI)-linked proteins including alkaline phosphatase, trehalase, GP330, a 95 kDa brush-border protein, leucine aminopeptidase, and the P-glycoprotein product of the MDR gene. Some of these proteins are decreased in quantity or activity, such as alkaline phosphatase and trehalase, but not in their polarized distribution. Of the proteins studied, few are mislocalized to the basolateral membranes in ADPKD and ARPKD but examples include the Na^+K^+2Cl cotransporter and secreted proteases, including cathepsins B and L. Several proteins, however, have a specific mislocalization to apical plasma membranes in cyst epithelia. These include NaK-ATPase, ankyrin, fodrin, E-cadherin, EGF receptor, calpactins I and II, c-met (the HGF receptor), and AQP-CHIP. Some of these changes are typical of secretory epithelia which further attests to a causative role in the pathogenesis of cyst formation in ADPKD and ARPKD.

These features have led us to examine potential unifying underlying cellular mechanism(s) which might be responsible for such a wide range of cellular changes in genetic cystic disease. One hypothesis might implicate a fundamental defect in the intracellular protein sorting machinery. Current attention is focused on a set of proteins, the Rab GTPases, which are homologous to Ras proteins and play key roles as master regulators of membrane trafficking via vesicular transport of proteins through each of the specifica stages of the secretory pathway and in endocytic membrane recycling pathways (Zerial and Stenmark 1993). Different and specific Rab proteins have been identified and include those responsible for endoplasmic reticulum to Golgi, *cis* to medial Golgi, medial to *trans* Golgi, and *trans* Golgi to plasma membrane transport. In addition, specific Rab proteins are associated with polarized vesicular transport, such as Rab 8, which is associated with *trans* Golgi to basolateral membrane transport, and Rab 17, which is epithelial cell-specific. Rab proteins have been determined to function via interconversion between GDP- and GPT- bound forms to control transport vesicle docking and/or fusion with their cognate target membrane sequences. This conversion is in turn mediated via Rab-specific GTPase-

Table 6.3 Polarity of membrane proteins in human autosomal dominant PKD

Apical no change
GPI-linked
Alkaline phosphatase
Trehalase
Leucine aminopeptidase
GP330
alpha 95 kDa
MDR P-glycoprotein
Carbonic anhydrase IV
Amiloride-sensitive Na$^+$ uptake
AQP-CD

Basal to apical
Na$^+$-K$^+$ ATPase
Fodrin
Ankyrin
E-cadherin
EGFR
Calpactin
c-Met
AQP-CHIP

Intracellular to apical
Cathepsin B
Cathepsin H
TIMP
Gelatinase A

Apical to basal
Na$^+$-K$^+$-2Cl$^-$
Cathepsin B + L secretion

Basal no change
HSPG
Collagen IV
Laminin
Integrin (alpha-6)
Band 3
Transferrin receptor

AQP, aquaporin; EGFR, epidermal growth factor; GPI, glycosyl phosphatidylinositol; HSPG, heparan sulphate proteoglycan; MDR, multidrug resistance.

activating proteins (GAPs), which then confers additional specificity to the processes (Pfeffer 1994). It is conceivable that a mutation affecting the integrity of one or more of these processes, might well lead to abnormalities of polarized membrane protein distribution typified by ADPKD and ARPKD cysts. Suggestive evidence in this regard has been the identification of the tuberous sclerosis (TSC-2) gene which has homology with a GAP protein. Recent analysis of some Rab proteins in normal and ADPKD and ARPKD tissue sections by immunostaining analysis in our laboratory has implicated quantitative alterations in the distribution of Rab 5 and Rab 8 which are involved in plasma membrane to endsome recycling and TGN to basolateral membrane sorting, respectively.

Ischaemia

Although renin expression is increased in the ADPKD kidney and thought to be associated with alterations in the vascularization in this disease, no indications of renal tubular injury are found in surgical specimens. Ischaemic injury in the kidney leads to ultrastructural and functional alterations in predominantly proximal tubule epithelium, including alterations in plasma membrane protein distribution and abnormalities in the actin-cytoskeleton (Fish and Molitoris 1994). Careful collection of surgical material for subsequent immunostaining and comparison with defined epithelial cell cultures and detailed ultrastructural analysis has shown that the alterations in ADPKD and ARPKD epithelium are quite distinct from those seen in ischaemic injury (Wilson *et al.* 1986; Falkenstein *et al.* 1994). Ultrastructural alterations characteristic of renal tubule ischaemic injury include clubbing and internalization of the microvilli of the brush border and membrane blebbing, none of which are seen in ADPKD and ARPKD where brush-border microvilli vary in density, presumably related to the tubule cell type of origin, but are normal and externally directed into the lumen. Although in early-stage ADPKD kidneys, light microscopy suggests some fragmentation of cells, particulary in those cysts with proximal tubule morphology, electron microscopy reveals that these fragmentation bodies contain normal densities of cytoplasm and organelles including mitochondria and endoplasmic reticulum, thus showing no resemblance to blebbed membranes characteristic of ischaemic castes or to apoptotic bodies. Changes in the actin cytoskeleton have also been characterized during ischaemic renal tubule damage and include disruption of the microvillar actin core and of the apical circumferential actin network leading to formation of perinuclear aggregates (Leiser and Molitoris 1993). Although the actin cytoskeleton has been well-studied and shown to undergo alterations in ADPKD, none of those changes seen during ischaemia have been documented, but rather an overabundance and increases in intracellular cytoplasmic microfilament bundles (Falkenstein *et al.* 1993). Likewise, disruptions in the membrane cortical cytoskeleton, including degradation of ankyrin and fodrin which have been documented in ischaemic injury, are not seen in ADPKD, where there is not only increased intensities of staining for ankyrin and fodrin but also an apical mislocation and co-localization with Na-K ATPase.

Na-K ATPase shows a clear disruption of polarity after ischaemic damage, which is characterized as a loss of restriction to the basolateral membrane domain and a redistribution to both apical and basolateral domains (Molitoris 1985). Likewise, alkaline phosphatase is redistributed equally throughout the basolateral and apical domains. Together with ultrastructural analysis, these changes are concluded to be due to a breakdown of the integrity of the molecular fence function of the tight junctions and desmosomes (Fish and Molitoris 1994; Mandel *et al.* 1993). In ADPKD, the mislocalization of

Na-K ATPase to the apical membrane is quite specific and asymmetric in that no staining or function is associated with the basolateral membrane domains. Also, alkaline phosphatase polarity is not altered, and no loss of structural or functional integrity of intercellular tight junctions or desmosomes have been seen in ADPKD. Finally, the maintenance of the specific mispolarized Na-K ATPase and EGF receptors in ADPKD and ARPKD epithelial cells *in vitro*, grown through several passages in oxygenated substrate-replete conditions, further confirms that these alterations in ADPKD and ARPKD are genetically determined intrinsic properties of those cells. In contrast, normal renal tubule epithelial cells *in vitro* show exclusively basolateral distribution of these proteins.

Apoptosis

Recent studies have suggested that apoptosis plays a more important role in renal morphogenesis than was formerly recognized (Coles *et al.* 1993). *In vitro*, *in vivo*, and WT-1 double 'knockout' mouse studies have shown that the metanephric mesenchyme is programmed to apoptose unless induced to condense and differentiate by the ingrowth of the ureteric bud (Coles *et al.* 1993; Koseki *et al.* 1992; Kreidberg *et al.* 1993). The bcl-2 gene has been shown to inhibit apoptosis and bcl-2-deficient mice develop renal cysts (Veis *et al.* 1993). Little analysis of apoptosis has been carried out in ADPKD kidneys. Although no characteristic apoptotic morphological profiles have been reported, there is some evidence of increased endonuclease activity in early-stage ADPKD disease. This may correlate with reports of SGP-2 expression in cpk mice (Harding *et al.* 1991), although its gene product, clusterin, is not always considered a truly specific marker for apoptosis. Interpretation of these findings will therefore await further studies.

Development and differentiation

The epithelial cells lining ADPKD and ARPKD cysts are clearly polarized in their overall structure, have distinct sets of integral membrane proteins in their apical and basolateral domains and have morphologically and functionally intact intercellular tight junctions at their apical aspect. Both in early-and end-stage disease there are clearly morphological as well as functional differences in cyst-lining epithelial cells in comparison to their normal nephron epithelial cell types of origin. It is important, however, to recognize that there is considerable cellular heterogeneity both between cysts and within cysts even in the later stages of disease. Certain changes in cell structure suggest a progressive loss of features of terminal differentiation in that clear discriminations between principal and intercalated cell morphologies can be made more easily in early-stage than in end-stage ADPKD. However, immunostaining, functional, and cyst fluid analyses have clearly shown that major differences are retained into end-stage disease, allowing discrimination between cysts with proximal, loop of Henle, distal, or collecting tubule origin. For instance, the proximal tubule markers AQP-CHIP, GP330, and gamma-glutamyl transpeptidase, and the distal tubule markers of low molecular weight keratin, vinculin, and AQP-CD are retained in subsets of cysts through to endstage disease. Other differentiated properties, such as villi of proximal tubule brush borders, microvilli, alkaline phosphatase, trehalase, Na–glucose transport, are lost or substantially reduced. This would suggest more specific mechanisms than a progressive gradual dedifferentiation to a 'generic' epithelial cell state.

Several lines of evidence suggest similarities between major features of ADPKD and ARPKD epithelia with fetal renal tubule epithelia (Wilson *et al.* 1992; Falkenstein *et al.* 1993). Although this seems obvious in the case ARPKD, which is clearly an abnormality of renal development and lethal *in utero* or shortly after birth, this is less intuitive for ADPKD. Detailed ultrastructural and immunolocalization analyses of normal fetal, normal adult, ADPKD, and ARPKD kidney epithelia *in vivo* and *in vitro* at the light and electron micro-scope levels have shown several striking structural and functional similarities between fetal and ADPKD. These include actin filament overabundance, glyco-gen deposition, lamellar body accumulation, apically located Na-K ATPase, and apical EGF receptors. In addition, the Na-K ATPase beta-2 isoform has been cloned from human fetal kidneys and its expression shown to be associated with early developing proximal tubules which exhibit apical membrane localization of the protein. An identical expression and distribution pattern is seen ADPKD cyst epithelia where Na-K ATPase beta-2 isoform mRNA is also detected in cells which exhibit apical mislocalization of the Na-K ATPase protein complex. This has led to the hypothesis that retention of a fetal phenotype or failure to complete the full transcriptional programme of polarization of membrane pro-teins could be the fundamental mechanism which results in the dramatic con-sequences that lead to cyst formation in ADPKD (Wilson *et al.* 1992). This would then suggest that an inherited mutation in one allelle of the PKD-1 gene leads to alterations in the developmental programme determining induction, differentiation, and polarization events that typify nephrogenesis. The effects appear to be relatively mild, affecting a subset of nephrons causing them to expand by proliferation and secretion without onset of clinical symptoms of renal functional decline until a substantial degree of cystic enlargement and tissue destruction has occurred.

In addition to the similarities in ultrastructure, and presence of apical Na-K ATPase and apical EGF receptors, additional features characteristic of fetal human kidneys have been detected in ADPKD and ARPKD kidneys (Table 6.4). These include aberrant expression of PCNA-DNA polymerase-delta, consistent with a high proliferative potential and aberrant expression of the transcription factors Pax-2 and WT-1, both of which are normally under strict temporal regulation during renal development. Additional similarities may be associated with growth factor-signal transduction pathways and include high levels of expression of membrane tyrosine and serine-threonine protein kinases and apical mislocation of calpactins which have EFG repeats and are substrates

Table 6.4   Expression of fetal proteins in ADPKD and ARPKD.

	Fetal	Adult	ADPKD	ARPKD
Apical Na-K ATPase	+	–	+	+
	a_1b_2	a_1b_1	a_1b_2	a_1b_2
Apical EGF receptor	+	–	+	+
Apical calpactin	+	–	+	ND
PCNA-DNA polymerase-delta	+	–	+	+
PAX-2 expression	+	–	+	+
WT-1 expression	+	–	+	+
Phosphotyrosine	++	±	++	++
ERK-1	++	±	++	++
Apical AQP-CHIP	++	±	++	++
Glycogen	+	–	+	+
Microfilaments	+	–	+	
Lamellar bodies	+	–	+	+
Albumin	+	–	+	ND

AQP, oquaporin; ND, not done; WT, Wilms' tumour.

for the EGF receptor. Finally, a predominantly apical localization of the AQP-CHIP water channel is characteristic of fetal, ADPKD and ARPKD epithelia. These studies suggest that several normal features of fetal kidneys are also seen in ADPKD and ARPKD and have led to our working hypothesis that cyst formation is the result of a faulty transcriptional programme of regulation of renal tubule polarization associated with the acquisition of the final terminally differentiated phenotype of the highly segmented nephron.

Conclusions

The pathogenesis of cyst formation is a complex and multifactorial process. A comparison of animal and experimental models with human genetic entities of ADPKD, ARPKD, and medullary cystic disease shows that renal cyst formation is a relatively common response to mutation or manipulation and it is likely that several different mechanisms can result in a superficially common change. On closer examination, each disease entity is also characterized by its own set of distinct features. Some common general themes are, however, associated with renal cyst formation and include abnormalities in matrix regulation, aberrant cell proliferation, epithelial secretion, and mispolarization of epithelial membrane proteins. The extent and fine details of each of these types of change varies with disease entity, experimental, or therapeutic intervention. Identification of the ADPKD-1 gene has not yet yielded insight into the underlying biological mechanism controlling these changes but current knowledge favours a developmental disregulation of the programming of normal epithelial cell polarization events.

Note added in proof

Since this manuscript was first written (July 1994), the structure of the full length CDNA for PKD-1 has been determined. It predicts a membrane protein with a long extracellular tail and multifunctional domains (American PKD Consortium (1995). *Hum. Molec. Genet.*, **4**, 575-82; International PKD Consortium (1995). *Cell*, **81**, 289-8; Hughes, J., Ward, C., Peral, B., Aspinwall, R., Clark, K., San Millan, J., Gamble, V., and Harris, P. C. (1995). *Nature Genetics*, **10**, 151-9). Expression studies using riboprobes and peptide antibodies derived against the putative plasma membrane domain of the PKD-1 protein have localized the mRNA and the protein to ADPKN cyst epithelia, where it is upregilated by comparison to normal adult kidneys where it is restricted to the inner medullary collecting ducts. A role for PKD-1 in the normal developmental regulation of renal epithelial differentiation and polarization is suggested by the high levels of expression of the PKD-1 mRNA and protein in the ureteric bud structures of the developing human kidney at 12 to 16 weeks' gestation (Qian, F., O'Sullivan, E., Germino, G., and Wilson, P. D. (1995). PKD-1 expression is developmentally regulated and is abnormal in renal cystic epithelia. *Nature Genetics*, in press; Onuchic, L. F., Herbert, R., Wilson, P. D., and Germino, G. G. (1995). Polycystin, the PKD-1 gene product, is developmentally regulated and overexpressed in ADPKD cystic epithelia. *J. Clin. Invest.*, under review).

References

Albeda, S. M. and Buck, C. A. (1990). Integrins and other cell adhesion molecules. *FASEB Journal*, **4** 2868–80.

Angeli, A., Bradlow, L., Chasalow, F. I., and Dogliotti, L. (1990). Biochemistry of breast cyst fluid: correlations with breast cancer risk. *Annals of the New York Academy of Science*, **586**, 1–295.

Avner, E. D., Sweeney, W. E., and Nelson, W. J. (1992). Abnormal sodium pump distribution during renal tubulogenesis in congenital murine polycystic kidney disease. *Proceedings of the National Academy of Sciences USA*, **89**, 7447–51.

Baert, L. (1978). Hereditary polycystic kidney disease (adult form): a microdissection study of two cases at an early stage of the disease. *Kidney International*, **13**, 519–25.

Bell, J. I., *et al.* (1986). Human epidermal growth factor precursor: cDNA sequence, expression *in vitro* and gene organization. *Nucleic Acids Research* **14**, 853–67.

Bernstein, J., Evan, A. P., and Gardner, K. J. (1987). Epithelial hyperplasia in human polycystic kidney diseases. Its role in pathogenesis and risk of neoplasia (Review). *American Journal of Pathology*, **129**, 92–101.

Burrow, C. R. and Wilson, P. D. (1993). A putative Wilms tumor-secreted growth factor activity required for primary culture of human nephroblasts. *Proceedings of the National Academy of Sciences USA*, **90**, 6066–70.

Burrow, C. R. and Wilson, P. D. (1994). Renal progenitor cells: problems of definition, isolation and characterization. *Experimental Nephrology*, **2**, 1–12.

Calvet, J. P. (1993). Polycystic kidney disease — primary extracellular matrix abnormality or defective cellular differentiation. *Kidney International*, **43**, 101–8.

Candiano, G., *et al.* (1992). Extracellular matrix formation by epithelial cells from human polycystic kidney cysts in culture. *Virchows Archiv für Pathologische Anatomie, B,* **63**, 1–9.

Carone, F. A., Hollenberg, P. F., Nakamura, S., Punyarit, P., Glogowski, W., and Flouret, G. (1989*a*) Tubular basement membrane change occurs pari passu with the development of cyst formation. *Kidney International,* **35**, 1034–40

Carone, F. A., Nakamura, S., Schumacher, B. S., and Punyarit, P. K. D. (1989*b*). Cyst-derived cells do not exhibit accelerated growth or feature of transformed cells in *in vitro. Kidney International,* **35**, 1351–7

Chiquet-Ehrisman, R., Mackie, E. J., Pearson, C. A., and Sakakura, T. (1986). Tenascin: an extracellular matrix protein involved in tissue interactions during fetal development and oncogenesis. *Cell,* **47**, 131–9.

Chung, C. Y. and Erickson, H. P. (1994). Cell surface annexin II is a high affinity receptor for the alternatively spliced segment of tenascin-C. *Journal of Cell Biology,* **126**, 539–48.

Coles, H. S. R., Burne, J. F., and Raff, M. C. (1993). Large-scale normal cell death in the developing rat kidney and its reduction by epidermal growth factor. *Development,* **118**, 777–84.

Cowley, B. J., Smardo, F. J., Grantham, J. J., and Calvet, J. P. (1987). Elevated c-myc protooncogene expression in autosomal recessive polycystic kidney disease. *Proceedings of the National Academy of Sciences USA,* **84**, 8394–8.

Cuppage, F. E., Huseman, R. A., Chapman, A., and Grantham, J. J. (1980). Ultrastructure and function of cysts from human adult polycystic kidneys. *Kidney International,* **17**, 372–81.

Daoust, M. C., Bichet, D., and Somlo, S. (1993). A French Canadian family with autosomal dominant polycystic kidney disease unlinked to ADPKD 1 and ADPKD 2. *Journal of the American Society of Nephrology,* **4**, 262.

Devuyst, O., Burrow, C. R., Smith, B. L., Agre, P., Knepper, M. A. and Wilson, P. D. (1995). Expression of aquaporins 1 and 2 during human nephrogenesis and in autosomal dominant polycystic kidney disease. *Am. J. Physiol.,* under review.

Dressler, G. R., Wilkinson, J. E., Rothenpieler, U. W., Patterson, L., Williams-Simons, L., and Westphal, H. (1993). Deregulation of Pax-2 expression in transgenic mice generates severe kidney abnormalities. *Nature,* **362**, 65–7.

Du, J. and Wilson, P. D. (1991). Increased distribution of uvomorulin to apical membrane surface in autosomal dominant polycystic kidney disease. *Journal of Cell Biology,* **115**, 67a.

Du, J. and Wilson, P. D. (1994). Abnormal polarity of EGF receptors: a mechanism for autocrine stimulation of cyst epithelial proliferation in human autosomal dominant polycystic kidney disease. *American Journal of Physiology,* **269**, Cell. Physiol., **38**.

Du, J., Norman, J. T., and Wilson, P. D. (1991). EGF as an autocrine/paracrine regulator of aberrant cell proliferation in ADPKD. *Journal of the American Society of Nephrology,* **3**, 251.

Eckardt, K., *et al.* (1989). Erythropoietin in polycystic kidneys. *Journal of Clinical Investigation,* **84**, 1160–6.

Ekblom, P. (1992). Renal development. In *The kidney: Physiology and pathophysiology,* (ed. D. W. Seldin and G., Giebisch), pp. 475–501. Raven, New York.

Ekblom, P., Vestweber, D., and Kemler, R. (1986). Cell-matrix interactions and cell adhesion during development. *Annual Review of Cell Biology,* **2**, 27–47.

Eng, E., Wilson, P. D., Racusen, L., and Burrow, C. R. (1994) Aberrant Pax-2-expression in human autosomal dominant polycystic kidney disease epithelia. *Journal of the American Society of Nephrology*, **5**, 621.

Erickson, H. P. and Bouirdon, M. A. (1989). Tenascin: an extracellular matrix protein prominent in specialized embryonic tissues and tumors. *Annual Review of Cell Biology*, **5**, 71–92.

Evan, A. P. and McAtter, J. A. (1990). Cyst cells and cyst walls. In *The cystic kidney*, (ed. K. D. Gardner and J. Bernstein) pp. 21–42. Kluwer, Boston.

Falkenstein, D., Burrow, C. R., Gatti, L., Hartz, P. A., and Wilson, P. D. (1993). Expression of fetal proteins in human polycystic kidney disease epithelia. *Journal of the American Society of Nepthrology*, **4**, 813.

Falkenstein, D., Burrow, C. R., Norman, J. T., Hartz, P. A., and Wilson, P. D. (1994). Abnormalities in membrane protein polarity, enzyme and ion secretion in human autosomal recessive polycystic kidney disease. *Journal of the American Society of Nephrology*, **5**, 621.

Faraggiana, T., Bernstein, J., Strauss, L., and Churg, J. (1985). Use of lectins in the study of histogenesis of renal cysts. *Laboratory Investigation*, **53**, 575–9. polycystic kidney disease. *Journal of the American Society Nephrology*, **3**, 1863–1870.

Fish, E. M. and Molitoris, B. A. (1994). Alterations in epithelial polarity and the pathogenesis of disease states. *New England Journal of Medicine* **330**, 1580–8.

Foxall, P., Price, R. G., Jones, J. K., Neild, G. H., Thompson, F. D., and Nicholson, J. K. (1992). High resolution proton magnetic resonance spectroscopy of cyst fluids from patients with polycystic kidney disease. *Biochimica Biophysica Acta*, **1138**, 305–14.

Fryer, A. E., *et al.* (1987). Evidence that the gene for tuberous sclerosis is on chromosome 9. *Lancet*, **1, 659–61**

Fushimi, K., Uchida, S., Hara, Y., Hirata, Y., Marumo, F., and Sasaki, S. (1993). Cloning and expression of apical membrane water channel of rat kidney collecting tubule. *Nature*, **361**, 549–52.

Gardner, K. D., Burnside, J. S., Elzinga, L. W., and Locksley, R. M. (1991). Cytokines in fluids from polycystic kidneys. *Kidney International*, **39**, 718–24.

Graham, P. C. and Lindop G. B. (1988). The anatomy of the renin-secreting cell in adult polycystic kidney disease. *Kidney International*, **33**, 1084–90.

Granot, Y., Van Putten, V., Przekwas, J., Gabow, P. A., and Schrier, R. W. (1990). Intra- and extracellular proteins in human normal and polycystic kidney epithelial cells. *Kidney International*, **37**, 1301–9.

Grantham, J. J. (1993). Fluid secretion, cellular proliferation and the pathogenesis of renal epithelial cysts. *Journal of the American Society of Nephrology*, **3**, 1843–57.

Hammel, R. L. and Wilson, P. D. (1989). Loss of Na-dependent glucose transport in adult human polycystic kidney disease derived apical membrane vesicles. *Kidney International*, **37**, 225.

Hanaoka, K., Schwiebert, E. M., Wilson, P. D., and Guggino, W. B. (1994). cAMP-activated chloride conductance in autosomal dominant polycystic kidney disease (ADPKD) cells in culture. *Journal of the American Society of Nephrology*, **5**, 286.

Harding, M. A., Chadwick, L. J., Gattone, V. H., and Calvet, J. P. (1991). The SGP-2 gene is developmentally regulated in the mouse kidney and abnormally expressed in collecting duct cysts in polycystic kidney disease. *Development Biology*, **146**, 483–90.

Hartz, P. A. and Wilson, P. D. (1994). Lysosomal proteinase abnormalities in autosomal dominant polycystic kidney disease. *American Journal of Physiology* (submitted).

Hartz, P. A. and Wilson, P. D. (1995). Functional defects in lysosomal enzymes in autosomal deminant polycystic kidney disease: abnormalities in synthesis, molecular processing, polarity and secretion, *Biochem. & Molec. Medicine*, under review.

Heptinstall, R. H. (1992). *Pathology of the kidney*, pp. 124–47. Little, Brown, Boston.

Hjelle, J. T., *et al.* (1990). Autosomal recessive polycystic kidney disease: characterization of human peritoneal and cystic kidney cells *in vitro* . *American Journal of Kidney Diseases*, **15**, 123–36.

Hughson, M. D., Hennigar, G. R., and McManus, J. F. (1980). Atypical cysts, acquired renal cystic disease, andrenal cell tumors in end stage dialysis kidneys. *Laboratory Investigation*, **42**, 475–80.

Kelley, K. A., Agarwal, N., Reeders, S., and Herrup, K. (1991). Renal cyst formation and multifocal neoplasia in transgenic mice carrying the Simian virus 40 early region. *Journal of the American Society of Nephrology*, **2**, 84–97.

Klingel, R., Storkel, S., and Dipplod, W. (1991). Autosomal dominant polycystic kidney disease. *In vitro* culture of cyst-lining epithelial cells. *Virchows Archiv B Cell Pathology*, **61**, 189–99.

Klingel, R., Dippold, W., Storkel, S., Meyer, K., and Kohler, H. (1992). Expression of differentiation antigens and growth-related genes in normal kidney, autosomal dominant polycystic kidney disease and renal cell carcinoma. *American Journal of Kidney Diseases*, **19**, 22–30.

Klingel, R., Ramadori, G., Schuppan, D., Knittel, T., zum Buschenfelde, K., M., and Kohler, H. (1993). Coexpression of extracellular matrix glycoproteins undulin and tenascin in human autosommal dominant polycystic kidney disease. *Nephron*, **65**, 111–18.

Koseki, C., Herzlinger, D., and Al-Awqati, Q. (1992). Apoptosis in metanephric development. *Journal of Cell Biology*, **119**, 1327–33

Kovacs, J., Carone, F., Liu, Z. Z., Nakumara, S., Kumar, A., and Kanwar, Y. S. (1994). Differential growth factor-induced modulation of proteoglycans synthesized by normal human renal versus cyst-derived cells. *Journal of the American Society of Nephrology*, **5** ,47–54.

Kreidberg, J. A., *et al.* (1993). WT-1 is required for early kidney development. *Cell*, **74**, 679–91.

Kuo, N. (1991). A role for acidic fibroblast growth factor in the fibroblast proliferative defect of autosomal dominant polycystic kidney disease. *Journal of Cell Biology*, **115**, 418a.

Kuo, N. and Wilson, N. (1990). Mitogenic effects of growth factors in human renal fibroblasts during normal development, ageing and polycystic kidney disease. *Journal of the American Society of Nephrology*, **1**, 723.

Kuo, N. and Wilson, O. D. (1994). Acidic FGF and hyperproliferation of fibroblasts from human autosomal dominant polycystic kidney disease. *Journal of Cellular Physiology*.

Kuo, N., Norman, J. T., and Wilson, P. D. (1995). Acidic EGF regulation of hyperproliferation of fibroblasts in human autosomal dominant polycystic kidney disease. *J. Cell Physiol.*, under review.

Lakshmanan, J. and Eysselein, V. (1993). Hereditary error in epidermal growth factor prohormone metabolism in a rat model of autosomal dominant polycystic kidney disease. *Biochemical and Biophysical Research Communications*, **197**, 1083–93.

Lakshmanan, J. and Fisher, D. A. (1993). An inborn error in epidermal growth factor prohormone metabolism in a mouse model of autosomal recessive polycystic kidney disease. *Biochemical and Biophysical Research Communications*, **196**, 892–901.

Leiser, J. and Molitoris, B. A. (1993). Disease processes in epithelia — the role of the actin cytoskeleton and altered surface membrane polarity. *Biochimica Biophysica Acta*, **1225**, 1–13.

Liu, Z. Z., Carone, F. A., Nakumara, S., and Kanwar, Y. S. (1992). Altered synthesis of proteoglycans by cyst-derived cells from autosomal-dominant polycystic kidneys. *American Journal of Physiology*, **263**, F697–704.

Mandel, L. J., Bacallao, R., and Zampighi, G. (1993). Uncoupling of the molecular 'fence' and paracellular 'gate' functions in epithelial tight junctions. *Nature*, **361**, 552–5.

Mangoo-Karim, R., *et al.* (1989). Renal epithelial fluid secretion and cyst growth: the role of cyclic AMP. *FASEB Journal*, **3**, 2629–32.

McAteer, J. A., Carone, F. A., Grantham, J. J., Kempson, S. A., Gardner, K. J., and Evan, A. P. (1988). Explant culture of human polycystic kidney. *Laboratory Investigation*, **59**, 126–36.

Milutinovic, J. and Agodoa, L. Y. (1983). Potential causes and pathogenesis in autosomal dominant polycystic kidney disease. *Nephron*, **33**, 139–44.

Milutinovic, J., *et al.* (1980). Autosomal dominant polycystic kidney disease: early diagnosis and data for genetic counselling. *Lancet*, **1**, 1203–6.

Molitoris, B., Wilson, P. D., Schrier, R. W., and Simon, F. R. (1985). Ischaemia induces partial loss of surface membrane polarity and accumulation of putative calcium ionophores. *Journal of Clinical Investigation*, **76**, 2097–2105.

Montesano, R. Matsumoto, K., Nakamura, T., and Orci, L. (1991*a*). Identification of a fibroblast-derived epithelial morphogen as hepatocyte growth factor. *Cell*, **67**, 901–8.

Montesano, R., Schaller, G., and Orci, L. (1991*b*). Induction of epithelial tubular morphogenesis *in vitro* by fibroblast-derived soluble factors. *Cell*, **66**, 697–711.

Murphy, G. and Reynolds, J. J. (1993). Extracellular matrix degradation. In *Connective tissue and its heritable disorders*, pp. 287–316. Wiley-Liss, New York.

Muther, R. S. and Bennett, W. M. (1981). Cyst fluid antibiotic concentrations in polycystic kidney disease: differences between proximal and distal cysts. *Kidney International*, **20**, 519–22.

Nelson, W. J. and Hammerton, R. W. (1989). A membrane-crytoskeletal complex containing Na⁺K⁺-ATPase, ankyrin and fodrin in Madin–Darby canine kidney (MDCK) cells. Implications for the biogenesis of epithelial cell polarity. *Journal of Cell Biology*, **108**, 893–902.

Nelson, W. J., Shore, E. M., Wang, A. Z., and Hammerton, R. W. (1990). Identification of a membrane-cytoskeletal complex containing the cell adhesion molecule uvomorulin (E-cadherin), ankyrin, and fodrin in Madin–Darby canine kidney epithelial cells. *Journal of Cell Biology*, **110**, 349–57.

Nielsen, S., Smith, B. L., Christensen, E. I., Knepper, M. A., and Agre, P. (1993). CHIP28 water channels are localized in constitutively water-permeable segments of the nephron. *Journal of Cell Biology*, **120**, 371–383.

Norman, J. T., Gatti, L., and Wilson, P.D. (1993). Abnormal matrix metalloproteinase regulation in human autosomal dominant polycystic kidney disease. *Journal of the American Society of Nephrology*, **4**, 819.

Norman, J., Kuo, N., Gatti, L., Orphanides, C., and Wilson, P. D. (1994). Changes in interstitial fibroblast growth and extracellular matrix metabolism in human autosomal dominant polycystic kidney disease. *Proceedings ISN Forefronts in Nephrology*.

Osathanondh, V. and Potter, E. L. (1964). Pathogenesis of polycystic kidneys: historical survey; survey of results of microdissection. *Archives of Pathology*, **77**, 459.

Pardee, A. B. (1989). G1 events and regulation of cell proliferation. *Science*, **246**, 603–8.

Pelletier, J., Breuning, W., Li, F. P., Haber, D., Glaser, T., and Housman, D. E. (1991). WT1 mutations contribute to abnormal genital system development and hereditary Wilms' tumor. *Nature*, **353**, 431–4.

Perrone, R. D. (1985). In vitro function of cyst epithelium from human polycystic kidney. *Journal of Clinical Investigation*, **76**, 1688–91.

Pfeffer, S. (1994). Rab GTPases: master regulators of membrane trafficking. *Current Opinion in Cell Biology*, **6**, 522–6.

Preston, G. M. and Agre, P. (1991). Isolation of the cDNA for erythrocyte integral membrane protein of 28 kilodaltons: Member of an ancient channel family. *Proceedings of the National Academy of Sciences USA*, **88**, 11110–14.

Ritz, E., Zeier, M., Geberth, S., and Waldherr, R. (1993). Autosomal dominant polycystic kidney disease (ADPKD) — mechanisms of cyst formation and renal failure. *Australian and New Zealand Journal of Medicine*, **23**, 35–41.

Rodriguez–Boulan, E. and Nelson, W. J. (1989). Morphogenesis of the polarized epithelial cell phenotype. *Science*, **245**, 718–25.

Ruoslahti, R., Noble, N. A., Kagami, S., and Border, W. A. (1994). Integrins. *Kidney International*, **45**, S17–22.

Sherwood, A. C. and Wilson, P. D. (1990*a*). Actin cytoskeleton in autosomal dominant polycystic kidney disease (ADPKD) epithelial cells. *Kidney International*, **37**, 229.

Sherwood, A. C. and Wilson, P. D. (1990*2b*). Membrane phospholipid-protein interactions in autosomal dominant polycystic kidney disease. *Journal of the American Society of Nephrology*. **1**, 642.

Silva, F. G., Nadasdy, T., and Laszik, Z. , (1993). Immunohistochemical and lectin dissection of the human nephron in health and disease. *Archives of Pathology and Laboratory Medicine*, **117**, 1233–9.

Sorokin, L. Sonnenberg, A., Aumailley, M., Timpi, R., and Ekblom, P. (1990). Recognition of the laminin E8 cell-binding site by an integrin possessing the a6 subunit is essential for epithelial polarization in developing kidney tubules. *Journal of Cell Biology*, **111**, 1265–73.

Torres, V. E., *et al.* (1992). Synthesis of renin by tubulocystic epithelium in autosomal-dominant polycystic kidney disease. *Kidney International*, **42**, 364–73.

Torres, V. E., Keith, D. S., Offord, K. P., Kon, S. P., and Wilson, D. M. (1994). Renal ammonia in autosomal dominant polycystic kidney disease. *Kidney International*, **45**, 1745–53.

Trudel, M., D'Agati, V., and Costanti, F. (1991). C-myc as an inducer of polycystic kidney disease in transgenic mice. *Kidney International*, **39**, 665–71.

Veis, D. J., Sorenson, C. M., Shutter, J. R., and Korsmeyer, S. J. (1993). Bcl-2-deficient mice demonstrate fulminant lymphoid apoptosis, polycystic kidneys, and hypopigmented hair. *Cell*, **75**, 229–40.

Von der Mark, K., Von der Mark, H., and Goodman, S. (1993). Cellular responses to extracellular matrix. *Kidney International*, **41**, 632–40.

Welling, L. W. and Welling, D. (1988). Theoretical models of cyst formation and growth. *Scanning Microscopy*, **2**, 1097–1102.

Wilson, P. D. (1991*a*). Aberrant epithelial cell growth in autosomal dominant polycystic kidney disease. *American Journal of Kidney Diseases*, **16**, 634–87.

Wilson, P. D. (1991*b*). Cell Biology of human autosomal dominant polycystic kidney disease. *Seminars in Nephrology*, **11**, 607–16.

Wilson, P. D. (1991*c*). Monolayer cultures of microdissected renal tubule epithelial segments. *Journal of Tissue Culture Methods*, **13**, 137–42.

Wilson, P. D. (1991*d*). Tubulocystic epithelium. *Kidney International*, **39**, 450–63.

Wilson, P. D. and Burrow, C. R. (1992). Autosomal dominant polycystic kidney disease. *Advances in Nephrology*, **21**, 125–42.

Wilson, P. D. and Falkenstein, D. F. (1994). The pathology of human renal cystic disease. In *Current topics in pathology*, (ed. C. L. Berry and E. Grundmann). Springer, Berlin.

Wilson, P. D., Dillingham, M. A., Breckon, R., and Anderson, R. J. (1985). Defined human renal tubular epithelia in culture: growth, characterization and hormonal response. *American Journal of Physiology*, **248**, F436–43.

Wilson, P. D., Schrier, R. W., Breckon, R. D., and Gabow, P. A. (1986). A new method for studying human polycystic kidney disease epithelia in culture. *Kidney International*, **30**, 371–8.

Wilson, P. D., Sherwood, A. C., Palla, K., Du, J., Watson, R., and Norman, J. T. (1991). Reversed polarity of Na^+-K^+-ATPase: mislocation to apical plasma membranes in polycystic kidney disease epithelia. *American Journal of Physiology*, **260**, F420–30.

Wilson, P. D., Hreniuk, D., and Gabow, P. A. (1992). Abnormal extracellular matrix and excessive growth of human adult polycystic kidney disease epithelia. *Journal of Cellular Physiology*, **150**, 360–9.

Wilson, P. D., Du, J., and Kuo, N. (1993*a*). Tyrosine kinase receptor abnormalities in human autosomal dominant polycystic kidney disease (ADPKD): implications for growth factor signal transduction. *Journal of the American Society of Nephrology*, **4**, 505.

Wilson, P. D., Du, J., and Norman, J. T. (1993*b*). Autocrine, endocrine and paracrine regulation of growth abnormalities in autosomal dominant polycystic kidney disease. *European Journal of Cell Biology*, **61**, 131–8.

Wilson, P. D., Gatti, L., and Burrow, C. R. (1993*c*). Expression of the beta-2 isoform of NaK-ATPase during human renal development and in polycystic kidney disease. *Molecular Biology of the Cell*, **4**, 34a.

Wilson, P. D., Falkenstein, D., Gatti, L., Racusen, L., and Burrow, C. R. (1994). NaK-ATPase isoform expression patterns provide a mechanism for apical membrane localization in human fetal kidneys and in autosomal dominant polycystic kidney disease. *Journal of the American Society of Nephrology*.

Ye, M., Grant, M., Sharma, M., Elzinga, L., Swan, S., Torres, V. E., and Grantham, J. J. (1992). Cyst fluid from human autosomal dominant polycystic kidneys promotes cyst formation and expansion by renal epithelial cells in vitro. *Journal of the American Society of Nephrology*, **3**, 984–94.

Zeier, M., Fehrenbach, P., Geberth, S., Mohring, K., Waldherr, R., and Ritz, E. (1992). Renal histology in polycystic kidney disease with incipient and advanced renal failure. *Kidney International*, **42**, 1259–65.

Zerial, M. and Stenmark, H. (1993). Rab GTPasses in vesicular transport. *Current Opinion in Cell Biology*, **5**, 613–20.

PART II

Cystic renal disease: clinical spectrum

7

Classification of cystic kidneys

Klaus Zerres

Introduction

Renal cysts are common and have an important role in many areas of medicine. Cystic lesions may be hereditary, developmental, or acquired. At least about 5–10 per cent of all patients on dialysis suffer from cystic kidney diseases. In paediatric autopsy material, cystic changes of the kidneys are among the most common malformations, and the obstetrician is frequently confronted with renal cysts in prenatal ultrasound examination. Autosomal dominant polycystic kidney disease (ADPKD) is one of the most frequent inherited diseases with an incidence of about 1/1000 (Dalgaard 1957).

Our knowledge about cystic kidneys is incomplete despite the vast amount of literature available. The complex and sometimes contradictory nomenclature is often unhelpful, and to date, no generally accepted classification of cystic kidney diseases exists.

Any classification has to account for cystic disorders that have differing patterns of inheritance and differing natural histories, thus offering prognostic implications. Any classification should be appropriate clinically, radiographically, genetically, and morphologically. Similarities in morphology, but differences in genetics and pathogenesis, make classification difficult. As postulated by Bernstein (1990), a classification needs the contribution of all disciplines.

Many attempts have been undertaken to classify cystic disorders. Important contributions have been made by pathologists such as Edith Louise Potter who summarized her work in the well-known monograph of 1972, *Normal and abnormal development of the kidney*, and Jay Bernstein who contributed very much to the understanding of cystic disorders (Bernstein 1990). In their important paper 'Polycystic disease of kidneys and liver presenting in childhood,' Blyth and Ockenden (1971)were the first to point out that both the recessive and the dominant types of PKD are not limited to a particular age group. The authors described autosomal dominant PKD presenting in early childhood as well as autosomal recessive PKD in adolescence, and even in young adults. The authors' conclusion, which was based on genetic and patho-anatomical findings, has changed the view on PKD in children despite the fact that not all of the authors' conclusions are still valid.

Many classifications have been suggested by collaborations of clinicians, radiologists, pathologists, and geneticists. These have been helpful in practical applications but are subject to change as new evidence of heterogeneity become apparent. On the basis of the patho-anatomical system proposed by Potter, we have taken the genetic aspects into account (Zerres *et al.* 1984).

It has been a subject of controversy as to what should be regarded as the most rational basis of a generally accepted classification of cystic kidney disorders. As we have learned from many other diseases, ultimate classifications are often based on the definition of the underlyling basic defects. Many inherited disorders have been classified in this way, although a phenotypic distinction of the defined entities is often not possible.

Although the basic defects of cystic disorders are still not known, the recent advances in genetics are important contributions for a rational classification. It can be predicted that basic defects will be discovered in the near future by positional cloning in molecular genetic research. As a further step, genotype–phenotype analyses will help to define genetic entities more clearly, which has been shown strikingly with the two different dominant types of PKD.

Value and limitations of a patho-anatomically orientated classification

It has been a matter of controversial debate whether a patho-anatomically orientated classification is still of any value. The most well-known classification by Osathanondh and Potter, known as the Potter classification (Potter 1972), is of limited value for clinical practice. Not all types defined by Potter represent clinical entities. This, and the semantic confusion with term 'Potter syndrome' or 'Potter phenotype' (see below), caused this classification to be unpopular. This opinion, however, is not justified — a patho-anatomically orientated classification gives the definition of cystic lesions, which can be different from disease entities.

The value of a patho-anatomically classification has recently been shown by Gillessen-Kaesbach *et al.* (1993). These authors described a disorder with characteristic face, microcephaly, brachymelia, congenital heart defect, cystic kidneys, and liver involvement indistinguishable from those in the autosomal recessive type. In addition, the children demonstrated a distinct phenotype that allows us to define this disorder (Gillessen-Kaesbach *et al.* 1993). The authors correctly described the cystic lesion as 'cystic kidneys type Potter I'. The term 'autosomal recessive polycystic kidney disease' defines a different disease which recently has been mapped to chromosome 6p (Zerres *et al.* 1994).

Table 7.1 summarizes renal cystic disorders and syndromes with cystic kidneys as a major feature are listed in Table 7.5 (see below). Syndromes which may be associated with the Potter sequence are listed in Table 7.4 (see below).

In the following discussion, major disorders are discussed in the light of the definition rather than the clinical aspects.

Table 7.1 Classification of renal cystic disorders

1.1	Autosomal recessive polycystic kidney disease (cystic kidneys Potter type I)
1.2	Renal and hepatic changes Potter type I as part of a syndrome (see text)
2.	*Autosomal dominant polycystic kidney disease (cystic kidneys Potter type III)*
2.1	Localization on chromosome 16p (PKD1)
2.2	Localization on chromosome 4p (PKD2)
2.3	Localization as yet unknown (PKD3) – not on chromosone 16p nor 4p
3.	*Cystic dysplasia (of whole kidney or a segment)*
3.1	Sporadic, multifactorial
3.2	Adysplasia (AD)
3.3	With autosomal recessive inheritance (?)
3.4	With X-linked inheritance (?)
3.5	Renal-hepato-pancreatic dysplasia (AR)
3.6	Cystic dysplasia as part of a syndrome (see text)
4.	*Glomerulocystic disease*
4.1	Sporadic
4.2	Autosomal dominant hypoplastic form
4.3	Early manifestation of autosomal dominant polycystic kidney disease
4.4	Due to ureteral obstruction (cystic kidneys Potter type IV) (NI.)
4.3	Glomerulocystic disease as part of a syndrome (see text)
5.	*Simple cysts*
6.	*Acquired renal cysts*
7.	*Juvenile nephronophthisis/ Medullary cystic disease*
7.1	Juvenile nephronopthisis (AR)
7.2	Renal retinal dysplasia syndrome complex (AR)
7.3	Medullary cystic disease (AD)
8.	*Medullary sponge kidney (MSK)*
8.1	Sporadic
8.2	With autosomal dominant inheritance
8.3	With congenital hemihypertrophy (NI)
8.4	Early stages of polycystic diseases (AR and AD)
9.	*Extraparenchymal renal cysts*
9.1	Calyceal diverticulum
9.2	Parapelvic lymphangiectasis
9.3	Perinephric cyst

AR, autosomal recessive inheritance; AD, autosomal dominant inheritance; NI, not inherited.

Autosomal recessive polycystic kidney disease (ARPKD)

ARPKD has been clearly defined patho-anatomically (Table 7.2). Blyth and Ockenden (1971) proposed a classification of four different subtypes according to the proportion of dilated renal collecting ducts and the extent of hepatic fibrosis

Table 7.2   Criteria for classification of polycystic kidney disease and dysplasia

	Autosomal recessive PKD	Autosomal dominant PKD	Cystic dysplasia
Synonyms	Infantile polycystic disease.	Adult polycystic kidney disease.	Potter IIA (enlarged). Multicystic kidneys (enlarged).
	Potter I.	Potter III.	Potter IIB (hypoplastic).
Chromosomal localization	Chromosome 6p (PKD3)	Chromosome 16p (PKD1) 85%. Chromosome 4q (PKD2) 15%.	–
Kidney lesion as part of syndromes	Usually not (1 exception, see text).	Often as Potter III changes.	Frequent
Incidence	About 1/6000– 1/40 000.	About 1/1000.	Including all types; about 1/1000.
Pathology of kidney Macroscopic Shape	Reniform	Reniform	Usually loss of reniform shape.
Size	Enlarged. Only normal at the . beginning.	Enlarged. Only normal at the beginning	Ranging from hyperplastic to hypoplastic kidneys.
Symmetry	Symmetrical	Symmetrical. At the beginning asymmetrical even over a period of years.	Often asymmetrical. Symmetrical involvement often in case of Potter sequence.
Microscopic Location of cysts	Dilated collecting ducts. (90% or more perinatal group; 60% neonatal group; 25% infantile group; 10% juvenile group).	Cysts in all parts of nephron, including collecting ducts.	Usually complete loss of kidney architecture
Diameter of cysts	At onset up to 2 mm, with longer survival up to ? cm.	At onset small, later very different, up to several cm.	Different, up to several cm.

Table 7.2 *Continued*

	Autosomal recessive PKD	Autosomal dominant PKD	Cystic dysplasia
Connective tissue	Usually not increased	Usually not increased, in later stages slight increase.	Increased.
Primitive ducts	None	None	Present
Cartilage	None	None	Nearly pathognomonic but not always present.
Pathology of urinary tract	No other malformations.	No other malformations.	Additional malformations, frequent ureteral obstruction.
Liver changes	Congenital hepatic fibrosis.	In about 1/3 of adult cases 'cystic liver'. Rare in children.	None
Associated symptoms	Cystic pancreas (rare).	Berry aneurysms. Cardiac valvular abnormalities. Thoracic aortic aneurysms.	Very often different associated malformations.
Main clinical manifestations	Neonatal period: respiratory distress. With prolonged survival, renal insufficiency and portal hypertension (highly variable).	Usual onset 3rd–5th , decade, sometimes in children, very rare in newborns with respiratory distress, and renal insufficiency. Pain and enlargement of kidneys, proteinuria, haematuria, hypertension, nephrolithiasis, urinary infection, cerebral haemorrhage. Milder course in PKD2. Childhood onset probably only in PKD1.	Variable: latent (unilateral involvement) or Potter sequence. Frequently symptoms from additional malformations.

Table 7.2 *Continued*

	Autosomal recessive PKD	Autosomal dominant PKD	Cystic dysplasia
Urography	Delayed excretion of contrast medium up to many hours. Radiolucent linear areas in cortex and medulla representing slender cystic structures. With increasing age, urogram similar to that observed in ADPKD.	Round areas of lucency, kidney' enlarged, scalloping of renal outlines, calices elongated and distorted, flask-shaped deformity of calyces, longitudinal axis of kidney displaced. In rare young cases, observed in ARPKD.	Usually 'silent kidneys (contrast medium absent). Occasional calcifications absence of renal outlines.
Ultrasound	Increased echogenicity of renal parenchyma throughout cortex and medulla. In later stages, single cysts.	Cysts of different size in cortex and medulla, with early manifestation sometimes not distinguishable from AR type.	Loss of reniform shape, conglomerate cysts of different size up to several cm in diameter.
Risk for siblings	25%	50% (In extremely rare cases of spontaneous mutation no risk.)	Unknown, usually below 10%. (In rare cases autosomal recessive, autosomal dominant, or X-linked inheritance.)
Risk for children	Below 1% (Unless non-affected parent is not related to the affected person, or no case in her/his family.)	50%	Usually below 10%. (in rare cases of autosomal inheritance up to 50%)
Manifestation in affected family members	Often similar course in siblings.	Variable. Often similar in the same family, Recurrence of early manifestations possible.	Variable. In same family renal agenesis, dysplasia, cortical cysts, and hydronephrosis possible.

Table 7.2   *Continued*

	Autosomal recessive PKD	Autosomal dominant PKD	Cystic dysplasia
Parental kidneys	No change.	Demonstration of 1 affected parent (unless parents are too young to demonstrate cystic changes in ultrasound). Rare cases of spontaneous mutation.	Unilateral agenesis or dysplasia up to about 10% in one per cent.
Prenatal diagnosis	By ultrasound: increased echogenicity, enlargement oligohydramnios. Often visible only in the second half of pregnancy. Biochemical methods not confirmed. In informative families by linkage analysis.	In rare cases by ultra-sound. In inform families, by linkage analysis. Problems of genetic heterogeneity. In single families, direct analysis of mutations.	Possible early in pregnancy, by ultrasound.
Potter sequence	Rare	Rare	Present in bilateral cases.

(Table 7.3). The analysis of affected siblings clearly shows that the proposed scheme is an oversimplification. In a series of 20 sibships with at least two affected children we have recently shown that, according to the proposed sub-classification of Blyth and Ockenden, 12 patients were assigned to the perinatal, 9 to the neonatal, 13 to the infantile, and 8 to the juvenile subtype of ARPKD. In 11 of 20 families different subtypes among affected siblings were observed. In

Table 7.3   Manifestation of autosomal recessive polycystic kidney disease according to the Blyth and Ockenden (1971) classification

Type	Percentage (%) of dilated renal tubules	Extent of hepatic fibrosis	Life span
Perinatal	≥ 90	Minimal	Hours
Neonatal	60	Mild	Months
Infantile	20	Moderate	Up to 10 yrs
Juvenile	<10	Gross	Up to 50 yrs or more

seven families, affected siblings belonged to adjacent subtypes and therefore cannot be regarded as appropriate in distinguishing genetic groups of ARPKD as suggested by Blyth and Ockenden (Deget *et al.* 1995). There are affected siblings demonstrating a much wider range of symptoms than those proposed by Blyth and Ockenden (1971). The extent of hepatic fibrosis is more variable, ranging from patients with hepatic involvement in early childhood to young adults without any clinical signs of liver involvement. (Zerres 1992; Neumann *et al.* 1988; Guay-Woodford *et al.* 1995). Linkage results so far provide no evidence of genetic heterogeneity among different clinical manifestations (Zerres *et al.* 1994).

Gillessen-Kaesbach *et al.*'s (1993) recently described syndrome clearly represents a rare disorder different from ARPKD. Potter type I cystic kidneys have been reported in a patient with Ehlers–Danlos syndrome (Mauseth *et al.* 1977). Further observations are necessary to classify this association.

Congenital hepatic fibrosis (CHF)/Caroli syndrome

CHF is a prerequisite for the diagnosis of the recessive from of PKD. Whether there is an isolated form of 'pure' congenital hepatic fibrosis without kidney involvement is not clear. Cases of CHF with only mild kidney involvement may be manifestations of ARPKD. Liver histology in CHF may not be distinguishable from that found in several syndromes associated with cystic kidneys such as Meckel syndrome, Jeune syndrome, short-rib-polydactyly syndromes, retinal-renal-dysplasia syndromes, and renal-hepatic-pancreatic dysplasia (see Zerres *et al.* 1984). With the exception of a case of trisomy C (Blair 1976), all these syndromes follow an autosomal recessive mode of inheritance.

It is clearly established that ADPKD can be associated with CHF (Tazelaar *et al.* 1984; Matzuda *et al.* 1990; Cobben *et al.* 1990). Caroli syndrome and 'adult polycystic kidney disease' also probably belong in this catagory (Jordon *et al.* 1989).

Gross cystic dilatation of the intrahepatic biliary tree is usually called Caroli syndrome. The frequent association with ARPKD is well established (Lieberman *et al.* 1971; Blyth and Ockenden 1971; Murray-Lyon *et al.* 1973; Bernstein *et al.* 1975). Presumably, ARPKD and Caroli disease are closely overlapping syndromes in which an abnormal developmental involvement of different levels of the biliary tree by the same pathogenetic mechanism could result in two different spectra or stages of a single disease (Nakanuma *et al.* 1982).

Observations of medullary sponge kidney (MSK) with congenital hepatic fibrosis are usually classified as a mild manifestation of ARPKD (Reilly and Neuhauser 1960; Unite *et al.* 1973).

The association of liver and pancreatic involvement with cystic changes in the kidneys is notable. Bernstein *et al.* (1987) summarize more than 10 disorders with the combination of renal cystic dysplasia and biliary dysgenesis, and in most cases, pancreatic dysplasia. These hereditary conditions indicate evidence of a pathogenetic link.

Autosomal dominant polycystic kidney disease (ADPKD)

ADPKD is a well-characterized condition (Table 7.2). The recently defined two different genetic types led to the description of different phenotypes, with the non 16p-linked cases demonstrating a usually milder phenotype (Parfrey *et al.* 1990). There is evidence of a third ADPKD locus (PKD 3)(Daoust *et al.* 1995). The gene locus for PKD 3 still has to be mapped.

Autosomal dominant polycystic kidney disease in children

Rare cases of ADPKD can present with clinical symptoms in early childhood. Prenatal diagnosis by ultrasound has been described (Zerres *et al.* 1982; Main *et al.* 1983). Kääriäinen (1988) has estimated that about 2 per cent of gene carriers of ADPKD can present in early childhood. Results of linkage studies in families with early onset PKD are compatible with chromosome 16p linkage (Gal *et al.* 1989).

It is important to be aware that the clinical picture in many cases of early onset ADPKD cannot be distinguished from ARPKD, with enlarged kidneys and increased echogenicity. The ultrasongraphic image of kidney lesions in cases of Meckel syndrome can also be indistinguishable (Zerres *et al.* 1988). A positive family history in terms of an affected parent is one of the major criteria for the diagnosis of ADPKD in a child.

Clinical studies in ADPKD families with children affected by early manifestations clearly demonstrate that there is a recurrence risk which has been estimated to be about 45 per cent of possible gene carriers (Zerres *et al.* 1993). The basic mechanism for early onset is still unknown.

Polycystic liver disease

Whether 'polycystic liver disease' is a disorder different from ADPKD is still a controversial point (Sotaniemi *et al.* 1979; Berrebri *et al.* 1982; Karhunen and Tenhu 1986). Our analysis of pedigrees with polycystic liver disease indicate that it is unlikely that it represents a different entity. Linkage studies are in preparation.

Unilateral adult polycystic kidney disease

Kossow and Meek (1982) described a non-familial case of 'unilateral adult polycystic kidney disease' in a 79-year-old woman. Clinically, the contralateral kidney revealed no abnormalities. However, the classification of this case is not possible without further information. In each case of unilateral polycystic kidney type Potter III, it must be remembered that, initially, ADPKD can be asymmetric for many years (Anton and Abramowsky 1982).

Cystic dysplasia

Cystic dysplasia can usually be diagnosed without difficulty (Table 7.2). This disorder seems to represent an unspecific reaction of the kidney towards disturbances in early development. Dysplastic lesions can be found as a result of exogeneous influences or as a part of genetic and non-genetic syndromes. The genetic basis of cystic dysplasia is still unclear. It is usually thought that the genetic basis is multifactorial with only a very low recurrence risk in isolated cases (Carter *et al.* 1979; Al Saadi *et al.* 1984; Roodhooft *et al.* 1984; Bankier *et al.* 1985). In several families, however, the familial pattern is compatible with autosomal recessive inheritance (Cain *et al.* 1974; Schinzel *et al.* 1978), or possible X-linked inheritance (Pashayan *et al.* 1977). In addition, it can be certain that a dominant condition with a varying degree of agenesis/dysplasia called 'adysplasia' exists (Buchta *et al.* 1973; McPherson *et al.* 1987). The condition is characterized by a highly variable kidney involvement ranging from normal kidneys in gene carriers and unilateral dysplasia or agenesis, to severe phenotypes with variable bilateral involvement leading to the Potter sequence as a consequence of severe oligo-/anhydramnios. Furthermore, the Mayer–Rokitansky–Küster anomaly can sometimes be found in affected females (Opitz 1987).

Renal dysplasia as a feature of defined syndromes

There are numerous conditions where renal dysplasia is a feature of well-defined syndromes. Winter and Baraitser (1990) listed 28 syndromes with 'renal dysplasia' in their identification program. The Australian program, POSSUM (version 1991) lists 86 syndromes with 'dysplastic/cystic-dysplastic kidneys'. The renal lesions in some of these syndromes do not fulfil the diagnostic criteria of dysplasia. In addition, the term 'dysplasia' is sometimes used to describe an undefined renal lesion.

The pathogenesis of the renal lesion is unknown in the majority of these syndromes but it can be speculated that the mechanism is non-specific, similar to others often found in common malformation syndromes (e.g. heart defects or cleft palate). Some of the more important syndromes with dysplasia as a major feature are discussed in more detail below.

Renal-hepatic-pancreatic dysplasia

The combination of renal, hepatic, and pancreatic dysplasia was first described by Ivemark *et al.* (1959), and more recent cases have been described by Crawfurd (1978), Carles *et al.* (1988), and Bernstein *et al.* (1987). The renal lesion consists of cystic dysplasia, with abnormally differentiated ducts, deficient nephron differentiation, and glomerular cysts. The hepatic abnormality consists of enlarged portal areas containing numerous elongated biliary 'profiles' with a tendency for perilobular fibrosis. Some patients have intrahepatic bile duct proliferation, which is clinically often diagnosed as Caroli syndrome. The pancreatic abnormality is characterized by fibrosis and cysts, with a diminution of parenchymal tissue (Bernstein *et al.* 1987). The occurrence of the disease in siblings of patients without signs of kidney or liver involvement in their parents gives evidence of autosomal recessive inheritance.

VATER association

This acronym describes a non-random association of *v*ertebral defects, imperforate *a*nus, *t*racheo-*o*esophageal fistula with oesophageal atresia, *r*enal, and *r*adial defects. Additional features have also been described. Renal anomalies can be found in more than 50 per cent of cases. The clinical spectrum ranges from uni- and/or bilateral agenesis/dysplasia to hydronephrosis (Quan and Smith 1973).

The VATER association is usually a sporadic condition, but it is of interest that there is a very similiar syndrome with CNS malformations (most frequently hydrocephalus due to aqueduct stenosis) which follows an autosomal recessive mode of inheritance (Briard *et al.* 1884; Evans *et al.* 1989).

Branchio-oto-renal dysplasia

The association of branchial arch anomalies (pre-auricular pits, branchial fistulas), hearing loss, and renal hypoplasia constitutes the branchio-oto-renal syndrome first described by Melnick *et al.* (1975) and further delineated by Fraser *et al.* (1978). About two-thirds of patients demonstrate cystic dysplasia. The condition follows an autosomal dominant mode of transmission with variable expression. The gene responsible has recently has been mapped to chromosme 8q (Smith *et al.* 1992).

Chromosomal disorders

Cystic dysplasia is a common feature in numerical and structural chromosomal aberrations, and numerous reports have been published. The most common aberrations with associated defects of ureteral developmental and metanephric induction and differentiation (renal agenesis, fused kidneys, vesico-ureteral reflux, ureteral duplication, ureteropelvic junction obstruction, and the spectrum of cystic dysplastic renal abnormalities) include trisomies 21 (Down syndrome), 13 (Pätau syndrome), 18 (Edwards syndrome), monosomy X (Turner syndrome), and 4p- syndrome (Wolf–Hirschhorn syndrome) (Fryns 1987; Gilbert and Opitz 1979). In the event of further abnormalities or malformations, a chromosomal disorder should always be excluded.

Potter sequence

The term 'Potter sequence' ('Potter syndrome', 'Potter phenotype') describes a fetal or neonatal phenotype of different aetiology due to the influence of a long-standing intra-uterine an- or oligohydramnios. The genetic interpretation depends on the underlying renal pathology. In a child with the Potter sequence the morphology of the kidney should be investigated carefully, supplemented by investigation of non-renal defects and chromosome analysis. Curry *et al.* (1984) reviewed the underlying conditions and summarized more than 50 conditions

Table 7.4   Selected syndromes and diseases which may be associated with the Potter sequence

Disorder	Inheritance
Autosomal recessive PKD	AR
Autosomal dominant PKD	AD
Renal agenesis, dysplasias, or combination	See text
Meckel syndrome	AR
VATER association	Usually NI
Caudal regression syndrome	Usually NI
Cerebro-oculo-facio-skeletal syndrome	AR
Fraser crypthopthalmos syndrome	AR
Branchio-oto-renal syndrome	AD
Prune belly syndrome	Different
Chromosomal disorders	–

AR, autosomal recessive; AD, autosomal dominant; NI, not inherited.

that can present with a Potter phenotype. The underlying conditions can be non-genetic and genetic in origin. All modes on inheritance have been described (see also Table 7.4).

Glomerulocystic kidneys

The terminology used for heterogeneous group has led to considerable confusion. In the American literature the term 'glomerulocystic disease' has often been used to denote early manifestations of ADPKD, but, to avoid confusion, should no longer be used.

Although the condition is usually sporadic, a rare distinct familial form with hypoplastic kidneys following autosomal dominant inheritance has been described by Rizzoni *et al.* (1982). In other cases, it is less clear whether there are additional entities (for a review see Carson *et al.* 1987).

Glomerulocystic changes can be found in several syndromes, for example tuberous sclerosis (Stapelton *et al.* 1980; Bernstein *et al.* 1986), orofaciodigital syndrome (Stapleton *et al.* 1982), trisomy 13, and Zellweger syndrome (see Bernstein 1990).

In cystic kidneys, Potter type IV, cortical cysts are typical findings. Due to urethral obstruction and increase of urine, the pressure extends in a retrograde manner to be exerted against the ampullae present at the end of the last generation which become enlarged. According to Potter (1972) her type IV occurred as a result of urethral occlusion. Depending on the time and extent of obstruction, dysplastic, or hydronephritic changes can be found indicating their close pathogenetic relation (Potter 1972; Zerres *et al.* 1984).

Simple cysts

These cysts are common findings in the ageing population. They are usually unilocular, often cortical with some distortion of the renal contour, and increase in number with increasing age. Simple cysts are acquired, probably due to infarction and obstruction of tubules. Single cysts can be confused with early stages of other cystic diseases. Ravine *et al.* (1993) recently examined 729 individuals and found nil prevalence in those aged 15–29 years, 1.7 per cent in those aged 30 to 49 years, 11.5 per cent in those aged 50 to 70 years, and 22.1 per cent in those aged 70 or more years. The prevalence of bilateral renal cysts (at least one cyst in each kidney) was 1 per cent in those aged 30–49 years, 4 per cent in those aged 50–70 years, and 9 per cent in those aged 70 or more years.

Acquired renal cystic disease (ARCD)

This common disorder was first defined by Dunnill and co-workers in 1977. The authors described multiple renal cysts occurring in haemodialysis patients whose original illness had not been cyst-related. Dunnill *et al.* pointed out that ARCD is a bilateral cystic disorder that develops in kidneys with end-stage renal disease.

The diagnostic criteria differ from the presence of at least one cyst in either kidney (Ishikawa *et al.* 1980; Bommer *et al.* 1980; Mickisch *et al.* 1984) to at least five cysts (Levine *et al.* 1984).

The incidence of ARCD in patients undergoing haemodialysis is 40–50 per cent in different reports of autopsy and surgical specimens, and in clinical studies. The occurrence of acquired cystic disease depends on the duration of haemodialysis, whether the patient has had a successful renal transplantation, and whether the subject is male or female. The incidence, however, does not depend on the patient's age, treatment, or the nature of the underlying renal disease (Ishikawa *et al.* 1990).

The patho-anatomical diagnosis 'cystic kidneys' in a patient with chronic renal impairment can be misinterpreted as being 'polycystic kidney disease', which can cause problems with regard to the genetic interpretation in affected families (Zerres *et al.* 1985).

Juvenile nephronopthisis/medullary cystic disease

These diseases, initially described as two different disorders, define a heterogeneous group of disorders rather than a single entity. At least two forms are recognized on the basis of inheritance and clinical presentation, a juvenile recessive form and an adult dominant form.

The kidneys are shrunken and scarred, resembling those seen in chronic pyelonephritis. In the majority of the cases, the cysts are located in the medullary and corticomedullary region of the kidney. Microdissection studies revealed the nephron to be altered by multiple diverticules, strikingly heterogeneous in size, and affected by cysts only along the distal convoluted tubular segments. Intra- and periglomerular fibrosis, hyalinosis, and interstitial and peritubular connective tissue have been documented. Waldherr *et al.* (1982) argue that the combination of the sclerosing tubulo-interstitial nephropathy with the typical clinical findings (e.g. chronic renal insufficiency, polyuria and/or polydipsia, hyposthenuria, anaemia, and growth retardation) are characteristic for the final diagnosis even in the absence of cysts.

Linkage studies have localized a gene for familial nephronophthisis to chromosome 2p, which could be excluded in cases of Senior–Loken syndrome (Antignac *et al.* 1993).

Senior–Loken syndrome

Senior *et al.* (1961) and Loken *et al.* (1961) first described the association of the nephronopthisis–medullary cystic disease complex and a pigmentary retinopathy. It is not clear whether the coexistence of other features, such as hepatic fibrosis, define distinct entities or represent different manifestations of the same disorder (Waldherr *et al.* 1982).

Kidney involvement resembling that of juvenile nephronophthisis can be observed in other conditions, such as asphyxiating thoracic dystrophy (Gruskin *et al.* 1974) or Bardet–Biedl syndrome (Hurley *et al.* 1975).

Multilocular cystic disease

The term 'multilocular' is related to the gross anatomical appearence of the lesion. The smooth external surface of the tumour and the absence of normal renal tissue in the septa of the locules distinguish it clearly from other renal cystic lesions and from most congenital cystic diseases of the kidney.

In 1951, Powell and co-workers defined eight criteria for the diagnosis of multilocular cystic disease:

(1) the lesion is unilateral;
(2) the lesion is solitary;
(3) the lesion is multilocular;
(4) cysts do not communicate with the renal pelvis;
(5) locules do not communicate with each other;
(6) locules are lined with epithelium;
(7) interlobular septa do not contain renal parenchyma; and
(8) surrounding renal tissue is normal except for compression.

Boggs and Kimmelstiel (1956) reported two cases and emphasized the presence of minimal renal tissue in the interlocular septa in one of these cases. This resulted in a modification of the criterion (7) of Powell *et al.* (1951) as an exclusion of cases with fully developed nephrons in the septa of the cyst.

The pathogenesis of multilocular cysts is controversial, the debate involves whether the lesion is a neoplasm or cyst. Theories of the pathogenesis of this entity include a developmental defect, harmatomata formation, dysplasia, a benign variant of Wilms' tumour, or a partial or total differentiated nephroblastoma (for review see Kissane 1990; Castillo *et al.* 1991).

Medullary sponge kidney (MSK)

This disorder is characterized by the presence of dilated collecting ducts and tubules in one or more renal pyramids. The condition was originally described by Lenarduzzi (1939) but has been defined by Cacci and Ricci in 1948. Abeshouse and Abeshouse (1960) and Kuiper (1976) gave comprehensive reviews of the condition. The true incidence is unknown, the prevalence in patients undergoing excretory urography is approximately 0.5 per cent. In patients with nephrolithiasis, the prevalence has been estimated at up to nearly 20 per cent.

MSK is probably a developmental anomaly. Supporting evidence includes the histological appearance of the lesion, the lack of progression in the absence of complications, and the occasional presence of embryonic tissue. Coexisting anomalies of the urinary tract are frequent, and there are numerous reports of congenital hemihypertrophy (Harris *et al.* 1981), which has been reported in as many as 25 per cent of patients.

MSK is asymptomatic unless complicated by nephrolithiasis, haematuria, or infection. The onset of symptoms often occurs during childhood or the second decade of life; occasionally as late as the sixth decade. Hypercalciuria has a prevalence of 40–50 per cent in MSK.

Despite the observation that some families with vertical transmission suggests autosomal dominant inheritance (Kuiper 1971) it has been assumed that most cases have no hereditary basis. This conclusion, however, must be interpreted with caution. Family studies encounter two problems: (1) diagnostic: the disorder is frequently asymptomatic and the diagnosis can be difficult; and (2) differentiation from the 'papillary blush', which is usually considered as a normal variant. Reports of autosomal recessive inheritance are not convincing (see Kuiper 1976).

As has been mentioned, the observation of MSK and congenital hepatic fibrosis can be regarded as mild manifestations of ARPKD (Reilly and Neuhauser 1960; Unite *et al.* 1973). Cases of simultaneously occurring MSK and ADPKD as reported by several authors (Nemoy and Forsberg 1968; Hockley *et al.* 1978; Abreo and Steele 1982) should be regarded as manifestations of ADPKD with more pronounced medullary involvement (e.g. in an early stage of development of ADPKD).

There are occasional reports of MSK in Ehlers–Danlos syndromes (Spence and Singleton 1972; Levine and Michael 1967; Morris *et al.* 1985)

Cystic kidneys associated with other syndromes

Cystic changes in the kidneys are common findings in many malformation syndromes. The *London Dysmorphology Database* (Winter and Baraitser 1990), is one of the syndrome-identification programs with records of about 2000 disorders summarized under 'multiple renal cysts', 49 conditions of 'renal agenesis', 50 of 'renal dysplasia', and 28 well-defined syndromes. The Australian POSSUM database (1991) contains records for 1783 syndromes and lists 108 with 'agenesis/ hypoplastic', 86 with 'dysplastic/cystic dysplastic', and 24 with 'polycystic'. The kidney lesion is not clearly defined in many syndromes. The different number of syndromes with a defined kidney lesion in the two programs underline the difficulties in determining that cystic lesions are associated with a syndrome. However, it is evident that cystic changes are common findings in malformation syndromes (see Table 7.5). The renal involvement is often very mild and the pathological classification may therefore be difficult or even impossible. Nearly all patho-anatomical types can be found in clearly defined syndromes: changes indistinguishable from those found in autosomal recessive and autosomal dominant PKD (Potter types I and III), dysplasia (type Potter II), medullary sponge kidney, juvenile nephronophthisis, and glomerulocystic disease. These findings emphasize that cystic changes can be the result of many different underlying basic defects so that a specific pathology of cystic lesions alone does not point towards a disease entity (Zerres *et al.* 1984).

Table 7.5   Selected syndromes associated with cystic kidneys

Disorder	Inheritance
Meckel syndrome	AR
Jeune syndrome	AR
Short-rib-polydactyly syndromes	AR
Zellweger syndrome	AR
Tuberous sclerosis	AD
von Hippel–Lindau syndrome	AD
VATER association	usually NI
Retinal-renal-dysplasia syndromes	AR
Renal-hepatic-pancreatic dysplasia	AR
Fryns' syndrome	AR
Different chromosomal disorders	–
Oral-facial-digital syndrome I	XL
Bardet–Biedl syndrome	AR
Kaufman–McKusick syndrome	AR
Hypothalamic hamartoma syndrome	NI?
Lissencephaly syndromes	Variable
Prune belly syndrome	NI?
Ehlers–Danlos syndromes	Variable
Branchio-oto-renal syndrome	AD
Roberts syndrome	AR
DiGeorge syndrome	Variable
Smith–Lemli–Opitz syndrome	AR

AR, autosomal recessive; AD, autosomal dominant; NI, not inherited; XL, X-linked.

Extraparenchymal cysts

The terms 'pyelogenic cyst', 'peripelvic cyst', and 'calyceal diverticulum' are synonymous, the last being the most accurate description of the abnormality. Parapelvic cyst is often synonymous with parapelvic lymphatic and parapelvic lymphangiectasia. Parapelvic lymphangiectasia is common in transplanted kidneys, secondary to lymphatic obstruction. The perinephric cyst is a collection of fluid around the kidney, known variously as hygroma perirenalis, perirenal effusion, hydrocele renalis, and pararenal pseudocyst. Perinephric cysts in childhood are usually subcapsular effusions secondary to urinary tract obstruction. They may in adults lie between the capsule and renal cortex, or between the capsule and perinephric fat. They are believed to result principally from extravasation of urine secondary to either trauma or urinary obstruction (see Bernstein 1990).

References

Abeshouse, B. S. and Abeshouse, G. A. (1960). Sponge kidney: A review of the literature and report of five cases. *Journal of Urology*, **84**, 252–67.

Abreo, K. and Steele, T. H. (1982). Simultaneous medullary sponge and adult polycystic kidney disease. *Archives of Internal Medicine*, **142**, 163–5.

Al Saadi, A. A., et al. (1984). A family study of renal dysplasia. *American Journal of Medical Genetics*, **19**, 669–77.

Antignac, C., et al. (1993). A gene for familial juvenile nephronophthisis (recessive medullary cystic kidney disease) maps to chromosome 2p. *Nature Genetics*, **3**, 342–5.

Anton, P. A. and Abramowsky, C. R. (1982). Adult polycystic renal disease presenting in infancy: a report emphasizing the bilateral involvement. *Journal of Urology*, **128**, 1290–1.

Bankier, A., De Campo, M., Newell, R., Rogers, J. G., and Danks, D. M. (1985). A pedigree study of perinatally lethal renal disease. *Journal of Medical Genetics*, **22**, 104–11.

Bernstein, J. (1990). A classification of renal cysts. In *The cystic kidney* (ed. K. D. Gardner and J. Bernstein), pp. 147–70. Kluwer, Dordrecht.

Bernstein, J. Viranuvatti, V., and Broyer, J. L. (1975). What is Caroli's disease? *Gastroenterology*, **63**: 417–9.

Bernstein, J., Robbins, T. O., and Kissane, J. M. (1986). The renal lesion in tuberous sclerosis. *Seminars in Diagnostic Pathology*, **3**, 97–105.

Bernstein, J., et al. (1987). Renal-hepatic-pancreatic dysplasia: a syndrome reconsidered. *American Journal of Medical Genetics*, **26**, 391–403.

Berrebi, G., Erickson, R. P., and Marks, B. W. (1982). Autosomal dominant polycystic liver disease: a second family. *Clinical Genetics*, **21**, 342–7.

Blair, J. D. (1976). Trisomy C and cystic dysplasia of kidneys, liver and pancreas. *Birth Defects*, **XII**, 139–49.

Blyth, H. and Ockenden, B. G. (1971). Polycystic disease of kidneys and liver presenting in childhood. *Journal of Medical Genetics*, **8**, 257–84.

Boggs, L. K. and Kimmelstiel P. (1956). Benign multilocular cystic nephroma: report of two cases of so-called multilocular cyst of the kidney. *Journal of Urology*, **76**, 530–41.

Bommer, J., Waldherr, R., van Kaick, G., Strauss, L., and Ritz, R. (1980). Acquired renal cysts in uremic patients — in vivo demonstration by computed tomography. *Clinical Nephrology*, **14**, 299–303.

Briard, M. L., *et al.* (1984). Association vacterl et hydrocéphalie: une nouvelle entité familiale. *Annales de Genetique*, **27**, 220–3.

Buchta, R. M., Viseskul, C., Gilbert, E. F., Sarto, G. E., and Opitz, J. M. (1973). Familial bilateral renal agenesis and hereditary renal adysplasia. *Zeitschrift für Kinderheilkunde*, **115**, 111–29.

Cacci, R. and Ricci, V. (1948). Sur une rare maladie kystique multiple des pyramides rénales, le 'rein en eponge'. *Journal d'urologie et de Nephrologie*, **55**, 497–519.

Cain, D. R., Griggs, D., Lackey, D. A., and Kagan, B. M. (1974). Familial renal agenesis and total dysplasia. *American Journal of Diseases of Children*, **128**, 377–80.

Carles, D., Serville, F., Dubecq, J. P., and Gonnet, J. M. (1988). Renal, pancreatic and hepatic dysplasia sequence. *European Journal of Pediatrics*, **147**, 431–2.

Carter, C. O., Evans, K., and Pescia, G. (1979). A family study of renal agenesis. *Journal of Medical Genetics*, **16**, 176–88.

Carson, R. W., Bedi, D., Cavallo, T., and DuBose, T. D. (1987). Familial adult glomerulocystic kidney disease. *American Journal of Kidney Diseases*, **9**, 154–65.

Castillo, O. A., Boyle, E. T., and Kramer, S. A. (1991). Multilocular cysts of kidney. *Urology*, **37**, 156–62.

Cobben, J. H., Breuning, M. H., Schloots, C., ten Kate, L. P., and Zerres, K. (1990). Congenital hepatic fibrosis in autosomal-dominant polycystic kidney disease. *Kidney International*, **38**, 880–5.

Crawfurd, Md', A. (1978). Renal dysplasia and asplenia in two sibs. *Clinical Genetics*, **14**, 338–44.

Curry, C. J. R., Jensen, K., Holland, J., Miller, L., and Hall, B. D. (1984). The Potter sequence: A clinical analysis of 80 cases. *American Journal of Medical Genetics*, **19**, 679–702.

Dalgaard, O. Z. (1957). Bilateral polycystic disease of the kidney: a follow-up of two hundred eighty-four patients and their families. *Acta Medica Scandinavica* (Suppl.), 328.

Deget, F., Rudnik-Schöneborn, S., Zerres, K., and members of the Arbeitsgemeinschaft für Pädiatrische Nephrologie, (1995). Course of autosomal recessive polycystic kidney disease (ARPKD) in siblings. A clinical comparison of 20 sibships. *Clinical Genetics*, **47**, 248–53.

Daost, M. C. Reynolds, D. M. Bichet, D. G., Sorulo, S. (1995). Evidence for a third genetic locus /or autosomal dominant polycystic kidney disease. *Genomics*, **25**, 733–6.

Dunnill, M. S., Millard, P. R., and Oliver, D. (1977). Acquired cystic disease of the kidneys: a hazard of long-term intermittent maintenance hemodialysis. *Journal of Clinical Pathology*, **30**, 868–877.

Evans, J. A., Stranc, L. C., Kaplan, P., and Hunter, A. G. W. (1989). VACTERL with hydrocephalus: further delineation of the syndrome(s). *American Journal of Medical Genetics*, **34**, 177–82.

Fraser, F. C., Ling, D., Clogg, D., and Nogrady, B. (1978). Genetic aspects of the BOR syndrome: Branchial fistulas, ear pits, hearing loss and renal anomalies. *American Journal of Medical Genetics*, **2**, 241–52.

Fryns, J. P. (1987). Chromosomal anomalies and autosomal syndromes. *Birth Defects*, **23**, 7–32.

Gal, A., *et al.* (1989). Childhood manifestation of autosomal dominant polycystic kidney disease: no evidence for genetic heterogeneity. *Clinical Genetics*, **35**, 13–19.

Gilbert, E. and Opitz, J. (1979). Renal involvement in genetic-hereditary malformation syndromes. In *Nephrology*, (ed. J. Hamburger, J. Crosnir, and J.-P. Grünfeld), pp. 909–44. Wiley, New York.

Gillessen-Kaesbach, G., Meinecke, P., Garrett, C., Padberg, B., C., Rehder, H., and Passarge, E. (1993). New autosomal recessive lethal disorder with polycystic kidneys type Potter I, characteristic face, microcephaly, brachymelia, and congenital heart defect. *American Journal of Medical Genetics*, **45**, 511–8.

Gruskin, A. B., Baluarte, H. J., Cote, M. L., and Elfenbein, I. B. (1974). The renal disease of thoracic asphyxiant dystophy. *Birth Defects*, X, 44–50.

Guay-Woodford, L. M. *et al.* (1995). The severe perinatal form of autosomal recessive polycystic kidney disease maps to chromosome 6p 21.1–p12: implications for genetic counselling, *American Journal of Human Genetics*, **56**, 1101–7.

Harris, R. E., Fuchs, E. F., and Kaempf, M. J. (1981). Medullary sponge kidney and congenital hemihypertrophy: case report and literature review. *Journal of Urology*, **126**, 676–8.

Hockley, B., J., Robinson, M. F., Tucker, W. G., and Lawrence, J. R. (1978). Combined polycystic and medullary sponge renal disease. *Australasian Radiology*, **22**, 315–18.

Hurley, R, M., Dery, P., Nogrady, M. B., and Drummond, K. N. (1975). The renal lesion of the Laurence–Moon–Biedl syndrome. *Journal of Pediatrics*, **87**, 206–9.

Ishikawa, I. (1990). Acquired renal cystic disease. In *The cystic kidney*, (ed. K. D. Gardner and J. Bernstein), pp. 351–77. Kluwer, Dordrecht.

Ishikawa, I., *et al.* (1980). Development of acquired cystic disease and adenocarcinoma of the kidney in glomerulonephritic chronic hemodialysis patients. *Clinical Nephrology*, **14**, 1–6.

Ivemark, B. J., Oldfelt, V., and Zetterström, R. (1959). Familial dysplasia of kidneys, liver and pancreas. A probably genetically determined syndrome. *Acta Paediatrica Scandinavica*, **48**, 1–11.

Jordon, D., Harpaz, N., and Thung, S. N. (1989). Caroli's disease and adult polycystic kidney disease: a rarely recognized association. *Liver*, **9**, 30–5.

Kääriäinen, H. (1988). Polycystic kidney disease in children: differential diagnosis between dominantly and recessively inherited forms. Medical thesis. University of Helsinki.

Karhunen, P. J. and Tenhu, M. (1986). Adult polycystic liver and kidney diseases are separate entities. *Clinical Genetics*, **30**, 29–37.

Kissane, J. M. (1990). Multilocular cystic renal lesions — malformations, benign nephromas or differentiated Wilms tumors? In *The cystic kidney*, (ed. K. D. Gardner and J. Bernstein), pp. 413–36. Kluwer, Dordrecht.

Kossow, A. S. and Meek, J. M. (1982). Unilateral adult polycystic kidney disease. *Journal of Urology*, **127**, 297–300.

Kuiper, J. J. (1971). Medullary sponge kidney in three generations. *New York State Journal of Medicine*, **71**, 2665–9.

Kuiper, J. J. (1976). Medullary sponge kidney. In *Cystic diseases of the kidney*, (ed. K. D. Gardner and J. Bernstein), pp. 151–71. Wiley, New York.

Lenarduzzi, G. (1939). Reperto pielografico poco commune (di-latazione delle vie urinarie intrarenali). *Radiologico Medica (Torino)*, **26**, 346–7.

Levine, A. S. and Michael, A. F. (1967). Ehlers-Danlors syndrome with renal tubular acidosis and medullary sponge kidney. *Journal of Pediatrics*, **71**, 107–13.

Levine, E., Grantham, J. J., Slusher, S. L., Greathouse, J. L., and Krohn, B. P. (1984). CT of acquired cystic kidney disease and renal tumors in long-term dialysis patients. *American Journal of Roentgenology*, **142**, 125–31.

Lieberman, E., Salinas-Madrigal, L., Gwinn, J. L., Brennan, L. P., Fine R. N., and Landing, B. H. (1971). Infantile polycystic disease of the kidneys and liver: clinical, pathological and radiological correlations and comparison with congenital hepatic fibrosis. *Medicine (Baltimore)*, **50**, 277–318.

Loken, A. C., Hansen, O., Halvorsen, S., and Jolsten, N. J. (1961). Hereditary renal dysplasia and blindness. *Acta Paediatrica Scandinavica*, **50**, 177–84.

Main, D., Mennuti, M. T., Cornfeld, D., and Coleman, B. (1983). Prenatal diagnosis of adult polycystic kidney disease. *Lancet*, **II**, 337–8.

Matzuda, O., *et al.* (1990). Polycystic kidney of autosomal dominant inheritance, polycystic liver and congenital hepatic fibrosis in a single kindred. *American Journal of Nephrology*, **10**, 237–41.

Mauseth, R., Liberman, E., and Heuser, E. T. (1977). Infantile polycystic disease of the kidneys and Ehlers–Danlos syndrome in an 11-year-old patient. *Journal of Pediatrics*, **90**, 81–3.

McPherson, E., *et al.* (1987). Dominantly inherited renal adysplasia. *American Journal of Medical Genetics*. **26**, 863–72.

Melnick, M., Bixler, D., Silk, K., Yune, H., and Nance, W. E. (1975). Autosomal dominant branchio-oto-renal dysplasia. *Birth Defects*, **XI**, 121–8.

Mickisch, O., Bommer, J., Bachmann, S., Waldherr, R., Mann, J. F. E., and Ritz, E. (1984). Multicystic transformation of kidneys in chronic renal failure. *Nephron*, **38**, 93–9.

Morris, R. C., Yamauchi, H., Palubinskas, A. J., and Howenstine, J. (1965). Medullary sponge kidney. *American Journal of Medicine*, **38**, 883–92.

Murray-Lyon, I. M., Ockenden B. G., and Williams, R. (1973). Congenital hepatic fibrosis — is it a single clinical entity? *Gastroenterology*, **64**, 653–6.

Nakanuma, Y., Terada, T., Otha, G., Kurachi, M., and Matsubara, F. (1982). Caroli's disease in congenital hepatic fibrosis and infantile polycystic disease. *Liver*, **2**, 346–54.

Nemoy, N. J. and Forsberg, L. (1968). Polycystic renal disease presenting as medullary sponge kidney. *Journal of Urology*, **100**, 407–11.

Neumann, H. P. H., *et al.* (1988). Late manifestation of autosomal-recessive polycystic kidney disease in two sisters. *American Journal of Nephrology*, **8**, 194–7.

Opitz, J. M. (1987). Vaginal atresia (von Mayer–Rokitansky–Küster or MRK anomaly) in hereditary renal adysplasia (HRA) (Editoral comment). *American Journal of Medical Genetics*, **26**, 873–6.

Pafrey, P. S., *et al.* (1990). The diagnosis and prognosis of autosomal dominant polycystic kidney disease. *New England Journal of Medicine*, **323**, 1085–90.

Pashayan, H. M., Dowd, T., and Nigro, A. V. (1977). Bilateral absence of the kidneys and ureters. Three cases reported in one family. *Journal of Medical Genetics*, **14**, 205–9.

POSSUM (Pictures of Standard Syndromes and Undiagnosed Malformations), Version 3.0 (1991). The Murdoch Institute for Research into Birth Defects, 1100 Parkville, 3052 Melbourne, Australia.

Potter, E. L. (1972). *Normal and abnormal development of the kidney*. Year Book Medical, Chicago.

Powell, T., Shackman, R., and Johnson, H. D. (1951). Multilocular cysts of the kidney. *British Journal of Urology*, **23**, 142–52.

Quan, L. and Smith, D. W. (1973). The VATER association. *Journal of Pediatrics*, **82**, 104–7.

Ravine, D., Gibson, R. N. Donlan, J., and Sheffield, L. J. (1993). An ultrasound renal cyst prevalence survey: specificity data for inherited renal cystic diseases. *American Journal of Kidney Disease*, **22**, 803–7.

Reilly, H. and Neuhauser, E. B. D. (1960). Renal tubular ectasia in cystic disease of the kidneys and liver. *American Journal of Radiology*, **84**, 546–54.

Rizzoni, G., Loirat, C., Levy, M., Milanesi, C., Zachello, G., and Mathieu, H. (1982). Familial hypoplastic glomerulocystic kidney. A new entity? *Clinical Nephrology*, **18**, 263–8.

Roodhooft, A. M., Birnholz, J. C., and Holmes, L. B. (1984). Familial nature of congenital absence and severe dysgenesis of both kidneys. *New England Journal of Medicine*, **310**, 1341–5.

Schinzel, A., Homberger, C., and Sigrist, T. (1978). Case report: bilateral renal agenesis in 2 male sibs born to consanguineous parents. *Journal of Medical Genetics*, **15**, 314–6.

Senior, B., Friedmann, A. I., and Braudo, J. I. (1961). Juvenile, familial nephropathy with tapetoretinal degeneration. A new oculorenal dystrophy. *American Journal of Ophthalmology*, **52**, 625–33.

Smith, R. J. H., *et al.* (1992). Localization of the gene for branchiootorenal syndrome to chromosome 8q. *Genomics*, **14**, 841–4.

Sotaniemi, E. A., Luoma, P. V., Järvensivu, P. M., and Sotaniemi, K. A. (1979). Impairment of drug metabolism in polycystic non-parasitic liver disease. *British Journal of Clinical Pharmacology*, **8**, 331–5.

Spence, H. M. and Singleton, R. (1972). What is a sponge kidney disease and where does it fit in the spectrum of cystic disorders? *Journal of Urology*, **107**, 176–83.

Stapleton, F. B., Johnson, D., Kaplan, G. W., and Griswold, W. (1980). The cystic renal lesion in tuberous sclerosis. *Journal of Pediatrics*, **97**, 574–9.

Stapleton, F. B., Bernstein, J., Koh, G., Roy, S., and Wilroy, R. S. (1982). Cystic kidneys in a patient with oral-facial-digital syndrome type I. *American Journal of Kidney Diseases*, **1**, 288–93.

Tazelaar, H. D., Payne, J. A., and Patel, N. S. (1984). Congenital hepatic fibrosis and asymptomatic familial adult-type polycystic kidney disease in a 19-year-old woman. *Gastroenterology*, **86**, 757–60.

Unite, I., Maitem, A., Bagnasco, F. M., and Irwin, G. A. L. (1973). Congenital hepatic fibrosis associated with renal tubular ectasia. *Radiology*, **109**, 565–70.

Waldherr, R., Lennert, T., Weber, H. P., Födisch, H. J., and Schärer, K. (1982). The nephronophthisis complex. *Virchows Archiv für Pathologische Anatomie*, **349**, 235–54.

Winter, R. M. and Baraitser, M. (1990). *London dysmorphology database*. Oxford Medical Databases, Oxford University Press.

Zerres, K. (1992). Autosomal recessive polycystic kidney disease. *Clinical Investigator*, **70**, 794–801.

Zerres, K., Weiss, H., Bulla, M., and Roth, B. (1982). Prenatal diagnosis of an early manifestation of autosomal dominant adult-type polycystic kidney disease. *Lancet*, **II**, 988.

Zerres, K., Völpel, M. C., and Weiss, H. (1984). Cystic kidneys. Genetics, pathologic anatomy, clinical picture, and prenatal diagnosis. *Human Genetics*, **68**, 104–35.

Zerres, K., Albrecht, R., and Waldherr, R. (1985). Acquired cystic kidney disease — a possible pitfall in genetic counselling. *Human Genetics*, **71**, 267–9.

Zerres, K., Hansmann, M., Mallman, R., and Gembruch, U. (1988). Autosomal recessive polycystic kidney disease. Problems of prenatal diagnosis. *Prenatal Diagnosis*, **8**, 215–29.

Zerres, K., Rudnik-Schönebron, S., Deget, F. and members of the German Working Group on Paediatric Nephrology (1993). Childhood onset autosomal dominant polycystic kidney disease in sibs: clinical picture and recurrence risk. *Journal of Medical Genetics*, **30**, 583–8.

Zerres, K., *et al.* (1994). Mapping of the gene for autosomal recessive polycystic kidney disease (ARPKD) to chromosome 6p21-cen. *Nature Genetics*, **7**, 429–32.

8

Diagnostic imaging of renal cystic diseases

Bernard F. King and Jane S. Matsumoto

Introduction

Renal cysts are the end result of many disorders. Diagnostic imaging findings do allow for a method of classification that correlates well with the various pathological entities and provides a practical approach to the evaluation of cystic diseases (Zerres *et al.* 1984; Bernstein 1990; Torres 1990).

Benign renal cysts are the most common renal masses encountered in diagnostic imaging. Approximately 50 per cent of individuals over the age of 50 will have renal cysts on autopsy (Kissane 1974). Therefore, because of the frequent finding of renal cysts on imaging studies, an efficient and accurate radiologic diagnosis is extremely important to differentiate these benign-appearing renal cysts from more significant renal masses. These cysts are non-neoplastic and rarely produce symptoms and, therefore, rarely require therapy.

'Polycystic kidney disease' is a term that encompasses autosomal recessive polycystic kidney disease (ARPKD) and autosomal dominant polycystic kidney disease (ADPKD). These two types of inheritable polycystic kidney disease can usually be easily identified on diagnostic imaging studies, but differentiation from each other and from other renal cystic diseases may sometimes be difficult, especially in neonates and young children.

Three disorders are associated with multiple renal neoplasms and renal cysts: acquired renal cystic disease (ARCD), tuberous sclerosis complex (TSC), and von Hippel–Lindau disease (VHL). Cysts may be the earliest presentation of TSC and VHL, and recognition of the correct diagnosis is essential in these patients. ARCD in patients on long-term dialysis is an indicator that they may also develop multiple bilateral adenomas and carcinomas.

There are rare types of renal cystic disease such as localized cystic disease, glomerulocystic disease, oro-facio-digital syndrome type I, cystic disease associated with malformation syndromes, and medullary cystic disease that may present with unusual but typical imaging findings that can aid in the correct diagnosis of the disease.

Finally, there are many diseases of the kidneys that may mimic renal cystic disease. A multiloculated cystic nephroma is a benign, focal, cystic neoplasm of the kidney that can often be confused with focal cystic disease of the kidney or possibly even a cystic renal cell carcinoma. Cystic Wilms' tumours in children and lymphoma in adults can often mimic polycystic kidney disease if diagnostic imaging is not done properly. Rarely, renal artery aneurysms and arteriovenous malformations can mimic focal cystic disease. Finally, various abscesses and infectious processes can present as cystic-appearing masses of the kidney.

Therefore, it is important to understand the various specific imaging findings in these renal cystic diseases in order to provide an accurate diagnosis and prognosis in these patients in whom the clinical findings and diagnosis may not be certain.

Benign renal cysts

Benign renal cysts are most commonly unilocular and arise in the cortex. These cysts usually bulge from the renal surface. Less commonly, these cysts can arise in the medulla and bulge into the parapelvic region. These cysts vary from a few millimetres up to as large as 20–30 centimetres in diameter. The cyst wall is usually very thin and imperceptible in diagnostic imaging studies. The fluid in these simple cysts is usually clear with a yellow tinge and has chemical features of a plasma transudate.

The frequency of benign renal cysts increases with age (Laucks and McLachlan 1981; Tada *et al.* 1983). According to a recent sonographic study, the occurrence of renal cysts is nil in individuals with normal renal function less than 30 years old, in 1.7 per cent of those 30–49 years old, in 11.5 per cent of those 50–70 years old, and in 22.1 per cent of those older than 70 years of age. Therefore, renal cysts in patients under the age of 30 should be considered abnormal and investigations to identify an underlying renal disorder are warranted (Ravine *et al.* 1993).

Plain film of the abdomen

Very few renal cysts can be appreciated on routine abdominal plain film examinations. Occasionally, a large cyst can be detected as a mass arising from the kidney. An unequivocal diagnosis of a simple cyst can never be made on a plain film, and further evaluation is always indicated to exclude a solid neoplasm.

Excretory urography

Depending on its size and location, a renal cyst is usually identifiable on an excretory urogram when nephrotomograms are performed. Because a renal cyst does not contain any blood vessels, and because the cyst does not concentrate iodinated contrast material, it will appear as a relatively radiolucent, well-defined, round mass on the nephrotomograms within the renal parenchyma. However, renal cell carcinoma can produce a similar finding on excretory urography, and in all cases, ultrasound correlation must be done of any renal mass identified on excretory urography to exclude the possibility of renal cell carcinoma.

Ultrasonography

A confident diagnosis of a simple renal cyst can be made on an ultrasound (US) examination. The sonographic criteria for a simple, uncomplicated, benign renal cyst should include:

(1) the absence of internal echoes;
(2) a strong, sharply defined, distant wall with smooth, distinct margins;
(3) acoustic enhancement; and
(4) a spherical or slightly ovoid shape (Fig. 8.1A) (Lingard and Lawson 1979).

If a renal mass on US meets the criteria for a simple, uncomplicated cyst, no further investigations need to be performed.

Proper positioning of the patient, as well as proper imaging technique, is necessary to provide the best acoustic window for optimal imaging of the renal cyst. This often requires the proper use of the appropriate transducer (liner vs. sector) as well as the frequency of the transducer used (i.e. 3.5, 5, and 7 MHz). Sonographic evaluation of renal cysts may be difficult in certain patients where body habits precludes adequate sound transmission to the kidneys. In addition, the left kidney can be difficult to image in some patients because of the lack of

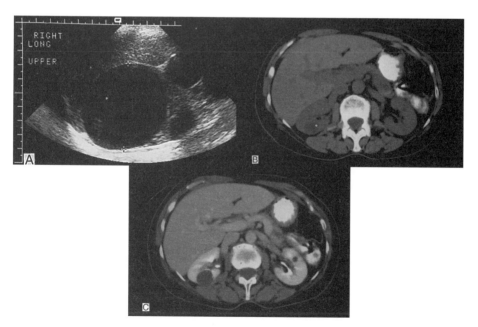

Fig. 8.1 (A) Longitudinal US of the upper pole of the right kidney demonstrating a simple cyst arising from the upper pole of the right kidney. (B) Non-contrast-enhanced CT scan of another patient through the kidneys demonstrating a simple cyst in the mid portion of the right kidney and a small cyst in the left kidney. (C) Contrast-enhanced CT scan of the same patient more clearly identifying the cysts in both kidneys.

an adequate acoustic window (i.e. liver). Therefore, caution should be exercised when evaluating renal masses in the left kidney, particularly the upper pole of the left kidney where an adequate acoustic window can be difficult to obtain.

Computed tomography

A correct computed tomography (CT) technique is necessary for adequate evaluation of renal masses. Specifically, when performing a renal CT, it is optimal to obtain images of the kidney prior to the administration of iodinated intravenous (IV) contrast media. The kidneys are then evaluated again utilizing intravenous iodinated contrast to enhance the renal parenchyma (Fig. 8.1B,C). Renal cysts are usually sharply marginated on CT and are round, smooth, and homogeneous with a low density compared to renal parenchyma (McClennan *et al.* 1979). Attenuation numbers (CT numbers) near that of water (–10 to +20) are necessary to make the diagnosis of a benign simple cyst. Attenuation of the renal cyst does not increase after the administration of IV contrast media. The cyst wall is very thin and usually imperceptible on CT. Strict adherence to proper CT technique and these criteria can result in accuracy of diagnosing simple renal cysts that approaches 100 per cent (Balfe *et al.* 1982).

Potential pitfalls of CT diagnosis include small cysts which are completely intrarenal and may appear to have the same CT attenuation numbers as a solid mass because of the partial volume effect. In these cases, thin section (5 mm) CT is recommended for evaluation.

Magnetic resonance imaging

On T-1 weighted magnetic resonance images (MRI), a simple benign cyst appears as a round or slightly oval, homogeneous, low-intensity mass. On T-2 weighted images, the cyst will be homogeneous, and its signal intensity will be high. Following the administration of intravenous gadolinium contrast agents, the normal kidney parenchyma will enhance tremendously, whereas the cyst will not enhance at all. On T-1 weighted gadolinium-enhanced images, the cyst will be relatively black compared to the high signal intensity renal parenchyma. This sharp contrast in signal intensity makes gadolinium-enhanced MRI T-1 weighted images an extremely useful tool in the evaluation of renal cystic disease. In fact, in our experience gadolinium-enhanced MRI of the kidney is more sensitive in the detection of renal cysts than US or CT.

Angiography

Angiographic criteria for a simple, benign renal cyst include vascular displacement by the cyst and the absence of any vascularity within the renal cyst. Intra-arterial epinephrine may be helpful in appreciating subtle neovascularity, which could be due to a cystic renal neoplasm. However, because of the widespread availability of non-invasive imaging modalities, such as sonography, angiography is no longer used routinely to diagnose simple, benign renal cysts.

Atypical renal cysts

A simple benign renal cyst can become complicated by haemorrhage, infection, or rupture. These atypical cysts do not meet the diagnostic criteria for simple cysts and can be similar in appearance to some cystic renal neoplasms. Because of this, these 'complex' atypical cysts often require further imaging evaluation to assure the benign nature of the mass. Bosniak has devised a classification of renal cysts to aid in the differentiation of benign cysts from cystic neoplasms (see Table 8.1) (Bosniak 1991*a*,*b*). Utilizing this classification of complex cysts, one can usually categorize benign cysts in category I or II, which require no intervention. Complex cysts that fall into category III are most often benign; however, surgical exploration is often needed to exclude the small likelihood of malignancy. Category IV lesions are highly suspicious for cystic or necrotic carcinoma and usually warrant a radical nephrectomy.

Haemorrhagic cysts

Haemorrhagic simple renal cysts refer to any cystic renal mass filled primarily with blood. Approximately 6 per cent of simple cysts are complicated by haemorrhage which is usually the result of trauma, varicosity's in the cyst wall, or a bleeding disorder (Jackman and Stevens 1974). A perirenal haematoma may result from a rupture of a haemorrhagic cyst. The ruptured haemorrhagic cyst can be difficult to differentiate from a small haemorrhagic neoplasm (Gibson 1954). The radiologic findings of a haemorrhagic cyst depend on the chronicity and degree to which the haemorrhage is organized.

Table 8.1 Bosniak's classification of renal cysts

Category I   Benign simple cysts
Thin, imperceptible wall on CT
Smooth wall on US
Water density on CT
No internal echoes on US
Increased through sound transmission on US

Category II   Benign minimally complicated cysts
Peripherally located small calcifications
Thin calcification in a wall or septum
No soft tissue mass
Septations are thin
No portion of the mass or septation enhances

Category III   Indeterminate cystic masses
Thick-walled septations, thick-walled cysts, large clumped calcifications, portions of the septations enhance with IV contrast

Category IV   Cystic renal cell carcinoma
Predominantly solid mass with cystic components
Definite solid component associated with one or more cysts

On an excretory urogram, an acute haemorrhagic cyst presents as a lucent mass and is indistinguishable from a simple cyst. As a haemorrhagic cyst matures, it becomes a chronic haemorrhagic cyst and frequently results in calcifications either peripheral or central within septations of the cyst. The chronic haemorrhagic cyst may often have a thick wall.

On sonographic examination, an acute haemorrhagic cyst may be impossible to differentiate from a solid mass because of the internal echoes of the recently clotted blood. Later, the clot will undergo lysis, and the cyst may be impossible to differentiate from an uncomplicated simple cyst. Eventually, internal echoes representing debris will be noted on the ultrasound. The chronic haemorrhagic cyst again may frequently demonstrate a thick calcified wall and/or may be multiloculated.

After acute haemorrhage into a cyst, a CT scan without IV contrast will demonstrate a homogeneous mass in the kidney with increased attenuation within the renal cyst. This increased attenuation will give a denser appearance of the haemorrhagic cyst as compared to renal parenchyma. As the blood liquefies and organizes, there may be a decrease in attenuation within the cyst and a subsequent increase in wall thickness. Again, old haemorrhages can result in cyst wall calcification that is easily identified on CT scans.

Magnetic resonance imaging of haemorrhagic cysts can be readily demonstrated. Although the appearance of haemorrhage within a cyst may vary with age on MRI, most haemorrhagic cysts on T-1 weighted images will reveal increased signal intensity as well as increase signal intensity on T-2 weighted images (Fig. 8.2A–C). One must exercise caution on MRI in that a small haemorrhagic solid renal cell carcinoma may have similar MRI characteristics as a haemorrhagic renal cyst.

The diagnosis of a benign haemorrhagic renal cyst is one of exclusion. Any clinical or radiologic findings that suggest malignancy require further evaluation and/or follow-up. In rare cases, surgical exploration may be required to exclude the possibility of renal malignancy.

Calcified cysts

Approximately 1–3 per cent of renal cysts are calcified (Daniel *et al.* 1972). Calcification in simple renal cysts is usually dystrophic and most likely is related to prior haemorrhage and/or infection. On plain film, the calcification is usually peripheral and curvilinear, but when viewed en face on a plain film, it may appear within the mass or may appear as punctate or amorphous calcification. Sonographic evaluation of renal cyst calcification is often difficult and unreliable owing to the shadowing and reverberation artefacts. CT scanning is the most sensitive and accurate technique for detecting and characterizing calcification within a renal cyst. CT is often able to characterize adequately and accurately the cyst calcification as benign and to exclude the possibility of any associated solid neoplasm with the calcification. Calcification is rarely visualized utilizing MRI; therefore, MRI is not recommended in the evaluation of any calcified renal cystic mass.

Confident radiologic differentiation of a calcified simple cyst from a cystic calcified renal cell carcinoma can be difficult. Features suggesting renal cell carcinoma include:

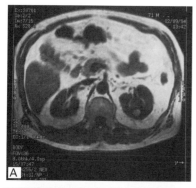
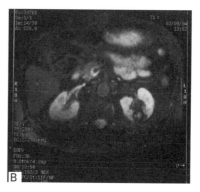
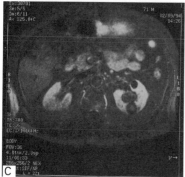

Fig. 8.2 (A) T-1 weighted MRI through the left kidney demonstrating a small cyst in the mid portion of the left kidney with increased signal intensity consistent with a haemorrhagic cyst. Smaller cyst in the anterior portion of the left kidney is barely visualized. (B) T-2 weighted MRI through the same kidney demonstrating the bright signal coming from the left haemorrhagic cyst and dark rim of the cyst consistent with haemosiderin deposition. The bright, small, benign cyst in the anterior portion of the left kidney is barely discernible from renal parenchyma. (C) Contrast-enhanced T-1 weighted fat saturated MRI image through the left kidney again demonstrating the haemorrhagic cyst in the mid portion of the left kidney with increase signal in the cyst. The benign cyst in the anterior portion of the left kidney is more clearly identified on this contrast-enhanced study.

(1) an associated soft tissue mass or soft tissue nodule;
(2) pre-contrast CT density greater than that of water;
(3) contrast enhancement on CT; and
(4) neovascularity on angiographic examination.

Infected renal cysts

A simple benign renal cyst may become infected by haematogenous dissemination, ascending infection, surgical manipulation, or puncture. Flank pain and fever may occur, but symptoms are often non-specific. Imaging studies often reveal a cystic renal mass that frequently has a thick wall. Occasionally, gas or a fluid level may be seen when the cyst is infected. Generally speaking, a thick wall on CT or US, air fluid level, debris fluid level, or inhomogeneous appearance of cyst fluid are key features that should suggest an infected renal cyst.

Nuclear medicine studies have demonstrated increased accumulation of [111]Indium-labelled white blood cells or increased activity of [67]Gallium in the region of an infected renal cyst. This is particularly helpful in polycystic kidney disease (Rothermel *et al.* 1977).

Parapelvic renal cysts

The parapelvic compartment of the kidney surrounds the pyelocalyceal collecting system and communicates immediately with the perinephric space. This parapelvic region is best termed the renal sinus. The contents of the renal sinus include the lymphatic channels emanating from the kidney, nerves, and renovascular structures all surrounded by fibroareolar fatty tissue. Renal sinus cysts have been termed 'peripelvic cysts', 'parapelvic cysts', and 'parapelvic lymphatic cysts'. Parapelvic renal cysts may be solitary or multiple. Multiple cysts frequently fill the sinus and surround the entire collecting system causing a pattern of effacement and stretching of the renal pelvis and infundibula. This condition has been termed 'polycystic disease of the renal sinus' (Vela Navarrete and Garcia Robledo 1983) and 'parapelvic or peripelvic lymphangiectasia' (Murray and McLellan 1991).

The pathogenesis of renal sinus cysts has not been definitively established. Most renal sinus cysts arise from dilated or obstructed renal sinus lymphatic channels. This origin is supported by the microscopic finding of endothelial lining that resembles that of lymphatic channels (Elkin and Bernstein 1969; Deliveliotis and Kavadis 1969; Dubilier and Evans 1958). Rarely, cysts in the renal sinus may be due to regressive changes in the adipose tissue due to localized vascular disease and/or atrophy due to recent wasting (Barrie 1953; Hellweg 1954).

Most renal sinus cysts occur in the fifth and sixth decades and are almost always asymptomatic and detected as incidental radiographic findings. Occasionally, compression of the renal pelvis or collecting system may cause pain from hydronephrosis. Rarely, stone formation and infection can also occur in the renal collecting system. Although extremely rare, renovascular hypertension has been reported in cases of a cyst expanding in the tight confines of the renal sinus and compressing renal arterial supply (Chan and Kodroff 1980; Scholl 1948).

When a mass is identified on excretory urography compressing the renal pelvis and infundibula, the differential diagnosis is usually between a simple parapelvic renal cyst and a solid or cystic parapelvic mass (Table 8.2) (Cover *et al.* 1988). Sonography is an excellent, non-invasive technique used to confirm that the mass is a simple renal sinus cyst. Occasionally, renovascular lesions (aneurysms, varices, arteriovenous malformations) may appear cystic in the region of the renal sinus but usually contain blood flow on colour Doppler sonography. If ultrasonography is equivocal, CT or MRI may be helpful for further evaluation.

Multiple, bilateral renal sinus cysts can mimic hydronephrosis on ultrasound (Fig. 8.3 A–D) (Cronan *et al.* 1982). This can be important in certain patients

Table 8.2 Differential diagnosis of masses of the renal sinus

---

Arising from structures transversing the sinus
Aneurysmal dilation of the renal artery
Varix of the renal vein
Diverticula of the renal pelvis

Arising within or from the sinus
Parapelvic cyst
Renal sinus lipomatosis
Resorptive cyst
Parapelvic pseudocyst

Arising from structures or tissue not ordinarily within the sinus
Cystic disease of the parenchyma (simple, polycystic, and others)
Neoplasm (transitional cell epithelioma, renal cell carcinoma, and others)
'Pseudotumour'

---

who present with renal insufficiency in whom renal ultrasound is being carried out to exclude urinary obstruction. Therefore, it may be necessary to do an excretory urogram or a CT scan with IV contrast to clearly differentiate multiple renal sinus cysts from a dilated obstructed collecting system. Bilateral renal sinus cysts can also mimic polycystic kidney disease on excretory urography (mild renal enlargement, effacement, and splaying of the renal pelvis and calyces) but this diagnosis can be easily excluded by ultrasonography or CT scan.

Perirenal cysts

These cysts are uncommon and like the parapelvic cysts are thought to be of lymphatic origin. Actually, parapelvic and perirenal cysts frequently coexist, which is consistent with the anatomy and dual exit of the renal lymphatic system (Meredith *et al.* 1988; Schwarz *et al.* 1993). The term 'renal lymphangiomatosis' has been used to describe the cystic dilatation of these lymphatic spaces. This can be caused by a congenital or acquired obstruction of the renal lymphatics and aggravated by conditions known to be result in an increased renal lymphatic flow.

Perirenal pseudocyst

Perirenal cysts should be differentiated from perirenal pseudocysts, which are due to extravasation of urine into the perirenal fat or a result of trauma or urinary obstruction. Contrary to the perirenal cysts or lymphangiomas, the wall of these pseudocysts consists of fibrous tissue without an endothelial lining (Meyers 1975).

Multicystic dysplastic kidney (MCDK)

Multicystic dysplastic kidney (MCDK) is one of the most common abdominal masses in the neonate (Kirks *et al.* 1985). It occurs in approximately 1 in 4300

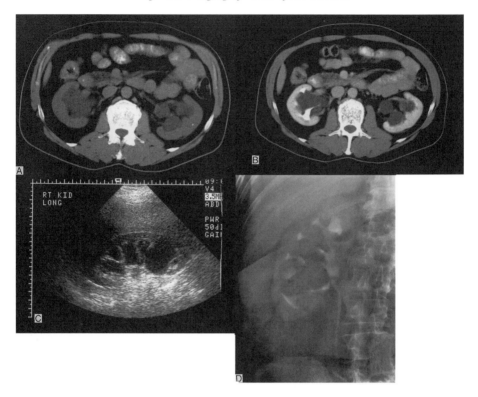

Fig. 8.3 (A) Non-enhanced CT scan of the kidneys demonstrating fluid-like areas within both parapelvic regions of the kidneys. (B) Contrast-enhanced CT scan of the same patient demonstrating parapelvic renal cysts compressing the right renal collecting system and left hydronephrosis due to a left ureteropelvic junction obstruction. (C) Longitudinal US of the right kidney suggesting hydronephrosis. (D) Excretory urogram of the same patient demonstrating parapelvic cyst compression of the right renal collecting system with no evidence of hydronephrosis.

births and is usually diagnosed during the first year of life (Gordon *et al.* 1988). MCDK is not an hereditary condition but is thought to be a developmental anomaly secondary to a segmental atresia of the renal collecting system. MCDK is categorized into two types of atresia: infundibulopelvic and hydronephrotic (Griscom *et al.* 1975; Vinocur *et al.* 1988). MCDK is usually unilateral; when bilateral, it is lethal and presents as Potter's syndrome (Fig. 8.4A,B). Before the advent of routine obstetrical sonography, most infants with MCDK presented with an asymptomatic abdominal mass. Currently, most cases of MCDK are discovered during prenatal sonography.

MCDK, although variable in size, has a characteristic sonographic appearance. It is composed of a cluster of multiple cysts that are variable in size and number. Most of these cysts do not communicate, although some may. The cysts have sharply defined thin walls and are anechoic. There may be a small amount of soft tissue adjacent to or between cysts but there is no recognizable normal renal parenchyma. Rarely, MCDK may develop in a renal variant such as an ectopic, duplicated, or crossed fused ectopic kidney. The normal reniform contour is often lost in MCDK. The ureter is not usually identified. Duplex Doppler evaluation has documented either no flow or flow with markedly abnormal waveforms in the renal arteries of MCDK (Hendry and Hendry 1991).

Renal scintigraphy with DMSA or DTPA characteristically demonstrates no uptake. In a few cases there may be minimal, faint uptake on delayed images. This is of doubtful significance if the sonographic appearance is classical for MCDK. Rarely, it may be difficult to differentiate a severe ureteropelvic junction obstruction (UPJ) from a MCDK. Communication between an enlarged central medially positioned renal pelvis and the symmetrically dilated and evenly distributed calyces are the features which differentiate a UPJ obstruction from the variably sized randomly positioned non-communicating cysts of MCDK. Sonography and renal scintigraphy are the imaging modalities of choice for diagnosis of MCDK. Uncommonly, CT, excretory urography, or cyst puncture may be helpful if there are atypical features or presentation.

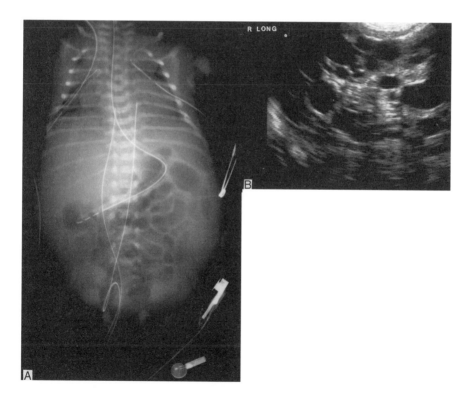

Fig. 8.4 New-born with Potter's syndrome. Chest and abdomen plain film (A) demonstrates bilateral abdominal flank masses, small lung volumes, and pneumothoraces with bilateral chest tubes. Sonography demonstrated a 'Swiss cheese' appearance of both kidneys (B) consistent with bilateral multicystic dysplastic kidneys.

MCDK is a dynamic entity which changes over time both prenatally and during the first years of life (Vinocur *et al.* 1988; Avni *et al.* 1986; Pedicelli *et al.* 1986; Strife *et al.* 1993; Rickwood *et al.* 1992; Mesrobian *et al.* 1993; Hashimoto *et al.* 1986). The majority of MCDK regress and involute within the first few years of life. The cysts become smaller in size and number. Eventually, the cysts may totally disappear with minimal renal dysplastic tissue remaining in the renal fossa. Often, no residual renal tissue is identified (Fig. 8.5A–C). Less commonly, MCDK may remain the same size or enlarge during the first years of life. There has been documentation of in utero involution with apparent unilateral renal agenesis at the time of birth. Except in a typical cases, a non-surgical approach to MCDK is generally indicated.

Compensatory hypertrophy of the contralateral kidney is expected. There are genitourinary abnormalities of the contralateral side in 20–50 per cent of patients (Vinocur *et al.* 1988; Strife *et al.* 1993; Atiyeh *et al.* 1992). The most common abnormalities are ureterovesical reflux and ureteropelvic junction obstruction. A voiding cysto-urethrogram for evaluation of reflux should be a part of the radiologic investigations.

There is no known predisposition of MCDK to malignant degeneration (Gordon *et al.* 1988; Menster *et al.* 1994; Noe *et al.* 1989). The natural history of MCDK is still under evaluation. Long-term follow-up is needed to evaluate the current trend of non-surgical management and a MCDK Registry was established in 1986 for this purpose (Wacksman and Phipps 1993).

Autosomal recessive polycystic kidney disease (ARPKD)

There is a spectrum of radiographic findings in ARPKD that reflects the variable clinical presentation (see Chapter 9). The radiographic characteristics change over time correlating with the evolving pathological process (McDonald and Avner 1991; Gagnadoux *et al.* 1989; Premkumar *et al.* 1988; Melson *et al.* 1985). As more cases are being detected earlier due to routine in utero sonography and screening of at-risk family members a greater variation in appearance and clinical course is being appreciated.

Ultrasound

Sonography is the study of choice in evaluating infants and children with suspected ARPKD. It offers superb morphological detail with no radiation and relative low cost. Renal enlargement is a characteristic feature of ARPKD. The kidneys may be mildly to massively enlarged. Renal enlargement is most often symmetric although rare cases of asymmetric enlargement are reported (Kogutt *et al.* 1993). As the child grows, the kidneys may grow or stabilize in size. With progression of renal disease, fibrosis and reactive tissue may develop resulting in an overall decrease in renal size (McDonald and Avner 1991; Gagnadoux *et al.* 1989; Liebermann *et al.* 1971). Normal renal size does not preclude a diagnosis of ARPKD (Kääriäinen *et al.* 1988). Reniform shape is usually maintained but

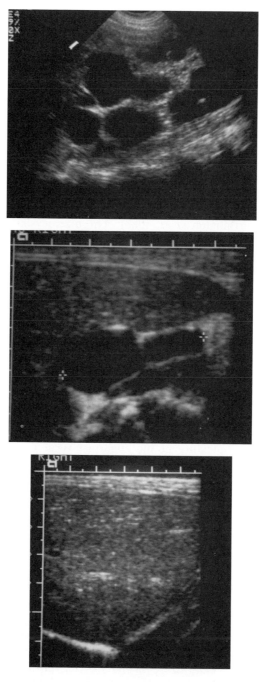

Fig. 8.5 Progression of multicystic dysplastic kidney. At birth, the MCDK is as large as a normal kidney and is composed of multiple cysts (A). At 1 year of age, the MCDK is much smaller and contains only two cysts (B). At 2 years of age, there is no residual cysts or tissue discernible in the renal fossa (C).

the contours may be ill defined. It may be difficult to differentiate the outline of the abnormal renal parenchyma from perirenal soft tissue because of similar echogenicity (Boal and Littlewood Teele 1980).

Cases presenting in the perinatal period characteristically have renal parenchymal echotexture which is inhomogeneously increased (Fig. 8.6) (McDonald and Avner 1991; Gagnadoux *et al.* 1989; Kääriäinen *et al.* 1988, Wernecke *et al.* 1985). Corticomedullary differentiation with hypoechoic medullary pyramids is usually absent. The inhomogeneous bright echotexture is thought due to the myriad of renal tubular microcysts resulting in multiple interfaces for the ultrasound beam. With the advent of high-energy ultrasound transducers, many of these tiny, 2–5 mm, cysts are now able to be resolved (Wernecke *et al.* 1985). Macrocysts greater than 1 cm are uncommon but are occasionally seen and are not incompatible with a diagnosis of ARPKD (Fig. 8.7) (Boal and Littlewood Teele 1980; Worthington *et al.* 1988). The macrocysts become more common with age (MacDonald and Avner 1991; Liebermann *et al.* 1971; Boal and Littlewood Teele 1980; Wernecke *et al.* 1985).

There is a growing appreciation of the variations in appearance of ARPKD at presentation and over time due to earlier detection. A subcapsular rim of normal hypoechoic cortex may be present (Melson *et al.* 1985). The medullary pyramids may be hypoechoic at birth but over time become hyperechoic and indistinguishable from the adjacent renal parenchyma (Fig. 8.8A,B). Focal areas of increased echogenicity may predominate within the medullary pyramids simulating nephrocalcinosis (Fig. 8.9) (Herman and Siegel 1991). There may be prominence of the renal pelvis and calyces due to distortion by the abnormal renal parenchyma, but no true hydronephrosis. Calcifications are not a feature of early ARPKD, but with renal fibrosis and failure, dystrophic calcification may occur. Calcifications may be difficult to detect on sonography due to the heterogeneous bright echotexture of the abnormal renal parenchyma (Lucaya *et al.*

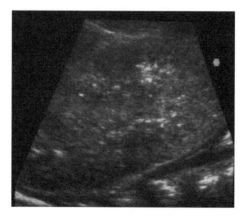

Fig. 8.6 Ten-month-old with hypertension diagnosed with ARPKD. The kidneys were mildly enlarged, reniform in contour, and increased in echotexture.

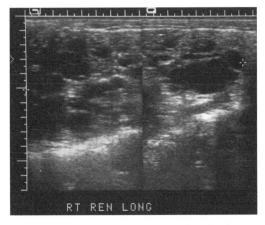

Fig. 8.7 Massively enlarged kidney with a multitude of micro- and macrocysts in a young child with ARPKD.

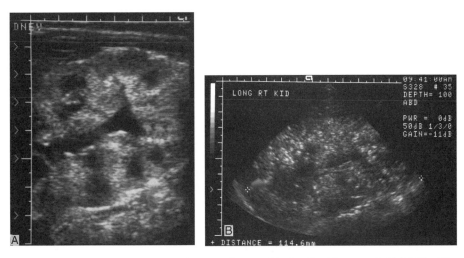

Fig. 8.8 Screening sonogram of a new-born with family history of ARPKD. The kidneys are enlarged and hyperechoic with preservation of the hypoechoic medullary pyramids (A). At 3 years of age there is diffuse increased echogenicity with loss of cortical medullary differentiation (B).

1993).

Sonographic evaluation of the liver is important in the radiologic evaluation of ARPKD. Hepatic involvement with ductal ectasia is an inherent component of the genetic disease process. While ultrasound may initially demonstrate normal hepatic echotexture, with development of periportal fibrosis, the hepatic echotexture will be coarsened or increased. Hepatic involvement may be diffuse or patchy in nature. Mild biliary dilatation and thickened or echogenic ductal walls

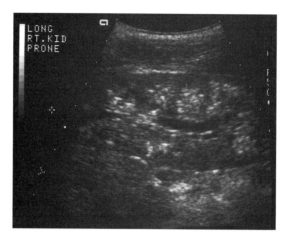

Fig. 8.9   There are multiple speckled areas of increased echogenicity predominantly in the regions of the medullary pyramids in both kidneys in a young child with ARPKD. This appearance may mimic nephrocalcinosis.

may develop. Small hepatic cysts ranging in size from millimetres to a few centimetres may develop. These cysts are commonly noted in the posterior aspect of the liver. Splenomegaly occurs with the development of portal hypertension.

Excretory urography

Excretory urograms (ExU) are no longer commonly done in the evaluation of ARPKD but may offer valuable information especially in atypical cases. In severe cases with little or no renal function, the nephrogram will be absent or delayed by hours. The classical appearance on ExU in infants or young children is that of symmetrically enlarged kidneys with a striated nephrogram (Fig. 8.10) (Melson *et al.* 1985; Kääriäinen *et al.* 1988; Childton and Cremin 1981). There are multiple linear striations radiating out from the medullary pyramids to the cortex. The collecting systems may be faintly opacified due to poor renal function. When visualized, the calyces may be midly blunted and the pelvis may be prominent but there is no true hydronephrosis.

The ExU on children with less extensive renal involvement may show only nephromegaly and tubular estasia of the medullary pyramids.

Computed tomography

If the renal function is adequate to allow use of intravenous contrast, the kidneys and liver are well evaluated with CT. In classical cases, the ExU equivalent of the striated nephrogram is present with streaky linear enhancement extending from the medullary pyramids out toward the cortex within significantly enlarged kidneys (Fig. 8.11A,B). Small streaky lucent areas are interspersed between the

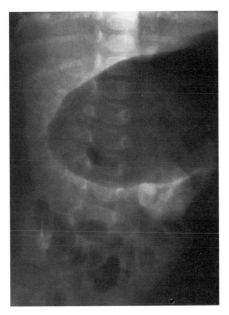

Fig. 8.10 Neonatal excretory urogram demonstrating characteristic appearance of ARPKD with massively enlarged kidneys and a streaky mottled nephrogram.

striations of the nephrogram. There are commonly a few well-defined cysts ranging in size from 5 mm to 1 cm. Although there may be a few macrocysts larger than 1 cm, the smaller cysts predominate (Fig. 8.12). The size and number of these cysts may be better appreciated on CT than with sonography. Although the cysts may increase in size and number with age, there is not the plethora of macrocysts typically seen in ADPKD.

As the child grows, renal enlargement is not as prominent a feature as in ADPKD. The kidneys may actually decrease in size with diminishing renal function and development of fibrosis. At end-stage the kidneys may not be discernibly different from other kidneys with long-standing dysfunction. Small speckled areas of dystrophic renal calcification may also develop with age (Lucaya *et al.* 1993).

In those patients with less extensive renal involvement, the kidneys may be normal in appearance or midly enlarged with a few scattered small cysts. Hepatic fibrosis may predominate in these patients. Hepatic involvement may already be present during infancy but may not manifest clinically until later in childhood or adolescence. The liver may appear normal initially. Over time, small hepatic cysts and mild biliary dilatation may develop. The biliary dilatation may become fairly extensive with development of multiple areas of ectatic dilatation resembling Caroli's disease. Hepatic enhancement tends to be fairly uniform as hepatocellular function is normal. Splenomegaly and varices reflect development of portal hypertension secondary to the periportal fibrosis.

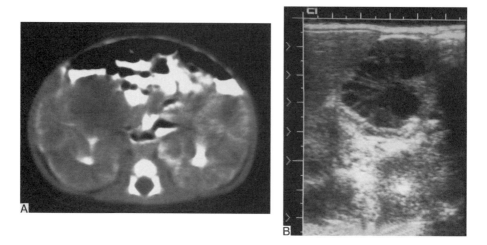

Fig. 8.11 (A) Abdominal CT of a 1-year-old with ARPKD. The kidneys are markedly enlarged with a striated nephrogram of the renal cortex. (B) Sonographic evaluation of the 3 cm low density mass in the upper medial pole of the right kidney demonstrated a complex cyst with internal radial septations.

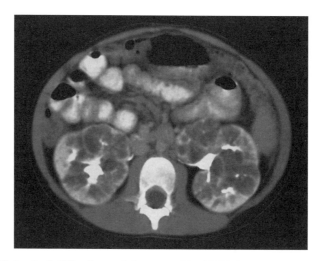

Fig. 8.12 Abdominal CT of an adolescent with ARPKD. The kidneys, while prominent, are not massively enlarged. There are multiple micro- and macrocysts with some distortion of the renal pelvis and calyces.

Magnetic resonance imaging

MRI evaluation may be especially helpful in those children with poor renal function, unable to tolerate intravenous contrast medium (Fig. 8.13). T-1 images with gadolinium and T-2 images in an axial and a coronal plan will demonstrate renal size, cyst size and number, the amount of normal renal parenchyma, biliary dilatation, splenic size, and the amount and location of varices.

Differential diagnosis

The wide variability in the clinical presentation and course of ARPKD is reflected in the range of radiographic appearance at diagnosis and during progression of the disease (McDonald and Avner 1991; Gagnadoux *et al.* 1989; Premkumar *et al.* 1988; Melson *et al.* 1985, Kääriäinen *et al.* 1988; Wernecke *et al.* 1985; Worthington *et al.* 1988; Childton and Cremin 1981). While the appearance of symmetrically enlarged echogenic kidneys is characteristic of ARPKD it is not absolutely specific for it. Both ADPKD and the much less common glomerulocystic kidney disease (GCD) can present in the neonate with enlarged echogenic kidneys (Premkumar *et al.* 1988; Pretorius *et al.* 1987). Some characteristics of sonography, ExU, and CT (see Table 8.3) may be helpful (initially), but sometimes it can be very difficult to differentiate renal cystic diseases in the neonate on the basis of their radiographic appearance alone (Worthington *et al.* 1988; Fitch and Stapleton 1986; McAlister *et al.* 1979; Cole *et al.* 1987; Cole 1990). Family history and screening are a vital part of the investigations of the infant with cystic renal disease.

The appearance of the kidneys and liver over time will help confirm the diagnosis in most cases of ARPKD. With diminished renal function the kidneys tend to decrease in size and will not continue enlarging as in ADPKD. The multiple small cysts in ARPKD may grow slightly over time but do not show

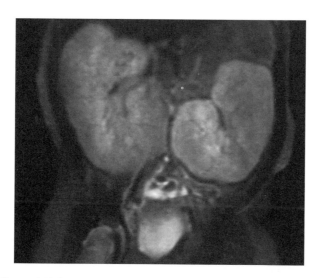

Fig. 18.13 Coronal T-2 weighted MRI of a 1-year-old with ARPKD. The kidneys are massively enlarged with a lobular reniform contour.

Table 8.3   Differential diagnosis of ARPKD and ADPKD in children by imaging techniques

Ultrasound	Excretory urogram	Computed tomography
ARPKD	**ARPKD**	**ARPKD**
KIDNEYS	KIDNEYS	KIDNEYS
Infancy:		
Enlarged	Enlarged	Enlarged
Inhomogeneously echogenic	Prolonged striated	Striated nephrogram
Pyramids may be visible	nephrogram	Delayed excretion
Usually no cysts	Delayed excretion	Multiple tiny cysts
		Few macrocysts
Childhood:		
Diffusely increased echogenicity		
Multiple tiny cysts		
Few macrocysts		
Pyramids not visible		
LIVER		
Normal or mildly coarsened parenchymal echotexture		
Few hepatic macrocysts		
SPLEEN		
Normal size or enlarged		
ADPKD	**ADPKD**	**ADPKD**
KIDNEYS	KIDNEYS	KIDNEYS
Infancy	*Infancy and childhood*	*Infancy*
Normal size and echotexture	Normal size	Normal size
Rarely will present with enlarged echogenic kidneys	Normal prompt nephrogram Normal calyces and pelvis	Normal density and collecting system
Childhood and adolescence	*Adolescence*	*Childhood and adolescence*
Small well-defined cysts which increase in size and number with age	Increasing size Prompt nephrogram Few well-defined masses	Enlarging size Few well-defined small cysts which increase in
Renal size increases over time	(cysts) which increase in size and number with age	size and number with age Normal renal parenchymal
	Calyces and pelvis may be distorted due to cysts	enhancement Cysts may distort calyces and pelvis

the progression in size and number that occurs in ADPKD. In those with stable renal function the congenital hepatic fibrosis becomes the dominant clinical problem in ARPKD.

In contrast, as a child with ADPKD grows, the kidneys take on the more classical appearance of enlarged kidneys with an increasing number and size of macrocysts. Hepatic cysts do not usually develop before adolescence. Congenital hepatic fibrosis has been reported in a few patients with ADPKD, although it is a much more dominant feature of ARPKD (Lipschitz *et al.* 1993; Cobben *et al.* 1990). While GCD, a non-inherited renal cystic disease, can mimic ARPKD, its usual presentation is of homogeneously enlarged kidneys with prominent subcapsular cortical cysts (McAlister *et al.* 1979).

Other uncommon renal cystic diseases of childhood include Meckel's syndrome (dysencephalia splanchnocystica), prenatal metabolic dysplasias (e.g. cerebro-oculo-hepato-renal syndrome of Zellweger and glutaric aciduria type II) TSC, von Hippel–Lindau syndrome, and medullary cystic disease. Infants with Beckwith–Wiedemann syndrome may have bilaterally enlarged kidneys which are not cystic or obstructed. The remaining differential diagnostic list for bilaterally enlarged, non-hydronephrotic kidneys in infants and young children includes processes which are usually unilateral but uncommonly, can involve both kidneys. These processes include bilateral nephroblastomatosis or Wilms' tumour, multicystic dysplastic kidneys, renal vein or artery thrombosis, acute pyelonephritis, or non-obstructed duplication. Most of these entities can be differentiated from cystic kidney disease by the clinical presentation and radiographic appearance.

Autosomal dominant polycystic kidney disease (ADPKD)

The diagnostic imaging findings of ADPKD vary depending on the age of presentation and degree of involvement. The minimal sonographic criteria to make a diagnosis of ADPKD in an individual with a 50 per cent risk of carrying the ADPKD gene have been recently revised by Ravine *et al.* (1994): two cysts in individuals less than 30 years old, two cysts on each kidney in those 30–59 years old, and four cysts on each kidney in individuals over age 60. With minimal disease, the size of the kidneys are normal, its surfaces are smooth, and small cysts are detected in both kidneys. As the size and number of cysts increase, they will enlarge the kidney without necessarily distorting the renal contour (Fig. 8.14A–C). With continued involvement, the cysts project beyond the renal margin resulting in a bosselated contour. With advanced disease, the parenchyma is almost completely replaced by innumerable cysts. Patients with ADPKD2 have fewer cysts than patients with ADPKD1 (Ravine *et al.* 1992) Cysts vary in size from barely visible on imaging studies to large diameters of up to 10 cm or more. The cysts are usually uncomplicated containing clear, straw-coloured fluid. However, haemorrhage or proteinaceous debris on one or more cysts is not uncommon on imaging studies (Fig. 8.15). Asymmetry and the number and size of cysts may be seen between the two kidneys (Fig. 8.16). True unilateral ADPKD is extremely rare.

With age, cystic disease of the liver develops in the majority of patients with ADPKD and is more severe in women than in men (see Chapter 21). Approximately 10 per cent of ADPKD patients have cysts in the pancrease, and less than 5 per cent have splenic cysts. In addition, cysts of the ovary, seminal vesicle, epididymis, pituitary gland, arachnoid, and pineal body have also been reported.

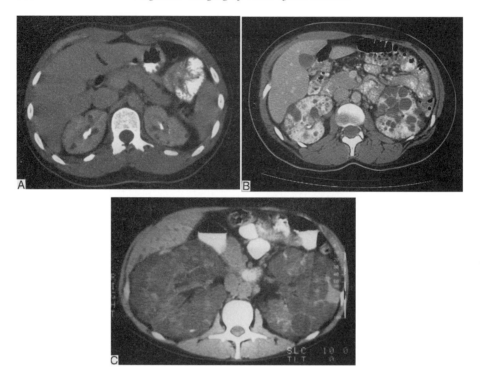

Fig. 8.14 (A) Contrast-enhanced CT scan of the kidneys in a patient with mild ADPKD. (B) Another patient with moderate ADPKD (C) Another patient with advanced ADPKD.

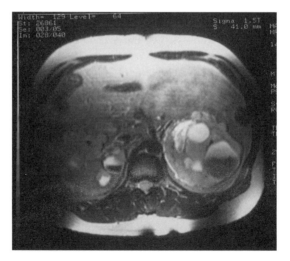

Fig. 8.15 T-2 weighted MRI of the kidneys in a patient with ADPKD. Note at least one cyst in both kidneys with layering haemorrhagic debris which has low signal intensity.

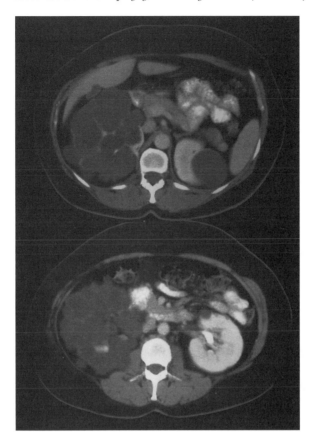

Fig. 8.16 CT scans at different levels in the same patient with ADPKD. Note the massive advanced involvement of the right kidneys with only minimal involvement of the left kidney.

Renal and liver cysts in patients with ADPKD can become infected. Infected cysts can be difficult to identify on imaging studies. If a cyst contains gas or a fluid debris level on CT, US, or MRI, the diagnosis of infected renal cyst should be considered. If these findings are not present, a nuclear medicine examination may be necessary to identify an infected cyst.

The diagnosis of other complications and associated pathology within the distorted anatomy of a polycystic kidney may be particularly challenging and can be missed unless adequate imaging techniques are used properly. CT is very useful in diagnosing stones (including uric acid stones, which occur with increased frequency in ADPKD), hydronephrosis, and neoplasms (Levine *et al.* 1981; Torres *et al.* 1988, 1993; Keith *et al.* 1994). MRI with gadolinium enhancement is particularly useful in difficult cases to diagnose obstruction or associated malignancies.

Excretory urography

The plain film of the abdomen is often normal in early stages of ADPKD. However, as the disease progresses, enlarged kidneys are often the initial finding. In fact, as the kidneys enlarge, it is generally difficult to trace the entire renal outline on a plain abdominal film in patients with ADPKD. Renal calculi may be difficult to differentiate from parenchymal calcifications.

During an excretory urogram in a patient with ADPKD, the nephrogram is characterized by numerous, smoothly marginated radiolucencies throughout the cortex and medulla in both kidneys which are often enlarged. The appearance has been likened to that of Swiss cheese (Fig. 8.17). Young, asymptomatic patients frequently have enlarged kidneys with smooth outlines and normal collecting systems. As the disease progresses the contour becomes lobulated and the calyces are often elongated, effaced, and somewhat displaced by the multiple large cysts. Occasionally, a large cyst may obstruct one or more calyces resulting in caliectasis. Rarely, cysts that have ruptured in the collecting system may fill with contrast media on the excretory urogram. Precalyceal tubular estasia can be detected in 15 per cent of the patients.

Retrograde pyelography

Retrograde pyelography is rarely indicated in the investigation of ADPKD. It may be necessary for the evaluation of a possible transitional cell epithelioma of the renal pelvis. In these cases, prophylactic antibiotics should be administered to prevent a serious kidney infection. Retrograde pyelography demonstrates splaying, effacement and displacement, and occasional dilatation of the pelvis and calyces.

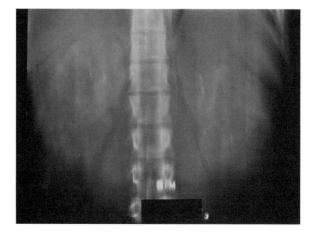

Fig. 8.17 Nephrotomogram of the kidneys after contrast administration in a patient with ADPKD demonstrating multiple cysts.

Ultrasonography

In utero and during the fist year of life, the sonographic appearance of the kidneys (enlarged and with increased echogenicity) may be indistinguishable from ARPKD and other renal cystic diseases. The presence of discrete cysts in these patients suggests a diagnosis of ADPKD. The appearance of ADPKD in older children and adults on sonography is usually that of enlarged kidneys containing multiple cysts. Because of the nature of the ultrasound beam, it is often difficult to identify renal margins on one particular sonogram image (Fig. 8.18). Therefore, it is often difficult to measure renal size exactly and, at times, further evaluation to characterize the kidneys for size and parenchyma may be necessary. The size of the cysts on ultrasound varies tremendously. Cysts that contain haemorrhage or infection may contain echogenic debris, and there may be a debris fluid level.

Computed tomography

CT is the most valuable, cost-effective way of evaluating the parenchyma in patients with ADPKD. Computed tomography should be performed without IV contrast first to detect any calcifications that may be present (Fig. 8.19). There is a correlation between renal calcifications and renal insufficiency in ADPKD patients. If not contraindicated, the non-enhanced study should be followed by a CT scan with IV contrast (Levine and Grantham 1981). Contrast enhancement facilitates the visualization of the preserved renal parenchyma and the distinction between parenchymal calcifications and stones within the collecting system. Renal cysts on CT are round to oval, vary in size, and are homogeneously scattered throughout the cortex and medulla. In the early stages, the kidney is of normal

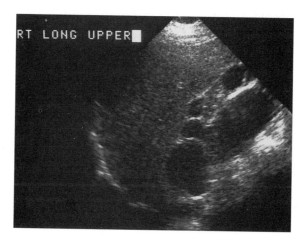

Fig. 8.18 Longitudinal ultrasound of the right kidney demonstrating multiple large cysts in a patient with ADPKD.

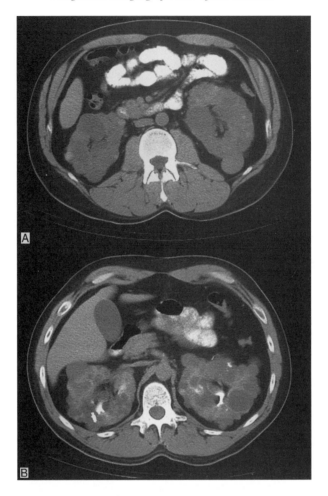

Fig. 8.19 (A) Non-contrast-enhanced CT scans through the kidneys in a patient with ADPKD. Note the small cysts with increased density. These small cysts contain areas of haemorrhage. (B) Contrast-enhanced CT scan of the same patient demonstrating the number, size, and location of the cysts more clearly following contrast administration. Also note the small areas of calcified cysts in the anterior portion of the left kidney and the posterior aspect of the right kidney.

size and contour on CT with scattered cysts throughout both kidneys. As the disease progresses, the size and number of the cyst and the renal volumes increase. The density of the cyst should be that of water on CT. However, it is common to see one or multiple cysts in each kidney with increased density. This is most often due to haemorrhage, but it can also be due to proteinaceous material within the cyst that results in increased cyst density (Levine and Grantham 1985).

When an ADPKD patient presents with acute flank pain, one of the concerns is acute haemorrhage into a cyst or from a cyst into the perinephric space.

Because high-density cysts are common (seen in up to 75 per cent of ADPKD patients), and are often multiple, it may be difficult to attribute acute flank pain to a particular haemorrhagic cyst. The presence of haemorrhage outside the cyst within the renal parenchyma or in the perinephric space helps identify the probable cause of the flank pain (Fig. 8.20) (Levine and Grantham 1981).

An infected cyst may have a thick, irregular wall with an increased density of the cyst fluid on CT. Localized thickening of Gerota's fascia may also occur, but this is a non-specific finding. Gas within a cyst is a helpful finding in the diagnosis of an infected renal cyst. Rarely, infected renal cysts can go on to develop perinephric or paranephric abscesses.

CT or excretory urography is most useful in evaluating ADPKD patients with unexplained deterioration of renal function. CT and excretory urography are particularly more specific than ultrasonography for the differentiation of hydronephrosis from centrally located cysts.

CT is also extremely useful in the detection of the uncommon occurrence of concomitant polycystic kidney disease and renal cell carcinoma. Pre- and post-contrast CT images are necessary for the proper identification of concomitant renal tumours.

Magnetic resonance imaging

MRI offers unique advantages in the evaluation of patients with ADPKD. Specifically, MRI is most useful in difficult problem-solving cases of flank pain, infection, and/or suspicion of concomitant renal cell carcinoma (Leung *et al.* 1984; Levine and Grantham 1987).

All MRI examinations of the kidneys in patients with ADPKD should involve T-1 and T-2 weighted images without gadolinium contrast media and T-1

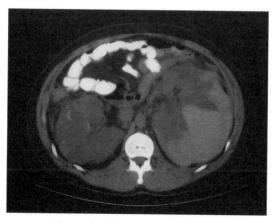

Fig. 8.20 Non-contrast-enhanced CT scan through the kidneys in a patient with ADPKD. There is a large area of increased density surrounding the left kidney consistent with perinephric haemorrhage due to a ruptured haemorrhagic cyst.

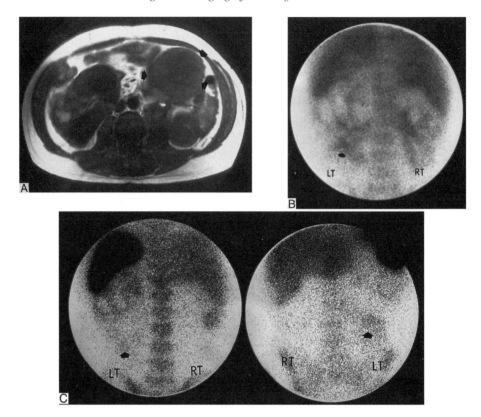

Fig. 8.21 (A) T-1 weighted MRI through the lower poles of both kidneys in a patient with ADPKD. The scan demonstrates a thick-walled cyst with increased signal in the mid portion of the left kidney. (B) [67]Gallium study demonstrating increased activity in the region of the left kidney corresponding to the area of the thick-walled cyst on CT. (C) [111]Indium white blood cell study of the same patient again demonstrating increased activity in the region of the left kidney in the region of the patient's infected cyst.

weighted images of the kidneys following gadolinium enhancement. Gadolinium-enhanced T-1 weighted images of the kidneys with fat suppression offers the best tissue contrast of all imaging studies and often identifies abnormal debris and cysts fluid that is not appreciated on CT scans. Pre- and post-gadolinium enhanced images of the kidneys are vital for the proper identification of thick-walled cysts in patients who may have an infected cyst because of the superior contrast resolution (Fig 8.21). Gadolinium-enhanced images are also essential in the rare circumstance where renal cell carcinoma is concomitant with ADPKD (Fig. 8.22).

Magnetic resonance urography

MR urography is a new technique that can provide coronal imaging of the renal collecting systems and ureters similar to conventional urography without the use

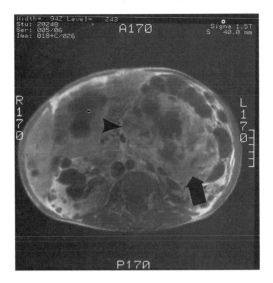

Fig. 8.22 Gadolinium-enhanced T-1 weighted MRI through the level of the kidneys in a patient with known ADPKD. Note the large irregular cystic mass arising from the anterior portion of the left kidney. This was found to represent a necrotic renal cell carcinoma at the time of surgery.

of iodinated contrast. MR urography may be helpful in patients with impaired renal function in whom urinary obstruction is a concern.

Magnetic resonance angiography

MR angiography is another new technique that can provide non-invasive imaging of the renal arteries without the use of IV contrast. MR angiography can also be utilized to measure renal blood flow (Wolf *et al.* 1993).

Angiography

Angiography in ADPKD is rarely used today but can be utilized for the evaluation of patients with significant haemorrhage for possible embolization of the bleeding vessel. The angiographic appearance in patients with ADPKD demonstrates stretching and displaced intrarenal arterial branches by the numerous cysts. The nephrogram is characterized by a variable number of avascular masses giving the so-called 'Swiss cheese' appearance. In some cases, angiography can be utilized to investigate neovascularity that might suggest renal cell carcinoma.

Radionuclide imaging

Renal cysts in ADPKD patients do not accumulate radionuclides employed for renal scintigraphy, and therefore, appear as multiple photopenic masses. If an infected cyst is clinically suspected, an [111]indium-labelled white blood cell study or a [67]gallium citrate scan may be valuable in defining specific infected cysts (Fig 8.21). An [111]indium-labelled white blood cell study is more sensitive and specific than a [67]gallium study. These studies may need to be done in conjunction with a regular technetium DTPA renal study to provide a normal background of activity in the kidney to subtract from the [111]indium-labelled white blood cell study or the [67]gallium citrate study.

Diagnostic imaging investigations

Advanced disease in ADPKD patients is readily apparent using any renal imaging modality. Early diagnosis in relatives, on the other hand, is important for genetic counselling. In view of its non-invasiveness, low cost, general availability, and lack of ionizing radiation, ultrasonography is probably the best imaging modality suited for screening the family of ADPKD patients.

CT, however, is ideally suited for further evaluation of the disease, assessment of severity and prognosis, and for detecting complications such as infections or abscess formation, heamorrhage, calculi, perinephric infection, coexistent tumour, and urinary tract obstruction. Because of its high sensitivity, as compared to ultrasonography, it is the best imaging modality for the screening of potential living, related transplant donors for patients with ADPKD.

MRI appears to play a role in ADPKD patients with complications, such as infection or tumour, when CT or nuclear medicine has been unable to adequately answer certain clinical questions. Again, MRI should be carried out without and with gadolinium enhancement for maximal benefit. In addition, coronal and sagittal imaging of the kidneys in these patients is extremely useful in appreciating the extent and degree of disease.

Differential diagnosis

Because of the wide variety of findings in ADPKD patients and the differing age groups at presentation, it is possible that ADPKD can be confused with other cystic disease of the kidneys.

Multiple simple renal cysts can occasionally be difficult to differentiate from ADPKD in patients who have a significant number of renal cysts. In this case, it is paramount to correlate with a thorough family history and to investigate the presence of cysts in other organs and other extrarenal manifestations of the disease. These factors will be helpful in differentiating the patient with multiple renal cysts from the patient with mild ADPKD.

Cystic kidney disease can occur in patient with tuberous sclerosis complex (TSC) (Narla *et al.* 1988). In fact, some children presenting with cystic kidney disease will be mistakenly diagnosed as having ADPKD when, in fact, a closer evaluation of the patient and their imaging studies will reveal the diagnosis of TSC (see Chapter 11). ARPKD may be indistinguishable from ADPKD in neonates or very young children (see p. 207). A knowledge of the family history is extremely important in differentiating the two diseases, as is the development of a typical appearance of ADPKD on later imaging studies. Von Hippel–Lindau (VHL) disease is also transmitted as an autosomal dominant trait and can present with multiple renal cysts (see Chapter 12).

Acquired cystic disease is a phenomenon that occurs in patients with prolonged uraemia or on long-term dialysis. These kidneys are generally much smaller than those of patients with ADPKD. Patients with acquired renal cystic disease can also have multiple solid renal tumours (adenomas or carcinomas).

Other renal cystic diseases that may be confused with ADPKD include localized cystic disease of the kidneys, oro-facio-digital syndrome type I, and pluricystic renal disease. These entities will be discussed later in the chapter.

Lymphoma can also present a confusing picture of multiple, low-density, renal masses. In fact, the most common presentation of lymphoma in the kidneys is multiple low-density renal masses. If proper attention is not made to the exact density of the lesions on CT, the multiple, low-density masses could be mistaken for multiple renal cysts. In addition, lymphomatous lesions of the kidneys are notoriously very hypoechoic on ultrasound, and if close attention is not paid to proper gain settings, these hypoechoic masses in the kidney could be mistaken for anechoic renal cysts. Lymphoma involvement of the kidneys is often associated with retroperitoneal adenopathy, and other manifestations of lymphoma.

Renal cystic disease associated with multiple renal neoplasms

Acquired renal cystic disease

Acquired renal cystic disease (ARCD) is a well-recognized entity characterized by multiple bilateral renal cysts in patients with chronic renal failure (Levine *et al.* 1984) and may be associated with serious complications such as retroperitoneal haemorrhage and renal cell carcinoma (see Chapter 10).

Sonography, CT, and MRI are useful imaging modalities for evaluating ARCD and its complications. Sonography may not be sensitive enough to detect the presence of small cysts in small hyperechoice kidneys or to identify solid tumours in the middle of diffusely cystic kidneys. For these patients, CT is the most efficacious technique for the diagnosis of ARCD (Fig. 8.23). CT scans should be obtained without and with contrast enhancement. On pre-contrast studies, cyst wall calcification and high density haemorrhagic cysts are commonly seen. The renal solid tumours that occur in these patients may be very small and difficult to detect unless high resolution, 5 mm slice imaging is performed. Because many of these patients are already on chronic dialysis, the use of iodinated contrast should not be a contraindication during the examination. MRI before and after gadolinium enhancement is as good as or superior to CT

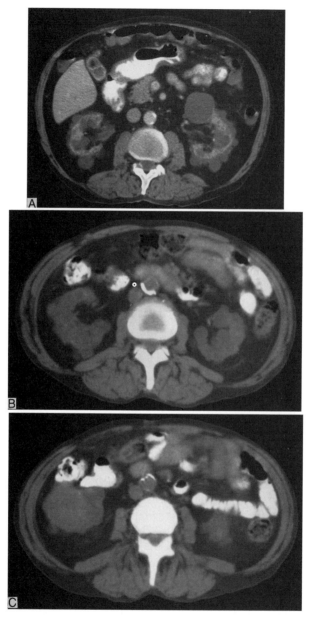

Fig. 8.23 (A) Contrast-enhanced CT scan of the kidneys in a patient with known ARCD. Note the peripheral nature of many of the cysts. (B) Non-contrast-enhanced CT scan through the kidneys in another patient with ARCD. Note the small calcifications associated with the many cysts. (C) Inferior CT scan through the lower pole of the right kidney of another patient. Note the solid mass arising from the lower pole of the right kidney which was found to be a renal cell carcinoma.

for the diagnosis of ARCD and its complications and can be used when the administration of intravenous radiologic contrast is contraindicated.

Tuberous sclerosis complex

Tuberous sclerosis complex (TSC) is a autosomal dominant multisystem disease that affects the kidneys (Gomez 1988). The most frequent renal findings in TSC patients are angiomyolipomas, renal cysts, and renal cell carcinomas (see Chapter 11).

Renal cystic disease in TSC patients can occur in the first year of life, whereas angiomyolipomas do not appear until later. The vast majority of patients with TSC and renal cystic disease have just 1–5 cysts in either one or both kidneys. Some patients with TSC and renal cysts present with a polycystic appearance, often at a young age (less than 5 years), without angiomyolipomas, with hypertension and, at times, renal insufficiency (Torres *et al.* 1994; Best *et al.* 1993). At a later age, the coexistence of renal cystic and angiomyolipomas is pathognomonic for TSC.

Renal, patients with TSC can present with perinephric or peripelvic lymphangiectasia (Fig. 8.24A,B). This rare cystic manifestation in the kidneys results from hamartomatous smooth muscle hypertrophy in lymphatic channels resulting in lymphatic obstruction (Torres *et al.* 1995). Retroperitoneal lymphangiomatous cysts not involving the kidneys can also be observed in these patients.

Von Hippel–Lindau disease

Von Hippel–Lindau (VHL) disease is transmitted by an autosomal dominant gene and affects multiple organs (see Chapter 12).

Renal cell carcinoma occurs in 35–40 per cent of patients with VHL. The tumours are usually bilateral and multiple. Most tumours are less than 3 cm in size. Renal cysts occur in about 76 per cent of patients (Levine *et al.* 1982). The renal cysts are usually small, multiple and bilateral (Fig. 8.25A,B). Such small cysts may be the earliest signs of VHL, and their detection is helpful in genetic counselling. Cysts usually range in size from 0.5 to 3.0 cm in size. They mainly involve the renal cortex and do not result in renal enlargement. Most cysts are lined by cuboidal epithelium; however, it is well known that clear cell carcinomas often arise from these cyst walls. In fact, some cysts in VHL are really cystic carcinomas (Lee *et al.* 1977).

CT scanning has been utilized in most patients with VHL to detect the multiple cysts and possible solid neoplasms in the kidneys. It is paramount to perform the CT scan of the kidneys without and then with IV contrast to determine the density of the lesions prior to and after the enhancement of contrast. Such density measurements allow for accurate assessment of cystic vs. solid masses. However, because of partial volume effects, CT scanning may not be able to differentiate cystic from solid masses when both cysts and solid masses

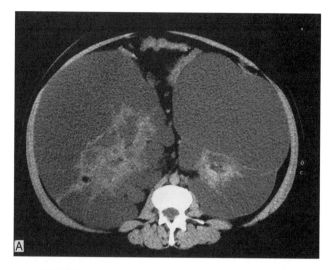

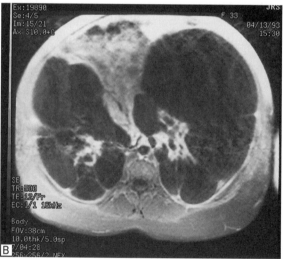

Fig. 8.24 (A) Contrast-enhanced CT scan of a patient with known TSC and perinephric lymphangiectasia. Note the low-density, small angiomyolipoma in the right kidney and the multiple, large, cystic spaces surrounding and compressing the parenchyma of both kidneys. (B) Gadolinium-enhanced T-1 weighted MRI of the same patient again demonstrating the multiple, large, perinephric lymphatic cysts compressing and distorting the parenchyma of both kidneys.

are less than 1 cm in size. Because of this, thin section (5 mm) CT or fast CT scanners (spiral or electron beam) may be necessary to detect small lesions.

MRI without and with gadolinium enhancement has proven to be a useful examination in selected patients for determining the exact size and number of multiple, small, solid, and cystic lesions in the kidney. Because of the dramatic contrast differences between enhancing renal parenchyma and enhancing solid

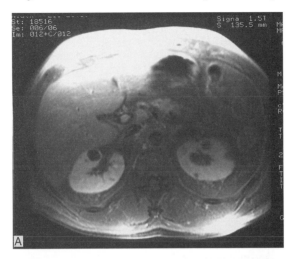

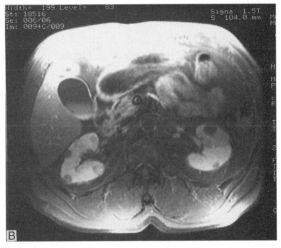

Fig. 8.25 (A) Gadolinium-enhanced MRI through the kidneys in a patient with VHL demonstrating multiple, non-enhancing cysts in both kidneys. (B) Gadolinium-enhanced MRI of the same patient at a lower level. Note the solid-appearing enhancing lesion in the medial aspect of the right kidney which was found to represent a renal cell carcinoma. Also note the small cystic renal cell carcinoma in the posterior aspect of the right kidney as well as the small benign-appearing cyst in the lateral portion of the right kidney. Finally, there is a small enhancing solid tumour in the anterior aspect of the right kidney. Small cysts are also noted in the left kidney.

tumours as compared to black, non-enhancing cysts, MRI is the most accurate means for determining the size and number of multiple cysts and solid lesions in the kidneys (Choyke *et al.* 1992). Several medical centres have turned to MRI in the routine follow-up of these patients because of the inherent superior contrast resolution.

Miscellaneous renal cystic disease

Localized cystic disease

Localized cystic disease of the kidney results in multiple simple cysts localized to one portion of the kidney (Fig. 8.26) This form of cystic disease is not genetically transmitted and is not a forme fruste of ADPKD. It is considered benign and is not associated with renal failure. It can be confused with multi-loculated cystic nephroma. However, there is no capsule between the cluster of cysts and renal parenchyma as is seen in multiloculated cystic nephroma. In addition, there are often several small parenchymal cysts not contained in the main cluster (Cho *et al.* 1979; Bosniak 1986).

Glomerulocystic kidney disease

Glomerular cysts can occur in a variety of cystic diseases such as ADPKD, TSC, oro-facio-digital syndrome type I and a number of malformation and dysplastic syndromes (Fig. 8.27) (Bernstein and Landing 1989; Bernstein 1993). Glomerulocystic kidney disease is used to describe a poorly defined disease or group of diseases characterized by the predominance of glomerular cysts, absence of or minimal tubular involvement, and lack of urinary tract obstruction, renal dysplasia or evidence of a recognizable cystic disease or malformation syndrome. Most initially described cases that met this definition were infants or young children, without a family history of renal disease, presenting with enlarged kidneys or variable degrees of renal insufficiency. Less often, glomerulocystic kidney disease has been diagnosed in adults in whom it appears to be inherited as an au-

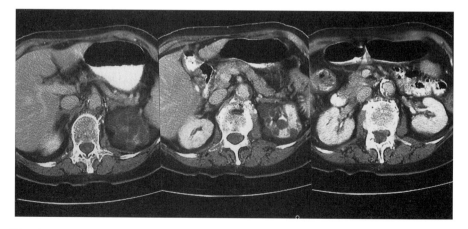

Fig. 8.26 Contrast-enhanced CT scans at various levels through both the right and left kidneys. Note the localized cystic disease involving the upper pole of the left kidney. The lower pole of the left kidney and the right kidney are free of cystic disease.

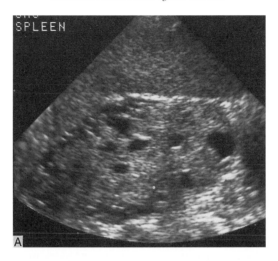

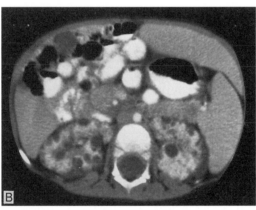

Fig. 8.27 (A) Longitudinal ultrasound of the right kidney in a 6-year-old boy with multiple malformations and glomerulocystic disease of the kidneys. Note the parenchymal and subcapsular cortical cysts. (B) Enhanced CT scan of the kidneys in the same patient demonstrating the cortical and subcapsular cysts.

tosomal dominant trait. Because glomerular cysts are often small, high resolution ultrasound and very thin section CT may be needed for their detection. The kidneys may be enlarged but maintain their normal contour. The natural history of this disease is not known (Carson *et al.* 1987; Bernstein 1993).

Oro-facio-digital syndrome type I

These patients may have kidneys indistinguishable from and often wrongly diagnosed as adult-type polycystic kidneys (Fig. 8.28) (Kennedy *et al.* 1991; Curry *et al.* 1992).

Pluricystic renal disease

Renal cysts are also encountered in many malformation syndromes due to sporadic defects (see Chapter 7).

Medullary cystic disease

The terms 'medullary cystic disease' or 'medullary cystic disease complex' refers to a group of similar diseases in which the basic lesion is a progressive tubulo-interstitial nephritis with secondary glomerulosclerosis and medullary cystic formation. Medullary cystic disease is an important cause of end-stage renal failure in children and a less common cause in adults. The childhood form of the disease is classically inherited as an autosomal recessive disorder and is frequently associated with a variety of extrarenal abnormalities such as congenital hepatic fibrosis, retinitis pigmentosa (Senior's syndrome), and skeletal malformations. The adult form of the disease is inherited as an autosomal dominant disease and is not associated with extrarenal abnormalities. A renal disease consistent with medullary cystic disease frequently occurs in two autosomal recessive syndromes, the Laurence–Moon–Bardet–Biedl syndrome (Srinivis *et al.* 1983; Gourdol *et al.* 1984; Linné *et al.* 1986) and Alström's syndrome (Cantani *et al.* 1985). The Laurence–Moon–Bardet–Biedl syndrome is characterized by obesity, polydactyly, retinitis pigmentosa, mental retardation, and hypogenitalism. Renal involvement is very common and consists of tubulo-interstitial nephritis and caliectasis, often with cystic spaces communicating with the collecting system. Alström's syndrome is characterized by obesity, diabetes mellitus, retinitis pigmentosa, and nerve deafness.

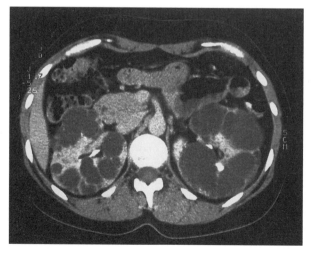

Fig. 8.28 Contrast-enhanced CT scan through the kidneys in a patient with known oro-facio-digital syndrome type I with multiple cysts in both kidneys.

Excretory urography will demonstrate poor visualization of normal or small kidneys with smooth contours. On occasion, medullary cysts may be identified as small lucencies in the medullary portions of the kidneys. Fan-shaped or striated, late-appearing, persistent nephrograms limited to the medullary portions of the parenchyma have also been described. High-frequency ultrasound will demonstrate small hyperechoic kidneys, and occasionally one may see small, fluid-filled, medullary cysts as well as small smooth kidneys with increased echogenicity. These small cysts can be identified in 90 per cent of patients with medullary cystic disease.

Computer tomography demonstrates kidneys that are bilaterally small and smooth, and the cysts are confined to the medulla or corticomedullary junction. Because the cysts are often small and completely surrounded by parenchyma, thin slices and fast scan times are needed for optimal visualization. Suspected cases of medullary cystic disease should be initially evaluated with high resolution ultrasound or thin section CT.

Although medullary cystic disease can be confused with acquired renal cystic disease (ARCD), the differentiation is made by identifying cysts only in the medulla of the kidneys in patients with medullary cystic disease, whereas ARCD also involves the cortex.

Medullary sponge kidney

On excretory urography, the mildest form of medullary sponge kidney (MSK) is the demonstration of discrete linear densities in one or more papillae. This results in a 'brush border' on urographic films and is often referred to as benign tubular ectasia. In moderate cases of MSK, the linear densities are more prominent and often contain calcifications resulting in medullary nephrocalcinosis. On the intravenous urogram, these foci of medullary calcifications are surrounded by contrast media. In more advanced cases, one can see gross deformity of the papillae with beaded or striated cavities on excretory urography. Calcifications are often large and numerous (Abeshouse and Abeshouse 1960; Davidson 1985).

Although excretory urography remains the mainstay of diagnosis, other imaging modalities may reveal unique findings. Sonographic findings include hyperechoic pyramids with or without acoustic shadowing. The visualization of the cystic dilatation of the distal collecting tubules is beyond the spatial resolution of sonography (Glazer *et al.* 1982). Computed tomography may demonstrate nephrocalcinosis or extracalyceal contrast accumulations within papillae (Boag and Nolan 1988).

Diseases that mimic renal cystic disease

Multilocular cystic nephroma

A multilocular cystic nephroma is an uncommon, benign cystic renal tumour. It tends to occur in young males less than 4 years of age or adult women. It is important to understand the nature of this rare benign tumour in order to avoid confusion with a cystic renal cell carcinoma or a multiloculated cyst that had been previously complicated by a haemorrhage or infection. A multiloculated cystic nephroma should be unilateral and should be solitary with a well-defined capsule which encompasses all the cyst (Fig. 8.29). Within this well-defined capsule should be multiple cystic areas with uniform thin wall thickness. There should be no solid mass associated within the capsular margins of this multi-loculated cystic mass (Madewell *et al.* 1983).

Despite strict adherence to the above features, it may be difficult to differentiate a multiloculated cystic nephroma from a cystic renal cell carcinoma. Therefore, many of these patients unfortunately have to undergo nephrectomy for definite evaluation.

CT without and with IV contrast or MRI without and with gadolinium contrast are the most helpful imaging modalities to characterize this mass. Sonography can also be utilized but may often not be able to visualize all portions of the mass because of a limited acoustic window and the size of these masses. The image findings on excretory urography are not reliable enough to differentiate from a cystic renal cell carcinoma or even a solid renal mass.

Cystic renal cell carcinomas

Most renal cell carcinomas contain small cystic areas. These cystic areas are often due to necrosis within a highly vascular tumour. However, sometimes a cystic component predominates, and such lesions are called cystic renal cell carcinomas. These cystic masses in the kidney can be misdiagnosed as benign simple or complex cysts. This is potentially harmful since simple cysts are not

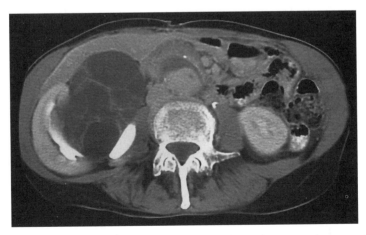

Fig. 8.29 Contrast-enhanced CT scan of the kidneys demonstrating a multilocular cystic nephroma arising from the perihilar region of the right kidney. Note the multiple internal septations surrounded by a well-defined capsule.

usually evaluated further. There are three pathological and radiologic patterns of cystic renal cell carcinoma: unilocular, multilocular, and discrete.

Unilocular cystic renal cell carcinoma usually results from extensive necrosis of previously solid renal cell carcinoma, although it may rarely be due to intrinsic cystic growth, such as in cyst adenocarcinomas. This type of cystic renal cell carcinoma is most common and is seen in about 50 per cent of renal cell carcinomas. Excretory urography is usually non-specific, and sonography and CT are best utilized in this type of mass. Sonography and CT generally show a fluid-filled mass which does not fulfil the simple criteria for a simple cyst (Fig. 8.30) (Charboneau *et al.* 1983). However, on CT the cystic tumour content may have a fluid attenuation value.

Multilocular renal cell carcinomas are composed of multiple, variably sized, irregular, non-communicating, fluid-filled, cystic spaces (Feldberg and vanWaes 1982). These locules can contain variable amounts of new and old blood and can be difficult to distinguish from a multilocular cystic nephroma which is usually a benign lesion.

Discrete mural tumour nodules in a cystic mass are the third pattern seen in cystic renal cell carcinomas (Foster *et al.* 1985). In this type of pattern, a tumour arises in the wall of a pre-existing simple renal cyst. In order to detect this rare presentation, meticulous technique must be applied to the evaluation of all potential simple renal cysts to exclude any nodular aspect to the cyst wall. This tumour nodule can be evaluated with ultrasound or CT guided needle biopsies if necessary. Angiographic evaluation can also be utilized to look for neovascularity in the tumour nodule.

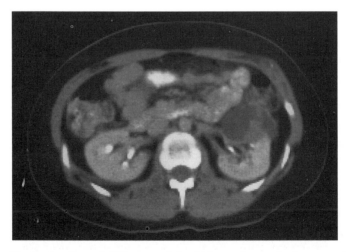

Fig. 8.30 Contrast-enhanced CT scan of the kidneys demonstrating a septated cystic renal cell carcinoma arising from the anterior portion of the left kidney. Note the thick nodular wall within the cystic mass which differentiates this mass from other benign cystic masses, such as a multiloculated cystic nephroma.

Cystic Wilms' tumours

Occasionally, Wilms' tumours can be multifocal and involve both kidneys. Although these tumours are often low in density on CT scans, they generally enhance and can confidently be identified as multiple solid lesions. Rarely, marked cystic change within multiple tumours or within a large Wilms' tumour may lead to the misinterpretation of a kidney or kidneys as polycystic kidneys (DeCampo 1986). Close attention to pre- and post-contrast enhanced images is paramount in order to clarify solid tissue components in polycystic kidneys that could represent solid Wilms' tumours.

Lymphoma

Secondary renal involvement of lymphoma generally occurs due to dissemination of pre-existing lymphoma. The appearance of multiple lymphomatous nodules in both kidneys can mimic that of ADPKD on excretory urography. Because lymphoma is markedly hypoechoic on ultrasound and very low density on CT, it is possible to misinterpret multiple lymphomatous masses in the kidneys as cystic lesions. Close attention to proper gain and power settings on ultrasound, as well as CT density, is important to avoid misdiagnosing renal lymphoma as multiple renal cysts.

Aneurysms and fistulas

Although most renal artery aneurysms occur in the proximal 1–2 cm of the renal artery, some renal artery aneurysms occur near the hilum of the kidney and can mimic cystic renal masses or renal sinus cysts. On ultrasound, the aneurysm may satisfy all the criteria for a simple renal cyst; however, one must always consider the use of Doppler to rule in or rule out blood flow within the cystic mass. If blood flow is demonstrated on Doppler, the diagnosis of a renal artery aneurysm can be made confidently (Lewis *et al.* 1989).

Arteriovenous malformations within the renal parenchyma can also appear as cystic renal masses. Generally, the cystic renal masses appear serpiginous in shape and nature and may be confused with a dilated calyx or collecting system. Again, the use of Doppler allows for definitive diagnosis of an arteriovenous malformation by demonstrating blood flow within the cystic spaces.

Infectious diseases

Many infectious processes of the kidneys can be mistaken for complex cystic masses, and important clinical information can be extremely valuable in order to make accurately the diagnosis of cystic infectious masses.

Echinococcal disease can result in cystic masses within the kidneys. Hydatid disease is predominantly found in sheep- and cattle-raising areas world-wide. It is divided into two major varieties: the less common multilocular or alveolar variety (*Echinococcus multilocularis*) and the more common unilocular or cystic hydatid disease (*Echinococcus granulosus*). These cysts in both types of varieties may or may not be calcified. Multiple ring-shaped calcifications within a larger calcified lesion suggest the presence of daughter cysts. The CT and sonographic appearances of renal hydatid cysts may appear as round, anechoic cysts with somewhat thicker than normal cyst walls. Mural irregularity and calcification may also be seen. As the cysts mature, daughter cysts are developed and the CT and ultrasound appearance may be that of a multilocular structure with curvilinear septa within the cysts. Daughter cysts may arrange themselves peripherally around the mother cysts.

Bacterial abscesses

Although the vast majority of renal infections undergo resolution with proper treatment, progression of the infection sometimes occurs that can result in renal abscesses. Two types of renal abscesses can develop. The first is a progression of focal bacterial pyelonephritis into liquefactive necrosis. The second type of renal abscess is often due to hematogenous spread of virulent bacteria such as Staphylococcus, Streptococcus, or Enterobacteriaceae.

Renal abscesses are usually easy to differentiate from simple benign cysts because of higher attenuation values of the abscess fluid and usually a thick wall on CT. A renal abscess on ultrasound has a typical sonographic appearance of a round, thick-walled hypoechoic mass containing internal echoes. Gas may be present within a renal abscess on both ultrasound and CT. Rarely, renal abscesses will have a thin wall and may be anechoic. In such cases, percutaneous needle aspiration of the cyst fluid may be necessary to rule in or rule out a renal abscess. In addition, haemorrhagic cysts, infected cysts, or necrotic neoplasms may each display the sonographic findings found in renal abscesses. Therefore, clinical correlation with laboratory and clinical findings is paramount.

References

Abeshouse, B. S. and Abeshouse, G. A. (1960). Sponge kidney: A review of the literature and a report of five cases. *J. Urol.*, **84**, 252–66.

Atiyeh, B., Husmann, D., and Baum, M. (1992). Contralateral renal abnormalities in multicystic-dysplastic kidney disease. *J. Pediatr.*, **121**, 65–7.

Avni, E. F., Thoua, Y., Lalmand, B., Didier, F., Droulle, P., and Schulman, C. C. (1986). Multicystic dysplastic kidney: evolving concepts — *in utero* diagnosis and post-natal follow-up by ultrasound. *Ann. Radiol.*, **29**, 663–8.

Balfe, D. M., McClennan, B. L., Stanley, R. J., Weyman, P. J., and Sagel, S. S. (1982). Evaluation of renal masses considered indeterminate on computed tomography. *Radiology*, **142**, 421–8.

Barrie, H. J. (1953). Paracalyceal cysts of the renal sinus. *Am. J. Pathol.*, **29**, 985–91.

Bernstein, J. (1990). A classification of renal cysts. In *The cystic kidney*, (ed. K. D. Gardner Jr and J. Bernstein), pp. 147–70. Kluwer, Dordrecht.

Bernstein, J. (1993). Glomerulocystic kidney disease — nosological considerations. *Pediatr. Nephrol.*, **7**, 464–70.

Bernstein, J. and Landing, B. H. (1989). Glomerulocystic kidney disease. *Prog. Clin. Biol. Res.*, **305**, 27.

Best, D. L., King, B. F., Hattery, R. R., Torres, V. E. and Gomez, M. R. (1993). Spectrum of findings in renal cystic disease associated with tuberous clerosis (Abstract). *RSNA*, Chicago, IL.

Boag, G. S., and Nolan, R. (1988). CT visualization of medullary sponge kidney. *Urol. Radiol.*, **9**, 220.

Boal, D. K. and Littlewood Teele, R. (1980). Sonography of infantile polycystic kidney disease. *Am J. Roentgenol.*, **135**, 575–80.

Bosniak, M. A. (1986). The current radiological approach to renal cysts. *Radiology*, **158**, 1–10.

Bosniak, M. A. (1991*a*) Differentiating between benign and malignant cystic lesions of the kidney (Abstract). *Radiology*, **181**, 293.

Bosniak, M. A. (1991*b*) Difficulties in classifying cystic lesions of the kidney. *Urol. Radiol.*, **13**, 91.

Cantani, A., Bellioni, P., Bamonte, G., Salvinelli, F., and Bamonte, M. T. (1985). Seven hereditary syndromes with pigmentary retinopathy. *Clin. Pediatr.*, **24**, 578–83.

Carson, R. W., Bedi, D., Cavallo, T., and DuBose, T. D. Jr (1987). Familial adult glomerulocystic kidney disease. *Am. J. Kidney Dis.*, **9**, 154–65.

Chan, J. C. M. and Kodroff, M. B. (1980). Hypertension and hematuria secondary to parapelvic cyst. *Pediatrics*, **65**, 821–2.

Charboneau, J. W., Hattery, R. R., Ernst, E. C., James, E. M., Williamson, B. Jr. and Hartman, G. W. (1983). Spectrum of sonographic findings in 125 renal masses other than benign simple cysts. *AJR*, **140**, 87–94.

Childton, S. J. and Cremin, B. J. (1981). The spectrum of polycystic disease in children. *Pediatr. Radiol.* **11**, 9–15.

Cho, K. J., Thornbury, J. R., Bernstein, J., Heidelberger, K. P., and Walter, J. F. (1979). Localized cystic disease of the kidney: angiographic-pathologic correlation. *AJR*, **132**, 891–5.

Choyke, P. L., *et al.* (1992). *AJR*, **159**, 1229.

Cobben, J. M., Breuning, M. H., Schoots, C., ten Kate, L. P., and Zerres, K. (1990). Congenital hepatic fibrosis in autosomal-dominant polycystic kidney disease. *Kidney Internat.*, **38**, 880–5.

Cole, B. R. (1990). Autosomal recessive polycystic kidney disease. In *The cystic kidney*, (ed. K. D. Gardner Jr and J. Bernstein), pp. 327–50. Kluwer, Boston.

Cole, B. R., Conley, S. B., and Stapleton, F. B. (1987). Polycystic kidney disease in the first year of life. *J. Pediatr.*, **111**, 693–9.

Cover, D. E., Torres, V. E., Hattery, R. R., and Berquist, T. H. (1988). Bilateral hemorrhagic parapelvic pseudocysts. *Am. J. Kidney Dis.*, **11**, 343–8.

Cronan, J. J., Amis, E. S. Jr, Yoder, I. C., Kopans, D. B., Simeone, J. F., and Pfister, R. C. (1982). Peripelvic cysts: An impostor of sonographic hydronephrosis. *J. Ultrasound. Med.*, **1**, 229–36.

Curry, N. S., Milutinovic, J., Grossnickle, M., and Munden, M. (1992). Renal cystic disease associated with orofaciodigital syndrome. *Urol. Radiol.*, **13**, 153–7.

Daniel, W. W. Jr, Hartman, G. W., Witten, D. M., Farrow, G. M., and Kelalis, P. P. (1972). Calcified renal masses: A review of 10 years experience at the Mayo Clinic. *Radiology*, **103**, 503–8.

Davidson, A. J. (1985). *Radiology of the kidney*, pp. 398–402. Saunders, Philadelphia, PA.

DeCampo, J. F. (1986). Ultrasound of Wilms' tumor. *Pediatr. Radiol.*, **16**, 21–4.

Deliveliotis, A. and Kavadis, C. (1969). Parapelvic cysts of the kidney: Report of seven cases. *Br. J. Urol.*, **41**, 386–93.

Dubilier, W. and Evans, J. A. (1958). Peripelvic cysts of the kidney. *Radiology*, 71, 404–8.

Elkin, M. and Bernstein, J. (1969). Cystic diseases of the kidney; Radiological and pathological considerations. *Clinical Radiology* 20, 65–82.

Feldberg, M. A. and van Waes, P. F. (1982). Multilocular cystic renal cell carcinoma. *AJR*, 138, 953–5.

Fitch, S. J. and Stapleton, F. B. (1986). Ultrasonographic features of glomerulocystic disease in infancy: similarity to infantile polycystic kidney disease. *Pediatr. Radiol.*, 16, 400–2.

Foster, W. L., Halvorsen, R. A., and Dunnick, N. R. (1985). The clandestine renal cell carcinoma: Atypical appearances and presentations. *Radiographics*, 5, 175–92.

Gagnadoux, M.-F., Habib, R., Levy, M., Brunelle, F., and Broyer, M. (1989). Cystic renal diseases in children. *Adv. Nephrol.*, 18, 33–58.

Gibson, T. E. (1954). Interrelationship of renal cysts and tumors. Report of three cases. *J. Urol.* 71, 241–52.

Glazer, G. M., Callen, P. W., and Filly, R. A. (1982). Medullary nephrocalcinosis: Sonographic evaluation. *AJR*, 138, 55–7.

Gomez, M. R. (ed.) (1988). *Tuberous sclerosis*, (2nd edn). Raven, New York.

Gordon, A. C., Thomas, D. F. M., Arthur, R. J., and Irving, H. C. (1988). MCDK: Is nephrectomy still appropriate? *J. Urol.* 140, 1231–4.

Gourdol, O., *et al.* (1984). L' Atteinte renale dans le syndrome de Laurence–Moon–Bardet–Biedl. *Pediatrie*, 39, 175–81.

Griscom, N. T., Vawter, G. F., and Felles, F. X. (1975). Pelvi-infundibular atresia: the usual form of multicystic kidney: 44 unilateral and 2 bilateral cases. *Semin. Roentgenol.*, 10, 113–23.

Hashimoto, B. E., Filly, R. A., and Callen, P. W. (1986). Multicystic dysplastic kidney in utero: changing appearance on US. *Radiology*, 159, 107–9.

Hellweg, G. (1954). Über Hiluscysten der Nieren. *Virchows Arch A*, 325, S98–108.

Hendry, P. J. and Hendry, G. M. A. (1991). Observations on the use of Doppler ultrasound in multicystic dysplastic kidney. *Pediatr. Radiol.*, 21, 203–4.

Herman, T. E. and Siegel, M. J. (1991). Pyramidal hyperechogenicity in autosomal recessive polycystic kidney disease resembling medullary nephrocalcinosis. *Pediatr. Radiol.*, 21, 270–1.

Jackman, R. J., and Stevens, G. M. (1974). Benign hemorrhagic renal cysts. Nephrotomography, renal arteriography and cyst puncture. *Radiology*, 110, 7–13.

Kääriäinen, H., Jääskeläinen, J. Kivisaari, L., Koskimies, O., and Norio, R. (1988). Dominant and recessive polycystic kidney disease in children: classification by intravenous pyelography, ultrasound, and computed tomography. *Pediatr. Radiol.*, 18, 45–50.

Keith, D. S., Torres, V. E., King, B. F., Zincke, H. and Farrow, G. M. (1994). Renal cell carcinoma in autosomal dominant polycystic kidney disease. *J. Am. Soc. Nephrol.*, 4, 1661–9.

Kennedy, S. M., Hashida, Y., and Malatack, J. J. (1991). Polycystic kidneys, pancreatic cysts, and cystadenomatous bile ducts in the oral-facial-digital syndrome type I. *Arch. Pathol. Lab. Med.*, 115, 519–23.

Kirks, K. R., Rosenberg, E. R., Johnson, D. G., and King, L. R. (1985). Integrated imaging of neonatal renal masses. *Pediatr. Radiol.*, 15, 147–56.

Kissane, J. M. (1974). Congenital malformations. In *Pathology of the kidney*, (ed. R. H. Hepinstall), pp. 69–119. Little, Brown, Boston.

Kogutt, M. S., Robichaux, W. H., Boineau, F. G., Drake, G. K., and Simonton, S. C. (1993). Asymmetric renal size in autosomal recessive polycystic kidney disease: a unique presentation. *Am. J. Roentgenol.*, **160**, 835–6.

Laucks, S. P. Jr and McLachlan, M. S. F. (1981). Aging and simple cysts of the kidney. *Br. J. Radiol.*, **54**, 12–14.

Lee, K. R., Wulfsberg, E., and Kepes, J. J. (1977). Some important radiological aspects of the kidney in Hippel–Lindau syndrome: The value of prospective study in an affected family. *Radiology*, **122**, 649–53.

Leung, A. W., Bydder, G. M., Steiner, R. E., Bryant, D. J., and Young, I. R. (1984). Magnetic resonance imaging of the kidney. *AJR*, **143**, 1215–27.

Levine, E. and Grantham, J. J. (1981). The role of computed tomography in the evaluation of adult polycystic kidney disease. *Am. J. Kidney. Dis.*, **1**, 99–105.

Levine, E. and Grantham, J. J. (1985). High-density renal cysts in autosomal dominant polycystic kidney disease demonstrated by CT. *Radiology*, **154**, 477–82.

Levine, E. and Grantham, J. J. (1987). Perinephric hemorrhage in autosomal dominant polycystic kidney disease: CT and MR findings. *J. Comput. Assist. Tomogr.*, **11**, 108.

Levine, E., Slusher, S. L., Grantham, J. J., and Wetzel, L. H. (1981). Natural history of acquired renal cystic disease in dialysis patients: A prospective longitudinal CT study. *AJR*, **156**, 501–6.

Levine, E., Collins, D. L., Horton, W. A., and Schimke, R. N. (1982). CT screening of the abdomen in von Hippel–Lindau disease. *AJR*, **139**, 505–10.

Levine, E., Grantham, J. J., Slusher, S. L., Greathouse, J. L., and Krohn, B. P. (1984). CT of acquired cystic kidney disease and renal tumors in long-term dialysis patients. *AJR*, **142**, 125–31.

Levine, E., Cook, L. T., and Grantham, J. J. (1985). Liver cysts in autosomal dominant polycystic kidney disease. Clinical and computed tomographic study. *AJR*, **145**, 229–33.

Lewis, B. D., James, M. E., Charboneau, J. W., Reading, C. C., and Welch, T. J. (1989). Current applications of color Doppler imaging in the abdomen and extremities. *Radiographics*, **9**, 599–631.

Lieberman, E., Salinas-Madrigal, L., Gwinn, J. L., Brennan, L. P., Fine, R. N., and Landing, B. H. (1971). Infantile polycystic disease of the kidneys and liver; clinical, pathological, and radiological correlations and comparison with congenital hepatic fibrosis. *Medicine*, **50**, 277–318.

Lingard, D. A. and Lawson, T. L. (1979). Accuracy of ultrasound in predicting the nature of renal masses. *J. Urol.*, **122**, 724–7.

Linné, T., Wikstad, I., and Zetterström, R. (1986). Renal involvement in the Laurence–Moon–Biedl syndrome. *Acta. Paediatr. Scand.* **75**, 240–4.

Lipschitz, B., Berdon, W. E., Defelice, A. R., and Levy, J. (1993). Association of congenital hepatic fibrosis with autosomal dominant polycystic kidney disease. Report of a family with review of literature. *Pediatr. Radiol.*, **23**, 131–3.

Lucaya, J., Enriquez, G., Nieto, J., Callis, L., Garcia Peña, P., and Dominguez, C. (1993). Renal calcifications in patients with autosomal recessive polycystic kidney disease: prevalence and cause. *Am. J. Roentgenol.*, **160**, 359–62.

Madewell, J. E., Goldman, S. M., and Davis, C. J. Jr (1983). Multilocular cystic nephroma: A radiographic pathologic correlation of 58 patients. *Radiology*, **146**, 309.

McAlister, W. H., Siegel, M. J., Shackelford, G. D., Askin, F., and Kissane, J. M. (1979). Glomerulocystic kidney. *Am. J. Roentgenol.*, **133**, 536.

McClennan, B. L., Stanley, R. J., Melson, G. L., Levitt, R. G., and Sagel, S. S. (1979). CT of the renal cyst: Is cyst aspiration necessary? *AJR*, **133**, 671–5.

McDonald, R. A. and Avner, E. D. (1991). Inherited polycystic kidney disease in children. *Sem. Nephrol.* **11**, 632–42.

Melson, G. L., Shackelford, G. D., Cole, B. R., and McClennan, B. L. (1985). The spectrum of sonographic findings in infantile polycystic kidney disease with urographic and clinical correlations. *J. Clin. Ultrasound.*, **13**, 113–19.

Menster, M., Mahan, J., and Koff, S. (1994). Multicystic dysplastic kidney. *Pediatr. Nephrol.*, **8**, 113–15.

Meredith, W. T., Levine, E., Ahlstrom, N. G., and Grantham, J. J. (1988). Exacerbation of familial renal lymphangiomatosis during pregnancy. *AJR*, **151**, 965–6.

Mesrobian, H. -G. J., Rushton, H. G., and Bulas, D. (1993). Unilateral renal agenesis may result from in utero regression of multicystic renal dysplasia. *J. Urol.*, **150**, 793–4.

Meyers, M. A. (1975). Uriniferous perirenal pseudocyst: New observations. *Radiology*, **117**, 539–45.

Murray, K. K. and McLellan, G. L. (1991). Renal peripelvic lymphangiectasia: Appearance at CT. *Radiology*, **180**, 455–6.

Narla, L. D., Slovis, T. L., Watts, F. B., and Nigro, M. (1988). The renal lesions of tuberous sclerosis (cysts and angiomyolipomas): Screening with sonography and computerized tomography. *Pediatr. Radiol.* **18**, 205–9.

Noe, H. N., Marshall, J. H. and Edwards , O. P. (1989). Nodular renal blastema in the multicystic kidney. **142**, 486–8.

Pedicelli, G., Jequier, S., Bowen, A. D., and Boisvert, J. (1986). Multicystic dysplastic kidneys: spontaneous regression demonstrated with US. *Radiology*, **160**, 23–6.

Premkumar, A., Berdon, W. E., Levy, J., Amodio, J., Abramson, S. J., and Newhouse, J. H. (1988). The emergence of hepatic fibrosis and portal hypertension in infants and children with autosomal recessive polycystic kidney disease. *Pediatr. Radiol.*, **18**, 123–9.

Pretorius, D. H., Lee, M. E., Manco-Johnson, M. L., Weingast, G. R., Sedman, A. B., and Gabow, P. A. (1987). Diagnosis of autosomal dominant polycystic kidney disease *in utero* and in the young infant. *J. Ultrasound Med.*, **6**, 249–55.

Ravine, D., *et al.* (1992). Phenotype and genotype heterogeneity in autosomal dominant polycystic kidney disease. *Lancet*, **340**, 1330–3.

Ravine, D., Gibson, R. N., Donlan, J. and Sheffield, L. J. (1993). An ultrasound renal cyst prevalence study: specificity data for inherited renal cystic diseases. *Am. J. Kidney Dis.*, **22**, 803–7.

Ravine, D., Gibson, R. N., Walker, R. G., Sheffield, L. J., Kincaid-Smith, P., and Danks, D. M. (1994). Evaluation of ultrasonographic diagnostic criteria for autosomal dominant polycystic kidney disease. *Lancet* **343**, 824–7.

Rickwood, A. M. K., Anderson, P. A. M., and Williams, M. P. L. (1992). Multicystic renal dysplasia detected by prenatal ultrasonography. Natural history and results of conservative management. *Br. J. Urol.*, **69**, 538–40.

Rothermel, F. J., Miller, F. J., Sanford, E., Drago, J., Rohner, T. J. (1977). Clinical and radiographic findings of focally infected polycystic kidneys. *Urology*, **9**, 580–5.

Scholl, A. J. (1948). Peripelvic lymphatic cysts of the kidney. *JAMA*, **136**, 4–7.

Schwartz, A., Lenz, T., Klaen, R., Offermann, G., Fiedler, V., and Nussberger, J. (1993). Hygroma renale: pararenal lymphatic cysts associated with renin dependent hypertension. *J. Urol.* **150**, 953–7.

Srinivas, V., Winsor, G. M., and Dow, D. (1983). Urologic manifestations of Laurence–Moon–Biedl syndrome. *Urology*, **21**, 581–3.

Strife, J. L., Souza, A. S., Kirks, D. R., Strife, C. F., Gelfand, M. J., and Wacksman, J. (1993). Multicystic dysplastic kidney in children: US follow-up. *Radiology*, **186**, 785–8.

Tada, S., Yamagishi, J., Kobayashi, H., Hata, Y., and Kobari, T. (1983). The incidence of simple renal cyst by computed tomography. *Clin. Radiol.*, **34**, 437–9.

Torres, V. E. (1990). Genetics of renal cystic diseases. In *Inheritance of kidney and urinary tract diseases*, (ed. A. Spritzer and E. D. Avner), pp. 178–219. Kluwer, Dordrecht.

Torres, V. E., Erickson, S. B., Smith, L. H., Wilson, D. M., Hattery, R. R., and Segura, J. W. (1988). The association of nephrolithiasis and autosomal dominant polycystic kidney disease. *Am. J. Kidney Dis.*, **11**, 318–25.

Torres, V. E., Wilson, D. M., Hattery, R. R., and Segura, J. W. (1993). Renal stone disease in autosomal dominant polycystic kidney disease. *Am. J. Kidney Dis.*, **22**, 513–19.

Torres, V. E., King, B. F., Holley, K. E., Blute, M. L., and Gomez, M. R. (1994). The kidney in the tuberous sclerosis complex. *Adv. Nephrol.*, **23**, 43–70.

Torres, V. E., *et al.* (1995). Extrapulmonary lymphangioleiomyomatosis and lymphangiomatous cysts in tuberous sclerosis complex. *Mayo Clinic Proceedings*, **70**, 641–8.

Vela Navarrete, R. and Garcia Robledo, A. (1983). Polycistic disease of the renal sinus: structural characteristics. *J. Urol.*, **129**, 700–3.

Vinocur, L., Slovis, T. L., Perlmutter, A. D., Watts, F. B. Jr, and Chang C.-H. (1988). Follow-up studies of multicystic dysplastic kidneys. *Radiology*, **167**, 311–15.

Wacksman, J. and Phipps, L. (1993). Report of the Multicystic Kidney Registry: Preliminary Findings. *J. Urol.*, **150**, 1870–2.

Wernecke, K., Heckemann, R., Bachmann, H., and Peters, P. E. (1985). Sonography of infantile polycystic kidney disease. *Urol. Radiol.*, **7**, 138–45.

Worthington, J. L., Shackelford, G. D., Cole, B. R., Tack, E. D., and Kissane, J. M. (1988). Sonographically detectable cysts in polycystic kidney disease in newborn and young infants. *Pediatr. Radiol.*, **18**, 287–93.

Zerres, K., Volpel, M. C., and Weiss, H. (1984). Cystic kidneys: genetics, pathologic anatomy, clinical picture, and prenatal diagnosis. *Hum. Genet.*, **68**, 104.

9

Autosomal recessive polycystic kidney disease: clinical and genetic profiles

Lisa M. Guay-Woodford

Introduction

Autosomal recessive polycystic kidney disease (ARPKD) is an inherited malformation complex that involves the kidney and the biliary tract. ARPKD encompasses a spectrum of clinical and histopathological manifestations. Yet, there are two invariant features: (1) fusiform dilatation of the renal collecting ducts; and (2) biliary dysgenesis associated with portal tract fibrosis (Bernstein and Slovis 1992). In the past, ARPKD has been variably referred to as infantile polycystic kidney disease, infantile polycystic disease of the kidneys and liver, sponge kidneys, microcystic kidney disease, and polycystic kidneys Potter type I (Zerres *et al.* 1984). While these designations were intended to describe either the predominant patient population or the key pathological features, they have tended to be more confusing than useful. For example, the clinical presentation of ARPKD can be delayed until adolescence or even adulthood (Kaplan *et al.* 1988; Neumann *et al.* 1988; Shaikewitz and Chapman 1993). Conversely, other clinically distinct polycystic kidney diseases can present in infancy (Cole *et al.* 1987; Kaplan *et al.* 1989*a*; Zerres *et al.* 1984). Therefore, the term 'ARPKD' is now generally preferred, because it reflects precise genetic description.

Exact incidence figures for ARPKD are not available. Estimates vary widely, ranging from 1/6000 live births in an American report to 1/40000 in the European literature (Bosniak and Ambos 1975; Zerres *et al.* 1984). The disparity in these estimates most likely results from differences in study populations and in study methodologies. Taking all available reports into account, the most representative incidence estimate is probably 1 to 2 per 10000 live births (Bernstein and Slovis 1992). Consistent with its autosomal recessive mode of inheritance, heterozygotes are unaffected and ARPKD is generally considered to have an equal sex distribution, although several reports cite a slightly increased prevalence in females (Bernstein and Slovis 1992; Gang and Herrin 1986; Kääriäinen 1987). Finally, although there is no conclusive evidence to suggest an ethnic predominance, review of the literature suggests that ARPKD occurs rarely in non-Caucasian populations (Kaplan *et al.* 1989*a*; Mattoo *et al.* 1994).

Embryology

Kidney

As in other mammals, human renal development is characterized by the successive formation of three distinct structures: the pronephros, the mesonephros, and the metanephros. The first two structures are transient and involute *in utero*. The metanephros gives rise to the definitive kidney (Saxen 1987).

Human metanephric kidney development begins at approximately four to five weeks gestation as a result of a complex set of mesenchymal–epithelial interactions between the ureteric bud and the metanephric mesenchyme. As shown in Fig. 9.1, the ureteric bud arises as an epithelial outgrowth of the mesonephric duct. As the ureteric bud extends dorsally and cephalad towards the metanephric mesenchyme, it divides dichotomously. These initial branches ultimately coalesce to form the renal pelvis and calyces (Osathanondh and Potter 1963; Evan and Larsson 1992).

Nephron formation begins at about the eighth week of gestation, as the ureteric bud branches induce the mesenchymal cells to begin a series of stereotypical changes (Fig. 9.2). Initially, the induced mesenchyme aggregates in a cap-like array around the advancing ureteric bud branches. Each condensed cellular mass becomes vesicular as its constituent cells undergo a mesenchymal to epithelial transformation, polarize, and form a lumen. The vesicular structures then progressively elongate to form S-shaped tubules. The lower portion of the tubule gives rise to the glomerular capsule. The remainder of the S-shaped structure differentiates into the proximal and distal tubule and the latter attaches to its associated ureteric bud branch. In a reciprocal fashion, the ureteric bud continues to divide dichotomously and its terminal branches differentiate into the collecting ducts. Newly formed branches of the ureteric bud contact uninduced cells of the metanephric mesenchyme and these in turn differentiate into the epithelial segments described above. Nephrogenesis proceeds in a centrifugal pattern, from the inner cortex to the periphery and is completed by 34 weeks gestation (Mugrauer *et al.* 1988; Osathanondh and Potter 1963; Evan and Larson 1992). The factors which direct terminal differentiation of the glomeruli and the tubular elements remain largely unknown.

Liver

Liver development similarly begins during the fourth week of human gestation. However, unlike the developing kidney where the ureteric bud invaginates a predetermined mesenchyme and induces an epithelial transformation, liver development is initiated when the ventral foregut mesenchyme undergoes an epithelial transformation and as a result, the hepatic diverticulum buds from the foregut wall (Desmet 1991). The cranial portion of this diverticulum gives rise to the hepatoblasts or hepatocyte precursor cells. Some of these hepatocyte precursors then migrate between the developing sinusoids to establish the architectural framework of the liver parenchyma (Desmet 1991). Data from morphological

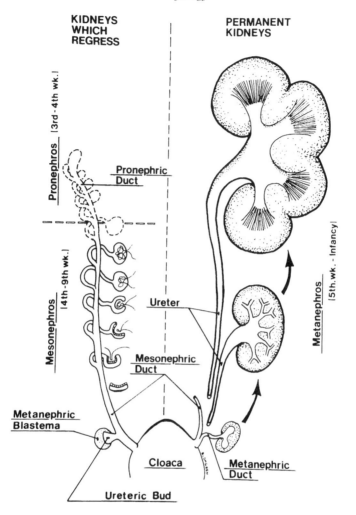

KIDNEYS WHICH REGRESS

PERMANENT KIDNEYS

Pronephros (3rd - 4th wk.)

Pronephric Duct

Mesonephros (4th - 9th wk.)

Ureter

Mesonephric Duct

Metanephric Blastema

Cloaca

Metanephric Duct

Ureteric Bud

Metanephros (5th. wk. - Infancy)

Fig. 9.1 *Mammalian renal development.* On the left, the initial events of pronephric and mesonephric development are illustrated. These structures involute early in gestation. As depicted on the right, the definitive kidney results from a series of reciprocal interactions between the ureteric bud and the metanephric blastema or mesenchyme. From Evan and Larssen (1992) with permission.

and immunohistochemical studies suggest that other hepatic precursor cells ultimately give rise to the intrahepatic biliary system (Desmet 1992). The caudal portion of the hepatic diverticulum develops into the common bile duct and the gallbladder (Desmet 1991).

The development of the intrahepatic biliary tree begins at about the eighth week of gestation. Hepatic precursor cells that lie adjacent to the hilar portal vein vessels undergo transformation to a biliary phenotype (Desmet 1992). This

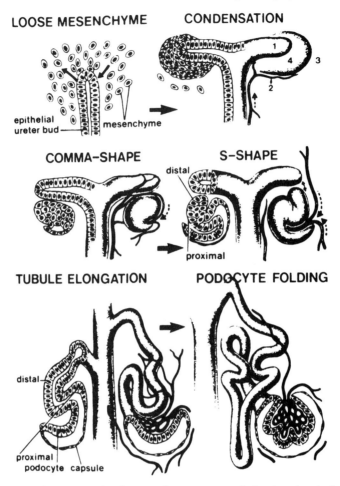

Fig. 9.2 *Schema for nephron development.* In response to inductive signals from the advancing ureteric bud branch, the metanephric mesenchyme is induced to undergo epithelial transformation (top left panel). In the condensation stage, the (1) ureteric bud branch, (2) the ingrowing blood vessels, (3) the uninduced mesenchyme, and (4) the induced mesenchyme are evident. Subsequently, the induced mesenchyme develops into a comma-shaped, then S-shaped structure, and the tubule elongates. At the lower portion of the tubule, the glomerular podocytes become folded and tortuous and the upper portion of tubule fuses with the ureteric bud branch. From Mugrauer *et al.* (1988) with permission.

sleeve-like layer of cells is then duplicated and extends toward the periphery along the smaller intrahepatic portal vein branches. As a result, the portal vein ramifications are surrounded by a double-layered sleeve of epithelial cells that are separated by a slit or plate-like lumen. Hammer designated this sleeve-like structure the 'ductal plate' (DP) (Jorgensen 1977).

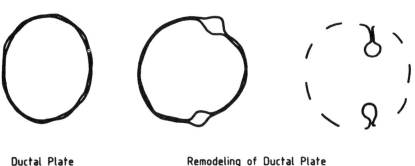

Ductal Plate   **Remodeling of Ductal Plate**

Fig. 9.3 *Schematic representation of ductal plate formation and remodelling.* A single layer of hepatocyte precursor cells surrounding the portal vein branch undergoes transformation to a biliary phenotype. The layer is duplicated and this double-layered sleeve is referred to as the 'ductal plate'. Short segments of the ductal plate dilate to form tubules and these are subsequently incorporated into the periportal mesenchyme. The remainder of the ductal plate involutes. From Desmet (1992) with permission.

Beginning at 12 weeks gestation and extending into the post-natal period, the DP undergoes progressive remodelling. This process begins at the hilum in the oldest DP and proceeds toward the periphery. As shown in Fig. 9.3, short segments of the double-layered sleeve dilate to form tubules. As they form, individual bile ductules are incorporated into the periportal mesenchyme that surrounds the portal vein branches (Desmet 1991; Van Eycken *et al.* 1988). In contrast, those hepatocyte precursor cells that are not associated with the differentiating DP and bile ductules eventually give rise to differentiated liver parenchymal cells (Desmet 1991; Van Eycken *et al.* 1988).

The genetic factor(s) which dictate the differentiation and remodelling of the DP remain to be elucidated. However, the available evidence suggests that biliary differentiation involves a series of interactions between the mesenchyme surrounding the portal vein branches and the DP epithelia (Desmet *et al.* 1990; Van Eycken *et al.* 1988; Shah and Gerber 1990). As a result, the DP is induced to form bile ductules, the ductules are incorporated into periportal mesenchyme and the non-tubular elements of the DP are absorbed. Thus, during successive periods of fetal life, DP remodelling leads to the formation of the intrahepatic biliary tree. The largest ducts are formed first, followed by the segmental, interlobular, and finally by the smallest bile ductules.

Pathogenesis

In ARPKD, the renal cystic lesion appears to be superimposed on normal kidney development. In an exquisitely detailed series of microdissection studies, Osathanondh and Potter determined that the number and distribution of collecting ducts and nephrons are normal in these kidneys (Osathanondh and Potter 1964). As shown schematically in Fig. 9.4, the tubular abnormality in ARPKD

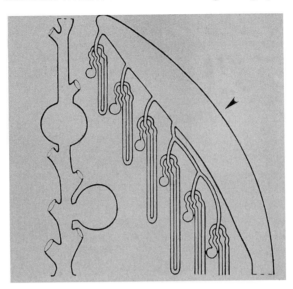

Fig. 9.4 *Schematic representation of the tubular lesion in ARPKD.* The cystic dilatation is confined to the collecting ducts (arrow), while the remainder of the nephron, including the glomerulus is structurally normal. From Potter (1972), with permission.

specifically involves fusiform dilatations of the collecting ducts. Electron microscopy studies have demonstrated that tubular obstruction is not involved in the pathogenesis (Osathanondh and Potter 1964, Kissane 1990). While the lesion involves all generations of collecting ducts, the terminal branches, including the cortical rays, are predominantly affected. Typically, the extent of the collecting duct involvement varies inversely with the age of presentation (Blyth and Ockenden 1971). In affected fetuses and neonates, 90 per cent of the collecting tubules are dilated, whereas, only 10 per cent are dilated in adolescents. By careful microdissection, a few connecting tubules, distal convoluted tubules, and ascending limbs were also found to be dilated. Furthermore, in some 30 per cent of nephrons, the angle of the loop of Henle contains a small cyst. The histopathological pattern has been termed polycystic kidneys, Potter type I (Osathanondh and Potter 1964). Interstitial, renal vascular, and glomerular abnormalities are not significant features of ARPKD (Osathanondh and Potter 1964).

In contrast, the biliary lesion appears to result from an early arrest or derangement in DP remodelling. This defect leads to the persistence of primitive bile duct configurations, or to what Jorgensen termed the 'ductal plate malformation' (DPM) (Jorgensen 1977). According to this paradigm, the DPM in ARPKD involves the 12th–20th week generations of the branching biliary epithelia (Desmet 1992). Desmet and others have postulated that the defective DP remodelling may induce variable degrees of necro-inflammation and destruction of immature intrahepatic bile ducts (Desmet 1992). Portal fibrosis is apparently a secondary consequence of the DPM. The remainder of the liver parenchyma develops normally. The defect in DP remodelling is also accompanied by portal vein branching abnormalities, resulting in a 'pollard willow' pattern of portal tract ramifications (Desmet 1992). Taken together, these events lead to the histopathological pattern referred to as congenital hepatic fibrosis (CHF).

Over the past 10–20 years, extensive experimental data have been generated regarding mechanisms of renal cyst formation. Based on these data, three working hypotheses have been proposed to account for renal cyst development. These include:

(1) tubule obstruction resulting in elevated tubular pressure;
(2) defective basement membrane assembly with resulting abnormalities in compliance; or
(3) dysregulated epithelial proliferation.

The weight of the experimental evidence from human and animal model studies suggests that a block in the terminal differentiation of the collecting duct epithelia leads to renal cyst development in recessive polycystic kidney disease (reviewed in Calvet 1993; Gattone and Grantham 1991). Similarly, the available evidence suggests that the biliary lesion in ARPKD results from an arrest in DP remodelling (Desmet 1992). Therefore, a proposed maturational arrest in both renal and biliary tubulo-epithelial differentiation could serve as a single unifying hypothesis to explain the development of renal cysts, the biliary dysgenesis, and the portal fibrosis that evolve in ARPKD.

Pathological anatomy

Kidney

The renal involvement in ARPKD is invariably bilateral and largely symmetrical, but the gross appearance of the kidneys varies depending on the age of presentation and the extent of cystic involvement.

In the affected neonate, the kidney weight can be as much as 10 times normal (Blyth and Ockenden 1971; Osathanondh and Potter 1964; Lieberman *et al.* 1971). Despite the large size, these kidneys retain a reniform configuration (Fig. 9.5A). The capsular surface is smooth and closely studded with 1–2 mm opalescent cysts. Cut section discloses that these cysts represent the cortical extension of fusiform collecting ducts that extend radially through the cortex (Fig. 9.5B). The medulla contains similarly dilated collecting ducts, but these are more often cut tangentially or transversely. Up to 90 per cent of the collecting ducts are involved and the corticomedullary junction is obscured. The renal pelvis, ureters, and bladder are structurally normal (Osathanondh and Potter 1964; Lieberman *et al.* 1971).

Microscopically, all cysts are lined with a single layer of nondescript cuboidal epithelium, typical of the collecting system. The collecting duct origin of the

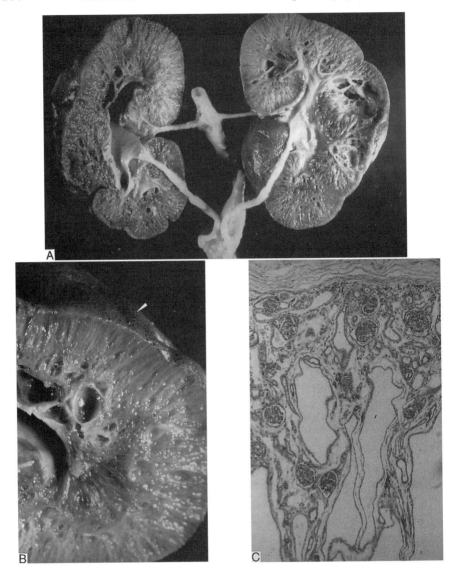

Fig. 9.5 *Renal pathology in ARPKD.* (A) The kidneys are symmetrically enlarged and maintain their reniform contour. The renal collecting system is structurally normal. (B) Cut section reveals the radially arrayed, cystic collecting ducts. These extend through the cortex and appear on the capsular surface as 1–2 mm opalescent cysts (arrow). (C) Microscopically, these dilated collecting ducts are radially oriented and run perpendicular to the renal capsule. While structurally normal, the glomeruli and remaining nephron segments are displaced into subcapsular wedges by the ectatic collecting ducts. (Courtesy of Dr Elizabeth Mroczek-Musulman, Department of Pathology, Children's Hospital of Alabama).

cysts has been confirmed by histochemical and lectin-binding studies (Faraggiana *et al.* 1985; Holthofer *et al.* 1990; Verani *et al.* 1989). The glomeruli and nephron segments proximal to the collecting ducts are structurally normal but, are often crowded between ectatic collecting ducts or displaced into subcapsular wedges (Fig. 9.5C) (Welling and Grantham 1991). In neonatal kidneys, there is little evidence of fibrosis. The presence of cartilage or other dysplastic elements suggests a diagnosis other than ARPKD.

In those who survive the perinatal period, the kidney size and extent of cystic involvement tend to be more limited (Blyth and Ockenden 1971; Osathanondh and Potter 1964). Typically, between 10 and 60 per cent of the collecting ducts are involved in these individuals. The cysts can expand up to 2 cm in diameter, assume a more spherical configuration, and be more irregularly distributed. These cystic changes are typically accompanied by progressive glomerular obsolescence, tubular atrophy, and interstitial fibrosis (Welling and Grantham 1991). As a result, the gross contour of the kidney becomes more irregular and a reduction in kidney size can occur. Based on a longitudinal analysis, Lieberman and co-workers reported that kidney size in affected patients peaks at 1 to 2 years of age, then gradually declines and stabilizes by 4 to 5 years of age (Lieberman *et al.* 1971). Prominent medullary ectasia persists, and in older children, may be the principle renal manifestation of ARPKD. Given this disease progression, ARPKD in older children may be mistaken for autosomal dominant polycystic kidney disease (ADPKD). In adults with medullary ectasia alone, the cystic lesion may be confused with medullary sponge kidney (Herrin 1989; Lieberman *et al.* 1971; Six *et al.* 1975).

Liver

Grossly, the liver in ARPKD can be either normal in size or somewhat enlarged and has a firm, almost gritty texture (Blyth and Ockenden 1971; Lieberman *et al.* 1971). On cut section, the liver is intersected by delicate fibrous septa which often link the portal tracts (Fig. 9.6A) (Summerfield *et al.* 1986). Microscopically, DPM is always found. The interlobular bile ducts are increased in number, rather tortuous in configuration and are often located along the periphery of the portal tract (Fig. 9.6B) (Alvarez *et al.* 1981; Bernstein *et al.* 1988; Desmet 1992). Few if any normal bile ducts are evident. There are varying degrees of portal fibrosis, hypoplasia of the small portal vein branches, and hepatic arteriolar prominence (Bernstein and Slovis 1992; Desmet 1992). Other abnormalities, such as degeneration of the biliary duct epithelium and mild cholestasis, are occasionally evident (Jorgensen 1977). However, the hepatocytes are not affected and liver synthetic function is usually unimpaired.

In the classic descriptions, the severity of the portal fibrosis and the associated pre-sinusoidal block ranges from minimal in infants to marked in older patients (Blyth and Ockenden 1971; Lieberman *et al.* 1971; Zerres *et al.* 1984). In the most severely affected patients, the extensive portal fibrosis and the occasional formation of fibrous septa may distort the lobular architecture of the liver (Gang

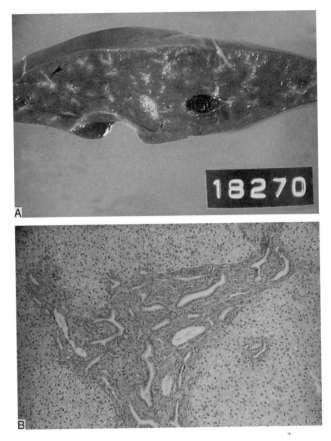

Fig. 9.6 *Biliary tract pathology in ARPKD.* (A) The liver can be either normal in size or somewhat enlarged. Cut section reveals delicate fibrous septa that connect the portal tracts (arrow). Otherwise, the liver parenchyma has a normal appearance. (B) Microscopically, the characteristic ductal plate malformation is evident. The interlobular bile ducts are increased in number, tortuous in their configuration, and often evident along the periphery of the ductal plate. The portal tract is expanded by fibrous tissue but there is no evidence of cirrhosis. (Courtesy of Dr Elizabeth Mroczek-Musulman, Department of Pathology, Children's Hospital of Alabama).

and Herrin 1986; Landing *et al.* 1980). However, the degree of fibrosis does not always correlate precisely with age and the biliary lesion may or may not be progressive (Welling and Grantham 1991). While bile ductules are often dilated, frank cysts are unusual. Yet, there are case reports of ARPKD associated with gross cystic dilatation of the entire intrahepatic biliary system, a condition otherwise referred to as Caroli's disease (Sung *et al.* 1992).

Clinical manifestations

The clinical spectrum of ARPKD is variable but the majority of cases present in infancy. In their classic report, Blyth and Ockenden unequivocally subdivided

ARPKD into four distinct phenotypes according to the age of presentation and the proportion of dilated renal collecting ducts: 90 per cent or more (perinatal); 60 per cent (neonatal); 25 per cent (infantile); and less than 10 per cent (juvenile) (Blyth and Ockenden 1971). They postulated that while the quantitative extent of renal cyst formation is variable in ARPKD, the cystic phenotype tends to breed true in families. Therefore, they proposed that these phenotypes were the result of four distinct genetic mutations. In this schema, the extent of hepatic fibrosis is inversely correlated with the age of presentation and the severity of renal involvement. More recent data suggests that ARPKD phenotypes are not so precisely circumscribed. In fact, numerous sibships have been reported in whom there are significant differences in the degrees of renal and hepatic involvement (Chilton and Cremin 1981; Gang and Herrin 1986; Herrin 1989; Kääriäinen 1988b; Kaplan et al. 1988, 1989a; Lieberman et al. 1971; Resnick and Vernier 1981). There are cases with early childhood onset in which severe liver involvement is predominant and other cases with the clinical onset of ARPKD in adulthood, but without evidence of portal hypertension (Zerres et al. 1984; Zerres 1992). Therefore, the rigid classification system of Blyth and Ockenden has limited clinical utility and is not genetically relevant.

Typically, ARPKD patients are identified either *in utero* or at birth. Prenatal diagnoses are made by routine screening fetal sonography or by serial monitoring in 'high-risk' pregnancies. Affected fetuses characteristically have enlarged echogenic kidneys and oligohydramnios due to poor renal output *in utero* (Mahony et al. 1984; Melson et al. 1985; Reuss et al. 1990). As a result of the oligoyhdramnios, these infants develop the 'Potter's phenotype', a syndrome consisting of pulmonary hypoplasia, a characteristic facies, and deformities of the spine and limbs (Fig. 9.7) (Osathanondh and Potter 1964; Potter 1964; Zerres et al. 1988). In addition, the massive abdominal distension due to nephromegaly and hepatosplenomegaly has resulted in birth dystocia (Blyth and Ockenden 1971). In affected neonates, the clinical course is most often characterized by respiratory insufficiency and death within the first few hours of life. These respiratory difficulties result from several factors including pulmonary hypoplasia, marked diaphragmatic elevation due to massive kidney enlargement, pneumothoraces, or even congestive heart failure. In contrast, while these neonates may have significant impairments in renal function, death from renal insufficiency is distinctly rare (Blyth and Ockenden 1971; Kääriäinen et al. 1988b; Kaplan et al. 1989a).

Severely affected neonates generally correspond to the 'perinatal group' defined by Blyth and Ockenden. However it is important to note that not all affected neonates die (Gang and Herrin 1986; Kääriänen et al. 1988b; Kaplan et al. 1989a). In fact, Kaplan et al. (1989a) reported that in those neonates whose respiratory status stabilized or improved, similar improvements occurred in their renal function and urine output. For those infants who survive the perinatal period, renal failure and hepatic involvement usually evolve, but there is wide variability in these manifestations.

Surviving neonates and infants generally have decreased glomerular filtration rates (GFR). However, Cole et al. (1987) reported that in a cohort of 17 patients who survived to 1 month of age, the GFR actually improved over the first 6

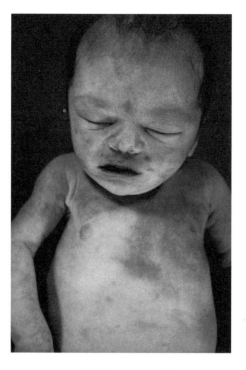

Fig. 9.7 *Potter's phenotype in an ARPKD infant.* The characteristic facies consists of widely set eyes, a prominent skin fold arising from the inner canthus, a beaked nose, mild retraction of the lower jaw, and large, low-lying ears with incomplete cartilaginous development. Contractures of the extremities, particularly of the lower extremities are commonly seen. (Courtesy of Dr Elizabeth Mroczek-Musulman, Department of Pathology, Children's Hospital of Alabama.)

months of life. These findings are consistent with renal maturation. In four of these 17 infants, the GFR was within the normal range at 12 months of age. GFR then decreased after the first year of the age. The decline in renal function was variable and some patients did not progress to end-stage renal disease (ESRD) until late childhood (Cole *et al.* 1987; Kääriäinen *et al.* 1988*b*).

Among perinatal survivors and those who present with ARPKD in infancy, hypertension is the most significant cause of morbidity and mortality (Rawhill and Reuben 1972). Recent studies have demonstrated that hypertension affects the majority of ARPKD patients and if not evident at initial presentation, it develops later in the clinical course (Herrin 1989; Kääriäinen *et al.* 1988*b*; Kaplan *et al.* 1989*a*; Zerres 1992). Severe hypertension frequently occurs in young infants and without early aggressive treatment, causes cardiac hypertrophy, congestive heart failure, and even death (Cole *et al.* 1987; Kaplan *et al.* 1989*a*).

The onset and severity of hypertension in ARPKD appear to be independent of glomerular abnormalities, interstitial fibrosis, or reductions in GFR (Gang and Herrin 1986; Kääriänen *et al.* 1988*b*; Mattoo *et al.* 1994; Osathanondh and

Potter 1964). To date, the pathogenesis of hypertension remains undefined. Kaplan and co-workers reported plasma renin activity (PRA) was not elevated in each of eight hypertensive ARPKD infants studied and proposed that the hypertension resulted from intravascular volume expansion (Kaplan *et al.* 1989*a*). As supportive evidence, they cited the low serum sodium concentration, the low plasma aldosterone levels, and the blood pressure response to potent loop diuretics in these patients. Further review of their clinical data reveals that in a subset of hypertensive ARPKD infants who had urinary potassium and sodium concentrations measured, the $U_{K:Na}$ ratios were generally > 2 (Kaplan, personal communication). Taken together, these data suggest that there is an 'aldosterone-like' effect at the level of the collecting duct despite low to low–normal levels of plasma aldosterone. A collaborative group is currently investigating whether abnormalities in the regulation of sodium transport across the collecting duct effect the intravascular volume expansion described by Kaplan *et al.* and cause the hypertension seen in ARPKD (Guay-Woodford, unpublished data).

In addition to hypertension, tubular functional abnormalities are evident in ARPKD patients. Hyponatraemia is a prominent feature in infants with ARPKD (Anand *et al.* 1975; Kaplan *et al.* 1989*a*). Given the collecting duct lesion, the generally preserved GFR, and the absence of renal salt wasting, hyponatraemia in these infants appears to result from their inability to dilute their urine maximally (Kaplan *et al.* 1989*a*). Several studies have demonstrated that ARPKD patients are unable to dilute their urine below 95 mmol/kg or to concentrate their urine above 600 mmol/kg (Anand *et al.* 1975; Kääriäinen *et al.* 1988*b*; Kaplan *et al.* 1989*a*). For these infants, the severity of their low serum sodium may be further compounded by the low sodium content of breast milk and formula. In addition, net acid excretion may be reduced in these patients causing a mild metabolic acidosis (Anand *et al.* 1975; Kääriäinen *et al.* 1988*b*; Kaplan *et al.* 1989*a*). However, prior to the development of renal insufficiency, metabolic acidosis is not a significant clinical feature of ARPKD (Kääriäinen *et al.* 1988*b*).

Abnormal urinalyses are common in both the infant and older child with ARPKD. Microscopic or gross a haematuria, proteinuria, or pyuria have all been reported (Lieberman *et al.* 1971). Pyuria is the most common sediment abnormality. It can occur without demonstrable bacteriuria and in the absence of documented infection. In two retrospective studies, an increased incidence of urinary tract infection as evidenced by significant bacteriuria was demonstrated in ARPKD patients (Kääriäinen *et al.* 1988*b*; Zerres 1992). However, these were uncontrolled series and it remains controversial as to whether children with ARPKD have an increased risk of upper or lower tract urinary infections (McDonald and Avner 1991).

Infants and children who do not present in the perinatal period can pose a more challenging diagnostic problem. These children generally correspond to the 'neonatal and infantile groups' defined by Blyth and Ockenden and have a wide variety of clinical manifestations that prompt medical evaluation (see Table

Table 9.1   Initial clinical manifestations in infants presenting with ARPKD

Manifestation	Incidence (%)
Flank mass	71
Hepatomegaly	35
Splenomegaly	23
Spontaneous pneumothorax	35
Hypertension	18
Proteinuria	35
Haematuria	29

Modified from Cole *et al.* (1987).

9.1). Most common among these are abdominal distension or palpable flank masses (Cole *et al.* 1987; Kääriäinen *et al.* 1988*b*; Zerres 1992). In these patients, the decline in GFR progresses at variable rates and the consequences of renal insufficiency, such as growth failure, anaemia, and osteodystrophy become apparent (Anand *et al.* 1975; Kääriäinen *et al.* 1988*b*; Kaplan *et al.* 1989*a*). With advances in effective therapy for ESRD, these patient have prolonged survival and for many, the hepatic complications come to dominate the clinical picture (Gang and Herrin 1986; Premkumar *et al.* 1988; Kaplan *et al.* 1989*a*; Zerres *et al.* 1984).

The patients presenting with ARPKD in adolescence and adulthood may present the greatest diagnostic challenge. Typically, these patients have congenital hepatic fibrosis with relatively mild renal medullary ectasia. Their clinical manifestations are generally a function of their portal hypertension. As such, these patients generally correspond to the 'juvenile group' defined by Blyth and Ockenden. However, a note of caution is important. There are case reports of ARPKD patients whose clinical presentation in early childhood was dominated by severe liver involvement as well as patients who presented in adulthood without signs of portal hypertension (Kerr *et al.* 1961; Zerres 1992).

In the typical scenario, these children present between 5 and 13 years of age with the complications of presinusoidal portal hypertension, including hepatosplenomegaly, bleeding oesophageal varices, portal thrombosis, and enlargement of the gallbladder, as well as hypersplenism with consequent thrombocytopenia, anaemia and leucopenia (Alvarez *et al.* 1981; Lieberman *et al.* 1971; Summerfield *et al.* 1986). Since the hepatic lesion in ARPKD is generally confined to the biliary tree, hepatic synthetic function is usually preserved (Bernstein and Slovis 1992; Kaplan *et al.* 1989*a*; Summerfield *et al.* 1986). A review of the literature does not reveal any reported case fatalities due to primary hepatocellular failure. However, ascending cholangitis can be a serious complication in these patients and it can cause fulminant hepatic failure (Alvarez *et al.* 1981, 1982; Summerfield *et al.* 1986). Cholangitis has been reported in infants as young as a few weeks of age (Kääriäinen *et al.* 1988*b*).

Radiologic features

Kidney

In ARPKD, the classic intravenous pyelogram (IVP) reveals enlarged kidneys and delayed nephrograms with medullary streaking (Lieberman *et al.* 1971). While this mottled and prolonged nephrogram is typical for ARPKD, it cannot be regarded as pathognomonic. A similar IVP pattern can be seen in infants with either early manifestations of autosomal dominant polycystic kidney disease (ADPKD) or Meckel syndrome (Zerres 1992).

Over the past 10–15 years, real time sonography has replaced the IVP as the radiologic modality of choice for evaluating children with cystic kidney disease. The sonographic findings vary depending on the age of the patient and the severity of renal involvement (Kääriäinen *et al.* 1988*b*; Kaplan *et al.* 1989*a*; Premkumar *et al.* 1988). In an affected neonate, ultrasound reveals enlarged, usually symmetrical, diffusely echogenic kidneys (Fig. 9.8A) (Boal and Teele 1980; Wernecke *et al.* 1985).This increased echogenicity obscures the border of the kidney and causes poor demarcation among the cortex, medulla, and renal sinus. In some infants, an hypoechoic subcapsular rim of parenchyma has been reported and is considered to be a specific ultrasound feature of ARPKD (Currarino *et al.* 1989). With prolonged survival, the diffusely echogenic pattern changes. Typically, the medullary echogenicity increases and the renal size reduces with age (Fig. 9.8B) (Gang and Herrin 1986; Herrin 1989; Kaplan *et al.* 1989*a*). Single macroscopic cysts are often evident, but these are usually less than 2 cm in diameter (Kaplan *et al.* 1989*a*). Progressive fibrosis and the development of macroscopic cysts can alter the reniform contour. Consequently, the sonographic pattern of the kidneys may resemble that typical of ADPKD (Zerres 1992).

Taking these age-related changes into account, Herman and Siegel (1991) have classified the sonographic features of ARPKD into three distinct patterns. The first is seen primarily in infants and is characterized by an ultrasound pattern of pyramidal hyperechogenicity that resembles medullary nephrocalcinosis. Most neonates and infants have the classic sonographic pattern of enlarged kidneys and globally increased echogenicity that occasionally spares the outer 2–3 mm of cortex. In older children, a third pattern involving intense central echogenicity with a preserved rim of 8–14 mm of cortex is typically seen.

Liver

The liver in affected infants may be either normal in size or enlarged and usually is less echogenic than the kidneys (Cole *et al.* 1987; Kääriänen *et al.* 1988*a*). However, dilated intrahepatic bile ducts or decreased visualization of the peripheral portal veins due to fibrosis may be evident even in the neonate (Fig. 9.8C) (Kaplan *et al.* 1989*b*). With age, the portal fibrosis tends to progress (Gang and Herrin 1986; Kääriäinen *et al.* 1988*a*; Lieberman *et al.* 1971) In the older child, the abdominal ultrasound typically reveals massive he-

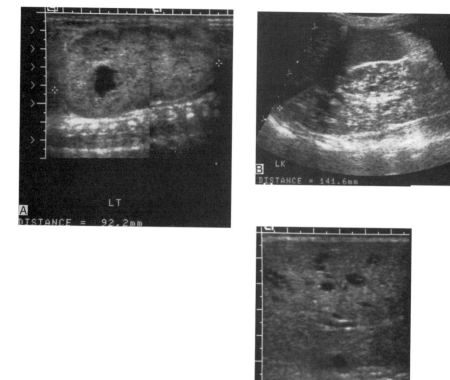

Fig. 9.8 *Sonographic features of ARPKD.* (A) On longitudinal view, the left kidney of a 1-month-old infant with ARPKD is symmetrically enlarged and measures 9.2 cm. In comparison, the normal age-adjusted renal length is 5 cm. Note the diffusely increased echogenicity and loss of the corticomedullary junction. The increased echogenicity is due to the multiple microcysts in the collecting ducts and the single 'cystic' structure (arrow) probably represents a macrocyst. (B) Renal sonogram from an adolescent with ARPKD demonstrates a generalized increase in parenchymal echogenicity but the medulla is relatively more echogenic. In addition, several macrocysts are evident. (C) Transverse view through an ARPKD liver reveals multiple 'cystic' areas due to the dilated bilary ducts. (Courtesy of Dr Jane C. Share, Department of Radiology, Children's Hospital, Boston.)

patosplenomegaly and a patchy pattern of increased hepatic echogenicity. In the presence of portal hypertension, Doppler flow studies of the portal vasculature reveal reversal of portal flow (Premkumar *et al.* 1988). Prominent intrahepatic bile duct dilatation suggests the presence of Caroli's disease (D'Agata *et al.* 1994; Premkumar *et al.* 1988; Sung *et al.* 1992).

Differential diagnosis

Sonographically and histologically, ARPKD is readily distinguished from cystic renal dysplasia (Bernstein and Slovis 1992; Blyth and Ockenden 1971; Lieberman *et al.* 1971). However, the sonographic pattern of uniform, enlarged kidneys with diffusely increased echogenicity may be seen in several disorders other than ARPKD. Most notably, *in utero* and in the perinatal period, both ADPKD and glomerulocystic disease can be clinically and sonographically indistinguishable from ARPKD (Anton and Abramowsky 1982; Farrell *et al.* 1984; fitch and Stapleton 1986). Table 9.2 shows the key characteristics which differentiate these disorders.

In addition, a number of other renal cystic diseases may have renal sonograms that are similar to ARPKD (see Table 9.3). Several of these disorders are associated with congenital hepatic fibrosis (Barnes and Opitz 1992; Bernstein 1987; Grossman and Seed 1966; Heptinstall 1992; Lipschitz *et al.* 1993; McDonald and Avner 1991; Pagon *et al.* 1982). However, for the most part, these renal cystic diseases occur in the context of multiple malformation syndromes. Less commonly, pyelonephritis, transient neonatal nephromegaly, neonatal contrast-induced nephropathy, nephroblastomatosis, and bilateral Wilm's tumour may have similar renal sonographic features as ARPKD (Avner *et al.* 1982; Stapleton *et al.* 1981; Kinoshita *et al.* 1986). Finally, the ultrasound findings of pyramidal hyperechogenicity in infants and medullary ductal ectasia in adults may suggest the diagnosis of medullary sponge kidney. While this disorder is sonographically similar, it is a generally non-heritable, isolated renal lesion that occurs more frequently in adult women. Therefore, the clinical context should readily distinguish ARPKD from medullary sponge kidney (Chilton and Cremin 1981; Hodgson *et al.* 1976).

For those patients with isolated renal cystic disease in whom the family history and the radiologic studies are inconclusive, histologic analysis of kidney and liver tissue is required to definitively establish the diagnosis of ARPKD (Cole *et al.* 1987; Gang and Herrin 1986; Kaplan *et al.* 1989*a*).

Table 9.2 Features that differentiate ARPKD, ADPKD, and glomerulocystic disease

	ARPKD	ADPKD	Glomerulocystic disease
Family history	+/− affected sibs	Affected parent	1. Parent with ADPKD 2. None; isolated entity 3. None; occurs as part of syndrome
Distribution of renal cysts	Collecting duct	Entire nephron	Bowman's space
Liver pathology	CHF	Rare CHF	None

CHF, Congenital hepatic fibrosis.

Table 9.3 Differential diagnosis of ARPKD

Genetic diseases	Renal cystic lesion	Associated with CHF
ADPKD	Along entire nephron	Rare
Glomerulocystic disease	Bowman's space	No
Juvenile nephronophthisis	Medullary cysts	Occasional
Tuberous sclerosis	Along entire nephron (eosinophilic hyperplastic epithelium)	Rare
Congenital hypernephronic nephromegaly with tubular dysgenesis		No
Cysts associated with multiple malformation syndromes:		
Meckel–Gruber syndrome	Cystic dysplasia	Yes
Ivemark syndrome	Cystic dysplasia	Yes
Jeune syndrome	Cystic dysplasia	Yes
Zellweger syndrome	Cystic dysplasia (primarily glomerular)	Yes and cirrhosis
Short-rib-polydactyly syndromes	Cystic dysplasia	Occasional
Vaginal atresia syndrome	Cystic dysplasia	Rare
Bardet–Biedl syndrome	Cystic dysplasia	Rare
Beckwith–Wiedemann syndrome	Cystic dysplasia or nephroblastomatosis	Rare
Trisomy 9 and 13	Cystic dysplasia	Rare
Glutaric aciduria type II	Cystic dysplasia	Rare

Nephropathies
Multicystic dysplastic kidneys
Pyelonephritis
Glomerulonephritis
Transient neonatal nephromegaly
Neonatal contrast-induced nephropathy
Nephroblastomatosis
Bilateral Wilms' tumour
Congenital nephrosis
Bilateral renal vein thrombosis
Leukaemia or lymphoma

CHF, congenital hepatic fibrosis.
Modified from Barnes and Opitz (1992); Glassberg *et al.* (1987); Heptinstall 1992; McDonald and Avner (1991); Zerres *et al.* (1984).

Prenatal diagnosis

At the present time, the fetal sonogram is the gold standard for the prenatal diagnosis of ARPKD. The diagnosis is suggested by sonographic findings that include enlarged echogenic kidneys, oligohydramnios, and absence of urine in the bladder (Fig. 9.9) (Habif *et al.* 1982; Nishi *et al.* 1991; Reuss *et al.* 1991). It is important to caution that even with state-of-the art technology, the sonogram is neither sensitive nor specific in diagnosing ARPKD. Typically, the sonographic features of ARPKD become evident between 16 and 26 weeks of gestation (Kaplan *et al.* 1989*b*; Reuss *et al.* 1991; Zerres *et al.* 1988). However, the sonographic abnormalities may not become evident until late in the third trimester (Argubright and Wicks 1987; Barth *et al.* 1992; Luthy and Hirsch 1985). *In utero*, sonography can not reliably distinguish ARPKD from ADPKD, glomerulocystic disease or Meckel syndrome. This imprecision is particularly important because ADPKD has been diagnosed as early as 16 weeks of gestation (Pretorius *et al.* 1987). Even with a classic fetal sonogram, the subsequent severity of ARPKD can not be predicted with any precision (Barth *et al.* 1992; Luthy and Hirsch 1985; Mahony *et al.* 1984). Thus, when counselling couples about pregnancies that are at risk for ARPKD, the discussion must take into account the limitations of sonographic evaluation.

Other maternal and fetal tests have been reported to be predictive of ARPKD. Preliminary data correlated elevated maternal alpha-fetoprotein levels with an increased risk of ARPKD (Townsend *et al.* 1988). But, further study has determined that this is a generally non-specific laboratory finding. Similarly, initial reports suggesting that increased amniotic fluid trehalase activity identified affected fetuses have not been confirmed (Morin *et al.* 1981).

Therefore, the potential for second trimester prenatal diagnoses of ARPKD should be approached with caution. However, in the light of recent genetic advances, DNA-based prenatal diagnosis may soon be available for at-risk pregnancies.

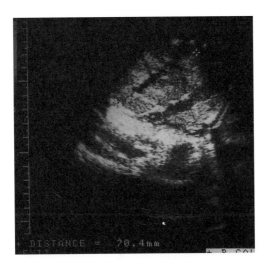

Fig. 9.9 *Late second trimester fetal sonogram.* Longitudinal scan of a 26-week fetus with ARPKD at reveals a massively enlarged and highly echogenic kidney. (Courtesy of Dr Jane C. Share, Department of Radiology, Children's Hospital, Boston).

Genetics

ARPKD

Given the autosomal recessive mode of inheritance, the parents of ARPKD children are obligate heterozygotes and each pregnancy has a 25 per cent recurrence risk. As noted previously, Blyth and Ockenden described the variable phenotypic manifestations of ARPKD. They subdivided their patients into four phenotypic groups and concluded that only one phenotype was expressed within a given family. Based on these analyses, they hypothesized that the four phenotypes are distinct disease entities caused by different mutant genes (Blyth and Ockenden 1971). Subsequent reviews of their cases make such a rigid genetic classification doubtful (Kaplan *et al.* 1989*a*). While the phenotypic expression within a given sibship is usually similar, numerous reports have identified discordant families with significant phenotypic variability within the sibship (Chilton and Cremin 1981; Gang and Herrin 1986; Herrin 1989; Kääriäinen *et al.* 1988*b*; Kaplan *et al.* 1989*a*; Lieberman *et al.* 1971; Resnick and Vernier 1981).

In an alternative genetic formulation, Zerres has proposed that ARPKD results from multiple allelism. The genetic model suggests that a few different mutant alleles of a single gene could account for both the relatively high level of phenotypic concordance within families as well as the broad range of phenotypes that is evident among different families (Zerres *et al.* 1984). The discordance in disease phenotypes that occur within some sibships may be explained by other non-mutant genes exerting a modifying influence on the expression of the ARPKD phenotype. Based on the available data, most investigators concur that ARPKD is a single gene disorder with a broad range of clinical and pathological manifestations (Cole *et al.* 1987; Gang and Herrin 1986; Kaplan *et al.* 1989*a*; Zerres *et al.* 1988).

A recent report in which Zerres and co-workers have mapped an ARPKD locus to the short arm of human chromosome 6 appears to confirm this hypothesis (Zerres *et al.* 1994). A series of strategies led to this map assignment. First, Zerres *et al.* excluded the possibility that ARPKD was the result of homozygosity at either the PKD1 or PKD2 locus (Wirth *et al.* 1987; Zerres *et al.* 1994). Secondly, the human syntenic regions for two mouse models of recessive polycystic kidney disease were excluded (Guay-Woodford *et al.* 1994; Zerres *et al.* 1994). Ultimately, using a genome scanning approach, these investigators found close genetic linkage between ARPKD and four chromosome 6p microsatellite markers (Zeres *et al.* 1994). These data positioned the ARPKD locus within a 13 cM region flanked by the markers TCTE1 and D6S294. None of the genes that have been mapped within this interval explains the pathogenesis of ARPKD.

Among the 27 families analysed, the full spectrum of renal and hepatic manifestations were manifest and no evidence of genetic heterogeneity was obtained. However, in the majority of these families, the affected children had milder forms of the disease with survival beyond the first year of life. Therefore, the authors cautioned that linkage must be confirmed for the severe perinatal form of the disease. In recent work, Guay-Woodford and co-workers have demonstrated that the severe perinatal phenotype of ARPKD is in fact linked to the same 6p interval (Guay-Woodford *et al.* 1994). Taken together, these data have important implications for DNA-based prenatal diagnoses. Studies are in progress to refine the ARPKD interval and identify optimally informative flanking markers for use in genetic analyse of pregnancies at risk.

Congenital hepatic fibrosis (CHF)

The current consensus holds that CHF is a developmental biliary abnormality rather than a single disease entity (Bernstein *et al.* 1988; Desmet 1992). Clinically and histopathologically, CHF is most commonly associated with ARPKD. Indeed, the finding of CHF is indispensable for the diagnosis of ARPKD (Blyth and Ockenden 1971; Lieberman *et al.* 1971). However, as noted in Table 9.3, CHF can be found in association with renal cystic disease in several different disorders, including Meckel syndrome, Jeune syndrome, different short-rib-polydactyly syndromes, Ivemark syndrome, vaginal atresia syndromes, and tuberous sclerosis. In addition, CHF has been observed in association with juvenile nephronophthisis and in rare cases of ADPKD (Boichis *et al.* 1973; Harris *et al.* 1986; Lipschitz *et al.* 1993). It remains a matter of some controversy as to whether the biliary lesion is identical in these different pathological conditions but, these findings suggest that several distinct gene defects are involved in the pathogenesis of CHF (Bernstein *et al.* 1988; Landing *et al.* 1980).

CHF may also be associated with other liver lesions such as Caroli's disease and choledochal cysts (Bernstein *et al.* 1988; Desmet 1992; Summerfield *et al.* 1986). In addition, there are case reports of Caroli's disease associated with ARPKD (Takehara *et al.* 1989; Sung *et al.* 1992). Therefore, some investigators have postulated that CHF and Caroli's disease represent overlapping syndromes in which abnormalities occur at different levels of the developing biliary tree (Desmet 1992).

It is controversial whether CHF occurs as an isolated hepatic lesion without associated renal cystic changes (Murray-Lyon *et al.* 1973). On the basis of histological and morphometric analyses, Landing *et al.* (1980) and later Helczynski *et al.* (1984) concluded that 'infantile polycystic disease' and 'CHF with medullary ductal ectasia' are two distinct diseases. Yet, the weight of family data from several studies suggest that the perinatal ARPKD phenotype and CHF with renal tubular ectasia are variable phenotypic expressions of a single gene defect (Gang and Herrin 1986; Kääriäinen *et al.* 1988*b*; Kaplan *et al.* 1989*a*). In separate studies, Kissane and Takehara and co-workers surveyed cohorts of patients with CHF and found that 50–80 per cent of these patients had medullary tubular dilatation (Kissane 1990; Takehara *et al.* 1989). In a cohort of 27 children who presented with CHF, Alvarez and co-workers detected obvious ARPKD or tubular ectasia in virtually all of the patients (Alvarez *et al.* 1981).

Based on these and other studies, Zerres has concluded that most, if not all patients with classic autosomal recessive CHF should be regarded as having ARPKD with limited renal tubular involvement (Zerres 1992). He postulates that the renal tubular abnormality in these patients involves minimal to subtle degrees of medullary tubular ectasia. In ARPKD, both the biliary lesion and the renal tubular lesion tend to progress. Therefore, in patients who present with CHF and no radiologic evidence of renal tubular abnormalities, the renal tubular lesion may become evident over time. The ARPKD locus has been mapped and there is no evidence of genetic heterogeneity among families with a broad spectrum of phenotypic manifestations (Zerres *et al.* 1994). Therefore, the hypothesis that classic CHF is a phenotypic variant of ARPKD rather than a distinct genetic disease can now be tested by genetic linkage analyses.

Management

In the 20 years since Blyth and Ockenden's seminal report, the survival of neonates with ARPKD has improved significantly due to advances in artificial ventilation and other supportive measures. However, it remains impossible to distinguish prospectively those neonates who can survive and those who have critical degrees of pulmonary hypoplasia incompatible with survival (Kääriäinen *et al.* 1988*b*; Sumfest *et al.* 1993). In a recent report, Sumfest *et al.* (1993) described the surgical management of three severely affected ARPKD infants. Each was diagnosed *in utero* and born with severe respiratory distress. Each underwent bilateral nephrectomies and began peritoneal dialysis shortly after birth. The authors postulated that two of the three survived because removal of the massively enlarged kidneys and improved fluid balance allowed optimal ventilation. Furthermore, they cautioned that because a phenomenon of rapid renal enlargement has been observed in some ARPKD neonates, bilateral nephrectomies are preferable to a unilateral approach. Other authors have advocated continuous arteriovenous haemofiltration to optimize the fluid balance in ARPKD infants and minimize pulmonary oedema, thereby allowing time to assess their long-term pulmonary prognosis (McDonald and Avner 1991).

For those children who survive the perinatal period, careful clinical monitoring is required. The most significant risk factor for morbidity and mortality is the development of hypertension. In those infants with severe hypertension, treatment with calcium channel blockers, beta blockers, and diuretics, particularly loop agents, are most efficacious. Although PRA are usually not elevated, those with refractory hypertension often respond to angiotensin-converting enzyme inhibitors (Kaplan *et al.* 1989*b*; McDonald and Avner 1991). In terms of tubular function, most children with ARPKD have a concentrating defect and thus risk significant dehydration during intercurrent illnesses. Of particular concern are illnesses associated with fever and tachypnoea, that in turn increase insensible water loss, and gastrointestinal infections which limit free water intake due to nausea and vomiting and/or cause diarrhoeal water loss (McDonald and Avner 1991). In those infants with severe polyuria, thiazide diuretics may be used to decrease distal nephron solute and water delivery. Metabolic acidosis is not a prominent clinical problem for infants with ARPKD. However, in order to optimize the linear growth in these patients, their acid–base balance should be closely monitored and supplemental bicarbonate therapy initiated as needed. Pyuria is relatively common in these patients, but its presence does not always indicate urinary tract infection (Kääriäinen *et al.* 1988*b*; McDonald and Avner l991; Zerres 1992). The clinical presentation and appropriately obtained urine cultures can confirm the diagnosis and guide antibiotic therapy. If a urinary tract infection is documented, a voiding cystourethrogram (VCUG) and renal ultrasound should be performed to ascertain whether vesico-ureteral reflux, ureteral obstruction or other upper tract abnormalities are present (Lebowitz and Mandell 1987).

Over the past decade, the treatment of chronic renal failure (CRF) in pae-diatric patients has dramatically improved. Linear growth, particularly in the first year of life, can be optimized by an aggressive nutritional programme that includes careful monitoring of caloric intake and administration of high-calorie formulas by nasogastric or gastrostomy tubes (Kim *et al.* 1991*b*). In addition, recent data suggest that recombinant growth hormone enhances growth in children with CRF (Fine *et al.* 1994). As a general rule, renal replacement therapy with dialysis or transplantation is indicated when children with CRF become symptomatic or when growth failure is refractory to medical management. For infants with ESRD, peritoneal dialysis is preferable for long-term therapy whereas, either peritoneal dialysis or haemodialysis are options for children who reach ESRD. Renal transplantation is the treatment of choice for paediatric ESRD patients. Based on a large paediatric transplant centre's experience, Kim and co-workers reported a one-year patient survival rate of 91 per cent (Kim *et al.* 1991*a*). Data from the recent North American Pediatric Renal Transplantation Cooperative Study demonstrate that allografts from living, related donors are preferable for paediatric transplant candidates (McEnery *et al.* 1993). As ARPKD is a recessive disorder, either parent may be a suitable kidney donor.

In addition to these general considerations, there are several specific issues for the ARPKD patient with ESRD. In some ARPKD patients, pre-transplant splenectomy may be indicated if there is marked leucopenia or thrombocytopenia due to severe hypersplenism (McDonald and Avner 1991). Native nephrectomies may be warranted in the neonate to ameliorate respiratory distress; in the infant to control refractory hypertension; or in infants and children with massively enlarged kidneys, to allow allograft placement. Finally, in immnuosuppressed ARPKD patients, bacterial cholangitis may present a particularly difficult diagnostic and therapeutic problem (McDonald and Avner 1991).

Close monitoring for the complications of portal hypertension is warranted in all ARPKD patients. Haematemesis or melaena suggest the presence of oesophageal varices. Endoscopy is indicated to assess the extent of variceal development and evaluate the efficacy of either sclerotherapy or variceal banding (D'Agata *et al.* 1994). The severity of portal hypertension and its progression can be monitored by serial ultrasound and Doppler flow studies (Kääriäinen *et al.* 1988*a*; Kapan *et al.* 1989*b*). Portacaval shunting may be indicated in some patients (McGonigle *et al.* 1981). Periodic monitoring for signs of hypersplenism is necessary, although splenectomy is seldom performed in patients other than transplant candidates. As noted, bacterial cholangitis may be a particularly difficult problem for the ARPKD patient. Unexplained fever with or without elevated transaminase levels suggests cholangitis and requires meticulous evaluation, often including a percutaneous liver biopsy, to make the diagnosis, and guide aggressive antibiotic therapy (Piccoli and Witzleben 1991).

As MacDonald and Avner note, ARPKD not only poses significant medical problems for the affected child, it imposes severe psycho-social stresses on the family. A management team composed of paediatric nephrologists, primary paediatricians, specialized nurses, nutritionists, and psycho-social support staff optimally provide comprehensive care for children with ARPKD and support for their families (McDonald and Avner 1991). In addition, parental support groups have proven to be uniquely capable of addressing parental concerns and the psycho-social stresses of ARPKD.

Prognosis

Given the paucity of long-term follow-up studies, the overall prognosis is difficult to determine in ARPKD. Prior to 1970, ARPKD was generally considered to be a lethal disease (Dalgaard 1957; Lundin and Olow 1961). In their classic report, Blyth and Ockenden distinguished the wide variability in ARPKD manifestations. Yet their findings, particularly for those patients presenting at birth, corroborated the dismal prognosis reported in previous studies (Blyth and Ockenden 1971). In 1971, Lieberman *et al.* (1971) reported that 8 of 14 infants who had presented with ARPKD in the first few months of life survived well into their childhood years. More recent studies have confirmed that survival in ARPKD is generally correlated with the age of presentation (Kääriäinen *et al.* 1988*b*; Kaplan *et al.* 1989*a*).

The most comprehensive prognostic analysis was reported by Kaplan *et al.* (1989*a*). They conducted a retrospective review of 55 ARPKD cases who had presented from 1950 to 1986. Of these 55 patients, 12 had been previously included in Blyth and Ockenden's study. Twenty-three (42 per cent) patients presented within the first month of life; 23 (42 per cent) presented between one month and one year; and nine patients (16 per cent) presented at greater than one year of age. The outcomes for 48 (87 per cent) patients were determined and 7 were lost to follow-up. Twenty-four patients died. Four died of respiratory failure as neonates and 13 died of renal failure, 6 of these before one year of age. The remainder died of sepsis, hypertension, or unrelated causes. Of note, 12 of the 23 patients who presented with ARPKD as neonates survived beyond 2 years of age. For this ARPKD patient cohort, the actuarial survival was calculated in two ways. Life-table survival rates calculated from birth revealed that 86 per cent were alive at three months, 79 per cent at one year, 51 per cent at 10 years and 46 per cent at 15 years. Calculations based on patients who survived to one year showed that 82 per cent were alive at 10 years and 79 percent at 15 years.

Data from other recent studies generally correspond with these findings. In a study of 17 ARPKD patients who had survived beyond the first month of life, Cole *et al.* (1987) found that only two died before one year of age and the remainder had a mean survival of 6.1 +/– 4.3 years. In a retrospective study, Kääriäinen *et al.* (1988*b*) studied a Finnish cohort that had presented between 1974 and 1983. Of 73 patients with ARPKD who presented in the neonatal period, only 18 survived beyond the first month of life and four more died before their first birthday. Of the 14 who survived beyond the first year of age, all were alive at the time the study was completed, with ages ranging from 2 to 23 years. In both these studies, respiratory failure was the primary cause of death in the neonatal period. Beyond the neonatal period, deaths were due to renal failure, systemic hypertension and sepsis as well as complications of bacterial cholangitis (Cole *et al.* 1987; Kääriäinen *et al.* 1988*b*).

Taken together, these studies suggest that the prognosis for ARPKD, particularly for those children who survive the first month of life, is far less bleak than the popular conception. Therefore, aggressive medical therapy is warranted for these infants (Cole *et al.* 1987). Continued progress in the management of neonates with respiratory insufficiency and infants with renal insufficiency as well as advances in solid organ transplantation should further reduce the morbidity and mortality associated with ARPKD.

References

Alvarez, F., Bernard, O., Brunelle, F., Hadchouel, M., Leblanc, A., Odievre, M., and Alagille, D. (1981). Congenital hepatic fibrosis in children. *Journal of Pediatrics*, **99**, 370–5.

Alvarez, F., Hadchouel, M., and Bernard, O. (1982). Latent chronic cholangitis in congenital hepatic fibrosis. *European Journal of Paediatrics*, **139**, 203–5.

Anand, S. K., Chan, J. C., and Lieberman, E. (1975). Polycystic disease and hepatic fibrosis in children. *American Journal of Diseases in Children*, **129**, 810–13.

Anton, P. A. and Abramowsky, C. R. (1982). Adult polycystic renal disease presenting in infancy: A report emphasizing the bilateral involvement. *Journal of Urology*, **128**, 1290–1.

Argubright, K. F. and Wicks, J. D. (1987). Third trimester ultrasonic presentation of infantile polycystic kidney disease. *American Journal of Perinatology*, **4**, 1–4.

Avner, E. D., Ellis, D., Jaffe, R., and Bowen, A. (1982). Neonatal radiocontrast nephropathy simulating infantile polycystic kidney disease. *Journal of Pediatrics*, **100**, 85–7.

Barnes, E. G. and Opitz, J. M. (1992). Renal abnormalities in malformation syndromes. In *Pediatric Kidney Disease*, (2nd edn), (ed. C. M. Edelmann), Vol. 2, pp. 1067–119. Little, Brown, Boston.

Barth, R. A., Guillot, A. P., Capeless, E. L., and Clemmons, J. W. (1992). Prenatal diagnosis of autosomal recessive polycystic kidney disease: Variable outcome within one family. *American Journal of Obstetrical Gynecology*, **166**, 560–7.

Bernstein, J. (1987). Hepatic involvement in hereditary renal syndromes. In *Birth defects original article series*, Vol. 23, pp. 115–30. March of Dimes Birth Defects Foundation Publishers, New York.

Bernstein, J. and Slovis, T. L. (1992). Polycystic diseases of the kidney. In *Pediatric kidney disease*, (2nd edn), (ed. C. M. Edelmann), Vol. 2, pp. 1139–53. Little, Brown, Boston.

Bernstein, J., Strickler, G. B., and Neel, I. V. (1988). Congenital hepatic fibrosis: Evolving morphology. *APMIS Suppl*, 4, 17–26.

Blyth, H. and Ockenden, B. G. (1971). Polycystic disease of kidneys and liver presenting in childhood. *Journal of Medical Genetics*, 8, 257–84.

Boal, D. K. and Teele, R. L. (1980). Sonography of infantile polycystic kidney disease. *American Journal of Radiology*, 135, 575–80.

Boichis, H., Passwell, J., David, R., and Miller, H. (1973). Congenital hepatic fibrosis and nephronophthisis. A family study. *Quarterly Journal of Medicine*, 42, 221–33.

Bosniak, M. A. and Ambos, M. A. (1975). Polycystic kidney disease. *Seminars in Roentgenology*, 10, 133–43.

Calvet, J. P. (1993). Polycystic kidney disease: Primary extracellular matrix abnormality or defective cellular differentiation? *Kidney International*, 43, 101–8.

Chilton, S. J. and Cremin, B. J. (1981). The spectrum of polycystic disease in children. *Pediatric Radiology*, 11, 9–15.

Cole, B. R., Conley, S. B., and Stapleton, F. B. (1987). Polycystic kidney disease in the first year of life. *Journal of Pediatrics*, 111, 693–9.

Currarino, G., Stannard, M. W., and Rutledge, J. C. (1989). The sonolucent cortical rim in infantile polycystic kidneys. *Journal of Ultrasound in Medicine*, 8, 571–4.

D'Agata, I. D. A., Jonas, M. M., Perez-Atayde, A. R., and Guay-Woodford, L. M. (1994). Combined cystic disease of the liver and kidney. *Seminar in Liver Disease*, 14, 215–28.

Dalgaard, O. Z. (1957). Bilateral polycystic disease of the kidneys: A follow-up study of 284 patients and their families. *Acta Medica Scandinavia* (Suppl.), 158, 1–255.

Desmet, V. J. (1991). Embryology of the liver and intrahepatic biliary tract, and an overview of malformations of the bile duct. In *The Oxford textbook of clinical hepatology*, (ed. N. McIntyre, *et al.*), Vol. 1, pp. 497–519. Oxford University Press.

Desmet, V. J. (1992). Congenital diseases of intrahepatic bile ducts: variations on the theme 'ductal plate malformation'. *Hepatology*, 16, 1069–83.

Desmet, V. J., Van Eycken, P., and Sciot, R. (1990). Cytokeratins for probing cell lineage relation in the developing liver. *Hepatology*, 12, 1249–51.

Evan, A. P. and Larsson, L. (1992). Morphologic development of the nephron. In *Pediatric kidney disease*, (2nd edn), (ed. C. M. Edelman), Vol. 2, pp. 19–48. Little, Brown, Boston.

Faraggiana, T., Bernstein, J., and Strauss, L. (1985). Use of lectins in the study of histogenesis of renal cysts. *Laboratory Investigation*, 53, 575–9.

Farrell, T. P., Boal, D. K., Wood, B. P., Dagen, J. E., and Rabinowitz, R. (1984). Unilateral abdominal mass: An unusual presentation of autosomal dominant polycystic kidney disease in children. *Pediatric Radiology*, 14, 349–52.

Fine, R. N., Kohaut, E. C., Brown, D., and Perlman, A. J. (1994). Growth after recombinant human growth hormone treatment in children with chronic renal failure: report of a multicenter randomized double-blind placebo-controlled study. Genentech Cooperative Study Group. *Journal of Pediatrics*, 124, 374–82.

Fitch, S. J. and Stapleton, F. B. (1986). Ultrasonographic features of glomerulocystic diseases in infancy: Similarity to infantile polycystic kidney disease. *Pediatric Radiology*, 16, 400–2.

Gang, D. L. and Herrin, J. T. (1986). Infantile polycystic disease of the liver and kidneys. *Clinical Nephrology*, **25**, 28–6.

Gattone, V. H. II and Grantham, J. J. (1991). Understanding human cystic disease through experimental models. *Seminars in Nephrology*, **11**, 617–31.

Glassberg, K. I., Stephens, F. D., and Lebowitz, R. L. (1987). Renal dysgenesis and cystic disease of the kidney: a report of the Committee on Terminology, Nomenclature and Classification, Section on Urology, American Academy of Pediatrics. *Journal of Urology*, **138**, 1085–92.

Grossmann, H. and Seed, W. (1966). Congenital hepatic fibrosis, bile duct dilatation, and renal lesion resembing medullary sponge kidney. (Congenital 'cystic' disease of the liver and kidneys). *Radiology*, **87**, 46–8.

Guay-Woodford, L. M., Hopkins, S. D., Muecher, G., and Zerres, K. (1994). The severe perinatal phenotype of ARPKD (autosomal recessive polycystic kidney disease) maps to chromosome 6p21-cen. *Journal of the American Society of Nephrology*, **5**, 624.

Habif, D. V. Jr, Berdon, W. E., and Yeh, M.-N. (1982). Infantile polycystic kidney disease: In utero sonographic diagnosis. *Radiology*, **142**, 475–7.

Harris, H. W., Carpenter, T. O., Shanley, P., Rosen, S., Levey, R. H., and Harmon, W. E. (1986). Progressive tubulointerstitial renal disease in infancy with associated hepatic abnormalities. *American Journal of Medicine*, **81**, 169–76.

Helczynski, L., Wells, T. R., Landing, B. H., and Lipsey, A. I. (1984). The renal lesion of congenital hepatic fibrosis: Pathologic and morphometric analysis, with comparison to the renal lesion of infantile polycystic disease. *Pediatric Pathology*, **2**, 441–55.

Heptinstall, R. H. (1992). *Pathology of the kidney*, (4th edn). Little, Brown, Boston.

Herman, T. E. and Siegel, M. J. (1991). Pyramidal hyperechogenicity in autosomal recessive polycystic kidney disease resembling medullary nephrocalcinosis. *Pathology Radiology*, **21**, 270–1.

Herrin, J. T. (1989). Phenotypic correlates of autosomal recessive (infantile) polycystic disease of kidney and liver; Criteria for classification and genetic counseling. In *Genetics of kidney disorders*, (ed. C. Bartsocas), pp. 45–54. Liss, New York.

Hodgson, H. J. F., Davies, D. R., and Thompson, R. P. H. (1976). Congenital hepatic fibrosis. *Journal of Clinical Pathology*, **29**, 11–16.

Holthofer, H., Kumpulainen, T., and Rapola, J. (1990). Polycystic disease of the kidney. Evaluation and classification based on nephron segment and cell-type specific markers. *Laboratory Investigation*, **62**, 363–9.

Jorgensen, M. J. (1977). The ductal plate malformation: a study of the intrahepatic bile-duct lesion in infantile polycystic disease and congenital hepatic fibrosis. *Acta Pathologica Microbiologica Scandinavia A* (Suppl.), **257**, 1–88.

Kääriäinen, H. (1987). Polycystic kidney disease in children: A genetic and epidemiological study of 82 Finnish patients. *Journal of Medical Genetics*, **24**, 474–81.

Kääriäinen, H., Jääskeläinen, J., Kivisaari, L., Koskimies, O., and Norio, R. (1988*a*). Dominant and recessive polycystic kidney disease in children: Classification by intravenous pyelography, ultrasound, and computed tomography. *Pediatric Radiology*, **18**, 45–50.

Kääriäinen, H., Koskimies, O., and Norio, R. (1988*b*). Dominant and recessive polycystic kidney disease in children: Evaluation of clinical features and laboratory data. *Pediatric Nephrology*, **2**, 296–302.

Kaplan, B. S., Kaplan, P., de Chadarevian, J.-P., Jequier, S., O'Regan, S., and Russo, P. (1988). Variable expression of autosomal recessive polycystic kidney disease and congenital hepatic fibrosis within a family. *American Journal of Medical Genetics*, **29**, 639–47.

Kaplan, B. S., Fay, J., and Shah, V. (1989*a*). Autosomal recessive polycystic kidney disease. *Pediatric Nephrology*, **3**, 49–9.

Kaplan, B. S., Kaplan, P., and Rosenberg, H. K. (1989*b*). Polycystic kidney diseases in childhood. *Journal of Pediatrics*, **115**, 867–80.

Kerr, D. N., Harrison, C. V., and Sherlock, S. (1961). Congenital hepatic fibrosis. *Quarterly Journal of Medicine*, **30**, 91–118.

Kim, M. S., Jabs, K., and Harmon, W. E. (1991*a*). Long-term patient survival in a pediatric renal transplantation program. *Transplantation*, **51**, 413–7.

Kim, M. S., Jabs, K., Spinozzi, N., and Harmon, W. E. (1991*b*). Growth in infants with chronic renal failure on conservative treatment. *Journal of the American Society of Nephrology*, **2**, 238a.

Kinoshita, T., Nakamura, Y., Kinoshita, M., Fukuda, S., Nakashima, H., and Hashimoto, T.(1986). Bilateral cystic nephroblastomas and Botryoid sarcoma in a child with Dandy-Walker syndrome. *Archives of Pathology in Laboratory Medicine*, **110**, 150–2.

Kissane, J. M. (1990). Renal cysts in pediatric patients. A classification and overview. *Pediatric Nephrology*, **4**, 69–77.

Landing, B. H., Wells, T. R., and Claireaux, A. E. (1980). Morphometric analysis of liver lesions in cystic diseases of childhood. *Human Pathology*, **11**, 549–60.

Lebowitz, R. L. and Mandell, J. (1987). Urinary tract infection in children: putting radiology in its place. *Radiology*, **165**, 1–9.

Lieberman, E., Salinas-Madrigal, L., and Gwinn, J. L. (1971). Infantile polycystic disease of the kidneys and liver: Clinical, pathological and radiological correlations and comparison with congenital hepatic fibrosis. *Medicine (Baltimore)*, **50**, 277–318.

Lipschitz, B., Berdon, W. E., Defelice, A. R., and Levy, J. (1993). Association of congenital hepatic fibrosis with autosomal dominant polycystic kidney disease. *Pediatric Radiology*, **23**, 131–3.

Lundin, P. M. and Olow, I. (1961). Polycystic kidneys in newborns, infants and children, a clinical and pathological study. *Acta Paediatrica*, **50**, 185–200.

Luthy, D. A. and Hirsch, J. H. (1985). Infantile polycystic kidney disease: observations from attempts at prenatal diagnosis. *American Journal of Medical Genetics*, **20**, 505–17.

Mahony, B. S., Callen, P. W., Filly, R. A., and Golbus, M. S. (1984). Progression of infantile polycystic disease in early prenancy. *Journal of Ultrasound in Medicine*, **3**, 277–9.

Mattoo, T. K., Khatani, Y., and Ashraf, B. (1994). Autosomal recessive polycystic kidney disease in 15 Arab children. *Pediatric Nephrology*, **8**, 85–7.

McDonald, R. A. and Avner, E. D. (1991). Inherited polycystic kidney disease in children. *Seminars in Nephrology*, **11**, 632–42.

McEnery, P. T., Alexander, S. R., Sullivan, K., and Tegani, A. (1993). Renal transplantation in children and adolescents: The 1992 Annual Report of the North American Pediatric Renal Transplant Cooperative Study. *Pediatric Nephrology*, **7**, 711–20.

McGonigle, R. J. S., Mowat, A. P., Bewick, M., Howard, E. R., Snowden, S. A., and Parson, V. (1981). Congenital hepatic fibrosis and polycystic kidney disease; role of porta-caval shunting and transplantation in three patients. *Quarterly Journal of Medicine*, **199**, 269–78.

Melson, G. L., Shackelford G. D., Cole, B. R., and McClennan, B. L. (1985). The spectrum of sonographic findings in infantile polycystic kidney disease with urographic and clinical correlations. *Journal of Clinical Ultrasound*, **13**, 113–19.

Morin, P. R., Potier, M., Dallaire, L., Melancon, S. M., and Boisvert, J. (1981). Prenatal detection of the autosomal recessive type of polycystic kidney disease by trehalase assay in amniotic fluid. *Prenatal Diagnosis*, **1**, 75–9.

Mugrauer, G., Alt, F. W., and Ekblom, P. (1988). N-mye proto-oncogene expression during organogenesis in the developing mouse as revealed by in situ hybridization. *Journal of Cell Biology*, **107**, 1325–35.

Murray-Lyon, I. M., Ockenden, B. G., and Williams, R. (1973). Congenital hepatic fibrosis — is it a single clinical entity? *Gastroenterology*, **64**, 653–6.

Neumann, H. P. H., *et al.* (1988). Late manifestation of autosomal-recessive polycystic kidney disease in two sisters. *American Journal of Nephrology*, **8**, 194–7.

Nishi, T., Iwasaki, M., Yamoto, M., and Nakano, R. (1991). Prenatal diagnosis of autosomal recessive polycystic kidney disease by ultrasonography and magnetic resonance imaging. *Acta Obstetrica Gynecologica Scandinavia*, **70**, 615–17.

Osathanondh, V. and Potter, E. L. (1963). Development of the human kidney as shown by microdissection. *Archives of Pathology*, **76**, 277–302.

Osathanondh, V. and Potter, E. L. (1964). Pathogenesis of polycystic kidneys. Type 1 due to hyperplasia of interstitial portions of the collecting tubules. *Archives of Pathology*, **77**, 466–73.

Pagon, R. A., Haas, J. E., and Blunt, A. H. (1982). Hepatic involvement in the Bardet-Biedl syndrome. *American Journal of Medical Genetics*, **13**, 373–81.

Piccoli, D. A. and Witzleben, C. L. (1991). Disorders of the intrahepatic bile ducts. In *Pediatric gastrointestinal disease*, (ed. W. A. Walker *et al.*), Vol. 2, pp. 1124–51. Decker, Philadelphia, PA.

Potter, E. L. (1946). Facial characteristics of infants with bilateral renal agenesis. *American Journal of Obstetrical Gynecology*, **51**, 885–8.

Potter, E. L. (1972). *Normal and abnormal development of the kidney*. Year Book Medical, Chicago.

Premkumar, A., Berdon, W. E., Levy, J., Amodio, J., Abramson, S. J., and Newhouse, J. H. (1988). The emergence of hepatic fibrosis and portal hypertension in infants and children with autosomal recessive polycystic kidney disease. *Pediatric Radiology*, **18**, 123–9.

Pretorius, D. H., Lee, M. E., Manco-Johnson, M. L., Weingast, G. R., Sedman, A. B., and Gabow, P. A. (1987). Diagnosis of autosomal dominant polycystic kidney disease in utero and in the young infant. *Journal of Ultrasound in Medicine*, **6**, 249–55.

Rawhill, W. J. and Rubin, M. I. (1972). Hypertension in infantile polycystic renal disease. *Clinical Pediatrics*, **11**, 232–5.

Resnick, J. and Vernier, R. L. (1981). Cystic disease of the kidney in the newborn infant. *Clinical Perinatology*, **8**, 375–90.

Reuss, A., Wladimiroff, J. W., Stewart, P. A., and Niermeijer, M. F. (1990). Prenatal diagnosis by ultrasound in pregnancies at risk for autosomal recessive polycystic kidney disease. *Ultrasound in Medicine and Biology*, **16**, 355–9.

Reuss, A., Wladimiroff, J. W., and Niermeyer, M. F. (1991). Sonographic, clinical and genetic aspects of prenatal diagnosis of cystic kidney disease. *Ultrasound in Medicine Biology*, **17**, 687–94.

Saxen, L. (1987). *Organogenesis of the kidney*. Cambridge University Press.

Shah, K. D. and Gerber, M. A. (1990). Development of intrahepatic bile ducts in humans; immunohistochemical study using monoclonal cytokeratin antibodies. *Archives of Pathology*, **114**, 597–600.

Shaikewitz, S. T. and Chapman, A. (1993). Autosomal recessive polycystic kidney disease: Issues regarding the variability of clinical presentation. *Journal of the American Society of Nephrology*, **3**, 1858–62.

Six, R., Oliphant, M., and Grossman, H. (1975). A spectrum of renal tubular ectasia and hepatic fibrosis. *Radiology*, **117**, 117–122.

Stapleton, F. B., Hilton, S., and Wilcox, J. (1981). Transient nephromegaly simulating infantile polycystic disease of the kidneys. *Pediatrics*, **67**, 554–9.

Sumfest, J. M., Burns, M. W., and Mitchell, M. E. (1993). Aggressive surgical and medical management of autosomal recessive polycystic kidney disease. *Urology*, **42**, 309–12.

Summerfield, J. A., Nagafuchi, Y., Sherlock, S., Cadafalch, J., and Scheuer, P. J. (1986). Hepatobiliary fibropolycystic diseases: a clinical and histological review of 51 patients. *Journal of Hepatology*, **2**, 141–56.

Sung, J. M., Huang, J. J., Lin, X. Z., Ruaan, M. K., Lin, C. Y., Chang, T. T., Shu, H. F., and Chow, N. H. (1992). Caroli's disease and congenital hepatic fibrosis associated with polycystic kidney disease. *Clinical Nephrology*, **38**, 324–8.

Takehara, Y., Takehara, M., Naijo, M., Kato, T., Nishimura, T., Isoda, H., and Kaneko, M. (1989). Caroli's disease associated with polycystic kidney: its non-invasive diagnosis. *Radiation Medicine*, **7**, 13–15.

Townsend, R. R., Goldstein, R. B., and Filly, R. A. (1988). Sonographic identification of autosomal recessive polycystic kidney disease associated with increased maternal serum/amniotic fluid alpha-fetoprotein. *Obstetrical Gynecology*, **71**, 1008–12.

Van Eyken, P., Sciot, R., and Callea, F. (1988). The development of the intrahepatic bile duct in man: a keratin–immunohistochemical study. *Hepatology*, **8**, 1586–95.

Verani, R., Walker, P., and Silva, F. G. (1989). Renal cystic disease of infancy: Results of histochemical studies. *Pediatric Nephrology*, **3**, 37–42.

Welling, L. W. and Grantham, J. J. (1991). Cystic and developmental diseases of the kidney. In *The kidney*, (4th edn), (ed. B. M. Brenner and F. C. Rector), pp. 1657–87. Saunders, Philadelphia, PA.

Wernecke, K., Heckemann, R., and Bachmann, J. (1985). Sonography of infantile poly-cystic kidney disease. *Urologic Radiology*, **7**, 138–45.

Wirth, B., Zerres, K., Fischbach, M., Claus, D., Neumann, H. P., Lenner, T. T., Brodehl, J., Neugebauer, M., Muller-Wiefel, D. E., Geisert, J., *et al.* (1987). Autosomal recessive and dominant forms of polycystic kidney disease are not allelic. *Human Genetics*, **77**, 221–2.

Zerres, K. (1992). Autosomal recessive polycystic kidney disease. *Clinical Investigation*, **70**, 794–801.

Zerres, K., Volpel, M.-C., and Weib, H. (1984). Cystic kidneys. Genetics, pathologic anatomy, clinical picture and prenatal diagnosis. *Human Genetics*, **68**, 124–67.

Zerres, K., Hansmann, M., and Mallmann, R. (1988). Autosomal recessive polycystic kidney disease. Problems of prenatal diagnosis. *Prenatal Diagnosis*, **8**, 215–19.

Zerres, K., *et al.* (1994). Mapping of the gene for autosomal recessive polycystic kidney disease (ARPKD) to chromosome 6p21-cen. *Nature Genetics*, **7**, 429–32.

Zerres, K., Mucher, G., and Rudnik-Schoneborn, S. (1994). Autosomal recessive poly-cystic kidney disease does not map to the second gene locus for autosomal dominant polycystic kidney disease on chromosome 4. *Human Genetics*, **93**, 697–8.

10

Acquired renal cystic disease

Eric P. Cohen

Simple cysts

The development of cysts in non-cystic kidneys has been recognized by pathologists for over a century (Simon 1847; Mallory 1914). Simple cysts of the kidney are more common in older subjects (Laucks and McLachlan 1981) and are uncommon under age 40. They are thus acquired in life, and probably not congenital. They are usually asymptomatic but may cause pain and may become infected. An association between simple cysts and hypertension has been noted, with reduction in blood pressure after cyst puncture or surgical cyst removal (Lüscher *et al.* 1986). This relation may derive from renin activation on the same side as the cyst, perhaps via compression and ischaemia. Simple cysts have also been associated with polycythaemia, and erythropoietic activity has been found in simple cyst fluid (Rosse *et al.* 1963). Simple cysts are easily identified by ultrasonography (US) or computed tomography (CT) scanning (Hartman 1989). Both imaging techniques are able to show the asymmetries or tissue bulges that may suggest an associated tumour or cancer.

Definition

Acquired renal cystic disease (ARCD) is the development of cysts in a previously non-cystic failing kidney. More than one cyst in each kidney will satisfy the criterion of 'multiple bilateral cysts' (Grantham and Levine 1985). The first detailed description of such cysts in failed kidneys was in 1847 (Simon 1847). Although so-called retention cysts in failed kidneys have long been known to pathologists, the modern rediscovery of cystic 'transformation' of end-stage kidneys was only published in 1977 (Dunnill *et al.* 1977). Pathologically, ARCD may be defined as 'replacement of 40 per cent or more of the renal parenchyma by multiple cysts'. (Feiner *et al.* 1981) and, radiologically, ARCD is four or more cysts per kidney by US or CT scanning (Narasimhan *et al.* 1986).

Morphology

Acquired cysts probably derive from the dilated tubules that are so common in chronically failing kidneys. Microdissection studies have shown continuity with

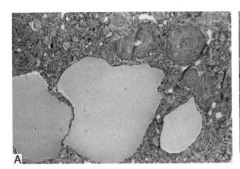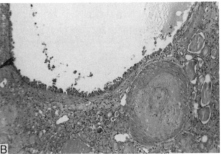

Fig. 10.1 (A) Photomicrograph (×100) of a portion of end-stage kidney with three acquired cysts. There is disruption of the normal kidney architecture, areas of dilated tubules containing casts, and multiple arterioles with marked intimal and medial hyperplasia. (B) Photomicrograph (×100) of a portion of cyst wall from the same patient. There is hyperplastic, dysplastic epithelium in the cyst wall. Severe intimal and medial hyperplasia is again evident in a small artery.

the proximal tubule in some cases (Feiner *et al.* 1981) and brush borders on the lining cells have been found by electron microscopy (Grantham and Levine 1985; Mickisch *et al.* 1984). Features of distal nephron epithelium have also been found (Mickisch *et al.* 1984). Histochemical studies using lectins and antibodies to specific kidney antigens showed cysts of both proximal and distal tubular origin (Deck *et al.* 1988). The cysts are typically lined with flattened epithelium but others have proliferative, even dysplastic appearing epithelium (Fig. 10.1A, B). Kidneys affected by ARCD may also show solid adenomas in 10–20 per cent of cases by histopathological examination (Hughson *et al.* 1980; Deck *et al.* 1988). These hyperplastic features suggest that end-stage kidneys are under the influence of proliferative stimuli (Grantham 1991). The latter are at least part of the basis for the adenocarcinomas that may form in end-stage kidneys, with or without acquired cysts. These adenocarcinomas are often typical clear cell renal cancer (Ishikawa *et al.* 1980; Ratcliffe *et al.* 1983; Turani *et al.* 1983; Gehrig *et al.* 1985) (Fig. 10.2). Recently, Ishikawa has emphasized that many of the tumours associated with ARCD have a papillary appearance (Ishikawa *et al.* 1993). He reported on 43 renal tumours resected from patients on haemodialysis, and found that half had papillary cancers, rather than the clear-cell type usually found in the general population. Using publications analysed earlier (Matson and Cohen 1990; Cohen 1993) as well as subsequent reports (Ishikawa *et al.* 1990, 1991*a,b*; Grantham 1991; Levine *et al.* 1991; Lien *et al.* 1991; Marcén *et al.* 1992; Ishikawa and Kovacs 1993), it is evident that 15 of 47 (32 per cent) of histopathologically reported cancers were of the papillary type.

Clinical features

The great majority of patients with ARCD have no symptoms related to the cysts. Haemorrhage, with urinary extension and gross haematuria, or retroperitoneal extension with pain and anaemia, is probably the most frequent

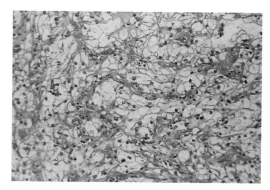

Fig. 10.2 Photomicrograph (×100) of a renal cell carcinoma in the same patient as in Fig. 10.2A. The clear cell morphology is evident. This patient began dialysis in 1979, underwent cadaveric kidney transplantation in 1981 and in 1982. This cancer was found in the right native kidney in 1991. The patient is currently alive without known residual disease, with a plasma creatinine of 97 μmol/l.

symptom. (Ratcliffe *et al.* 1983; Tielemans *et al.* 1983; Levine *et al.* 1987). A recent report has shown the development of renin-related hypertension after perinephric haemorrhage in a patient with ARCD (Bongu *et al.* 1994). Although it is usually asymptomatic, erythrocytosis (relative or absolute) may be the most frequent laboratory correlate of ARCD. This has been related to increased levels of plasma erythropoietin in dialysis patients with cysts as opposed to those without cysts (Edmunds *et al.* 1991). In that report, the average blood haemoglobin in those with cysts was 11 g/dl, and those without cysts was 8 g/dl, but it is not stated whether any of these patients were taking exogenous erythropoietin. Others have shown a direct correlation between years on dialysis, extent of cysts, and blood haemoglobin level (Goldsmith *et al.* 1982; Glicklich *et al.* 1990). The latter group was however unable to correlate haematocrit with cyst formation independently of time on dialysis.

Hypercalcaemia has been reported in one case of clear-cell adenocarcinoma initially without metastatic disease, and at a time when parathyroid hormone (PTH) was almost undetectable and vitamin D metabolite levels were not elevated (Thomson *et al.* 1985). Fever has been reported (Gehrig *et al.* 1985; Marcén *et al.* 1992). Other paraneoplastic syndromes, such as gonadotrophin or corticotrophin secretion that may accompany classical hypernephromas, have not been reported in cancers accompanying ARCD. Symptoms of metastatic disease including skin metastasis (Lien *et al.* 1991), chest metastasis (Ratcliffe *et al.* 1983; Almirall *et al.* 1989; Covarsi *et al.* 1991), and bony metastasis (Faber and Kupin 1987) have all been reported.

The physical examination of a patient with suspected ARCD and/or its complications is only rarely specific. A tumoral or haemorrhagic flank mass may be felt (Ratcliffe *et al.* 1983; Tielemans *et al.* 1983; Arias *et al.* 1986; Marcén *et al.* 1992). ARCD is not a systemic condition: non-renal cysts have not been reported in such patients (Grantham 1991).

Imaging

Simple cysts are readily imaged by ultrasonography (US) or computed tomography (CT) scanning (Hartman 1989). It could thus be predicted that the same techniques would be useful to define ARCD. CT scanning was shown to be effective already in 1980 (Ishikawa *et al.* 1980; Bommer *et al.* 1980). The first published report on the efficacy of US was in 1982 (Goldsmith *et al.* 1982). Comparative studies of CT and US soon followed (Narasimhan *et al.* 1986; Jabour *et al.* 1987; Taylor *et al.* 1989). These studies have shown that US is less sensitive than CT in the diagnosis of ARCD. What is of greater importance is whether these techniques will show the complications of ARCD, especially cancers. Gehrig *et al.* (1985) reported that US did not show a 2.5 cm diameter neoplasm that was shown by CT, and a similar occurrence was shown by others in the same year (Henson *et al.* 1985). Both US and CT did not show a 2 cm diameter native kidney cancer with metastases (Almirall *et al.* 1989). In another report, CT did not show an 8 cm diameter native cancer (Cho *et al.* 1984). On balance, either US or CT will generally suffice for the definition of ARCD and its complications. However, US alone does not entirely rule out cancer, so that contrast-assisted CT scanning should be used if doubt persists The use of intravenous contrast not only helps to define the renal parenchyma, but has been found to be safe in dialysis patients (Taylor *et al.* 1989; Levine *et al.* 1991).

Renal arteriography, still the 'gold standard' for renal cancer imaging in non-dialysis patients, is not usually indicated for the diagnosis of cancer in ARCD. This is because end-stage kidneys are hypovascular. Both cysts and tumours are well imaged by magnetic resonance imaging, but that technique is too expensive to justify routine use in ARCD.

Epidemiology

Acquired cysts have been labelled an artefact of organ replacement technology, and related to dialysis itself. However, careful analysis shows that acquired cysts may be present at onset of dialysis in 10–20 per cent of patients (Bommer *et al.* 1980; Matson and Cohen 1990). In retrospect this is not surprising, given the older data on cyst formation in failing kidneys. Single centre data (Ishikawa *et al.* 1980; Levine *et al.* 1991; Spiegel *et al.* 1991) as well as our synthesis of literature data (Fig. 10.3) show that acquired cyst formation is progressive with time on dialysis in an approximately linear fashion. Still, it is possible that the prevalence of ARCD does not really change until the third year of dialysis. That interpretation would fit with the notion that failed kidneys shrink during the first three years of dialysis, with subsequent but variable enlargement (Ishikawa *et al.* 1980).

ARCD may affect end-stage kidneys which have failed for a variety of diagnoses. Although an earlier report implied that ARCD might not develop in diabetic nephropathy (Thomson *et al.* 1988), subsequent studies have shown that diabetic nephropathy does not exclude the development of acquired cysts (Matson and Cohen 1990).

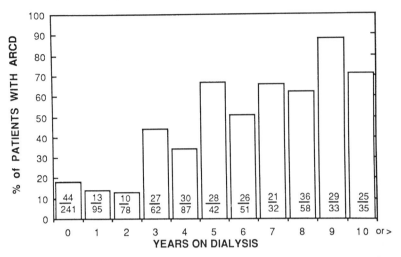

Fig. 10.3 Prevalence of acquired renal cystic disease with time of dialysis. The year of dialysis corresponds to the time up to and including the stated year. The number of patients studied in a given year yields the fraction seen at the bottom of each column, which is transformed to a percentage on the *y*-axis. The height of each column is proportional to the percentage of patients with ARCD in the indicated year. Reprinted from *Medicine* by permission. (Matson M. A. and Cohen E. P. (1990) Acquired cystic kidney disease: Occurrence prevalence, and renal cancers. *Medicine*, **69**(4), 217–826.)

In an autopsy study, it was found that the prevalence of ARCD was significantly greater in patients with nephrosclerosis compared to patients with other causes of renal failure (Miller *et al.* 1989). This was also noted by Deck *et al.* (1988). Overall, however, years of dialysis appears to be the strongest determinant of ARCD, which has been found in both haemo- and peritoneally dialysed patients (Katz *et al.* 1987; Thomson *et al.* 1988; Truong *et al.* 1988; Matson and Cohen 1990). Age *per se* does not seem to be a factor, because ARCD can occur in children with end-stage renal disease (Leichter *et al.* 1988). Being male is a risk factor for ARCD (Miller *et al.* 1989; Matson and Cohen 1990; Marco-Franco *et al.* 1991). Black patients are at greater risk for ARCD than whites by one analysis (Matson and Cohen 1990) but not for another (Miller *et al.* 1989). Finally, if prolonged uraemia is responsible for ARCD, then perhaps better dialysis might be associated with less ARCD. This was not the case in the only published attempt at correlation of ARCD with the dialysis index, Kt/V (Marco-Franco *et al.* 1991). At the Tassin dialysis unit, where very high dialysis delivery is achieved, ARCD is common after 10 years of dialysis (Charra, personal communication). Known associations or lack thereof are shown in Table 10.1.

Cross sectional studies have shown a lesser prevalence of ARCD in patients with successful kidney transplants (Minar *et al.* 1984; Thompson *et al.* 1986; Lien *et al.* 1993). One study showed regression of ARCD in two patients after successful kidney transplantation (Ishikawa *et al.* 1983). But kidney trans-

Table 10.1   Clinical features associated and not associated with ARCD in dialysis patients

Associated
Duration of dialysis
Male gender
Nephrosclerosis
Black race

Not associated
Age
Type of dialysis
Dialysis efficacy

plantation is not necessarily protective against ARCD, because the same group later showed an increase in native kidney cysts in 11 patients after kidney transplantation (Ishikawa *et al.* 1989, 1991*b*). Graft function may not be crucial for the development (or regression) of ARCD, because in the latter study, the average serum creatinine did not differ between those with cyst regression and those with cyst progression after transplant (113 vs. 121 µmol/l, P = n.s.). The graft itself may develop cysts, and an adenoma has been reported in a recent study of chronically rejected allografts (Chung *et al.* 1992). In past years, the common practice of pre-transplant native nephrectomy precluded concern about changes in native kidneys after transplantation. It has been shown that native kidney retention has been more and more common over the past twenty years (Fig. 10.4), which is a factor in the increased prevalence of ARCD in both dialysis and transplant patients (Matson and Cohen 1990). An additional influence may be the use of cyclosporine (CSA). In a series of 33 transplant patients with satisfactory graft function (average serum creatinine = 141 µmol/l), 9 per cent of patients not on CSA had ARCD, whereas 57 per cent of those on CSA had ARCD in their native kidneys (Lien *et al.* 1993).

Pathogenesis

The pathogenesis of ARCD remains uncertain. It is clear that ARCD is more common in patients who have been on dialysis for many years as opposed to just a few months. But it is not known precisely what aspect of renal failure causes the cystic changes. Proposed factors include accumulation of oxalate or other chemicals, the effects of interstitial scarring, secondary hyperparathyroidism, renotropic growth factors, and ischaemia (Dunnill *et al.* 1977; Grantham 1991).

   Oxalate does accumulate in chronically dialysed patients, and this accumulation dissipates after successful kidney transplantation (Worcester *et al.* 1994). Moreover, oxalate crystals are often found in acquired cysts (Dunnill *et al.* 1977; Fayemi and Ali 1980; Feiner *et al.* 1981; Turani *et al.* 1983), and, *in vitro*, oxalate is a proliferative stimulus for renal epithelium (Lieske *et al.* 1991). Ono and associates have shown that oxalate supplementation in subtotally nephrec-

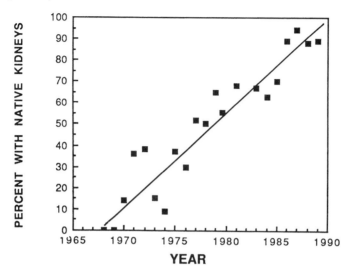

**NATIVE KIDNEY RETENTION IN FIRST TRANSPLANTS
(n=956)**

Fig. 10.4 Time-series plot of native kidney retention at first kidney transplant as a function of time in 956 patients undergoing kidney transplantation at the Medical College of Wisconsin Hospitals. The best-fit linear regression line is shown ($r = 0.9$). Reprinted from *Medicine* by permission. (Matson, M. A. and Cohen, E. P (1990). Acquired cystic kidney disease: Occurrence, prevalence, and renal cancers. *Medicine*, 69(4), 217–26.)

tomized rats may enhance cyst formation in that model (Ono *et al.* 1989). Clinically, however, the correlation of plasma oxalate and cyst formation in their haemodialysis patients is unimpressive (Fig. 10.5) and was also not evident in another analysis (Marco-Franco *et al.* 1991). Finally, acquired cysts were present without oxalate crystals in patients on dialysis for six months or less, and there were cysts with oxalate crystals in patients on dialysis for more than two years in the study of Deck *et al.* (1988), which suggests that oxalate deposition does not preceed acquired cyst formation.

The best known models of acquired cystic kidneys are those produced in rats by addition of diphenylamine (Thomas *et al.* 1957) or of diphenylthiazole to the diet (Carone *et al.* 1974). The latter model shows reversibility of cysts when diphenylthiazole is removed from the diet (Kanwar and Carone 1984). Clinically, phenolic compounds do accumulate in renal failure (Wardle and Wilkinson 1976) but it is not known whether these include diphenylamine or diphenylthiazole.

Interstitial fibrosis is usually extensive in end-stage kidneys, and in part accounts for the increased ultrasonic echogenicity of chronically failing kidneys (Hricak *et al.* 1982). It is possible that this fibrosis may contribute to ARCD via tubular obstruction (Dunnill *et al.* 1977). Experimental and clinical ureteral

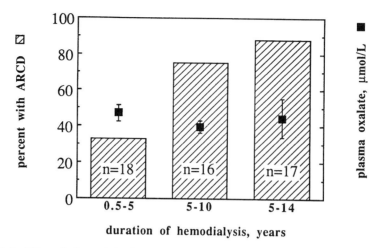

Fig. 10.5 The relation of ARCD to years on dialysis and concurrent plasma oxalate levels. The dialysis time is shown on the *x*-axis, in years, with the number of patients as 'n', within each column. The percentage of patients having ARCD is shown on the left-hand *y*-axis, and the average plasma oxalate (μmol/l, $\pm$ s.e.) on the right-hand *y*-axis. Although plasma oxalate levels are ~10 times normal, there is no clear relation to prevalence of ARCD. Data adapted from Ono *et al.* (1987).

obstruction have also been associated with cyst formation (Fetterman *et al.* 1974; Baert and Steg 1976). Mere obstruction might not, however, account for the proliferative features of ARCD.

Experimental cyst formation using normal human cortical epithelium may be promoted by cyclic AMP (Neufeld *et al.* 1992) and parathyroid hormone (PTH) may activate adenylate cyclase. It is possible that the common secondary hyper-parathyroidism of chronic renal failure might play a role in acquired cyst formation with emphasis on its possible ability to stimulate cyst fluid accumulation via activation of adenylate cyclase (Grantham 1991). However, these facilitory effects of PTH *in vitro* are seen at nanomolar concentrations, whereas mere picomolar concentrations are present in the blood of patients on dialysis.

Renotropic growth factors, long suspected to play a role in the hypertrophy that results from reduction in kidney mass, could explain the proliferative aspects of ARCD. A renal cell growth factor has been recently reported (Klotz *et al.* 1991). This factor was isolated from the sera of patients on dialysis, is a polypeptide or glycopeptide, and has a molecular weight of approximately 20 kDa. Only the proliferative aspects of ARCD would be explained by such a factor, and not the fluid accumulation and cyst enlargement. The progression of native kidney cyst formation in patients with functioning kidney transplants would also not be easily explained by such a factor, if it depends on a uraemic environment.

Cysts form in at least two experimental models of chronic renal failure, the subtotal nephrectomy model (Kenner *et al.* 1985) and in radiation nephropathy

(Moulder *et al.* 1993). High protein intake exacerbates the changes seen in the remnant model, which is reminiscent of the observations of sixty years ago that a 30 per cent protein diet leads to renal injury and cystic tubular dilatation in rats (Newburgh and Curtis 1928). However, these observations do not clarify the pathogenesis of ARCD in man.

The contribution of ischaemia to ARCD is increasingly recognized. Gross cysts have long been associated with so-called 'arteriosclerotic kidneys' (Mallory 1914; Allen 1962). Cystic changes in ischaemic single kidneys have been reported (Michel *et al.* 1987) but azotaemia was present in those rats. Experimentally, in a two-kidney one-clip model, addition of diphenylthiazole to the feed was associated with substantial enhancement of cystic changes on the clipped, ischaemic side (Torres *et al.* 1988). This appeared to be related to physiologically significant renal artery stenosis, because such enhancement did not occur in clipped animals without hypertension. In a clinical case report, severe renal artery stenosis was associated with ipsilateral ARCD and renal cell cancers (Sinsky *et al.* 1993). These authors suggested that long-term ischaemia was 'a major contributing factor in the development of ARCD and neoplasia'. Additional clinical support is provided by our report of five cases of severe uni-lateral renal ischaemia with same-side cyst formation, and with kidney function varying from normal to severely impaired (Cohen and Elliott 1990). Such a phe-nomenon might well explain the increasing frequency of simple cysts with age, given that vascular disease is more prevalent with increasing age. In addition, ARCD itself would then be easily explained by the severe arterial and arteriolar sclerosis so often seen in end-stage kidneys. We hypothesized (Fig. 10.6) that such ischaemia could act via the induction of local acidosis, the latter being a growth factor for renal cortical epithelium (Blumenthal *et al.* 1989). Chronic ischaemia might also play a role in the extensive interstitial fibrosis seen in end-stage kidneys (Ong and Fine 1994). While this hypothesis might explain the proliferative features of ARCD, it would not easily explain the cyst fluid accumulation. Nonetheless, the role of ischaemia in cyst formation is evident in the recent report of enhanced cyst formation in native kidneys of cyclosporine-treated renal transplant recipients (Lien *et al.* 1993). Cyclosporine has distinct vasoconstrictor properties, and has already been associated with renal interstitial fibrosis. Confirmation of these studies would add cyclosporine to the list of kidney cystogens.

These are few data on molecular mechanisms of acquired cyst formation. One report documented somewhat higher epidermal growth factor (EGF) levels in acquired cyst fluid compared to simple cyst fluid (Moskowitz *et al.* 1990), but there was no variation in plasma EGF according to extent of ARCD. Another bit of evidence for the importance of growth factors is the demonstration of renal epithelial overexpression of the c-erb B2 gene in cases of ARCD and ADPKD but not in normal kidneys or in simple cysts (Herrera 1991). This gene, located on chromosome 17, codes for a 185 kDa protein that is similar to EGF, a growth factor which may have mitogenic activity in ADPKD. Both of these studies may merely be the molecular counterpart of what has been known

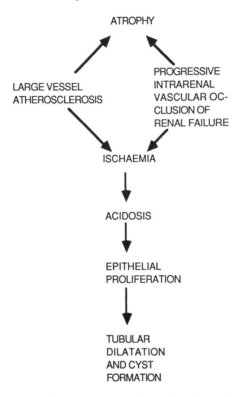

Fig. 10.6 Flow diagram showing the hypothetical relationship of renal ischaemia to acquired cyst formation. Kidney atrophy may result from vascular occlusion. Parenchymal acidosis might result from chronic progressive occlusion and, if sustained just short of causing cell death, could result in tubular cell proliferation. That could facilitate cyst formation and may contribute to the proliferative complications of acquired renal cystic disease, including adenoma and carcinoma. Reprinted from the *American Journal of Kidney Diseases* by permission. (Cohen and Elliott 1990.)

since the report of Dunnill and co-workers in 1977, that is, that ARCD has proliferative features.

Treatment

ARCD itself requires no treatment. End-stage kidneys that are larger than normal kidneys may be at greater risk for associated renal cancers (MacDougall *et al.* 1990). However, in the absence of symptoms, bleeding, or a radiologic mass, it is hard to justify a nephrectomy. The finding of a mass by CT scanning is 75 per cent predictive of a cancer (Taylor *et al.* 1993), so that nephrectomy is justified if a mass is found either because of symptoms or on screening. Bilateral nephrectomy should probably be carried out in that case, given that what is happening in one failed kidney is also apt to occur in its mate.

Older data show that bilateral nephrectomy in dialysis patients has a 3 to 4 per cent mortality in non-diabetic patients, which may increase to 15 per cent in diabetic patients (Matas *et al.* 1975; Yarimizu *et al.* 1978). As shown previously, native nephrectomy is less common now than in past years, which may account for the lack of updated statistics. Still, over the past six years, and for nine dialysis or transplant patients undergoing native nephrectomy at our centre, there have been no post-operative deaths (Cohen, unpublished data).

Screening for ARCD

Sarasin and co-workers have published their analysis of the utility of screening, in abstract form (Sarasin *et al.* 1991). In their analysis, there is little, if any patient benefit from a screening programme. It is true that screening for ARCD should probably not be done in dialysis patients who are substantially ill with other conditions. In those patients, attention to the immediate illness is indicated. Similarly, in patients who are unwell from inadequate dialysis, the first priority is to improve the quality of dialysis. But ARCD is much more common now than in years past, both because of native kidney retention and increasing numbers of dialysis patients. In addition, kidney transplantation with the use of cyclosporine may maintain, rather than decrease, the prevalence of ARCD. Screening for ARCD with imaging of native kidneys three years after start of dialysis, has been advised by more than one group (Leichter *et al.* 1988; Matson and Cohen 1990; Grantham 1991). If radiologic screening is not done, then clinicians should be alert for signs and symptoms which may suggest that ARCD and/or a complication has occurred. CT scanning remains the best imaging technique for ARCD and its complications, and bilateral nephrectomy is indicated if a mass is found in an end-stage kidney.

References

Allen, A. C. (1962). *The kidney*, p. 554. Grune & Stratton, New York.

Almirall, J., Mallofre, C., Campistol, J. M., Montoliu, J., Ribalta, T., and Revert, L. (1989). Metastatic renal cell carcinoma in a hemodialysis patient with acquired renal cystic disease. *Nephron*, **52**, 96–7.

Arias, M., de Francisco, A. L. M., Ruiz, L, Val, F., Gonzelez, M., and Zubimendi, A. (1986). Acquired renal cystic disease and renal adenocarcinoma in a long term renal transplant patient. *International Journal of Artificial Organs*, **9**, 271–2.

Baert, L. and Steg, A. (1976). Cystic changes in adult human kidneys after ureteral obstruction. *Urology*, **7**, 526–8.

Blumenthal, S. S., *et al.* (1989). Effect of pH on growth of mouse renal cortical tubule cells in primary culture. *American Journal of Physiology*, **257**, C419–26.

Bommer, J., Waldherr, R., VanKaick, G., Strauss, L., and Ritz, E. (1980). Acquired renal cysts in uremic patients — *in vivo* demonstration by computed tomography. *Clinical Nephrology*, **14**, 299–303.

Bongu, S., Faubert, P. F., Porush, J. G., and Gulmi, F. (1994). Uncontrolled hypertension and hyperreninemia after hemorrhage in a patient with end-stage renal disease and acquired renal cysts. *Journal of the American Society of Nephrology*, **5**, 22–26.

Brendler, C. B., Albertsen, P. C., Goldman, S. M., Hill, G. S., Lowe, F. C., and Millan, J. C. (1984). Acquired renal cystic disease in the end stage kidney: urological implications. *Journal of Urology*, **132**, 548–52.

Carone, F. A., Rowland, R. G., Perlman, S. G., and Ganote, C. E. (1974). The pathogenesis of drug-induced renal cystic disease. *Kidney International*, **5**, 411–21.

Cho, C., Friedland, G. W., and Swenson, R. S. (1984). Acquired renal cystic disease and renal neoplasms in hemodialysis patients. *Urologic Radiology*, **6**, 153–7.

Chung, W. Y., Nast, C. C., Ettenger, R. B., Danovitch, G. M., Ward, H. J., and Cohen, A. H. (1992). Acquired cystic disease in chronically rejected renal transplants. *Journal of the American Society of Nephrology*, **2**, 1298–1301.

Cohen, E. P. (1993). Epidemiology of acquired cystic kidney disease. In *Proceedings of the Fifth International Workshop on Polycystic Kidney Disease*, (ed. P. Gabow and J. Grantham), pp. 81–5. Polycystic Kidney Research Foundation, Kansas City.

Cohen, E. P. and Elliott, W. C. (1990). The role of ischemia in acquired cystic kidney disease. *American Journal of Kidney Diseases*, **15**, 55–60.

Covarsi, A., Rodriguez, A. M., Marigliano, N., and Novillo, R. (1991). Metastasizing renal cell carcinoma and acquired renal cystic disease in a hemodialysis patient. *American Journal of Nephrology*, **11**, 224–8.

Deck, M. A., Verani, R., Silva, F. G., Davis, L. D., and Cohen, A. H. (1988). Histogenesis of renal cysts in end-stage renal disease (acquired cystic kidney disease): an immunohistochemical and lectin study. *Surgical Pathology*, **1**, 391–406.

Dunnill, M. S., Millard, P. R., and Oliver, D. (1977). Acquired cystic disease of the kidneys: a hazard of long-term intermittent maintenance haemodialysis. *Journal of Clinical Pathology*, **30**, 868–77.

Edmunds, M. E., *et al.* (1991). Plasma erythropoietin levels and acquired cystic disease of the kidney in patients receiving regular haemodialysis treatment. *British Journal of Haematology*, **78**, 275–7.

Faber, M., and Kupin, W. (1987). Renal cell carcinoma and acquired cystic kidney disease after renal transplantation. *Lancet*, **1**, 1030–1.

Fayemi, A. O. and Ali, M. (1980). Acquired renal cysts and tumours superimposed on chronic primary kidney diseases. *Pathology Research and Practice*, **168**, 73–83.

Feiner, H. D., Katz, L. A., and Gallo, G. R. (1981). Acquired cystic disease of kidney in chronic dialysis patients. *Urology*, **17**, 260–4.

Fetterman, G. H., Ravitch, M. M., and Sherman, F. E. (1974). Cystic changes in fetal kidneys following ureteral ligation: studies by microdissection. *Kidney International*, **5**, 111–21.

Gehrig, J. J., Gottheiner, T. I., and Swenson, R. S. (1985). Acquired cystic disease of the end-stage kidney. *American Journal of Medicine*, **79**, 609–20.

Glicklich, D., Kutcher, R., Rosenblatt, R., and Barth, R. H. (1990). Time-related increase in hematocrit on chronic hemodialysis: uncertain role of renal cysts. *American Journal of Kidney Diseases*, **15**, 46–54.

Goldsmith, H. J., *et al.* (1982). Association between rising haemoglobin concentration and renal cyst formation in patients on long term regular haemodialysis treatment. *Proceedings of the European Dialysis and Transplant Association*, **19**, 313–18.

Grantham, J. J. (1991). Acquired cystic kidney disease. *Kidney International*, **40**, 143–52.

Grantham, J. J. and Levine, E. (1985). Acquired cystic disease: replacing one kidney disease with another. *Kidney International*, **28**, 99–105.

Hartman, D. S. (1989). *Renal cystic disease*. Saunders, Philadelphia, PA.

Henson, J. H. L., Al-Hilli, S., Penry, J. B., and Mackenzie, J. C. (1985). The development of acquired renal cystic disease and neoplasia in a chronic haemodialysis patient. *British Journal of Radiology*, **58**, 1215–17.

Herrera, G. A. (1991). C-erb B-2 amplification in cystic renal disease. *Kidney International*, **40**, 509–13.

Hricak, H., *et al*. (1982). Renal parenchymal disease: sonographic-histologic correlation. *Radiology*, **144**, 141–7.

Hughson, M. D., Hennigar, G. R., and McManus, J. F. A. (1980). Atypical costs, acquired renal cystic disease, and renal cell tumours in end stage dialysis kidneys. *Laboratory Investigation*, **42**, 475–80.

Ishikawa, I. and Kovacs, G. (1993). High incidence of papillary renal cell tumours in patients on chronic haemodialysis. *Histopathology*, **22**, 135–9.

Ishikawa, I., *et al*. (1980). Development of acquired cystic disease and adenocarcinoma of the kidney in glomerulonephritic chronic hemodialysis patients. *Clinical Nephrology*, **14**, 1–6.

Ishikawa, I., Yuri, T., Kitada, H., and Shinoda, A. (1983). Regression of acquired cystic disease of the kidney after successful renal transplantation. *American Journal of Nephrology*, **3**, 310–14.

Ishikawa, I., Shikura, N., Kitada, H., Yuri, T., Shinoda, A., and Nakazawa, T. (1989). Severity of acquired renal cysts in native kidneys and renal allograft with long-standing poor function. *American Journal of Kidney Disease*, **14**, 18–24.

Ishikawa, I., Saito, Y., Shikwa, N., Kitada, H., Shinoda, A., and Suzuki, S. (1990). Ten-year prospective study on the development of renal cell carcinoma in dialysis patients. *American Journal of Kidney Diseases*, **16**, 452–8.

Ishikawa, I., *et al*. (1991*a*). Renal cell carcinoma of the native kidney after renal transplantation. *Nephron*, **58**, 354–8.

Ishikawa, I., Shikura, N., and Shinoda, A. (1991*b*). Cystic transformation in native kidneys in renal allograft recipients with long-standing good function. *American Journal of Nephrology*, **11**, 217–23.

Jabour, B. A., *et al*. (1987). Acquired cystic disease of the kidneys. Computed tomography and ultrasonography appraisal in patients on peritoneal and hemodialysis. *Investigative Radiography*, **22**, 728–32.

Kanwar, Y. S. and Carone, F. A. (1984). Reversible changes of tubular cell and basement membrane in drug-induced renal cystic disease. *Kidney International*, **26**, 35–43.

Katz, A., Sombolos, K., and Oreopoulos, D. G. (1987). Acquired cystic disease of the kidney in association with chronic ambulatory peritoneal dialysis. *American Journal of Kidney Diseases*, **9**, 426–9.

Kenner, C. H., Evan, A. P., Blomgren, P., Aronoff, G. R., and Luft F. C. (1985). Effect of protein intake on renal function and structure in partially nephrectomized rats. *Kidney International*, **27**, 739–50.

Klotz, L. H., Kulkarni, C., and Mills, G. (1991). End stage renal disease serum contains a specific renal cell growth factor. *Journal of Urology*, **145**, 156–60.

Laucks, S. P. and McLachlan, M. S. F. (1981). Aging and simple cysts of the kidney. *British Journal of Radiology*, **54**, 12–14.

Leichter, H. E., *et al*. (1988). Acquired cystic kidney disease in children undergoing long-term dialysis. *Pediatric Nephrology*, **2**, 8–11.

Levine, E., Grantham, J. J., and MacDougall, M. L. (1987). Spontaneous subcapsular and perinephric hemorrhage in end-stage kidney disease: clinical and CT findings. *American Journal of Roentgenology*, **148**, 755–8.

Levine, E., Slusher, S. L., Grantham, J. J., and Wetzel, L. H. (1991). Natural history of acquired renal cystic disease in dialysis patients: a prospective longitudinal CT study. *American Journal of Roentgenology*, **156**, 501–6.

Lien, Y. H., Kam, I., Shanley, P. F., and Shröter, G. P. J. (1991). Metastatic renal cell carcinoma associated with acquired cystic kidney disease 15 years after successful renal transplantation. *American Journal of Kidney Diseases*, **18**, 711–15.

Lien, Y. H., Hunt, K. R., Siskind, M. S., and Zukoski, C. (1993). Association of cyclosporin A with acquired cystic kidney disease of the native kidneys in renal transplant recipients. *Kidney International*, **44**, 613–16.

Lieske, J. C., Walsh-Reitz, M. M., and Toback, F. G. (1991). Calcium-containing urinary crystals interact with renal tubular cells and induce proliferation. *Journal of the American Society of Nephrology*, **2**, 625.

Lüscher, T. F., Wanner, C., Siegenthaler, W., and Vetter, W. (1986). Simple renal cyst and hypertension: cause or coincidence? *Clinical Nephrology*, **26**, 91–5.

MacDougall, M. L., Welling, L. W., and Wiegmann, T. B. (1990). Prediction of carcinoma in acquired cystic disease as a function of kidney weight. *Journal of the American Society of Nephrology*, **1**, 828–31.

Mallory, F. B. (1914). *The principles of pathologic histology*, (1st edn), p. 572. Saunders, Philadelphia, PA.

Marcén, R., *et al.* (1992). Renal cell carcinoma of the native kidney in a female renal allograft patient without acquired cystic kidney disease. *Nephron*, **61**, 238–9.

Marco-Franco, J. E., *et al.* (1991). Oxalate, silicon, and vanadium in acquired cystic kidney disease. *Clinical Nephrology*, **35**, 52–8.

Matas, A. J., Simmons, R. L., Buselmeier, T. J., Najarian, J. S., and Kjellstrand, C. M. (1975). Lethal complications of bilateral nephrectomy and splenectomy in hemodialyzed patients. *American Journal of Surgery*, **129**, 616–20.

Matson, M. A. and Cohen, E. P. (1990). Acquired cystic kidney disease: occurrence, prevalence, and renal cancers. *Medicine*, **69**, 217–26.

Michel, J. B., *et al.* (1987). Consequences of renal morphologic damage induced by inhibition of converting enzyme in rat renovascular hypertension. *Laboratory Investigation*, **57**, 402–11.

Mickisch, O., Bommer, J., Bachmann, S., Waldherr, R., Mann, J. F. E., and Ritz, E. (1984). Multi-cystic transformation of kidneys in chronic renal failure. *Nephron*, **38**, 93–9.

Miller, L. R., Soffer, O., Nassar, V. H., and Kutner, M. H. (1989). Acquired renal cystic disease in end-stage renal disease: an autopsy study of 155 cases. *American Journal of Nephrology*, **9**, 322–8.

Minar, E., Tscholakoff, D., Zazgornick, J., Schmidt, P., Marosi, L., and Czembirek, H. (1984). Acquired cystic disease of the kidneys in chronic hemodialyzed and renal transplant patients. *European Urology*, **10**, 245–8.

Moskowitz, D. M., Bonar, S. L., and Patel, B. (1990). Acquired renal cystic disease and plasma epidermal growth factor in dialysis patients. *Journal of American Society of Nephrology*, **1**, 636.

Moulder, J. E., Fish, B. L., and Cohen, E. P. (1993). Treatment of radiation nephropathy with ace inhibitors. *International Journal of Radiation Oncology Biology and Physics*, **27**, 93–9.

Narasimhan, N., Golper, T. A., Wolfson, M., Rahatzad, M., and Bennett, W. M. (1986). Clinical characteristics and diagnostic considerations in acquired renal cystic disease. *Kidney International*, **30**, 748–52.

Neufeld, T. K., *et al.* (1992). *In vitro* formation and expansion of cysts derived from human renal cortex epithelial cells. *Kidney International*, **41**, 1222–36.

Newburgh, L. H. and Curtis, A. C. (1928). Production of renal injury in the white rat by the protein of the diet. *Archives of Internal Medicine*, **42**, 801–21.

Ong, A. C. M., and Fine, L. G. (1994). Loss of glomerular function and tubulointerstitial fibrosis: cause or effect? *Kidney International*, **45**, 345–51.

Ono, K., Yasukohchi, A., and Kikawa, K. (1987). Pathogenesis of acquired renal cysts in hemodialysis patients. *Transactions American Society of Artificial Internal Organs*, **33**, 245–9.

Ono, K., Ono, H., Ono, T., Kikawa, K., and Oh, Y. (1989). Acquired renal cysts in five-sixth nephrectomized rats: the role of oxalate deposits in renal tubules and renotropic factor. *Nephron*, **51**, 393–8.

Ratcliffe, P. J., Dunnill, M. S., and Oliver, D. O. (1983). Clinical importance of acquired cystic disease of the kidney in patients undergoing dialysis. *British Medical Journal*, **287**, 1855–8.

Rosse, W. F., Waldmann, T. A., and Cohen, P. (1963). Renal cysts erythropoietin, and polycythemia. *American Journal of Medicine*, **34**, 76–81.

Sarasin, F. P., Meyer, K. B., Wong, J. B., Pauker, S. G., and Levey, A. S. (1991). Screening for acquired cystic kidney disease. *Journal of the American Society of Nephrology*, **2**, 348.

Simon, J. (1847). On sub-acute inflammation of the kidney. *Medical-Chirurgical Transactions*, **30**, 141–64.

Sinsky, C. A., Dahlberg, P. J., and O'Connor, J. (1993). Unilateral acquired renal cystic disease and neoplasia in a patient with renal artery stenosis. *Urology*, **41**, 287–8.

Spiegel, D. M., Yuen-Ko, J. L., Hou, S. H., Brandt, T. D., and Grant, T. H. (1991). Incidence of renal cell carcinoma and natural history of acquired renal cystic disease in end-stage renal disease. *American Journal of Nephrology*, **11**, 166–7.

Taylor, A. J., Cohen, E. P., Erickson, S. J., Olson, D. L., and Foley, W. D. (1989). Renal imaging in long-term dialysis patients: a comparison of CT and sonography. *American Journal of Roentgenology*, **153**, 765–7.

Taylor, A. J., Cohen, E. P., Levine, E., and Grantham, J. J. (1993). Etiology of non-cystic renal masses in the end-stage renal disease kidney. *Proceedings of the 1993 American Roentgen Ray Society Meeting*, San Francisco.

Thomas, J. O., Cox, A. J., and DeEds, F. (1957). Kidney cysts produced by diphenylamine. *Stanford Medical Bulletin*, **15**, 90–3.

Thomson, B. J., Jenkins, D. A. S., Allan, P. L., Elton, R. A., and Winney, R. J. (1988). Acquired cystic disease of the kidney in patients with end-stage chronic renal failure: a study of prevalence and aetiology. *Nephrology, Dialysis, Transplantation*, **1**, 38–43.

Thompson, B. J., *et al.* (1986). Acquired cystic disease of the kidney: an indication for renal transplantation? *British Medical Journal*, **293**, 1209–10.

Thomson, B. J., Allan, P. L., and Winney, R. J. (1985). Acquired cystic disease of kidney: metastatic renal adenocarcinoma and hypercalcemia. *Lancet*, **1**, 502–3.

Tielemans, C. L., Collart, F. E., Hooghe, L., and Dratwa, M. (1983). Renal hematoma in a patient undergoing hemodialysis. *Archives of Internal Medicine*, **143**, 1623–5.

Torres, V. E., *et al.* (1988). Mechanisms affecting the development of renal cystic disease induced by diphenylthiazole. *Kidney International*, **33**, 1130–9.

Truong, L. D., Ansari, M. Q., Ansari, S. J., Wheeler, T. M., Mattioli, C. M., and Gillum, D. (1988). Acquired cystic kidney disease: occurrence in patients on chronic peritoneal dialysis. *American Journal of Kidney Disease*, **11**, 192–5.

Turani, H., Levi, J., Zevin, D., and Kessler, E. (1983). Acquired cystic disease and tumors in kidneys of hemodialysis patients. *Israel Journal of Medical Sciences*, **19**, 614–18.

Wardle, E. N. and Wilkinson, K. (1976). Free phenols in chronic renal failure. *Clinical Nephrology*, **6**, 361–4.

Worcester, E. M., Fellner, S. K., Nakagawa, Y., and Coe, F. L. (1994). The effect of renal transplantation on serum oxalate and urinary oxalate excretion. *Nephron*, **67**, 414–18.

Yarimizu, S. N., Susan, L. P., Straffon, R. A., Steward, B. H., Magnusson, M. O., and Nakamoto, S. S. (1978). Mortality and morbidity in pretransplant bilateral nephrectomy. *Urology*, **12**, 55–8.

11

Tuberous sclerosis complex

Vicente E. Torres

Introduction

Tuberous sclerosis complex (TSC) is an autosomal dominant disease that affects all tissues with the possible exception of the peripheral nervous system, meninges, and skeletal muscles. The term 'tuberous sclerosis complex' is preferred to tuberous sclerosis because it emphasizes the multiplicity of organs involved. Some of the lesions are so characteristic that they are considered diagnostic for the disease. Other lesions by themselves are not sufficient unless they are multiple, Table 11.1 (Gomez 1988*a*; 1991).

The lesions of TSC become clinically detectable by different ages (Gomez 1992). This is important to assess the significance of the absence of a certain lesion in individuals at risk. Cardiac rhabdomyomas are present at birth and

Table 11.1   Clinical findings leading to a diagnosis of tuberous sclerosis complex

Neurological (definite diagnosis: single with histological confirmation;
   multiple by imaging or ophthalmoscopy):
Cortical tuber
Subependymal glial nodule/giant cell astrocytoma
Retinal hamartoma

Dermatological (definite diagnosis)
Facial angiofibromas
Fibrous forehead plaque
Ungual fibroma
Shagreen patch (histological confirmation)

Visceral (presumptive diagnosis)*
Multiple renal angiomyolipomas
Multiple cardiac rhabdomyomas
Multiple renal cysts and an angiomyolipoma
Pulmonary lymphangioleiomyomatosis and a renal angiomyolipoma

Suggestive: hypomelanotic skin macules;
enamel pits; hamartomatous rectal polyps; ragiographic sclerotic
bone patches and cysts; angiomyolipoma of kidney, liver, adrenal or gonads; thyroid
adenoma (papillary or fetal type); infantile spasms

*Individuals with only these findings have borne children with TSC.

diminish in size and even disappear in subsequent years. Fibrous forehead plaques may be present at birth. White macules, which are not diagnostic by themselves, develop earlier than the other skin lesions and may also be present at birth. Facial angiofibromas appear after 3 years of age with a peak of onset around 10 years and rarely after 20 years. Subependymal giant cell astrocytomas develop between 5 and 15 years and stop growing after 20 years of age. Renal cysts, but not angiomyolipomas, can be observed in the first year of age.

The most common clinical presentations include neurological and skin manifestations. Other presenting manifestations include symptoms related to cardiac rhabdomyomas, renal angiomyolipomas, or pulmonary lymphangioleiomyomatosis (Fig. 11.1). Approximately 80 per cent of affected individuals have seizures and

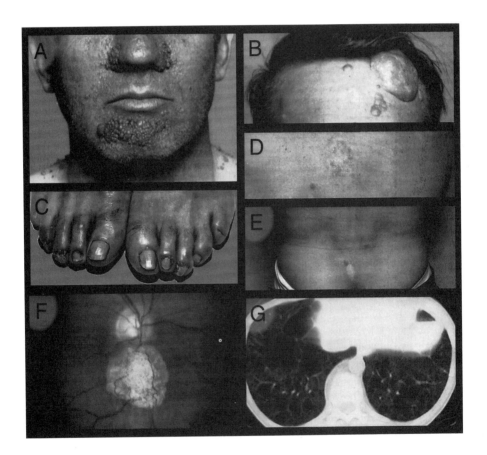

Fig. 11.1 Lesions of tuberous sclerosis complex: facial angiofibroma (A), forehead fibrous plaques (B), ungual fibromas (C), shagreen patch (D), hypomelanotic macule (E), retinal hamartoma (F), and CT of pulmonary lymphangioleiomyomatosis (G).

50 per cent have mental retardation (Torres *et al.* 1994). In affected individuals over five years of age, facial angiofibromas are found in 86 per cent, hypomelanotic macules in 78 per cent, ungual fibromas in 47 per cent, shagreen patches in 41 per cent, and forehead plaques in 26 per cent (Rogers 1988). Retinal hamartomas are present in 50 per cent of the patients (Robertson 1991). Cardiac rhabdomyomas occur in approximately 50 per cent of children with TSC with a higher frequency in the first two years of life (Watson 1991).

History

The first illustration of typical angiofibromas of TSC was probably by Rayer (1835), in his *atlas of skin diseases*. In 1862, von Recklinghausen described the presence of multiple cardiac 'myomata' and cerebral 'sclerosis' in an infant who died shortly after birth. The term 'tuberous sclerosis of the cerebral convolutions' was coined by Bourneville in 1880 when he described the potato-like hardening of the hypertrophic cerebral gyri in a 15-year-old epileptic, hemiplegic, and mentally defective girl. Bourneville also recognized the association of these cerebral lesions and kidney tumours. This patient also had facial angiofibromas which were mistaken for acne rosacea. In 1885 Balzer and Ménétrier described this lesion in detail under the name of 'adenoma sebaceum'. The same lesion was described five years later by Pringle in a 25-year-old woman with mental retardation (Pringle 1890). The diagnostic significance of the facial angiofibromas together with seizures and mental retardation was pointed out by Vogt in 1908. The histological features of renal angiomyolipoma were described in 1911 by Fischer in patients with TSC. It soon became clear that none of the elements of the classic Vogt's triad (seizures, mental retardation, and facial angiofibromas) is essential for the diagnosis of TSC. In 1914, Schuster reported a patient with facial angiofibromas and seizures but of normal intelligence. In 1920, Van der Hoeve described the retinal hamartomas of TSC and coined the term 'retinal phakoma'. Hypomelanotic macules were recognized by Critchley and Earl in 1932, and pulmonary cysts were described by Berg and Vejlens in 1939. Other associations listed in Table 11.1 have been described more recently.

Prevalence

Increasing recognition of mild forms of TSC and better case assessment explain why the prevalence of TSC in population-based service is now estimated at approximately 1/10000 as compared with 1/150000 in 1956 (Stevenson and Fisher 1956; Nevin and Pearce 1968; Singer 1971; Hunt and Lindenbaum 1984; Wiederholt *et al.* 1985; Sampson *et al.* 1989; Osborne *et al.* 1991; Shepherd *et al.* 1991; Ahlsén *et al.* 1994). Because the diagnosis of TSC is not made in many asymptomatic and some symptomatic subjects and because some patients with this disease have shortened life expectancies, these figures likely underestimate the prevalence of the TSC gene in the population at large and also at birth. The prevalence rates for Rochester, and Olmsted County, Minnesota are 1/9400 and 1/14 400, respectively (Wiederholt *et al.* 1985; Shepherd *et al.* 1991*a*). A study from Bristol, United Kingdom, suggests that the prevalence at birth may be as high as 1/5800 (Osborne *et al.* 1991). In a recent study from western Sweden, the prevalence of TSC was found to be 1/12 900 in the whole age cohort 0–20 years and 1/6800 in the 11- to 15-year-old age group (Ahlsén *et al.* 1994). The frequency of new mutations has remained constant at approximately 60–70 per cent. As cases with TSC with reduced expression are recognized, the frequency of seizures and mental retardation in the population-based studies has decreased.

Aetiology and pathogenesis

TSC is an autosomal dominant disease with a high mutation rate that appears to affect cell migration and differentiation in a variety of organs. It has been suggested that derivatives of the neural crest cells constitute the chief elements involved in the lesions of TSC (Johnson *et al.* 1991; Lallier 1991). A 'two-hit' hypothesis has been proposed to explain the variability of expression, focal character, and multiplicity of these lesions. The first hit would be an inherited germ cell mutation, while the second hit occurs later as a random new mutations or other chromosomal event. As in many other genetic diseases, the novel approach of reverse genetics has been applied to TSC. Linkage studies to a variety of genetic markers in different chromosomes indicate that TSC is genetically heterogeneous. There are at least two gene loci. The first one to be found is in chromosome 9q32q34 near the ABO blood group and *ABL* oncogene (Connor and Sampson 1991; Haines *et al.* 1991; Janssen *et al.* 1991). The second was discovered near the ADPKD1 locus in chromosome 16p13 (Kandt *et al.* 1992). Other gene loci reported to be in chromosome 11, 12, and 14 have not been confirmed in a majority of TSC patients by subsequent investigators (Fahsold *et al.* 1991; Kandt *et al.* 1991; Smith *et al.* 1991). The gene in chromosome 16p13.3 has been recently identified and sequenced (The European Chromosome 16 Tuberous Sclerosis Consortium 1993). Its protein product, which has been named tuberin, has a region of homology to the GTPase activating protein GAP3. GTPase activating proteins bind to Ras proteins, regulate their activity, and are involved in the control of cell proliferation and differentiation (Satoh *et al.* 1992). Two other recent observations have provided support to the neural crest derivation and two-hit hypothesis. The presence of cells in angiomyolipomas and in pulmonary and extrapulmonary lymphangioleiomyomatosis of melanoma-related antigens recognized by the antibody HMB-45 may reflect a neuro-ectodermal origin of these cells (Pea *et al.* 1991; Tsui *et al.* 1992; Bonetti *et al.* 1993; Torres *et al.* 1995). Loss of heterozygosity (allele loss on chromosome 16p13.3) has been demonstrated in a number of benign lesions from patients with TSC, including renal angiomyolipomas, one cardiac rhabdomyoma, one cortical tuber, and one giant cell astrocytoma (Green *et al.* 1994; Smith *et al.* 1993). In one of these cases, it was shown that the allele loss involved the allele inherited by the patient's unaffected daughter and, therefore, not affected by the germ line mutation. These observations are consistent with the hypothesis that the *TSC* gene is a tumour or growth suppressor gene.

Central nervous system

The main neurological manifestations of TSC include, by decreasing order of frequency seizures, mental retardation, intracranial hypertension, and focal neurological deficits (Gomez 1988*b*; Curatolo *et al.* 1991). The lesions of TSC in the CNS include cortical tubers, subependymal glial nodules, and giant cell astrocytomas. These lesions result from defects in the migration of neurone and glia precursors during embryonic development (Huttenlocher and Wollmann 1991). The more dysplastic cells remain in a subependymal location and give rise to the subependymal glial nodules and giant cell astrocytomas. Tracks of heterotopic neural astrocytes can extend from the periventricular zone throughout the subcortical white matter to the cerebral cortex. The cortical tubers contain a mixture of undifferentiated and more differentiated neurones and glia. The cortical tubers are thought to be responsible for the seizures and mental retardation. Only patients who have had seizures, especially in the first year of life, are mentally retarded (Gomez 1988*b*). The seizures can be generalized or less often partial. The most common generalized seizures are infantile spasms and tonic–clonic seizures. Symptoms of intracranial hypertension (headaches, nausea, vomiting, and personality changes) occur less frequently than seizures and mental retardation. The intracranial hypertension is caused by obstruction of the cerebrospinal fluid circulation caused by a giant cell astrocytoma situated near the foramen of Monro (Gomez 1988*b*). Focal neurological deficits, such as spastic hemiplegia and cerebellar signs, occur rarely. The early diagnosis and treatment of seizures in patients with TSC is essential to reduce the risk of mental deficits. While the treatment of seizures unique and not unique to childhood in TSC is beyond the scope of this chapter, it should be noted that the development of new anticonvulsant drugs, imaging techniques, and epilepsy surgery provide an opportunity to improve the condition of some of these patients (Bebin *et al.* 1993). The treatment of intracranial hypertension is either shunting or resection of the giant cell astrocytoma when feasible.

Skin

The skin lesions of TSC (Fig. 11.1) include facial angiofibroma, fibrous plaques, ungual fibromas, shagreen patches, and hypomelanotic macules (Rogers 1988). The first three are pathognomonic for TSC. The facial angiofibroma consists of red-to-pink papules or nodules with a smooth surface, symmetrically distributed over the central facial areas, particularly in the nasolabial folds and on the cheeks. In the first year of life, they may appear as a central facial flushing when the child cries. Well-developed angiofibromas may appear by the age of four years and the lesions may become more numerous and prominent at puberty. The fibrous plaques are large angiofibromas which appear as flesh-coloured plaques usually on the forehead or scalp. The ungual fibromas or Koenen's tumours are papular or nodular lesions arising from the nailbed and protruding around the nail groove or under the nail. They are more common on toes than fingers and they appear at or after puberty. Shagreen patches (from the French '*peau chagriné*' meaning 'skin with appearance of untanned leather') are usually found on dorsal body surfaces, particularly the lumbosacral area, and appear as skin-coloured rubbery plaques ranging in size from a few millimetres to a few centimetres. Hypomelanotic macules are the most frequent and earliest skin manifestations of TSC and is helpful to suspect the disease in individuals at risk but are not specific and by themselves are not diagnostic. Three types of hypomelanotic macules have been described: polygonal (like a thumbprint), the most common; lance-ovate (ash-leaf spot), the most characteristic; and confetti-like, rare but quite specific (Fitzpatrick 1991). The term 'poliosis' refers to hypomelanotic macules in the scalp with hypopigmented hairs. The hypomelanotic macules in TSC are usually numerous, asymmetrically distributed over the entire body, and best detected with the Wood's lamp. Angiofibromas can be treated by excisional surgery, dermabrasion or, if there is a significant vascular component, by yellow laser or argon laser therapy. Ungual fibromas are excised only when they cause pain or functional impairment. Treatment of the other skin lesions is rarely indicated.

Eye

Retinal astrocytic hamartomas occur in approximately half of the patients with TSC and in half of them the lesions are bilateral (Robertson 1991). The lesions are circular or oval and may be salmon-coloured and smooth surfaced or white, elevated, multinodular, and calcified (Fig. 11.1). Retinal hamartomas do not grow, but over the years they may become calcified. Visual loss is very rare and may be due to involvement of the fovea or to retinal detachment. Treatment is rarely indicated.

Heart

Cardiac rhabdomyomas are benign tumours that are often multiple, affect the ventricles more often than the atria, and are more frequently located in the ventricular septum (Burke and Virmani 1991). Recent echocardiographic studies indicate that the frequency of cardiac rhabdomyomas in TSC may be as high as 50–86 per cent during late pregnancy and 90 per cent below the age of two years (Jozwiak *et al.* 1994). During childhood, the rhabdomyomas tend to regress spontaneously. A rhabdomyoma-related clinical deterioration or death is rare. The symptoms can develop by one of three mechanisms: (1) obstruction to passage of blood by intracavitary tumours; (2) loss of contractility and congestive heart failure by replacement of myocardial tissue; and (3) arrhythmias including fetal bradycardia, ventricular tachycardia and fibrillation and the Wolff–Parkinson–White syndrome (Jayakar *et al.* 1986; Garson *et al.* 1987; Case *et al.* 1991). The treatment of patients with symptomatic cardiac rhabdomyomas is usually conservative, hoping for a regression of the lesions, but surgical removal can be considered in patients with severe haemodynamic obstruction or life-threatening arrhythmias resistant to other forms of therapy.

Lung

The pulmonary lesion of TSC is histologically indistinguishable from idiopathic pulmonary lymphangioleiomyomatosis (Lie 1991). It is estimated to occur in less than 1 per cent of patients, but its frequency may be higher with current imaging techniques (Hoffman 1991). It occurs predominantly in females. It is characterized by an abnormal proliferation of smooth muscle cells around the airways, blood vessels, and lymphatics resulting in obstructive airway disease, cysts, pneumothorax, chylothorax, hemoptysis, and pulmonary hypertension. Tissue obtained from pulmonary lymphangioleiomyomatosis often, but not always, express oestrogen and progesterone receptors (Graham *et al.* 1984; Schiaffino *et al.* 1989; Colley *et al.* 1989; Ohori *et al.* 1991). The chest X-ray commonly demonstrates diffuse interstitial infiltrates and hyperinflation, but the most sensitive imaging technique to detect this lesion is high resolution computed tomography (CT), which demonstrates the characteristic cysts throughout the lungs (Hoffman 1991). Most patients have gradual deterioration of pulmonary function which may result in respiratory failure. Selected patients with pulmonary lymphangioleiomyomatosis without TSC have benefited from oophorectomy, radioablation of the ovaries, or administration of progesterone, anti-oestrogens, or androgens (Garson *et al.* 1987). On this basis, some patients with TSC and progressive pulmonary lymphangioleiomyomatosis have also been treated with hormonal manipulation. In a review on pulmonary lymphangioleiomyomatosis, it was suggested that the administration of medroxyprogesterone acetate at a dose of 400–800 mg intramuscularly per month could be used as the initial treatment and that oophorectomy could be performed for patients not responding to this therapy (Taylor *et al.* 1990). Pregnancy and administration of oestrogens should be avoided in these patients. Patients with end-stage respiratory failure can be treated by a single lung transplantation.

Other organs

In addition to the kidneys, angiomyolipomas can occur in other organs such as the liver, adrenal gland, and gonads. As it is the case in the kidney, hepatic angiomyolipomas are more frequent in women than in men and most patients with hepatic angiomyolipomas do not have TSC (Nonomura *et al.* 1994). Hamartomatous rectal polyps are common in TSC. They may be potential useful clinical marker and cause no symptoms (Gould 1991). Skeletal abnormalities are also common, usually asymptomatic and consist of areas of sclerosis and

cyst-like lesions (Hoffman 1991). Pitted enamel hypoplasia of the teeth occurs frequently (Lydidakis and Lindbaum 1987). Extrapulmonary lymphangioleiomyomatosis with retroperitoneal, pelvic or perirenal lymphangiomatous cysts,
chylous ascites, and involvement of the uterus has been observed in association
with TSC and pulmonary lymphangioleiomyomatosis (Torres *et al.* 1995).
Involvement of medium-sized and large vessels, including aortic aneurysms, aortic
coarctation, and intracranial aneurysms may occur rarely in TSC (Lie 1991).

Renal involvement in tuberous sclerosis complex

The kidneys are frequently involved in TSC. The main renal manifestations of
TSC include angiomyolipomas, cysts, and renal cell carcinomas (Torres *et al.*
1994; Bernstein *et al.* 1986; Bernstein and Robbins 1991). Other renal neoplasms, interstitial renal disease, focal segmental glomerulosclerosis (FSGS),
peripelvic and perirenal lymphangiomatous cysts, glomerular microhamartomas,
vascular dysplasia, ureteropelvic junction obstruction, and renal malformations
are less often observed (Torres *et al.* 1994). Unfortunately, information on the
frequency of these manifestations in population-based studies of TSC is limited.
Of the 10 Olmsted County residents included in the study of Shepherd and co-
workers in 1991; two patients had renal angiomyolipomas; one patient had
increased renal echogenicity on sonography and hypertension; one patient had
multiple angiomyolipomas, cysts, and a renal cell carcinoma and underwent
unilateral nephrectomy, dialysis, and renal transplantation; three patients had
normal renal sonograms; and three patients did not have renal imaging studies
(Shepherd *et al.* 1991*a*). The importance of the kidney in TSC is reflected by
the fact that renal involvement is second only to the involvement of the central
nervous system as a cause of death in patients with TSC (Shepherd *et al.*
1991*b*). Of 403 patients with a diagnosis of TSC seen at the Mayo Clinic since
1940, 49 were known to have died. The cause of death was a brain tumour or
status epilepticus in 19; renal disease in 11; and pulmonary lymphangioleiomyomatosis in 4. Of the 11 patients with a renal cause of death; six died of renal
failure; three died of retroperitoneal hemorrhage (one on dialysis and two with
preserved renal function); and two died of metastatic renal cell carcinoma
(Shepherd *et al.* 1991*b*). Of the seven patients who had reached end-stage renal
failure at the time of death; three had large polycystic kidneys; two had small
contracted cystic kidneys; and two had experienced progressive renal
insufficiency following unilateral nephrectomies for angiomyolipomas (Torres
et al. 1994; Shepherd *et al.* 1991*b*). The details of the renal pathology in one
patient were not available.

Renal angiomyolipomas

Angiomyolipomas are benign tumours composed of abnormal thickened-wall
vessels that lack a well-developed internal elastic lamina and of varying amounts
of spindle smooth muscle-like cells and adipose tissue (Fig. 11.2) (Farrow *et al.*

1968). These tumours are benign but can be locally invasive, extending into perirenal fat or, more rarely, collecting system, renal vein, and even inferior vena cava and right atrium (Camúnez *et al.* 1987; Kutcher *et al.* 1982; Rothenberg *et al.* 1986). Lymph node and splenic involvements probably represent multicentricity of origin rather than metastases as long-term follow-up of patients with such presentations has not demonstrated tumour recurrence (Bloom *et al.* 1982; Hulbert and Graf 1983). Angiomyolipomas are found in about 0.3 to 2.1 per cent of kidneys at routine autopsy (Hajdu and Foote 1969; Reese and Winstanley 1958). With the availability and more frequent use of ultrasonography (US) and computed tomography (CT), small asymptomatic angiomyolipomas are now more often clinically diagnosed. Because these figures largely exceed both the frequency of symptomatic angiomyolipomas in the general population and the estimated prevalence of TSC, it is obvious that most patients with angiomyolipomas never have symptoms and do not have TSC. Symptomatic angiomyolipomas in patients without TSC are usually single and mainly found in middle-aged women (Blute *et al.* 1988; Heckl *et al.* 1987; Oesterling *et al.* 1986). On the other hand, angiomyolipomas in patients with TSC are usually multiple and bilateral (Steiner *et al.* 1993; Stillwell *et al.* 1987).

The histogenesis of the renal angiomyolipomas is not understood. In 1954, Inglis suggested that the spindle muscle-like cells in these tumours were immature Schwann's cells derived from the neural crest. The same author later retracted this hypothesis and suggested that these cells originate from pericytes

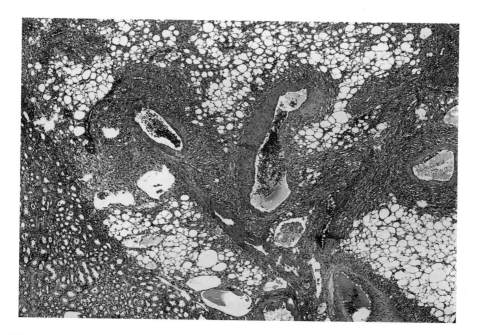

Fig. 11.2 Angiomyolipoma containing adipose tissue, abnormal vessels with thickened walls, and spindle, smooth muscle-like cells.

or modified smooth muscle cells (Inglis 1960). An electron microscopic study that suggested a similarity to blastic Schwann's cells and supported the first of these hypotheses has not been confirmed by later studies (Mori *et al.* 1971). On the other hand, many electron microscopic and immunohistochemical studies have provided strong support for the smooth muscle origin of the majority of spindle cells in the angiomyolipomas (Chalvardjian *et al.* 1978; Holm-Nielsen and Sørensen 1988; Perez-Atayde *et al.* 1981; Sun *et al.* 1975). Crystalloid structures have been described in these smooth muscle cells (Mukai *et al.* 1992). The nature of these crystalloids is not known, but they are not renin, as they do not stain with antirenin antiserum. Two recent observations have provided new support for the participation of neural crest cells in the pathogenesis of the renal angiomyolipomas. Pea and co-workers have consistently detected immunoreactivity with the melanocyte-related monoclonal antibody HMB-45 in a subset of cells comprising about 10 per cent of the tumour cell population in renal angiomyolipomas, but not in renal cell carcinomas, Wilms' tumours, and retroperitoneal sarcomas (Pea *et al.* 1991). In addition, Davidson and colleagues showed staining of cultured cells isolated from a renal angiomyolipoma in a patient with TSC with neuronal antibodies (Davidson *et al.* 1991). Possibly neural crest-derived cells could interact with surrounding cells through the secretion of growth factors, trophic factors, or neurotransmitters. Factor XIII$_a$ (a factor that stimulates the proliferation of fibroblasts and the formation of collagen matrix), for example, has been demonstrated in the stromal cells of a renal angiomyolipoma in a patient with TSC (Penneys *et al.* 1991).

Angiomyolipomas are extremely common in patients with TSC. At autopsy they are found in 40 to 80 per cent of the patients, but rarely before five years of age (Reed *et al.* 1963). The frequency and the size of angiomyolipomas increase with age as demonstrated by a study of 164 patients who were seen at the Mayo Clinic and had at least one renal CT or US (Torres *et al.* 1994) (Fig. 11.3). Angiomyolipomas were not observed in the first year of age, but were present in 37 per cent of the children between one and five years of age. After the age of five years, angiomyolipomas were observed in 41 per cent of males and 63 per cent of females. Women had more and larger angiomyolipomas than men. Small angiomyolipomas were most often cortical and frequently had a wedge-shaped appearance with the base of the wedge facing the surface of the kidney. As the lesions increase in size, they penetrate deeper into the renal parenchyma or become exophytic extending into the renal parenchyma or become exophytic extending into the perirenal fat. Thirty-three of 403 patients seen at Mayo Clinic had multiple studies over periods of time ranging from 3 to 13 years. New angiomyolipomas appeared in six patients with negative initial studies. An increase in the number and/or size of the angiomyolipomas were observed in 9 of 13 patients who already had lesions at the time of the initial evaluation. The rate of growth of the large lesion ranged from 1 to 12 mm per year, with a mean of 5 mm per year. It has been suggested that angiomyolipomas associated to TSC and angiomyolipomas greater than 4 cm in diameter are more likely to grow than sporadic or smaller lesions (Steiner *et al.* 1993).

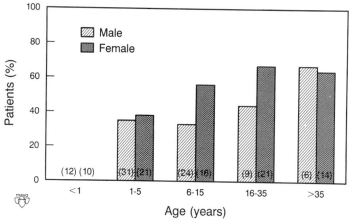

Fig. 11.3 Frequency of angiomyolipomas at the age of the first computed tomography or sonography in 164 patients with tuberous sclerosis complex. Reproduced by permission from Torres *et al.* (1994). *Advances in Nephrology*, **23**: 43–70.

The main manifestations of the renal angiomyolipomas relate to their potential for haemorrhage (haematuria, intratumoral, or retroperitoneal haemorrhage), and mass effect (abdominal or flank mass and tenderness, hypertension, renal insufficiency) (Blute *et al.* 1988; Heckl *et al.* 1987; Oesterling *et al.* 1986). An angiomyolipoma, even small and non-necrotic, can be a source of fever of unknown origin (Steiner *et al.* 1993). Tumour size correlates with the presence or absence of symptoms. Small angiomyolipomas are usually, but not always asymptomatic (Blute *et al.* 1988; Heckl *et al.* 1987; Oesterling *et al.* 1986). Microhaematuria is commonly reported in surgical studies (Reese and Winstanley 1958), but is rarely observed in patients with asymptomatic angiomyolipomas (Stillwell *et al.* 1987). There have been a number of reports of life-threatening gross haematuria or retroperitoneal haemorrhage during pregnancy, and it has been suggested that an increased blood volume may be a factor in causing these tumours to rupture and bleed (Torres *et al.* 1994; Lewis and Palmer 1985; Petrikovsky *et al.* 1990). As women have more numerous and larger angiomyolipomas than men, it seems likely that the hormonal changes associated with pregnancy also may play a role in the growth and risk for haemorrhage in this condition. Hypertension occurs less often in the patients with angiomyolipomas without cysts than in those with renal cysts with or without angiomyolipomas (Torres *et al.* 1994). The pathogenesis of hypertension associated with renal angiomyolipomas is not known. Immunohistochemical studies suggest that these tumours do not contain renin (Mukai *et al.* 1992). The possibility that the hypertension may be caused by compression of the adjacent kidney by the tumour and release of renin was suggested by the observation of patients whose hypertension was cured after removal of the tumour (Van Baal *et al.* 1989; Futter and Collins 1974). Nevertheless, the majority of patients with renal angiomyolipomas have normal blood pressure, and most of those with pre-existing hypertension remain hypertensive following the surgical removal of the angiomyolipoma (Blute *et al.* 1988). Peripheral renin activity in these patients has been normal or low, suggesting a volume-expanded state (Futter and Collins 1974; Green *et al.* 1990). Bilateral renal angiomyolipomas can destroy enough renal tissue to cause significant impairment of renal function. These patients with bilateral angiomyolipomas and an elevated serum creatinine also have low-grade proteinuria by urinalysis, suggesting the possible coexistence of hypertension and FSGS.

Prior to the introduction of US and CT, the pre-operative diagnosis of an angiomyolipoma could rarely be made with certainty because the angiographic characteristics of these lesions (serpentine vessels, saccular aneurysms, and puddling of contrast medium) are not specific and occasionally can be observed in malignant renal tumours (Heckl *et al.* 1987). The diagnosis of angiomyolipoma by any of these techniques requires the identification of fat in the tumour, increased echogenicity on US, and low attenuation of CT (Bosniak *et al.* 1988; Totty *et al.* 1981; Uhlenbrock *et al.* 1988). Therefore, the diagnostic accuracy depends on the amount of fat tissue in the tumour. US may be more sensitive than CT for detecting small angiomyolipomas because the fatty tissue is highly echogenic and lesions smaller than 1 cm may be difficult to diagnose on CT due to partial volume effect (Fig. 11.4). The use of 5-mm thin sections and un-enhanced scans improves the accuracy of CT in detecting fat in small lesions in which partial volume effect may be significant. On the other hand, the specificity of CT may be superior to that of US in differentiating small angiomyolipomas from perinephric or renal sinus fat. CT also may be superior to US for detecting small angiomyolipomas in a diffusely hyperechoic kidney (see Fig. 11.4). When the angiomyolipomas contain mainly smooth muscle and little fat, US may show a hypoechoic pattern, and CT may display a density comparable to carcinoma or normal renal tissue. More recently, magnetic resonance imaging (MRI) has been added to the evaluation of these tumours, and in some cases may be more sensitive in demonstrating the fat in the tumour (Ulenbrock *et al.* 1988). On MRI, the fat gives a high signal intensity in T-1 weighted images and an intermediate signal in T-2 weighted images (see Fig. 11.4). Occasionally, the distinction between an angiomyolipoma and a renal cell carcinoma cannot be reliably established by any imaging techniques. In this situation, US or CT-guided fine-needle aspiration biopsy has been proposed to help differentiate between a renal angiomyolipoma and a renal cell carcinoma and avoid surgical exploration (Sant *et al.* 1990; Tallada *et al.* 1994). At present, the safety and efficacy of this approach are not clearly defined, and our preference in this setting is to proceed with surgical exploration.

Renal angiomyolipomas are benign lesions and often require no treatment. The increased frequency and size of the angiomyolipomas in women and the reports of haemorrhagic complications during pregnancy suggest that female sex hormones may foster the growth of these lesions. It seems, therefore, reasonable to caution patients with multiple angiomyolipomas about the potential risks of

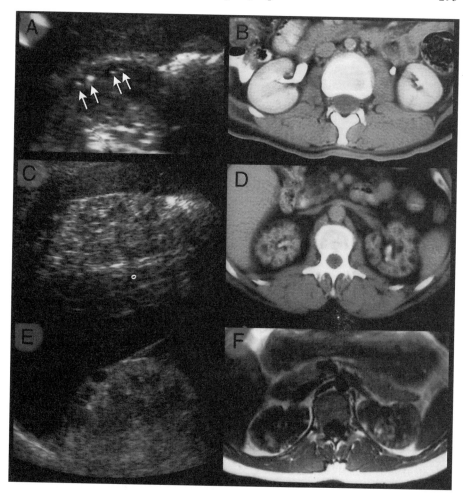

Fig. 11.4 Small angiomyolipomas detected by US (arrows in A), but not seen on contrast-enhanced CT (B). Hyperechoic kidney by US (C), containing numerous small angiomyolipomas detected by CT (D). Hyperechoic kidney by US (E) containing numerous small angiomyolipomas detected by MRI (F).

pregnancy and oestrogen administration. In pulmonary lymphangioleiomyomatosis, which is more life-threatening than multiple renal angiomyolipomas, oophorectomy, radioablation of the ovaries, progesterone administration, antioestrogens, and androgens have been used (Adamson *et al.* 1985; Banner *et al.* 1981; Bush *et al.* 1969; Clemm *et al.* 1987; El Allaf *et al.* 1984; McCarty *et al* 1980). Whether any of these treatment modalities has had any beneficial effect on the development and growth of the renal angiomyolipomas is not known. Because of the potential that angiomyolipomas have for growth and development of complications, annual re-evaluation with US or CT is necessary (Blute *et al.*

1988; Oesterling *et al.* 1986). Indications for intervention include symptoms such as pain or haemorrhage, growth with compromise of functioning renal parenchyma, and inability to exclude an associated renal cell carcinoma. Because angiomyolipomas greater than 4 cm in patients with TSC are more likely to grow and cause symptoms, some authors suggest that prophylactic intervention should be considered in these patients. (Steiner *et al.* 1993). When associated malignancy can be excluded, the treatment should be aimed to spare as much renal tissue as possible. Renal-sparing surgery, such as enucleation or partial nephrectomy, should be used (Blute *et al.* 1988; Oesterling *et al.* 1986). Some lesions, because of their size or central location, may be more amenable to selective arterial embolization (Earthman *et al.* 1986; Eason *et al.* 1979; Johnson *et al.* 1991; Van Baal *et al.* 1990). This procedure is often facilitated by the presence of one or more large hypertrophic feeding vessels. This technique has been found to be effective and safe, with a low rate of complications, including haemorrhage and infection.

Renal cysts

Cystic disease is the second most common renal manifestation of TSC (Bernstein *et al.* 1986; Bernstein and Robbins 1991; Stillwell *et al.* 1987; Robbins and Bernstein 1988). The number of cysts may range from one or few to innumerable and, in the absence of angiomyolipomas, macroscopically indistinguishable from polycystic kidney disease. Because cystic kidneys may be the presenting manifestation of TSC, this diagnosis should be considered in children with renal cysts and no family history of polycystic kidney disease (Steiner *et al.* 1993; Berant and Alon 1987; Wenzl *et al.* 1970). The renal cystic involvement in TSC is particularly prominent in certain families, suggesting genetic determinants that at present are not understood (Durham 1987; Mitnick *et al.* 1983; O'Callaghan *et al.* 1975).

The cysts in TSC develop from any segment of the nephron. When their number is limited and the size is small, they are predominantly cortical. In some cases, glomerular cysts may predominate (Bernstein and Robbins 1991; Saguem *et al.* 1992). Large epithelial cells may line the Bowman's capsules and cover the glomerular tufts. Bernstein has suggested that the epithelial lining of the cysts is distinctive and unique to TSC (Bernstein *et al.* 1986; Bernstein and Robbins 1991). The cells are large and acidophilic, and contain large, hyperchromatic nuclei with occasional mitotic figures. Papillary hyperplasia and adenomas are common.

Cysts were detected in 20 per cent of male and 9 per cent of female patients with TSC who were seen at the Mayo Clinic and had at least one renal CT or US (Torres *et al.* 1994). Their frequency increases with age, but in some patients extensive cystic disease is already present at birth and during the first year of life (Berant and Alon 1987; Dommergues *et al.* 1982; Miller *et al.* 1989; Stapleton *et al.* 1980; Wenzl *et al.* 1970; Moss and Hendry 1988).

The major clinical problem associated with severe cystic changes in TSC is the development of hypertension and renal failure (Torres *et al.* 1994; Okada *et al.* 1982). The clinical presentation of TSC with large cystic kidneys often with associated hypertension usually occurs early, during the first year of life or childhood (Berant and Alon 1987; Dommergues *et al.* 1982; Miller *et al.* 1989; Stapleton *et al.* 1980; Wenzl *et al.* 1970; Durham 1987; Mitnick *et al.* 1983; O'Callaghan *et al.* 1975; Saguem *et al.* 1992; Moss and Hendry 1988). The pathogenesis of the hypertension is not known, but the peripheral renin activity has been found to be elevated (Michel *et al.* 1983; Yu and Sheth 1985). Renal failure is likely to develop in many of these patients in the second or third decades of life. Whether the absence or strict control of hypertension has a favourable impact on the prognosis of these patients is not known.

The appearance of the cysts on US, CT or MRI is identical to that of benign simple cysts or polycystic kidney disease except for the frequent coexistence of angiomyolipomas (Torres *et al.* 1994; Bernstein *et al.* 1986; Bernstein and Robbins 1991). In the absence of angiomyolipomas, it may be impossible to differentiate radiologically demonstrated TSC from autosomal dominant polycystic kidney disease (Fig. 11.5). Approximately 10 per cent of TSC patients have hepatic angiomyolipomas, and 3 per cent have hepatic cysts (Torres *et al.* 1994).

The mainstay of the treatment for the cystic disease associated with TSC is strict control of the hypertension. Surgical decompression of these kidneys has been considered, but the experience available in patients with autosomal dominant polycystic kidney disease does not suggest that surgical decompression has, at least in the short term, a beneficial effect.

Renal cell carcinoma

At the turn of the century, an association between TSC and renal cell carcinoma was often noted. Later, this association was doubted because of the less-than-strict criteria used to diagnose renal cell carcinoma and the infrequency of metastases and deaths from malignancy in these patients. In the last 15 years, an increasing number of cases of renal cell carcinoma associated with TSC have been reported (Chan *et al.* 1983; Graves and Barnes 1986; Gutierrez *et al.* 1979; Lynne *et al.* 1979; Ohigashi *et al.* 1991; Taylor *et al.* 1989; Washecka and Hanna 1991; Hardman *et al.* 1993; Torres *et al.* 1994). The coexistence of an oncocytoma (Green 1987; Srinivas *et al.* 1985) or a leiomyosarcoma (Ferry *et al.* 1991; Kragel and Toker 1985; Fernandez *et al.* 1988) has been observed less often. In a review of 16 patients with TSC and renal cell carcinoma, 81 per cent of the patients were female, the median age at diagnosis was 28 years, and 43 per cent of the carcinomas were bilateral (Washecka and Hanna 1991). The natural history of renal cell carcinoma associated with TSC is not as benign as once believed. Nineteen to 50 per cent of the patients with TSC and renal cell carcinoma die of metastatic disease (Torres *et al.* 1994; Washecka and Hanna 1991).

Early detection is essential for the management of these patients. The association of renal cell carcinoma with TSC should be suspected in cases of enlarging lesions with no fatty tissue demonstrable by US, CT, or MRI (Fig. 11.6), and

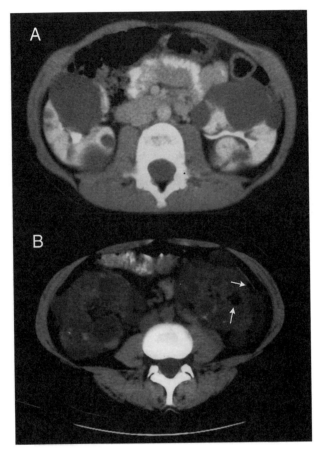

Fig. 11.5 Multiple bilateral renal cysts without angiomyolipomas demonstrated by contrast enhanced computed tomography in a 7-year-old boy with tuberous sclerosis complex (A). Multiple renal cysts and angiomyolipomas (arrows) in a 46-year-old woman with tuberous sclerosis complex (B).

when intratumoral calcifications, which occur very rarely in uncomplicated angiomyolipomas, are present (Honey and Honey 1977; Shapira *et al.* 1984; Suslavich *et al.* 1979; Weinblatt *et al.* 1987). In these cases, fine-needle aspiration biopsy or (preferably in our opinion) surgical exploration should be performed. Because of the frequent bilaterality of the lesions in TSC, renal-sparing surgery should be performed whenever possible (Blute *et al.* 1988; Oesterling *et al.* 1986).

Focal segmental glomerular sclerosis and interstitial fibrosis

Patients with TSC may have small, contracted kidneys (Fig. 11.7) with small angiomyolipomas or cysts which are diffusely hyperechoic on ultrasound (Torres

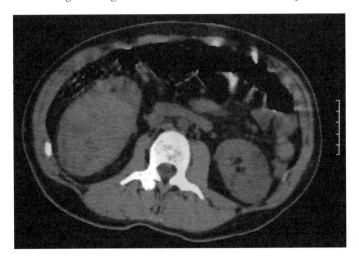

Fig. 11.6   Right renal cell carcinoma in a 23-year-old patient with tuberous sclerosis complex.

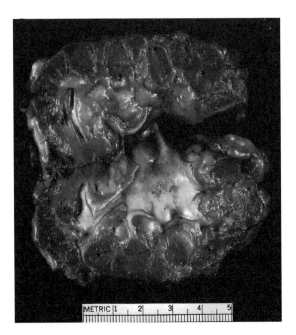

Fig. 11.7   Small contracted kidney in a 53-year-old patient with end-stage renal failure secondary to tuberous sclerosis complex. Multiple cortical cysts. Microscopic examination revealed multiple pseudo-encapsulated lesions consisting of smooth muscle cells and vascular elements, and segmental glomerulosclerosis with hyalinosis.

et al. 1994; Davidson *et al.* 1991; Hervé *et al.* 1982; Kleinknecht *et al.* 1976; Meyrier *et al.* 1980; Mirouze *et al.* 1963; Rosenberg *et al.* 1975; Schillinger *et al.*

1985, 1988). Clinically, these patients may have proteinuria and progressive renal insufficiency. Pathological examination of the kidneys reveals chronic interstitial nephritis with inflammatory cellular infiltrates, interstitial fibrosis, and FSGS. Some authors have observed a diffuse hyperplastic appearance of the interstitial stroma with areas of spindle cell, smooth muscle, and fibroblastic cells (Rolfes *et al.* 1985). The FSGS may result from renal mass reduction caused by angiomyolipomas, cysts, or interstitial fibrosis, with resulting hyperfiltration in the remnant glomeruli.

Other renal lesions

Perirenal and peripelvic lymphangiomatous cysts in patients with TSC probably represent dilatations and proliferations of intrinsically normal lymphatic channels in response to the obstructive effects of perilymphatic smooth muscle proliferation ('leiomyomatosis') (Torres *et al.* 1995). Intraglomerular microhamartomatous lesions of probable mesangial origin have been described (Nagashima *et al.* 1988). TSC can rarely involve medium-sized and large vessels, including the renal arteries, and few cases of renal artery stenosis have been reported (Rolfes *et al.* 1985). Of interest, because of their association with other renal cystic diseases such as autosomal dominant polycystic kidney disease, are the observations of intracranial aneurysms, Moya–Moya disease, aortic aneurysms, and valvular heart abnormalities (Lie 1991; Kleinknecht *et al.* 1976). Other renal abnormalities described in TSC are probably coincidental, although ureteropelvic junction stricture with hydronephrosis was noted in 11 per cent of patients in one series, and horseshoe kidneys have been noted in some case reports (Golji 1961; Oritz *et al.* 1990).

Treatment of renal failure in tuberous sclerosis complex

End-stage renal failure in TSC may occur by different mechanisms, including bilateral nephrectomies to treat life-threatening haemorrhages, polycystic kidneys, replacement of the renal tissue by angiomyolipomas, interstitial fibrosis, and FSGS (Torres *et al.* 1994; Manno *et al.* 1991). As the treatment of the central nervous system manifestations of this disease and life expectancy of these patients improve, renal failure will become a more important component of TSC. Both dialysis and renal transplantation prove an adequate means of survival, but the risk of haemorrhage and malignant degeneration in TSC poses special problems (Torres *et al.* 1994; Lynne *et al.* 1979; Anderson and Tannen 1969). Therefore, it is advisable that patients with TSC and end-stage renal failure undergo bilateral nephrectomies before entering a dialysis or renal transplantation programme.

References

Adamson, D., Heinricks, W. L., Raybin, D. M., and Raffin, T. A. (1985). Successful treatment of pulmonary lymphangiomyomatosis with oophorectomy and progesterone. *Am. Rev. Respir. Dis.*, **132**, 916–21.

Ahlsén, G., Gillberg, C., Lindblom, R., and Gillberg, C. (1994). Tuberous sclerosis in western Sweden. *Arch. Neurol.*, **51**, 76–81.

Anderson, D. and Tannen, R. L. (1969). Tuberous sclerosis and chronic renal failure. *Am. J. Med.*, **47**, 163–8.

Balzer, R. and Ménétrier, P. (1885). Etude sur un cas d'adénomes sébacés de la face et du cuir chevelu. *Arch. Physiol. Norm. Pathol. (Série III)*, **6**, 564–76.

Banner, A. S., *et al.* (1981). Efficacy of oophorectomy in lymphangioleiomyomatosis and benign metastasizing leiomyoma. *N. Engl. J. Med.*, **305**, 204–9.

Bebin, E. M., Gomez, M. R., and Kelly, P. J. (1993). Results of tuberectomy for intractable seizures. *Program of VI International Symposium on Tuberous Sclerosis Complex*, p. 26. Mayo Clinic, Rochester, MN.

Berant, K. M. and Alon, U. (1987). Polycystic kidneys as the presenting feature of tuberous sclerosis. *Helv. Paediatr. Acta*, **42**, 29–33.

Berg, G. and Vejlens, G. (1939). Maladie kystique du poumon et sclérose tubéreuse du cerveau. *Acta Paeditr (Uppsala)*, **26**, 16–30.

Bernstein, J. and Robbins, T. O. (1991). Renal involvement in tuberous sclerosis. *Ann. NY Acad. Sci.*, **615**, 36–49.

Bernstein, J., Robbins, T. O., and Kissane, J. M. (1986). The renal lesions of tuberous sclerosis. *Semin. Diagn. Pathol.*, **3**, 97–105.

Bloom, D. A., Scardino, P. T., Ehrlich, R. M., and Waismann, J. (1982). The significance of lymph nodal involvement in renal angiomyolipoma. *J. Urol.*, **128**, 1292–5.

Blute, M. L., Malek, R. S., and Segura, J. W. (1988). Angiomyolipoma: clinical metamorphosis and concepts for management. *J. Urol.*, **139**, 20–4.

Bonetti, F., *et al.* (1993). Transbronchial biopsy in lymphangiomyomatosis of the lung. *Am. J. Surg. Pathol.*, **17**, 1092–102.

Bosniak, M. A., Migibow, A. J., Hulnick, D. H., Horii, S., and Raghavendra, B. N. (1988). CT diagnosis of renal angiomyolipoma: the importance of detecting small amounts of fat. *Am. J. Roentgenol.*, **151**, 497–507.

Bourneville, D.-M. (1880). Sclérose tubéreuse des circonvolutions cérébrales: idiotie et épilepsie hémiplégique. *Arch. Neurologie*, **1**, 81–91.

Burke, A. P. and Virmani, R. (1991). Cardiac rhabdomyoma: a clinicopathologic study. *Mod. Pathol.*, **4**, 70–4.

Bush, J. K., McLean, R. L., and Sieker, H. O. (1969). Diffuse lung disease due to lymphangiomyolipoma. *Am. J. Med.*, **46**, 645.

Camúnez, F., *et al.* (1987). CT demonstration of extension of renal angiomyolipoma into the inferior vena cava in a patient with tuberous sclerosis. *Urol. Radiol.*, **9**, 152–4.

Case, C. L., Gillette, P. C., and Crawford, F. A. (1991). Cardiac rhabdomyomas causing superventricular and lethal ventricular arrhythmias in an infant. *Am. Heart J.*, **122**, 1484.

Chalvardjian, A., Kovacs, K., and Horvath, E. (1978). Renal angiomyolipoma: ultrastructural study. *Urology*, **12**, 717–20.

Chan, H. S. L., Daneman, A., Gribbin, M., and Martin, D. J. (1983). Renal cell carcinoma in the first two decades of life. *Pediatr. Radiol.*, **13**, 324–8.

Clemm, C., Jehn, U., Wolf-Hornung, B., Siemon, G., and Walter, G. (1987). Lymphangioleiomyomatosis: a report of three cases treated with tamoxifen. *Klin. Worchenschr.*, **65**, 391.

Colley, M. H., Geppert, E., and Franklin, W. A. (1989). Immunohistochemical detection of steroid receptors in a case of pulmonary lymphangioleiomyomatosis. *Am. J. Surg. Pathol.*, **13**, 803–7.

Connor, J. M. and Sampson, J. (1991). Recent linkage studies in tuberous sclerosis: chromosome 9 markers. *Ann. NY Acad. Sci.*, **615**, 265–73.

Critchley, M. and Earl, C. J. C. (1932). Tuberous sclerosis and allied conditions. *Brain*, **55**, 311–46.

Curatolo, P., Cusmai, R., Cortesi, F., Chiron, C., Jambaque, I., and Dulac, O. (1991). Neuropsychiatric aspects of tuberous sclerosis. *Ann. NY Acad. Sci.*, **615**, 8–16.

Davidson, M., Yoshidome, H., Stenroos, E., and Johnson, W. G. (1991). Neuron-like cells in culture of tuberous sclerosis tissue. *Ann. NY Acad. Sci.*, **615**, 196–210.

Dommergues, J. P., Pollet, F., Valayer, J., Roset, F., and Aicardi, J. (1982). Maladie polykstique rénale à révélation précoce: première manifestation d'une sclérose tubéreuse de Bourneville. *Arch. Fr. Pediatr.*, **39**, 31–2.

Durham, D. S. (1987). Tuberous sclerosis mimicking adult polycystic kidney disease. *Aus. NZ J. Med.*, **17**, 71–3.

Earthman, W. J., Mazer, M. J., and Winfield, A. C. (1986). Angiomyolipomas in tuberous sclerosis: subselective embolotherapy with alcohol, with long-term follow-up study. *Radiology*, **160**, 437–41.

Eason, A. A., Cattolica, E. V., and McGrath, T. W. (1979). Massive renal angiomyolipoma: Preoperative infarction by balloon catheter. *J. Urol.*, **121**, 360–1.

El Allaf, D., Borlee, G., Hadjoudj, H., Henrard, L., Marcelle, R., and Van Cauwenberge, H. (1984). Pulmonary lymphangioleiomyomatosis. *Eur. J. Respir. Dis.*, **65**, 147–52.

European Chromosome 16 Tuberous Sclerosis Consortium (1993). Identification and characterization of the tuberous sclerosis gene on chromosome 16. *Cell*, **75**, 1305–15.

Fahsold, R., Rott, H. D., Lorenz, P. (1991). A third gene locus for tuberous sclerosis is closely linked to the phenylalanine hydroxylase gene locus. *Hum. Genet.*, **88**, 85–90.

Farrow, G. M., Harrison, E. G., Utz, D. C., and Jones, D. R. (1968). Renal angiomyolipoma: a clinicopathologic study of 32 cases. *Cancer*, **22**, 564–70.

Fernandez de Sevilla, T., Muniz, R., Palou, J. Banus, J. M., Alegre, J., and Garcia, A. (1988). Renal leiomyosarcoma in a patient with tuberous sclerosis. *Urol. Int.*, **43**, 62–4.

Ferry, J. A., Malt, R. A., and Young, R. H. (1991). Renal angiomyolipoma with sarcomatous transformation and pulmonary metastases. *Am. J. Surg. Pathol.*, **15**, 1083–8.

Fischer, W. (1911). Die Nierentumoren bei der Tuberosen Hirnsklerose. *Zeigler Beitr. Path. Anat. Allg. Path.*, **50**, 235.

Fitzpatrick, T. B. (1991). History and significance of white macules, earliest visible sign of tuberous sclerosis. *Ann. NY Acad. Sci.*, **615**, 26–35.

Futter, N. G. and Collins, W. E. (1974). Renal angiomyolipoma causing hypertension: a case report. *Br. J. Urol.*, **46**, 485–7.

Garson, A. Jr, Smith, R. T., Moak, J. P., Kearney, D. L., Hawkins, E. P., and Titus, J. L. (1987). Incessant ventricular tachycardia in infants: myocardial hamartomas and surgical cure. *J. Am. Coll. Cardiol.*, **10**, 619–26.

Golji, H. (1961). Tuberous sclerosis and renal neoplasms. *J. Urol.*, **85**, 919–23.

Gomez, M. R. (1988*a*). Criteria for diagnosis. In *Tuberous sclerosis*, (2nd edn), (ed. M. R. Gomez), pp. 9–19. Raven, New York.

Gomez, M. R. (1988*b*). Neurologic and psychiatric features. In *Tuberous sclerosis*, (2nd edn), (ed. M. R. Gomez), pp. 21–36. Raven, New York.

Gomez, M. R. (1991). Phenotypes of the tuberous sclerosis complex with a revision of diagnostic criteria. *Ann. NY Acad. Sci.*, **615**, 1–7.

Gomez, M. R. (1992). The tuberous sclerosis complex, a prototype of hamartiosis and hamartomatosis. *J. Dermatol*, **19**, 892–6.

Gould, S. R. (1991). Hamartomatous rectal polyps are common in tuberous sclerosis. *Ann. NY Acad. Sci.*, **615**, 71–80.

Graham, M. L., Spelsberg, T. C., Dines, D. E., Payne, W. S., Bjornsson, J., Lie, J. T. (1984). Pulmonary lymphangiomyomatosis: with particular reference to steroid-receptor assay studies and pathologic correlation. *Mayo Clin. Proc.*, **59**, 3–11.

Graves, N. and Barnes, W. F. (1986). Renal cell carcinoma and angiomyolipoma in tuberous sclerosis: case report. *J. Urol.*, **135**, 122–3.

Green, A. J., Smith, M., and Yates, J. R. W. (1994). Loss of heterozygosity on chromosome 16p13.3 in hamartomas from tuberous sclerosis patients. *Nature Genet.*, **6**, 193–6.

Green, J. A. S. (1987). Renal oncocytoma and tuberous sclerosis. *S. African Med. J.*, **71**, 47–8.

Green, J. E., *et al.* (1990). Hypertension and renal failure in a patient with tuberous sclerosis. *S. African Med. J.*, **83**, 451–4.

Gutierrez, O. H., Burgener, F. A., and Schwartz, S. (1979). Coincident renal cell carcinoma and renal angiomyolipoma in tuberous sclerosis. *Am. J. Radiol.*, **132**, 848–50.

Haines, J. L. *et al.* (1991). Genetic heterogeneity in tuberous sclerosis: study of a large collaborative dataset. *Ann. NY Acad. Sci.*, **615**, 256–64.

Hajdu, S. I. and Foote, F. W. (1969). Angiomyolipoma of the kidney: report of 27 cases and review of the literature. *J. Urol.*, **102**, 396–401.

Hardman, J. A., McNicholas, T. A., Kirkham, N., and fletcher, M. S. (1993). Recurrent renal angiomyolipoma associated with renal carcinoma in a patient with tuberous sclerosis. *Br. J. Urol.*, **72**, 983–4.

Heckl, W., Osterhage, H. R., and Frohmüller, H. G. W. (1987). Diagnosis and treatment of renal angiomyolipoma. *Urol. Int.*, **42**, 201–6.

Hervé, J. P., *et al.* (1982). L'insuffisance rénale chronique de la sclérose tubérose de Bourneville. *J. Nephrol.*, **3**, 49–50.

Hoffman, A. D. (1991). Imaging of tuberous sclerosis lesions outside of the central nervous system. *Ann. NY Acad. Sci.*, **615**, 94–111.

Holm-Nielsen, P. and Sørenson, F. B. (1988). Renal angiomyolipoma: an ultrastructural investigation of three cases with histogenetic considerations. *AMPIS Suppl.*, **4**, 37–47.

Honey, R. J. and Honey, R. M. (1977). Tuberose sclerosis and bilateral renal carcinoma. *Br. J. Urol.*, **49**, 441–6.

Hulbert, J. C. and Graf, R. (1983). Involvement of the spleen by renal angiomyolipoma: metastasis or multicentricity? *J. Urol.*, **130**, 328.

Hunt, A. and Lindenbaum, R. H. (1984). Tuberous sclerosis: a new estimate of prevalence within the Oxford region. *J. Med. Genet.*, **21**, 272–7.

Huttenlocher, P. R. and Wollmann, R. L. (1991). Cellular neuropathology of tuberous sclerosis. *Ann. NY Acad. Sci.*, **615**, 140–8.

Inglis, K. (1954). The relation of the renal lesions to the cerebral lesions in the tuberous sclerosis complex. *Am. J. Pathol.*, **30**, 739–55.

Inglis, K. (1960). The nature and origin of smooth muscle-like neoplastic tissue in renal tumors of the tuberous sclerosis complex. *Cancer*, **3**, 602–11.

Janssen, L. A. J., *et al.* (1991). A comparative study on genetic heterogeneity in tuberous sclerosis: evidence for one gene on 9q34 and a second gene on 11q22-23. *Ann. NY Acad. Sci.*, **615**, 306–15.

Jayakar, P. B., Stanwick, R. S., and Seshia, S. S. (1986). Tuberous sclerosis and Wolff–Parkinson–White syndrome. *J. Pediatr.*, **108**, 259.

Johnson, W. G., Yoshidome, H., Stenroos, E. S., and Davidson, M. M. (1991). Origin of the neuron-like cells in tuberous sclerosis tissues. *Ann. NY Acad. Sci.*, **615**, 211–19.

Johnson, E., Sueoka, B. L., Spiegel, P. K., Richardson, J. R., and Heavey, J. A. (1991). Angiographic management of retroperitoneal hemorrhage from renal angiomyolipoma in polycystic kidney disease. *J. Urol.*, **145**, 1248–50.

Jozwiak, S., Kawalec, W., Dluzewska, J., Daszkowska, J., Mirkowicz-Malek, M., and Michalowicz, R. (1994). Cardiac tumours in tuberous sclerosis: their incidence and course. *Eur. J. Pediat.*, **153**, 155–7.

Kandt, R. S., *et al.* (1991). Linkage studies in tuberous sclerosis: chromosome 9?, 11?, or maybe 14! *Ann. NY Acad. Sci.*, **615**, 284–97.

Kandt, R. S., *et al.* (1992b). Linkage of an important gene locus for tuberous sclerosis to a chromosome 16 marker for polycystic kidney disease. *Nature Genet.*, **2**, 37–41.

Kleinknecht, D., Haiat, R., Frija, J., and Mignon, F. (1976). Sclérose tubéreuse de Bourneville avec bicuspidie aortique et insullisance rénale. *Nouv. Presse Médic.*, **5**, 1196–8.

Kragel, P. J. and Toker, C. (1985). Infiltrating recurrent renal angiomyolipoma with fatal outcome. *J. Urol.*, **133**, 90–1.

Kutcher, R., Rosenblatt, R., Mitsudo, S. M., Goldman, M., and Kogan, S. (1982). Renal angiomyolipoma with sonographic demonstrations of extension into the inferior vena cava. *Radiology*, **147**, 755–6.

Lallier, T. E. (1991). Cell lineage and cell migration in the neural crest. *Ann. NY Acad. Sci.*, **615**, 158–71.

Lewis, E. L. and Palmer, J. M. (1985). Renal angiomyolipoma and massive retroperitoneal hemorrhage during pregnancy. *West J. Med.*, **143**, 675–6.

Lie, J. T. (1991). Cardiac, pulmonary, and vascular involvements in tuberous sclerosis. *Ann. NY Acad. Sci.*, **615**, 58–70.

Lydidakis, N. A. and Lindenbaum, R. H. (1987). Pitted enamel hypoplasia in tuberous sclerosis patients and first-degree relatives. *Clin. Genet.*, **32**, 216–22.

Lynne, C. M., Carrion, H. M., Bakshandeh, K., Nadji, M., Russel, E., and Politano, V. A. (1979). Renal angiomyolipoma polycystic kidney, and renal cell carcinoma in patients with tuberous sclerosis. *Urology*, **14**, 174–6.

Manno, C., Claudatus, J., LaRaia, E., Savino, L., and Schena, F. P. (1991). Chronic renal failure for bilateral spontaneous kidney rupture in a case of tuberous sclerosis. *Am. J. Nephrol.*, **11**, 416–21.

McCarty, K. S. Jr, Mossler, J. A., McLelland, R., and Sieker H. O. (1980). Pulmonary lymphangiomyomatosis responsive to progesterone. *N. Engl. J. Med.*, **303**, 1461.

Meyrier, A., Rainfray, M., Roland, J., and Merlier, J. (1980). Sclérose tubéreuse de Bourneville avec insuffisance rénale chronique traitée par hémodialyse et transplantation. *Néphrologie*, **1**, 85–8.

Michel, J. M., Diggle, J. H., Brice, J., Mellor, D. H., and Small, P. (1983). Two half-siblings with tuberous sclerosis, polycystic kidneys and hypertension. *Dev. Med. Child Neurol.*, **25**, 239–44.

Miller, J. M., Gray, E. S., and Lloyd, D. L. (1989). Unilateral cystic disease of the neonatal kidney: a rare presentation of tuberous sclerosis. *Histopathology*, **14**, 529–32.

Mirouze, J., *et al.* (1963). L'urémie de la maladie de Bourneville (à propos de deux observations). *J. D'Urol. Néphrol.*, **69**, 639–47.

Mitnick, J. S., Bosniak, M. A., Hilton, S., Raghavendra, B. N., Subramanyam, B. R., and Genieser, N. B. (1983). Cystic renal disease in tuberous sclerosis. *Radiology*, 147, 85–7.

Mori, M., Ikeda, T., and Onoe, T. (1971). Blastic Schwann cells in renal tumor of tuberous sclerosis complex: an electron microscopic study. *Acta Pathol. Jap.*, 21, 121–9.

Moss, J. G. and Hendry, G. M. A. (1988). The natural history of renal cysts in an infant with tuberous sclerosis: evaluation with ultrasound. *Br. J. Radiol.*, 61, 1074–6.

Mukai, M., *et al.* (1992). Crystalloids in angiomyolipoma: 1. A previously unnoticed phenomenon of renal angiomyolipoma occurring at a high frequency. *Am. J. Surg. Pathol.*, 16, 1–10.

Nagashima, Y., Ohaki, Y., Tanaka, Y., Misugi, K., and Horiuchi, M. (1988). A case of renal angiomyolipomas associated with multiple and various hamartomatous microlesions. *Virchows Archiv Pathol Anat.*, 413, 177–82.

Nevin, N. C., and Pearce, W. G. (1968). Diagnostic and general aspects of tuberous sclerosis. *J. Med. Genet.*, 5, 273–80.

Nonomura, A., Mizukami, Y., and Kadoya, M. (1994). Angiomyolipoma of the liver: A collective review. *J. Gastroenterol.*, 29, 95–105.

O'Callaghan, T. J., Edwards, J. A., Tobin, M., and Mookerjee, B. K. (1975). Tuberous sclerosis with striking renal involvement in a family. *Arch. Intern. Med.*, 135, 1082–7.

Oesterling, J. E., Fishman, E. K., Goldman, S. M., and Marshall, F. F. (1986). The management of renal angiomyolipoma. *J. Urol.*, 135, 1121–4.

Ohigashi, T., Iigaya, T., and Hata, M. (1991). Coincidental renal cell carcinoma and renal angiomyolipomas in tuberous sclerosis. *Urol. Int.*, 47, 160–3.

Ohori, N. P., Yousem, S. A., Sonmez-Alpan, E., and Colby, T. V. (1991). Estrogen and progesterone receptors in lymphangioleiomyomatosis, epithelioid hemangioendotheliona and sclerosing hemangioma of the lung. *Am. J. Clin. Pathol.*, 96, 529–35.

Okada, R. D., Platt, M. A., and Fleishman, J. (1982). Chronic renal failure in patients with tuberous sclerosis: association with renal cysts. *Nephron*, 30, 85–8.

Oritz, Cabria, R., Blanco Parra, M., and Rodriguez de la Rua Roman, J. (1990). Esclerosis tuberosa patologia renal multiple presentacion de un caso. *Actas Urol. Espanolas*, 14, 310–13.

Osborne, J. P., Fryer A. and Webb, D. (1991). Epidemiology of tuberous sclerosis. *Ann. NY Acad. Sci.*, 615, 125–7. 1991

Pea, M., *et al.* (1991). Melanocyte marker AMB-45 is regularly expressed in angiomyolipoma in the kidney. *Pathology*, 23, 185–8.

Penneys, N. S., Smith, K. J., and Nemeth, A. J. (1991). Factor XIIIa in the hamartomas of tuberous sclerosis. *J. Dermatol. Sci.*, 2, 50–3.

Perez-Atayde, A. R., Iwaya, S., and Lack, E. E. (1981). Angiomyolipomas and polycystic renal disease in tuberous sclerosis: ultrastructural observations. *Urology*, 17, 607–10.

Petrikovsky, B. M., Vintzileos, A. M., Cassidy, S. B., and Egan, J. F. X. (1990). Tuberous sclerosis in pregnancy. *Am. J. Perinatol*, 7, 133–5.

Pringle, J. J. (1890). A case of congenital adenoma sebaceum. *Br. J. Dermatol*, 2, 1–14.

Rayer, P. F. O. (1835). *Traité theorique et pratique de maladies de la peau.*, (2nd edn). Baillière, Paris.

Reese, A. J. M. and Winstanley, D. P. (1958). The small tumour-like lesions of the kidney. *Br. J. Cancer*, **12**, 507–16.

Robbins, T. O., and Bernstein, J. (1988). Renal involvement. In *Tuberous sclerosis*, (2nd edn), (ed. M. R. Gomez), pp. 133–46. Raven, New York.

Robertson, D. M. (1991). Ophthalmic manifestations of tuberous sclerosis. *Ann. NY Acad. Sci.*, **615**, 17–25.

Rogers, R. S., III. (1988). Dermatologic manifestations. In *Tuberous sclerosis*, (2nd edn), (ed. M. R. Gomez), pp. 111–31. Raven, New York.

Rolfes, D. B., Towbin, R., and Bove, K. E. (1985). Vascular dysplasia in a child with tuberous sclerosis. *Pediatr. Pathol.*, **3**, 359–73.

Rosenberg, J. C., Bernstein, J., and Rosenberg, B. (1975). Renal cystic disease associated with tuberose sclerosis complex renal failure treated by cadaveric renal transplantation. *Clin. Nephrol.*, **4**, 109–12.

Rothenberg, D. M., Brandt, T. D., and D'Cruz, I. (1986). Computed tomography of renal angiomyolipoma presenting as right atrial mass. *J. Comput. Assist. Tomogr.*, **10**, 1054–6.

Saguem, M. H., Laarif, M., Remadi, S., Bozakoura, C., and Cox, J. N. (1992). Diffuse bilateral glomerulocystic disease of the kidneys and multiple cardiac rhabdomyomas in a newborn: relationship with tuberous sclerosis and review of the literature. *Pathol. Res. Pract.*, **188**, 367–73.

Sampson, J. R., Scahill, S. J., Stephenson, J. B., Mann, L., and Connor, J. M. (1989). Genetic aspects of tuberous sclerosis in the west of Scotland. *J. Med. Genet.*, **26**, 28–31.

Sant, G. R., Ayers, D. K., Bankoff, M. S., Mitcheson, H. D., and Ucci, A. A. Jr (1990). fine needle aspiration biopsy in the diagnosis of renal angiomyolipoma. *J. Urol.*, **143**, 999–1001.

Satoh, T., Nakafuku, M., and Kaziro, Y. (1992). Function of Ras as a molecular switch in signal transduction. *J. Biol. Chem.*, **267**, 24149–52.

Schiaffino, E., Tavani, E., Dellafiore, L., and Schmid, C. (1989). Pulmonary lumphangiomyomatosis Report of a case with immunohistochemical and ultrastructural findings. *Appl. Pathol.*, **7**, 265–72.

Schillinger, F., Montagnac, R., Grapin, J. L., Birembaut, P., and Hopfner, C. (1985). L'insuffisance rénale de al sclérose tubéreuse de Bourneville: une nouvelle forme d'atteinte glomérulaire par hyperfiltration? *Nephrologie*, **6**, 219–23.

Schillinger, F., Montagnac, R., Grapin, J. L., Schillinger, D., and Bressieux J. M. L. (1988). Le rein au cours de la sclérose tubéreuse de Bourneville. *Rev. Med. Intern.*, **9**, 61–6.

Schuster, P. (1914). Beiträge zur Klinik der tuberösen Sklerose des Gehirns. *Dtsch Z. Nervenheilk.*, **50**, 96–133.

Shapiro, R. A., Skinner, D. G., Stanley, P., and Edelbrock, H. H. (1984). Renal tumors associated with tuberous sclerosis: the case for aggressive surgical management. *J. Urol.*, **132**, 1170–4.

Shepherd, C. W., Beard, M., Gomez, M. R., Kurland, L. T., and Whisnant, J. P. (1991a). Tuberous sclerosis complex in Olmsted County, Minnesota, 1950–1989. *Arch. Neurol.*, **48**, 400–1.

Shepherd, C. W., Gomez, M. R., Lie, J. T., and Crowson, C. S. (1991b). Causes of death in patients with tuberous sclerosis. *Mayo Clin. Proc.*, **66**, 792–6.

Singer, K. (1971). Genetic aspects of tuberous sclerosis in a Chinese population. *Am. J. Hum. Genet.*, **23**, 33–40.

Smith, M., Yoshiyama, K., Wagner, C., Flodman, P., and Smith, B. (1991). Genetic heterogeneity in tuberous sclerosis: map position of the TSC2 locus on chromosome 11q and future prospects. *Ann. NY Acad. Sci.*, **615**, 274–83.

Smith, M., Handa, K., Wei, H., and Spear, G. (1993). Loss of heterozygosity for chromosome 16p13.3 markers in renal hamartomas from tuberous sclerosis patients (Abstract). *Am. J. Hum. Genet.*, **53**, 366.

Srinivas, V., Herr, H. W., and Hajdu, E. O. (1985). Partial nephrectomy for a renal oncocytoma associated with tuberous sclerosis. *J. Urol.*, **133**, 263–5.

Stapleton, F. B., Johnson, D., Kaplan, G. W., and Griswold, W. (1980). The cystic renal lesion in tuberous sclerosis. *J. Pediatr.*, **97**, 574–9.

Steiner, M. S., Goldman, S. M., Fishman, E. K., and Marshall, F. F. (1993). The natural history of renal angiomyolipoma. *J. Urol.*, **150**, 1782–6.

Stevenson, A. C. and Fisher, O. D. (1956). Frequency of epiloia in Northern Ireland. *Br. J. Prev. Soc. Med.*, **10**, 134–5.

Stillwell, T. J., Gomez, M. R., and Kelalis, P. P. (1987). Renal lesions in tuberous sclerosis. *J. Urol.*, **138**, 477–81.

Sun, C. N., White, H. J., and Bissada, N. K. (1975). Renal angiomyolipoma in a case of tuberous sclerosis and electron microscopy study. *Beitr. Path. Bd.*, **156**, 401–10.

Suslavich, F., Older, R. A., and Hinman, C. G. (1979). Calcified renal carcinoma in a patient with tuberous sclerosis. *Am. J. Radiol.*, **133**, 524–6.

Tallada, N., Martinez, S., and Raventos, A. (1994). Cystologic study of renal angiomyolipoma by fine-needle asporation biopsy: Report for four cases. *Diag. Cytopathol.*, **10**, 37–40.

Taylor, J. R., Ryu, J., Colby, T. V., and Raffin, T. A. (1990). Lymphangioleiomyomatosis Clinical course in 32 patients. *N. Engl. J. Med.*, **323**, 1254–60.

Taylor, R. S., Joseph, D. B., Kohaut, C., Wilson, E. R., and Bueschen, A. J. (1989). Renal angiomyolipoma associated with lymph node involvement and renal cell carcinoma in patients with tuberous sclerosis. *J. Urol.*, **141**, 930–2.

Torres, V. E., King, B. F., Holley, K. E., Blute, M. L., and Gomez, M. R. (1994). The kidney in the tuberous sclerosis complex. *Adv. Nephrol.*, **23**, 43–70.

Torres, V. E., et al. (1995). Extrapulmonary lymphangioleiomyomatosis and lymphangiomatous cysts in tuberous sclerosis complex. *Mayo Clin. Proc.*, **70**, 641–8.

Totty, W. G., McClennan, B. L., Melson, G. L., and Patel, R. (1981). Relative value of computed tomography and ultrasonography in the assessment of renal angiomyolipoma. *J. Comput. Assist. Tomogr.*, **5**, 173–8.

Tsui, W. M. S., Yuen, A. K. T., Ma, K. F., and Tse, C. C. H. (1992). Hepatic angiomyolipomas with a deceptive trabecular pattern and HMB-45 reactivity. *Histopathology*, **21**, 569–73.

Uhlenbrock, D., Fischer, C., and Beyer, H. K. (1988). Angiomyolipoma of the kidney: comparison between magnetic resonance imaging, computed tomography, and ultrasonography for diagnosis. *Acta Radiol.*, **29**, 523–6.

Van Baal, J. G., Fleury, P., and Brummelkamp, W. H. (1989). Tuberous sclerosis and the relation with renal angiomyolipoma: a genetic study on the clinical aspects. *Clin. Genet.*, **35**, 167–73.

Van Baal, J. G., et al. (1990). Percutaneous transcatheter embolization of symptomatic renal angiomyolipomas: a report of four cases. *Neth. J. Surg.*, **42**, 72–7.

Van der Hoeve, J. (1920). Eye symptoms in tuberous sclerosis of the brain. *Trans. Ophthalmol. Soc. UK*, **40**, 329–34.

Vogt, H. (1908). Zur Diagnostik der tuberösen Sklerose. *Z. Erforsch. Behandl. Jugendl. Schwachsinns.*, **2**, 1–12.

Von Recklinghausen, F. (1862). Ein Herz von einem Neugeborenen welches mehrere theils nach aussen, theils nach den Höhlen prominierende Tumoren (Myomen) trug. Verhandlungen der Gesellshaft für Geburtskunde, 25 März. *Monatschrift für Geburtskunde*, **20**, 1–2.

Washecka, R. and Hanna, M. (1991). Malignant renal tumors in tuberous sclerosis. *Urology*, **37**, 340–3.

Watson, G. H. (1991). Cardiac rhabdomyomas in tuberous sclerosis. *Ann. NY Acad. Sci.*, **615**, 50–7.

Weinblatt, M. E., Khan, E., and Kochen, J. (1987). Renal cell carcinoma in patients with tuberous sclerosis. *Pediatrics*, **80**, 898–903.

Wenzl, J. E., Lagos, J. C., and Albers, D. D. (1970). Tuberous sclerosis presenting as polycystic kidneys and seizures in an infant. *J. Pediatr.*, **77**, 673–6.

Wiederholt, W. C., Gomez, M. R., and Kurland, L. T. (1985). Incidence and prevalence of tuberous sclerosis in Rochester, Minnesota: 1950 through 1982. *Neurology*, **35**, 600–3.

Yu, D. T. and Sheth, K. J. (1985). Cystic renal involvement in tuberous sclerosis. *Clin. Pediatr.*, **24**, 36–9.

12

Von Hippel–Lindau disease

Virginia Michels

Introduction

Von Hippel–Lindau (VHL) disease is an autosomal dominant disorder characterized by central nervous system (CNS) and/or retinal haemangioblastomas, visceral cysts, renal cancer and, less frequently, pheochromocytoma, and pancreatic
cancer. Patients with VHL disease usually present with CNS or visual symptoms (Melmon and Rosen 1964). However, as physicians become more aware of
the value of family screening and as diagnostic technology advances, a greater
number of asymptomatic patients will be detected. In clinical series the age of
onset of symptoms has ranged from 4 (Fill *et al.* 1979) to 65 years (Melmon and
Rosen 1964). The mean age of death in various reported families is approximately 49 years (Lamiel *et al.* 1989; Latif *et al.* 1993). In another family, the
average age of the affected members, all still living, was 43 years (Lee *et al.*
1977), and survival to age 80 years has been reported (Lamiell *et al.* 1989).

Von Hippel-Lindau disease occurs in virtually all ethnic groups (Bickler *et al.*
1984; Go *et al.* 1984; Yimoyines *et al.* 1982). The incidence of the disease is approximately 1/40 000 (Neumann *et al.* 1989) to 1/100 000 (Maher *et al.* 1990).
The mutation rate has been estimated to be 1.8×10^7 to 4.4×10^6 per gene per
generation (Mahler *et al.* 1991; Vogel and Motulsky 1979).

History

Panas and Remy described a retinal haemangioblastoma in 1879, although they
did not recognize it as such. In 1894, Collins examined autopsy material and
speculated that the lesions originated in the capillaries; he also recognized their
hereditary nature. Von Hippel in 1904 outlined the progressive nature of the
retinal lesion, and in 1911 concluded that it was a haemangioblastoma which he
called 'angiomatosis retinae' (Melmon and Rosen 1964). Pye-Smith, in 1884, reported the autopsy findings of a cystic haemangioblastoma of the cerebellum in a
patient with renal and pancreatic cysts which he dismissed as coincidental (Dan
and Smith 1975). In 1911, one of von Hippel's original patients with retinal
lesions was found at autopsy to have a cerebellar tumour, hypernephromas, and
renal, pancreatic, and epididymal cysts (Melmon and Rosen 1964). Tresling, in
1920, reported for the first time a family with both retinal and cerebellar
tumours (Jeffreys 1975).

In 1926, the Swedish pathologist, Arvid Lindau (Obrador and Martin-Rodriguez 1977), published a monograph based on the findings in 40 patients, including 16 of his own, thus establishing the clinico-pathological constellation of this unique disorder. He recognized the histological similarities of the retinal and cerebellar haemangioblastomas (Jeffreys 1975), and noted they may be found in the medulla and cord in association with syringomyelia. Ten per cent of patients had multiple CNS tumours and in his own cases, 50 per cent had pancreatic cysts, 62 per cent renal cysts, 38 per cent 'benign renal hypernephroid tumours', and some had adrenal, epididymal, and liver adenomas (Campbell *et al.* 1978; Melmon and Rosen 1964). Schubach first used the term 'von Hippel–Lindau complex' to refer to this syndrome in 1927, and in 1929 Möller recognized the inheritance pattern as autosomal dominant (Jeffreys 1975; Melmon and Rosen 1964).

Clinical findings

Eye

The typical ocular lesion of VHL disease is the retinal haemangioblastoma, sometimes referred to as a retinal angioma, haemangioma, or 'angiomatosis retinae'. This benign tumour often is the earliest manifestation of VHL disease. The mean age at diagnosis is 21–28 years (Horton *et al.* 1976; Wing *et al.* 1981; Huson *et al.* 1986). However, retinal haemangioblastomas have been detected in children as young as 2 years (Ridley *et al.* 1986; Filling-Katz *et al.* 1991). Since new lesions have been detected in retinas previously examined and found to be normal, it is unlikely that the lesion is congenital; however, this does not preclude that the lesions arise from the proliferation of vascular epithelium vestiges (Augsburger *et al.* 1981).

The earliest clinically detectable retinal lesion is small red dot resembling an aneurysmal dilatation of retinal capillaries. As it grows, the lesion may appear as a flat or slightly elevated grey disc and later as a globular, orangish-red tumour of 0.5 mm to more than 1 cm in diameter (Fig. 12.1). The hallmark of this mature tumour is a pair of dilated tortuous vessels running between the lesion and the disc. The dilated afferent arteriole and efferent venule reflect significant arteriovenous shunting (Augsburger *et al.* 1981; Greenwald and Weiss 1984).

As the retinal haemangioblastomas frequently are located in the periphery, a careful search by indirect ophthalmoscopy may be needed to detect small lesions (Palmer 1972). Large lesions may be obscured by accumulated exudate on their surface and around their edges, resulting in gliosis (Augsburger *et al.* 1981). Occasionally, the lesions are associated with a cyst or may calcify (Melmon and Rosen 1964). The lesions progress at a variable rate, either rapidly over a few years, slowly over many years (Horton *et al.* 1976), or not at all (Augsburger *et al.* 1981). If multiple, the lesions may be at different stages. The lesions may leak, and fluid accumulates within or beneath the retina, between the lesion and the optic disc, or in the macular area. In the macula, this leakage may form an

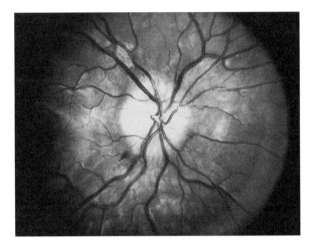

Fig. 12.1 Small retinal haemangioblastoma in a patient with von Hippel–Lindau disease.

'exudative mound', an exaggerated macular exudate next to an exudate-free between lesion and macula (Augsburger *et al.* 1981). Localized retinal detachment is a feature of all but the smallest tumours (Peyman *et al.* 1983). Retinal exudate and haemorrhage may result in reactive retinal inflammation and more extensive exudative retinal detachment, causing decreased visual acuity or blurred vision progressing to blindness (Melmon and Rosen 1964). Exophytic lesions that project into the vitreous may haemorrhage and also result in decreased vision (Augsburger *et al.* 1981).

The frequency of at least one retinal lesion in patients with VHL has varied between series, ranging from 24 per cent (Levine *et al.* 1983) to 73 per cent (Malek and Greene 1971). This variability reflects the intrinsic nature of the disease as well as the selection of subjects by age, clinical presentation, and method of study. Of those with VHL and eye lesions, 33–58 per cent (Melmon and Rosen 1964; Hardwig and Robertson 1984) had multiple lesions within one eye and 20–57 per cent had bilateral lesions (Peymann *et al.* 1983; Hardwig and Robertson 1984; Braffman *et al.* 1990).

Although small peripheral retinal haemangioblastomas frequently are asymptomatic, 16 per cent of patients in one large family had symptons (Horton *et al.* 1976). There are numerous reports of blindness (unilateral or bilateral) in patients in their twenties and several reports of 8- and 9-year-old children with blindness due to retinal haemangioblastoma (Atuk *et al.* 1979; Scully *et al.* 1978; Kupersmith and Bereinstein 1981). At the other end of the spectrum, patients with retinal lesions have remained asymptomatic past the age of 50 years (Peyman *et al.* 1983). In one series of ophthalmological patients with retinal involvement, 47 per cent had normal vision and 36 per cent had diminished vision to less than 20/200 (Hardwig and Robertson 1984). Leucocoria and strabismus in children are rare manifestations (Augsburger *et al.* 1981). Secondary changes resulted in cataracts, uveitis, painful glaucoma, or phthisis necessitating enucle-ation in 11 per cent of patients in one selected series (Hardwig and Robertson 1984).

Haemangioblastomas of the optic disc are rare (Ridley *et al.* 1986; Schlindler *et al.* 1975). In some instances, an incorrect initial diagnosis of papilloedema, which also may occur in VHL in association with a posterior fossa tumour, has been made. The disc lesions appear as well-circumscribed, reddish-orange, round or oval, elevated lesions obscuring part of the optic disc, usually temporally. Less commonly, the lesion is flat and grey with poorly defined margins extending from the disc into the retina. The most common symptom is visual loss resulting from chronic macular oedema or repeated vitreous haemorrhages. Intra-orbital optic nerve haemangioblastoma is even more rate (Seich *et al.* 1982).

The proportion of patients presenting with haemangioblastoma of the retina who have VHL is at least 10–20 per cent based on the number of patients who also have CNS tumours (Melmon and Rosen 1964; Wing *et al.* 1981), but may be as high as 86 per cent (Neumann and Wiestler 1991). All patients with retinal haemangioblastoma should be evaluated for other signs of VHL, and all patients with multiple retinal lesions should be considered to have VHL unless proven otherwise (Ridley *et al.* 1986).

The differential diagnosis of retinal angiomas includes diabetic micro-aneurysms (Greenwald and Weiss 1984) and multiple cavernous haemangiomas of the CNS and retina (Michels 1988). Secondary changes may mask the under-lying lesions and result in the misdiagnosis of Coat's exudative retinitis, for example (Melmon and Rosen 1964).

Retinal haemangioblastomas are composed of relatively well-formed capillaries and contain the same three cell types as do cerebellar tumours (Scully *et al.* 1978). The vascular channels leak fluid into the subretinal space, which results in lipid accumulation and retinal detachment (Greenwald and Weiss 1984).

Central nervous system

CNS haemangioblastomas are histopathologically benign tumours with morbidity and mortality due to space occupying effects. They occur most frequently in the cerebellum and spinal cord but also in the medulla oblongata and rarely in the cerebrum.

Cerebellar haemangioblastomas usually are located peripherally close to the pial surface in the hemispheres but also occur in the vermis or medulla (Lee *et al.* 1989). They occur in 50–79 per cent of autopsy-confirmed cases (Lamiell *et al.* 1989), and in 18 per cent (Green *et al.* 1986) to 52 per cent (Filling-Katz *et al.* 1991) of patients in various clinical series. They result in the first symptoms in 40 per cent of cases (Kadir *et al.* 1981), and in the past were the greatest cause of morbidity and mortality in VHL patients (Horton *et al.* 1976; Fill *et al.* 1979). However, with improved techniques for earlier detection of tumours and with improved surgical techniques, renal cell cancer now may be the leading cause of death (Latif *et al.* 1993).

The average age of onset of symptoms from cerebellar haemangioblastoma is approximately 30 years (Mahler *et al.* 1990) with an age range of 9–62 years (Huson *et al.* 1986; Hardwig and Robertson 1984). The lesion is said to be rare before puberty (Hellams *et al.* 1981) but there have been reports of 10-year-old children with papilloedema due to cerebellar haemangioblastoma (Hardwig and Robertson 1984). In series of consecutive patients presenting with CNS haemangioblastoma, 19–40 per cent were found to have VHL, although some of the patients had not been fully evaluated for other signs of VHL (Michels 1988; Neumann and Wiestler 1991; Maher *et al.* 1991).

The majority of patients (76 per cent) with cerebellar haemangioblastoma present with symptoms of increased intracranial pressure (Obrador and Martin-Rodriguez 1977). The symptoms usually worsen gradually but occasionally there is sudden onset due to bleeding into the tumour and rapid increase of intracranial pressure. Subarachnoid haemorrhage, an infrequent complication (Hellams *et al.* 1981), was suspected in some patients presenting with sudden onset of neck pain and stiffness (Mondkar *et al.* 1967).

Approximately 60–75 per cent (Obrador and Martin-Rodriguez 1977) of patients with cerebellar haemangioblastoma have signs of cerebellar dysfunction and/or increased intracranial pressure (Jeffreys 1975). The cerebellar signs are unilateral in half of these patients (Mondkar *et al.* 1967).

In various series of VHL patients, the incidence of spinal haemangioblastomas was 10 per cent (Blight *et al.* 1980) to 44 per cent (Filling-Katz *et al.* 1991). At post-mortem examination, spinal cord haemangioblastomas were found in 25–28 per cent, but many of these lesions had been asymptomatic and only 4 per cent had clinical symptoms. The mean age of diagnosis in patients whose lesions were detected during life was 25–35 years (Lamiell *et al.* 1989; Horton *et al.* 1976). The cord lesions are associated with syringomyelia in most cases (Horton *et al.* 1976). They may be located in any spinal segment including the conus medullaris (Kadir *et al.* 1981), although they are most common in the lower cervical and thoracic sites (Melmon and Rosen 1964). Initial symptoms may include loss of sensation and impaired proprioception. As cord compression progresses, weakness, muscle wasting, anaesthesia, sphincter disturbances, spasticity, and paraplegia may develop (Melmon and Rosen 1964). There has been at least one report of paraplegia of sudden onset due to a 'ruptured' cervical cord haemangioblastoma (Pearson *et al.* 1980).

In clinical series, haemangioblastomas of the brainstem occur in 18 per cent of patients (Filling-Katz *et al.* 1991). The medulla oblongata is involved in approximately 2.5 per cent of cases, often associated with syringobulbia (Blight *et al.* 1980; Fill *et al.* 1979). At autopsy they have been found in 17–25 per cent of VHL patients but most are asymptomatic (Lamiell *et al.* 1989). The mean age of diagnosis in symptomatic cases was 27–36 years (Lamiell *et al.* 1989; Horton *et al.* 1976).

Supratentorial haemangioblastomas are rare in VHL disease. In one review of 62 patients with supratentorial haemangioblastoma, 14.5 per cent were known to have VHL disease (Diehl and Symon 1981). These tumours were located in the pituitary (Dan and Smith 1975), the lateral wall and choroid plexus of the third ventricle, and in the parietal, occipitoparietal, temporal, or frontal lobes (Diehl and Symon 1981; Ishwar *et al.* 1971). Care must be taken to exclude the diagnosis of metastatic renal carcinoma when supratentorial lesions are detected, since the histology can be confusing, even to experienced pathologists (Richards *et al.* 1973).

There have been sporadic reports of meningioma (Melmon and Rosen 1964), ependymoma, intraventricular neuroblastoma (Ho 1983), and cerebellar astrocytoma (Ludmerer and Kissane 1981) in VHL disease.

Haemangioblastomas are benign neoplasms of endothelial origin with hypertrophied afferent and efferent cortical vessels (Lee *et al.* 1989). They usually are cystic and filled with xanthochromic fluid. A highly vascular nodule can be identified in the wall of the cyst and is usually in contact with the pia-arachnoid (Oliverona 1952). Approximately 20–32 per cent of lesions are solid (Melmon and Rosen 1964; Mondkar *et al.* 1967). They are sharply demarcated, not locally invasive, and do not metastasize. Lesions thought to show malignant spread have been reported (Mohan *et al.* 1976), but it is difficult to exclude multiple primary lesions or metastatic renal carcinoma, which histologically can be confused with haemangioblastoma. Approximately 80 per cent of tumours are located in the hemispheres, 13 per cent in the vermis, and 7 per cent in the 4th ventricle as they arise from the posterior medullary velum or occasionally from the floor or lateral margins (Olivecrona 1952). Solid lesions are more likely to be located at the inferior vermis (Gardeur *et al.* 1983).

Microscopically, the solid areas are composed of endothelial cells, pericytes, and stromal cells. These stromal cells may arise from undifferentiated mesenchyme as suggested by positive vimentin immunohistochemistry (Frank *et al.* 1989). There are numerous thin-walled vascular channels lined by plump endothelial cells that are separated by reticular and interstitial cells filled with abundant, vacuolated, lipid-rich citoplasm. The cyst walls are composed of neuroglia cells (Lee *et al.* 1989).

The haemangioblastomas located elsewhere in the CNS have a similar pathological appearance; they are more likely to be solid, although small cysts may be associated. Medulla and upper cord lesions are usually located posteriorly and are associated with syringobulbia or syringomyelia in up to 80 per cent of cases. Lesions in the sacral region and cauda equina are histologically different and may appear gelatinous or myxomatous (Melmon and Rosen 1964).

Kidney

The renal lesions of VHL disease include simple cysts, haemangiomas, benign adenomas, and most importantly, malignant hypernephromas. In clinical and autopsy series, 24–100 per cent had some type of renal lesion (Lamiell *et al.* 1989; Melmon and Rosen 1964).

In autopsy series, 42–88 per cent of patients with VHL had renal cysts (Lamiell *et al.* 1989). In clinical surveys up to 76 per cent of VHL patients had cysts, usually asymptomatic (Levine *et al.* 1983). Rarely, the renal cysts of VHL disease may be so extensive as to mimic polycystic kidney disease and cause renal failure (Michels 1988; Lamiell *et al.* 1980). The cysts vary in size from a few millimetres to more than 2 centimetres; they are bilateral in 60 per cent and frequently multiple (Ibrahim *et al.* 1989).

Renal haemangiomas occur in approximately 7 per cent of VHL patients at autopsy and virtually always are asymptomatic (Horton *et al.* 1976). In one clinical series, only 2 per cent of patients had a renal angioma when screened with abdominal computed tomography (CT) and ultrasound (US). Similarly, benign adenomas are asymptomatic with an incidence of 14 per cent at autopsy.

Renal clear-cell cancer (hypernephroma) is a major cause of morbidity and mortality. It is the most commonly symptomatic lesion of VHL disease, after cerebellar and retinal lesions. In autopsy series of VHL patients, 35–75 per cent had hypernephroma (Lamiell *et al.* 1989). The lesions are bilateral in 15 per cent (Ludmerer and Kissane 1981) to 75 per cent (Fill *et al.* 1979), and multiple in 40–87 per cent (Fill *et al.* 1979; Ibrahim *et al.* 1989). The frequency of malignant hypernephroma in clinical series is 25 per cent (Blight *et al.* 1980) to 45 per cent (Glenn *et al.* 1991), resulting in death in almost one-third (Horton *et al.* 1976). The average age of death from renal cancer was 44.5 years (Christenson *et al.* 1982). Symptomatic renal cancer tends to be one of the later clinical manifestations of VHL, being detected at a mean age of 41–45 years with a range of 19–69 years (Horton *et al.* 1976; Huson *et al.* 1986; Maher *et al.* 1990). In a literature review, 40 per cent of cases had metastases (Christenson *et al.* 1982). The tumours often can be diagnosed by CT when less than 3 cm in size, when they are unlikely to be invasive. Therefore, increased awareness of this lesion in VHL patients, with earlier detection, can result in successful removal before metastases occur.

The diagnosis of VHL disease must be considered in patients who present with renal cancer, particularly those who present at a young age, with a positive family history, or with multiple lesions. If the patient also has a cerebellar lesion, it must be appreciated that this may be a resectable haemangioblastoma rather than metastatic renal cancer with a poor prognosis (Broker *et al.* 1984).

Grossly, the renal cysts are greyish, translucent, and filled with clear fluid. They range in size from a few millimetres to over 1.5 centimetres (Christenson *et al.* 1982). Benign cysts are lined by a one to two cell layer of normal epithelium or atypical cuboidal hyperplastic epithelium (Blight *et al.* 1980). Some cysts are lined with clear cells or contain a nest of tumour cells beneath the cyst lining (Spencer *et al.* 1988); the presence of atypia or carcinoma does not correlate with the size of the cyst (Solomon and Schwartz 1988).

The solid tumours grossly are yellowish in colour with a well-defined capsule. The nodules may be solid or cystic are surrounded by a fibrous pseudocapsule. Some nodules are composed of loose fibrous tissue with occasional areas of myxoid degeneration (Christenson *et al.* 1982) or foci of calcification (Scully *et al.* 1978). Small (< 3 cm) cortical tumours are sometimes classified as adenomas, but this distinction based on size is somewhat arbitrary, and they probably represent the early stage of the malignant lesions (Ludmerer and Kissane 1981). This is supported by the finding that some of these nodules have a clear cell pattern typical of malignant hypernephroma and occasionally appear to be locally invading the pseudocapsule (Blight *et al.* 1980). Other solid lesions are hyalinized fibrotic nodules (Solomon and Schwartz 1988). The clear-cell renal tumours can invade veins and metastasize to the adrenal glands and CNS (Kadir *et al.* 1981). Immunohistochemical stains for vimentin and epithelial membrane antigen may be helpful in distinguishing cerebellar haemangioblastoma from intracranial metastatic renal cancer (Frank *et al.* 1989).

Pancreas

The pancreatic lesions of VHL disease include cysts, adenomas, haemangioblastomas, and malignancies.

Cysts of the pancreas are rare in the general population (Barkin *et al.* 1985), but are common in VHL disease, being detected in 9–29 per cent (Phytinen *et al.* 1982; Levine *et al.* 1983) by CT and in 40–72 per cent at autopsy (Lamiell *et al.* 1989; Jeffreys 1975). The great majority of these cysts are asymptomatic. The cysts frequently are multiple, and rarely replace most of the pancreas leading to diabetes mellitus or steatorrhoea (Hull *et al.* 1979; Fishman and Bartholomew 1979). The size of the cysts may be up to 10 cm in diameter and may cause displacement of the duodenum or abdominal distention (Jackaman 1984). Rarely, pancreatic disease is the first manifestation of the syndrome (Fill *et al.* 1979). Symptomatic pancreatic disease tends to cluster within certain VHL families (Fishman and Bartholomew 1979).

Benign angiomas and cystadenomas are found at autopsy in 7 per cent of VHL patients (Horton *et al.* 1976). These cystadenomas may be multilocular and asymptomatic; rarely they present as a palpable abdominal mass, cause abdominal pain, or obstruct the common bile duct. Pancreatic haemangioblastomas are very rare (Fill *et al.* 1979; Fishman and Bartholomew 1979).

Pancreatic cancer (cystadenocarcinoma or islet cell tumour) tends to cluster within certain VHL families (Cornish *et al.* 1984). In some families, 7.5–25 per cent (Lamiell *et al.* 1989; Binkovitz *et al.* 1990) had pancreatic cancer, but overall pancreatic cancer appears to be less common. There have been occasional reports of VHL patients with pancreatic 'apudomas' that produced vasoactive intestinal peptide and that were associated with hypercalcaemia (Mulshine *et al.* 1984).

Pancreatic cysts are lined by columnar epithelium consistent with ductal origin (Dan and Smith 1975). The pancreatic cystadenomas are the same histologically as the microcystic form of sporadic cystadenoma (Beerman *et al.* 1982).

Adrenal glands

Pheochromocytomas, benign adenomas, and less frequently, medullary cysts or cortical hyperplasia can occur in patients with VHL disease. The cysts and adenomas are asymptomatic and are found in 3 per cent of cases at autopsy (Horton *et al.* 1976). Small adenomas detected by CT also are common in the general population (Schimke 1990). Adrenal cortical hyperplasia has been found in 7 per cent of autopsy cases (Horton *et al.* 1976).

Pheochromocytomas tend to cluster within certain VHL families, so that in three large families involving more than 85 affected members, none had a pheochromocytoma (Go *et al.* 1984; Fill *et al.* 1979; Phytinen *et al.* 1982). However, in other families 17–92 per cent had pheochromocytomas (Horton *et al.* 1976; Atuk *et al.* 1979); more than one-third were not associated with high blood pressure when detected (Atuk *et al.* 1979). On average, approximately 3.5–17 per cent of VHL patients have pheochromocytomas (Christenson *et al.* 1982; Kiechle-Schwarz *et al.* 1989); 17–34 per cent are bilateral, although not always detected simultaneously (Atuk *et al.* 1979; Hoffman *et al.* 1982). The average age of diagnosis was 25–34 years with a range of 10–56 years (Horton *et al.* 1976; Huson *et al.* 1986; Atuk *et al.* 1979). Rarely, pheochromocytoma is the first manifestation of VHL disease. In one series, 19 per cent of patients presenting with pheochromocytoma had VHL (Neumann *et al.* 1993). By linkage studies, families with and without pheochromocytomas have defects within the same gene (Seizinger *et al.* 1991). The pheochromocytoma of VHL disease are histologically similar to sporadic lesions. Metastatic pheochromocytoma is extremely rare (Christenson *et al.* 1982).

Paragangliomas of the symptomatic chain are infrequently seen in VHL disease. In some families, not such lesions are found (Fill *et al.* 1979) while in other families 7 per cent had lesions incidentally detected at autopsy (Horton *et al.* 1976). It is extremely rare for these lesions to be functional or metastasize (Hoffman *et al.* 1982; Hull *et al.* 1982).

Since surgery or renal arteriography can trigger hypertensive crises in patients with pheochromocytomas, it is important to screen VHL patients prior to these procedures, particularly when a positive family history of pheochromocytoma is present. In the general population, up to 10 per cent of pheochromocytomas may be familial (Ludmerer and Kissane 1981); the diagnosis of VHL should be considered in these families.

Epididymis

Many males with VHL disease have benign and usually asymptomatic epididymal lesions, although occasionally fertility may be impaired (Lamiell *et al.* 1989). Simple cysts were reported in 7–27 per cent of patients (Horton *et al.* 1976; Fill *et al.* 1979). The size of the cysts ranges from 0.5 to 2.0 cm, and they may be detected as a painless mass (Blight *et al.* 1980).

Haemangiomas of the epididymis are rare (Malek and Greene 1971). Benign adenomas were seen in 3–26 per cent of patients at autopsy (Lamiell *et al.* 1989; Horton *et al.* 1976). Papillary cystadenomas may feel crystic or firm and frequently are asymptomatic, although they occasionally cause slight discomfort or pain. In one series of patients with bilateral lesions, the age of detection was from 18 to 28 years (Price 1971). In one series of patients with papillary cyst-adenomas, there were no further genital lesions or complications 1–15 years later. Patients with bilateral cysts or adenomas should be evaluated for VHL disease. However, because they are common, an epididymal cyst in a family member at risk is not sufficient by itself to make a diagnosis of VHL (Seizinger *et al.* 1991).

Cysts and cystadenomas frequently are present in the head of epididymis but also can occur in the spermatic cord. The cut surface of the cystadenoma appears spongy or multicystic, occasionally with a mural nodule. The well-circumscribed cystadenomas have three components: (1) papillary processes surfaced by epithelial cells; (2) ectatic ducts and microcysts lined by epithelial cells; and (3) fibrous stroma (Price 1971).

Other organs

Cysts in the liver were seen in 17 per cent of VHL patients in one autopsy series; none had been symptomatic (Horton *et al.* 1976). Liver cysts can be detected by CT and may be helpful in making the diagnosis of VHL. Less frequent are liver adenomas (3 per cent) and liver haemangiomas (7 per cent), which also are asymptomatic (Horton *et al.* 1976; Fill *et al.* 1979).

Asymptomatic spleen angiomas and cysts occur in 3–7 per cent of autopsied patients and are asymptomatic (Horton *et al.* 1976). Lung cysts and angiomas, omentum cysts, parametrial cysts, ovarian angiomas, broad ligament papillary cystadenomas, bone cysts and haemangiomas, bladder haemangioblastomas, and skin haemangiomas have been reported in patients with VHL disease (Scully *et al.* 1978; Horton *et al.* 1976; Melmon and Rosen 1964). These lesions are uncommon and asymptomatic, and many were detected at autopsy. The cysts in other visceral organs are not distinctive and are lined by epithelium (Scully *et al.* 1978). Bladder papillomas were present in von Hippel's original patient and have been noted subsequently (Melmon and Rosen 1964). There have been two cases of carcinoid tumour (in one case of the common bile duct) (Fellows *et al.* 1990). Single case reports exist of VHL patients with a variety of other lesions, such as adenocarcinoma of the ampulla of VATER (Fill *et al.* 1979), thyroid cancer (Reyes 1984), and papillary adenomas of the temporal bone (Levine 1985); some of these lesions may be coincidental.

Physical examination and investigations

The annual physical examination should include a careful neurological evaluation for signs of a cerebellar or spinal cord lesion. Opthalmological examination also should be performed annually and may reveal papilloedema as the first sign of cerebellar haemangioblastoma or retinal haemangioblastomas. Elevated blood pressure warrants investigation for pheochromocytoma. Apart from epididymal cysts, the remainder of the general physical examination usually is normal, as the pancreatic and renal cysts are rarely large enough to be palpated. The skin is not involved. A normal physical examination does not preclude the necessity for investigations.

The red blood cell count may be elevated in VHL patients who have cerebellar haemangioblastoma or renal cancer because of erythropoietin activity in cyst fluid (Trimble *et al.* 1991). The frequency of polycythaemia is approximately 10–20 per cent (Trimble *et al.* 1991). A normal red blood cell count never excludes the diagnosis of a significant tumour and should not replace imaging for VHL patients or their family members.

Patients with CNS tumours, particularly those involving the medulla and cord, may have elevated cerebrospinal fluid protein (Helle *et al.* 1980).

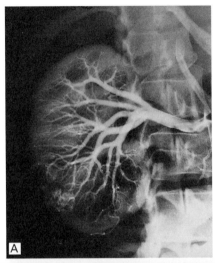

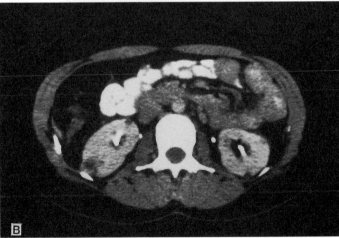

Fig. 12.2 Renal arteriogram (A) and CT (B) from a 33-year-old woman with von Hippel–Lindau disease illustrating a hypervascular mass in the right kidney and multiple bilateral small cysts.

Some patients with renal cancer have gross or microscopic haematuria, while others with extensive cancer have a normal urinalysis (Richards *et al.* 1973). Therefore, although patients with VHL should have a urinalysis as part of their annual evaluation, the absence of haematuria does not preclude the need for US or, preferably, CT of the abdomen (Fig. 12.2).

Twenty-four hour urine collections for epinephrine, norepinephrine, metanephrine, and vanillylmandelic acid also have been recommended to screen for pheochromocytoma (Christenson *et al.* 1982). This is particularly important for patients from families in which other members have had pheochromocytomas and for patients who are hypertensive or scheduled to have renal arteriography or surgery.

All patients who have, or who are suspected to have VHL disease should have CT or MRI of the head and MRI of the upper spine to search for haemangioblastomas. Early detection of tumours is important so that they may be monitored or surgically removed before secondary changes occur. Furthermore, surgical removal may be more difficult in some cases when the tumour and/or cyst is very large. The frequency for repeating CNS imaging is debatable. Some advocate a baseline evaluation with repeat studies only if symptoms or signs develop, while many advocate annual or semi-annual imaging.

Cerebellar haemangioblastomas have a typical appearance by CT; they are round, hypodense, cystic nodules sometimes surrounded by a hyperdense ring-like shadow after contrast injection (Baleriaux-Waha *et al.* 1978). CT with contrast is helpful in defining the intensely enhancing mural nodule within the cystic component, which facilitates its complete removal by the surgeon (Hellams *et al.* 1981). The less frequent, completely solid tumours are homogeneously isodense or hyperdense and enhance after contrast (Fig. 12.3). These

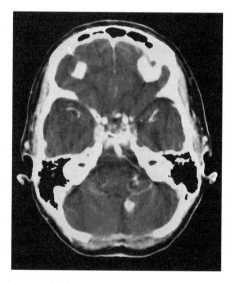

Fig. 12.3 Cerebellar haemangioblastoma in a patient with von Hippel–Lindau disease visualized by CT with intravenous contrast injection.

solid lesions are more apt to be located in the inferior vermis. Mass effect may cause obliteration of the fourth ventricle and hydrocephalus.

Magnetic resonance imaging (MRI) is useful for detection of cerebellar hae-mangioblastomas and may show smaller lesions than CT (Lee *et al.* 1989; Sato *et al.* 1988). The cystic portion of the tumour is sharply marginated with smooth borders and is isointense or of low intensity on T-1 weighted images and hyper-intense on T-2 weighted images compared to cerebrospinal fluid (Lee *et al.* 1989). The mural nodule, compared to surrounding gray matter, is isointense on T-1 weighted images and of high signal intensity on T-2 weighted images. When the lesions are over 1 cm in size, vessels may appear as serpentine areas of signal void at the periphery and within the tumour. The parenchyma adjacent to the cyst may have increased signal on T-2 weighted images compatible with oedema (Lee *et al.* 1989). The tumour nodule enhances after administration of intravenous gadolinium-diethylene triamine pentaacetic acid (Braffman *et al.* 1990) and the films should be taken immediately after contrast administration for the best results (Filling-Katz *et al.* 1989). In one series of VHL patients with haemangioblastomas, 19 lesions were detected by CT with contrast, 22 by plain MRI, and 31 by MRI with gadolinium-DTPA (Filling-Katz *et al.* 1989).

MRI with gadolinium-DTPA is also better than plain MRI for detecting spinal cord lesions, especially those associated with syringomyelia (Pearson *et al.* 1980) (Fig. 12.4). Angiograms may be helpful to better define the blood vessels connected to the lesion prior to surgical removal.

Visceral and epididymal cysts may be evident by US, MRI, or CT examina-tion (Dershaw 1985; Choyke *et al.* 1990). CT may be more sensitive and prob-

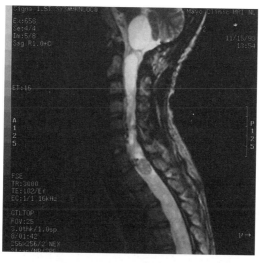

Fig. 12.4 Large spinal cord haemangioblastoma with syrinx in a patient with von Hippel–Lindau disease visualized by MRI with gadolinium-diethylene triamine pentaacetic acid.

ably is the method of choice, but the experience of the radiographer and sonographer can be taken into account (Sato *et al.* 1988). Renal cancer can remain undetected after intravenous pyelography with tomography (Campbell *et al.* 1978) and CT is useful for annual screening (Christenson *et al.* 1982). In general, renal cancers can be detected when less than 3 cm in size when they usually are non-invasive (Levine *et al.* 1983). In patients with suspicious pancreatic lesions by US or CT, angiography is helpful for diagnosis of cystadenocarcinoma (Lamiell *et al.* 1989). Annual investigation is recommended.

Use of fluorescein angiography of retinal lesions may be helpful to reveal typical early filling and late leakage of dye in the diagnosis of tiny or atypical lesions which are masked by secondary changes (Diehl and Symon 1981). Calcification or enhancement of retinal haemangioblastomas are occasionally noted by CT or MRI (Braffman *et al.* 1990).

Diagnostic criteria

The diagnosis should be made in a person with multiple central nervous system or retinal haemangioblastomas, or a single haemangioblastoma plus one of the other characteristic physical abnormalities or a family history of VHL disease. In some cases, the diagnosis may be warranted in a patient with a positive family history but without a central nervous system or retinal lesion, who has one or more of the less specific findings, with the exception of epididymal cysts which are too non-specific (Seizinger *et al.* 1991). It is important to make the diagnosis of VHL disease to ensure proper monitoring and early treatment of the patient and his family members, as well as for genetic counselling purposes.

Therapy

Cerebellar haemangioblastomas can be successfully removed surgically in 85–90 per cent of patients. The surgeon should carefully inspect the cyst walls to ensure that the mural nodule has been removed. Some patients with secondary hydrocephalus may require ventricular decompression by drainage prior to opening the posterior fossa. Rarely it is necessary to place a permanent shunt (Jeffreys 1975). Between 8 and 15 per cent (Jeffreys 1975; Obrador and Martin-Rodriguez 1977) of lesions recur, and recurrences are more frequent for solid tumours. However, it sometimes is difficult to distinguish between the true recurrence or a second primary tumour. Such 'recurrences' may occur up to 24 years later, but the average time interval is 5 years (Mondkar *et al.* 1967). Tumours in the 4th ventricle, medulla, and spinal cord are more difficult to remove completely, and decisions regarding surgery must be made on an individual basis.

In one case of bulbar haemangioblastoma not amenable to surgical treatment, radiation resulted in amelioration of symptoms and was said to have resulted in the appearance of planes of dissection that facilitated surgery (Helle *et al.* 1980). Radiotherapy also has been suggested for patients whose lesions are not amenable to complete surgical resection (Smalley *et al.* 1990).

Since surgical outcome can be improved by early detection of CNS tumours before surrounding oedema and secondary effects become severe, increased awareness of the diagnosis and screening of family members may lead to improved outcome.

If small, peripheral, and stable in size, retinal lesions may be serially observed to watch for retinal detachment and progressive visual impairment (Fill *et al.* 1979). Some recommend obliteration of all lesions by cryocoagulation or photocoagulation unless they are in or near the macula or disc (Augsburger *et al.* 1981). The latter lesions also may require treatment if they cause significant visual impairment. In general, small lesions ($< \frac{1}{2}$ disc diameter in size) respond well to therapy, lesions of 1 to $1\frac{1}{2}$ disc diameter in size respond satisfactorily but may require repeated treatments, and large lesions (> 2 disc diameters in size) respond poorly and treatment may result in further tractional detachment of the retina (Peyman *et al.* 1983).

It is probably safe to observe small renal cysts (Melmon and Rosen 1964). However, unroofing and gross examination of larger apparently simple cysts is not adequate to exclude microscopic foci of cancer (Christenson *et al.* 1982). Both cysts and solid tumours, particularly if detected when small, are usually surrounded by a pseudocapsule of compressed parenchyma and can be shelled out (Pearson *et al.* 1980). It probably is safe to monitor very tiny lesions (< 1 cm in diameter) for rapid growth (Kadir *et al.* 1981). It is important to spare renal tissue and perform partial nephrectomy when possible, particularly in patients with low tumour stage and grade. This conservative approach has led to prolonged survival in select cases that compares favourably to the alternative of nephrectomy requiring dialysis (Morgan and Zincke 1990; Frydenberg *et al.* 1993). Bilateral and multiple lesions are apt to be present or be detected subsequently. Patients with high grade and stage may warrant complete nephrectomy (Frydenberg *et al.* 1993). In one recent survey of 318 patients with VHL, 74 had kidney lesions. Mean age of diagnosis of kidney involvement was 38 years (range 16–68 years). Forty-eight of these patients had at least one focus of clear-cell carcinoma or atypical cyst resulting in unilateral conservative surgery in 4 cases, unilateral nephrectomy in 17 cases, unilateral nephrectomy with contralateral partial renal resection in 5 cases, and unilateral nephrectomy with contralateral tumour resection in 2 cases. Two additional patients had bilateral nephrectomy, while 13 had small tumours that were considered too small to warrant surgery or because of metastatic or other severe disease manifestations. After a mean follow-up of 3.7 years (range 0–16 years), 22 patients were alive. Of the 16 who had died: 3 died post-operatively after renal surgery; 4 died of renal cancer metastases; and 8 died of other manifestations of VHL (Richard *et al.* 1994). These results are similar to another series (Frydenberg *et al.* 1993) in which 19 patients were diagnosed with kidney disease at a mean of 40 years. Of 7 patients with unilateral disease: 6 had partial nephrectomy; and 1 had nephrectomy. Another 12 had bilateral disease; 1 had bilateral nephrectomy; 3 had bilateral partial nephrectomy; 4 had nephrectomy and contralateral partial nephrectomy; and 4 had unilateral nephrectomy. After a mean of 5 years of follow-up (range 3 months to 14 years), 10 had not evidence of disease; 7 died of renal disease; and 2 were alive with disease. In the few cases that present with extensive polycystic disease and renal failure requiring dialysis, nephrectomy should be performed since cancer may develop (Blight *et al.* 1980). In cases in which renal transplant is contemplated, care must be taken to avoid an affected but undiagnosed relative as donor.

Pancreatic lesions usually require no treatment (Melmon and Rosen 1964) except in the case of malignancy or when large cysts cause symptoms. Aspiration of a cyst resulted in relief of abdominal swelling in one patient (Jackaman 1984). In more extensive polycystic disease with diabetes mellitus and steatorrhoea, partial or complete pancreatectomy may be warranted (Fishman and Bartholomew 1979).

Genetic counselling

The autosomal dominant inheritance of VHL disease is firmly established. Non-penetrance in families who have been evaluated using modern techniques and in whom all pertinent family members had reached an age at which signs would have been expected is extremely rare (Go *et al.* 1984; Davies *et al.* 1994). Penetrance has been estimated as 0.96 by age 60 and 0.99 by age 70 years (Maher *et al.* 1991). Males and females are affected equally.

Any patient with a central nervous system or retinal haemangioblastoma should have a complete review of the family history and should be screened by CT or MRI of the head and upper spine, ophthalmological examination, and CT or US of the abdomen to look for other signs of VHL disease. If the family history is positive or a second characteristic lesion is identified, the diagnosis should be made. Such screening also should be done in patients who present with bilateral epididymal cysts or polycystic pancreas, and should be considered in patients presenting with pheochromocytomas, polycystic kidneys, or renal cancer, particularly when there is a suspicious family history or when the lesions are bilateral, multifocal, occur at an unusually young age, or are atypical in some other way.

Patients diagnosed as having VHL disease need an annual physical and oph-thalmological examination, a peripheral blood cell count, urinalysis and yearly CT or US of the abdomen. Evaluation of urinary catecholamines is reasonable, particularly if the patient is hypertensive or has a positive family history of pheochromocytoma. Initial imaging of the head is mandatory, but the necessity or frequency of subsequent monitoring is not clear since small asymptomatic lesions may not require immediate removal. Until further information is avail-able, annual or biennial CT or MRI of the head and upper spine may be reason-able (Huson *et al.* 1986). All affected patients should have genetic counselling and all first-degree relatives (parents, siblings, children) should have physical and ophthalmological examinations beginning at age 1–2 years (Ridley *et al.* 1986; Greenwald and Weiss 1984; Filling-Katz *et al.* 1991), imaging of the head and spine by around 10 years and imaging of the abdomen beginning at age 18 years (Levine *et al.* 1983). Although appropriate ages at which to begin screening family members has been delineated, it is not known at what age one can discontinue screening for at-risk members and assume they do not have the disease. Therefore, at the present time, screening must be continued indefinitely unless genetic studies demonstrate that the relative is not at risk.

Genetic counselling should be provided to inform the patient of the nature of the disease and to co-ordinate evaluation and treatment by other specialists; to ensure adequate subsequent evaluations; to document the family history and arrange for investigations of other family members; and to explain the inheritance pattern and discuss options for family planning. These options include accepting the 50 per cent chance that any child will be affected or remaining childless, adopting a child or, for affected males, artificial insemination of the wife with donor semen. *In vitro* fertilization of a donor egg implanted in an affected woman is another option, since there are no proven adverse effects of pregnancy on the disease. Prenatal or presymptomatic diagnosis using linked DNA restriction fragment length polymorphisms is possible for at least 74 per cent of subjects with a positive family history (Maher *et al.* 1992). Although linkage analysis cannot be used in sporadic cases or when DNA is not available from pertinent family members, approximately 15 per cent of patients with von Hippel–Lindau have a rearrangement within the gene that can be detected by direct DNA mutation analysis (Johns Hopkins DNA Diagnostic Laboratory, H. H. Kazazian 1994, personal communication). There are two support groups for von Hippel–Lindau patients, the von Hippel–Lindau Family Alliance (VHL 1993) and the von Hippel–Lindau Syndrome Foundation, Inc (VHL 1992).

Molecular genetics

The defective autosomal dominant gene that causes von Hippel–Lindau disease has been identified (Latif *et al.* 1993). The exact function of the gene product is unknown, but the gene is widely expressed in fetal and adult tissues. It is localized to chromosome 3p25-26. Flanking markers that bracket the VHL gene have been identified and are the basis for a useful genetic test for presymptomatic and prenatal diagnosis. In 38 VHL pedigrees there is no evidence thus far for non-allelic heterogeneity, even in families with a strong predisposition for pheochromocytomas (Seizinger *et al.* 1991; Richards *et al.* 1993). There are multiple different mutations that can occur in the gene. Approximately 15 per cent of mutations involve an intragenic rearrangement readily detectable by DNA analysis in a clinical setting (John Hopkins). On a research basis, mutations can be found in approximately 28 per cent of patients (Maher *et al.* 1993).

Loss of heterozygosity studies for alleles on 3p in renal cell carcinomas, pheochromocystomas, and haemangioblastomas from VHL patients show that the allelic loss is from the non-affected parental chromosome (Tory *et al.* 1989). This is consistent with the normal gene at the VHL locus acting as a tumour suppressor gene. Thus, at the molecular level this clinically dominant disease functions as an 'autosomal recessive oncogene' (Seizinger *et al.* 1988).

Microscopically visible chromosome abnormalities in renal cell carcinomas from both VHL patients and otherwise normal individuals frequently involve 3p. It recently has been determined that the VHL locus also is involved in isolated hereditary renal cancer in patients with the constitutional chromosome translocation t(3;8)(p14;q24). In addition, acquired somatic mutations in the von Hippel–Lindau gene play a role in sporadic renal cancers, as shown by loss of heterozygosity and mutation studies (Gnarra *et al.* 1994).

References

Atuk, N. O., *et al.* (1979). Familial pheochromocytoma, hypercalcemia, and von Hippel–Lindau disease: a ten year study of a large family. *Medicine*, **58**, 209–18.

Augsburger, J. J., Shields, J. A., and Goldberg, R. E. (1981). Classification and management of hereditary retinal angiomas. *International Ophthalmology*, **4**, 1–2, 93–106.

Baleriaux-Waha, D., *et al.* (1978). CT scanning for the diagnosis of the cerebellar and spinal lesions of von Hippel–Lindau disease. *Neuroradiology*, **14**, 241–4.

Barkin, J. S., Goldberg, H., and Bradley, E. L. (1985). Cysts and pseudocysts of the pancreas. In *Gastroenterology*, (ed. W. S. Haubrick, M. H. Kalser, J. L. A. Roth, F. Schaffner, and J. E. Berk), Vol. 6, pp. 41–5. Saunders, Philadelphia, PA.

Beerman, M. H. Fromkes, J. J, Carey, L. C., and Thomas, F. B. (1982). Pancreatic cystadenoma in Von Hippel–Lindau disease: an unusual cause of pancreatic and common bile duct obstruction. *Journal of Clinical Gastroenterology*, **4**, 537–40.

Bickler, S., Wile, A. G., Melicharek,. M., and Recher, L. (1984). Pancreatic involvement in Hippel-Lindau disease. *Western Journal of Medicine*, **140**, 280–2.

Binkovitz, L. A., Johnson, C. D., and Stephens, D. H. (1990). Islet cell tumors in von Hippel-Lindau disease: increased prevalence and relationship to the multiple endocrine neoplasias. *American Journal of Roentgenology*, **155**, 501–15.

Blight, E. M. Jr, Biggers, R. D., Soderdahl, D. W., Brossman, S. A., Lamiell, J. M., and Raleigh, E. N. (1980). Bilateral renal masses. *Journal of Urology*, **124**, 695–700.

Boker, D. K, Wassmann, H., and Solymosi, L. (1984). Multiple spinal haemangioblastomas in a case of Lindau's disease. *Surgical Neurology*, **22**, 439–43.

Braffman, B. H., Bilaniuk, L. T., and Zimmerman, R. A. (1990). MR of central nervous system neoplasia of the phakomatoses. *Semin-Roentgenology*, **25**, 198–217.

Campbell, D. R., Mason, W. F, and Standen, J. R. (1978). Renal arteriography in von Hippel–Lindau disease. *Journal of the Canadian Association of Radiology*, **29**, 243–6.

Choyke, P. L., *et al,* (1990). Von Hippel–Lindau disease: radiologic screening for visceral manifestations. *Radiology*, **174**, 815–20.

Christenson, P. J, Craig, J. P., Bibro, M. C., and O'Connell, K. J. (1982). Cysts containing renal cell carcinoma in von Hippel–Lindau disease. *Journal of Urology*, **128**, 798–800.

Cornish, D., Pont, A., Minor, D., Coombs, J. L., and Bennington, J. (1984). Metastatic islet cell tumor in von Hippel–Lindau disease. *American Journal of Medicine*, **77**, 147–50.

Dan, N. G. and Smith, D. E. (1975). Pituitary hemangioblastoma in a patient with von Hippel–Lindau disease. *Journal of Neurosurgery*, **42**, 232–5.

Davies, D. R., Norman, A. M., Whitehouse, R. W., and Evans, D. G. R. (1994). Non-expression of von Hippel–Lindau phenotype in a obligate gene carrier. *Clinical genetics*, **45**, 104–6.

Dershaw, D. D. (1985). Sonography of epididymal cystadenoma. *Urologic Radiology*, 7, 119–20.

Diehl, P. R. and Symon, L. (1981). Supratentorial intraventricular hemangioblastoma: case report and review of literature. *Surgical Neurology*, 15, 435–43.

Fellows, I. W., Leach, I. H., Smith, P. G., Toghill, P. J., and Doran, J. (1990). Carcinoid tumour of the common bile duct: a novel complication of von Hippel–Lindau syndrome. *Gut*, 131, 728–9.

Fill, W. L., Lamiell, J. M., and Polk, N. O. (1979). The radiographic manifestations of von Hippel–Lindau disease. *Diagnostic Radiology*, 133, 289–95.

Filling-Katz, M. R., *et al.* (1989). Radiologic screening for von Hippel–Lindau disease: the role of Gd-DTPA enhanced MR imaging of the CNS. *Journal of Computer Assisted Tomography*, 13, 743–55.

Filling-Katz, M. R., *et al.* (1991). Central nervous system involvement in von Hippel–Lindau disease. *Neurology*, 41, 41–6.

Fishman, R. S. and Bartholomew, L. G. (1979). Severe pancreatic involvement in three generations in von Hippel–Lindau disease. *Mayo Clinic Proceedings*, 54, 329–31.

Frank, T. S., Trojanowski, J. Q., Roberts, S. A., and Brooks, J. J. (1989). A detailed immunohistochemical analysis of cerebellar hemangioblastoma: an undifferentiated mesenchyma tumor. *Modern Pathology*, 2, 638–51.

Frydenberg, M, Malek, R. S., and Zincke, H. (1993). Conservative renal surgery for renal cell carcinoma in von Hippel–Lindau's disease. *Journal of Urology*, 149, 461–4.

Gardeur, D., Palmieri, A., and Mashaly, R. (1983). Cranial computed tomography in the phakomatoses. *Neuroradiology*, 25, 293–304.

Glenn, G. M., *et al.* (1991). Von Hippel–Lindau (VHL) disease: distinct phenotypes suggest more than one mutant allele at the VHL locus. *Human Genetics*, 87, 207–10.

Gnarra, J. R., *et al.* (1994). Mutations of the VHL tumour suppressor gene in renal carcinoma. *Nature Genetics*. 7, 85–90.

Go, R. C. P., Lamiell, J. M., Hsia, Y. E., Yuen, J. W.-M., and Paik, Y. (1984). Segregation and linkage analyses of von Hippel–Lindau disease among 220 descendants from one kindred. *American Journal of Human Genetics*, 36, 131–42.

Green, J. S., Bowmer, M. I., and Johnson, G. J. (1986). Von Hippel–Lindau disease in a Newfoundland kindred. *Canadian Medical Association Journal*, 134, 133–8.

Greenwald, M. J. and Weiss, A. (1984). Ocular manifestations of the neurocutaneous syndromes. *Pediatric Dermatology*, 2, 98–117.

Hardwig, P. and Robertson, D. M. (1984). Von Hippel–Lindau disease: a familial, often lethal multi-system phakomatosis. *Opthalmology*, 91, 263–70.

Hellams, S. E., Cohen, R. J., and Young, H. F. (1981). Cerebellar hemangioblastomas and von Hippel–Lindau syndrome. *Virginia Medicine*. 108, 42–5.

Helle, T. L., Conley, F. K., and Britt, R. H. (1980). Effect of radiation therapy on hemangioblastoma: a case report and review of the literature. *Neurosurgery*, 6, 82–6.

Ho, K.-L. (1983). Von Hippel–Lindau disease and neurogenous tumors (Letter to the editor). *Archives of Pathology and Laboratory Medicine*, 107, 48.

Hoffmann, R. W., Gardner, D. W., and Mitchell, F. L. (1982). Intrathoracic and multiple abdominal pheochromocytomas in von Hippel–Lindau disease. *Archives of Internal Medicine*, 142, 1962–4.

Horton, W. A., Wong, V., and Eldrige, R. (1976). Von Hippel–Lindau disease: clinical and pathological manifestations in nine families with 50 affected members. *Archives of Internal Medicine*, 136, 769–77.

Hull, M. T., Warfel, K. A., Muller, J., and Higgins, J. T. (1979). Familial islet cell tumors in von Hippel–Lindau's disease. *Cancer*, **44**, 1523–6.

Hull, M. T., Roth, L. M., Glover, J. L., and Walker, P. D. (1982). Metastatic carotid body paraganglioma in von Hippel–Lindau disease: an electron microscopic study. *Archives of Pathology and Laboratory Medicine*, **106**, 235–9.

Huson, S. M., Harper, P. S., Hourihan, M. D., Cole, G., Weeks, R. D., and Compston, D. A. (1986). Cerebellar haemangioblastoma and von Hippel–Lindau disease. *Brain*, **109**, 1297–310.

Ibrahim, R. E., Weinberg, D. S., and Weidner, N. (1989). Atypical cysts and carcinomas of the kidneys in the phacomatoses. A quantitative DNA study using static and flow cytometry. *Cancer*, **63**, 148–57.

Ishwar, S., Taniguchi, R. M., and Vogel, F. S. (1971). Multiple supratentorial hemangioblastomas: case study and ultrastructural characteristics. *Journal of Neurosurgery*, **35**, 396–405.

Jackaman, F. R. (1984). Polycystic pancreas: Lindau's disease. *Journal of the Royal College of Surgery (Edinburg)*, **29**, 121–2.

Jeffreys, R. (1975). Clinical and surgical aspects of posterior fossa haemangioblastomata. *Journal of Neurology, Neurosurgery and Psychiatry*, **38**, 105–11.

Kadir, S., Kerr, W. S. Jr, and Athanasoulis, C. A. (1981). The role of arteriography in the management of renal cell carcinoma associated with von Hippel–Lindau disease. *Journal of Urology*, **126**, 316–19.

Kiechle-Schwarz, M., Neumann. H. P., Decker, H. J., Dietrich, C., Wullish, B., and Schempp, W. (1989). Cytogenetic studies on three pheochromocytomas derived from patients with von Hippel–Lindau syndrome. *Human Genetics*, **82**, 127–30.

Kupersmith, M. J. and Berenstein, A. (1981). Visual disturbances in von Hippel–Lindau disease. *Annals of Ophthalmology*, **13**, 195–7.

Lamiell, J. M., Stor, R. A., and Hsia, Y. E. (1980). Von Hippel–Lindau disease stimulating polycystic kidney disease. *Urology*, **15**, 287–90.

Lamiell, J. M., Salazar, F. G., and Hsia, Y. E. (1989). Von Hippel–Lindau disease affecting 43 members of a single kindred. *Medicine (Baltimore)*, **68**, 1–29.

Latif, F., *et al.* (1993). Identification of the von Hippel–Lindau disease tumor suppressor gene. *Science*, **260**, 1317–20.

Lee, K. R., Wulfsberg, E., and Kepes, J. J. (1977). Some important radiological aspects of the kidney in Hippel–Lindau syndrome: the value of prospective study in an affected family. *Diagnostic Radiology*, **122**, 649–53.

Lee, S. R., Sanches, J., Mark, A. S., Dillon, W. P., Norman, D., and Newton, T. H. (1989). Posterior fossa hemangioblastomas: MR imaging. *Radiology*, **171**, 463–8.

Levine, E. (1985). Computed tomography of renal masses. *Critical Review in Diagnostic Imaging*, **24**, 91–200.

Levine, E., Weigel, J. W., and Collins, D. L. (1983). Diagnosis and management of asymptomatic renal cell carcinomas in von Hippel–Lindau syndrome. *Urology*, **21**, 1946–50.

Ludmerer, K. M. and Kissane, J. H. (1981). Renal mass in a man with von Hippel–Lindau disease. *American Journal of Medicine*. **71**, 287–97.

Maher, E. R., Yates, J. R., and Ferguson-Smith, M. A. (1990). Statistical analysis of the two stage model in von Hippel–Lindau disease, and in sporadic cerebellar haemangioblastoma and renal cell carcinoma. *Journal of Medical Genetics*, **27**, 311–14.

Maher, E. R., *et al.* (1991). Von Hippel–Lindau disease: a genetic study. *Journal of Medical Genetics*, **28**, 443–7.

Maher, E. R., *et al.* (1992). Presymptomatic diagnosis of von Hippel–Lindau disease with flanking DNA markers. *Journal of Medical Genetics*, **29**, 902–5.

Maher, E. R., *et al.* (1993). Molecular genetic analysis in the management of von Hippel–Lindau (VHL) disease (Abstract 16). *American Journal of Human Genetics*, (Suppl. No. 3), **53**.

Malek, R. S. and Greene, L. F. (1971). Urologic aspects of von Hippel–Lindau syndrome. *Journal of Urology*, **106**, 800–1.

Melmon, K. L. and Rosen, S. W. (1964). Lindau's disease: review of the literature and study of a large kindred. *American Journal of Medicine*. **36**, 595–617.

Michels, V. V. (1988). Investigative studies in von Hippel–Lindau disease. *Neurofibromatosis*, **1**, 159–63.

Mohan, J., Brownell, B., and Oppenheimer, D. R. (1976). Malignant spread of hemangioblastoma: report on two cases. *Journal of Neurology, Neurosurgery and Psychiatry*, **39**, 515–25.

Mondkar, V. P., McKissock, W., and Russell, R. W. R. (1967). Cerebellar haemangioblastomas. *British Journal of Surgery*, **54**, 45–9.

Morgan, W. R. and Zincke, H. (1990). Progression and survival after renal-conserving surgery for renal cell carcinoma: experience in 104 patients and extended follow up (Discussion). *Journal of Urology*, **144**, 852–7, 857–8.

Mulshine, J. L., Tubbs, R., Sheeler, L. R., and Gifford, R. W. Jr (1984). Case report: clinical significance of the association of the von Hippel–Lindau disease with pheochromocytoma and pancreatic apudoma. *American Journal of Medical Science*, **288**, 212–16.

Neumann, H. P, Eggert, H. R., Weigel, K., Friedburg, H., Wiestler, O. D., and Schollmeyer, P. (1989). Hemangioblastomas of the central nervous system. A 10-year study with special reference to von Hippel–Lindau syndrome. *Journal of Neurosurgery*, **70**, 24–30.

Neumann, H. P. H. and Wiestler, O. D. (1991). Clustering of features of von Hippel–Lindau syndrome: evidence for a complex genetic locus. *Lancet*, **337**, 1052–4.

Neumann, H. P. H., *et al.* (1993). Pheochromocytomas, multiple neoplasia type 2, and von Hippel–Lindau disease. *New England Journal of Medicine*, **329**, 1531–8.

Obrador, S. and Martin-Rodriguez, J. G. (1977). Biological factors involved in the clinical features and surgical management of cerebellar hemangioblastomas. *Surgical Neurology*, **7**, 79–85.

Olivecrona, H. (1952). The cerebellar angioreticulomas. *Journal of Neurosurgery*, **9**, 317–30.

Palmer, J. J. (1972). Haemangioblastomas: a review of 81 cases. *Acta Neurochirurgica (Wien)*, **27**, 125–48.

Pearson, J. C., Weiss, J., and Tanagho, E. A. (1980). A plea for conservation of kidney in renal adenocarcinoma associated with von Hippel–Lindau disease. *Journal of Urology*, **124**, 910–12.

Peyman, G. A., Rednam, K. R. V., Mottow-Lippa, L., and Flood, T. (1983). Treatment of large von Hippel tumors by eye wall resection. *Opthalmology*, **90**, 840–7.

Phytinen, J., Suramo, I., Lohela, P., and Mustonen. E. (1982). Abdominal ultrasonography and computed tomography in von Hippel–Lindau disease. *Annals of Clinical Research*, **14**, 172–6.

Price, E. B. Jr (1971). Papillary cystadenoma of the epididymis: a clinicopathologic analysis of 20 cases. *Archives of Pathology*, **91**, 456–70.

Reyes, C. V. (1984). Thyroid carcinoma in von Hippel–Lindau disease (Letter to the editor). *Archives of Internal Medicine*, **144**, 413.

Richards, F. M., *et al.* (1993). Detailed genetic mapping of the von Hippel–Lindau disease tumour suppressor gene. *Journal of Medical Genetics*, **30**, 104–7.

Richards, R. D., Mebust, W. K, and Schimke, R. N. (1973). A prospective study on von Hippel–Lindau disease. *Journal of Urology*, **110**, 27–30.

Richard, S., *et al*, (1994). Renal lesions and pheochromocytoma in von Hippel–Lindau disease. *Advances in Nephrology*, **23**, 1–27.

Ridley, M., Green, J., and Johnson, G. (1986). Retinal angiomatosis: the ocular manifestations of von Hippel–Lindau disease. *Canadian Journal of Ophthalmology*, **21**, 276–83.

Sato, Y., *et al.* (1988). Hippel–Lindau disease: MR imaging. *Radiology*, **166**, 241–6.

Schimke, R. N. (1990). Multiple endocrine neoplasia: how many syndromes? *American Journal of Medical Genetics*, **37**, 375–83.

Schindler, R. F., Sarin, L. K., and MacDonald, P. R. (1975). Hemangiomas of the optic disc. *Canadian Journal of Ophthalmology*, **10**, 305–18.

Scully, R. E., Galdabini, J. J., and McNeely, B. U. (1978). Case records of the Massachusetts General Hospital. *New England Journal of Medicine*, **298**, 95–101.

Seich, I., Miyagi, J., Kojho, N., Kuramoto, S., and Urehara, M. (1982). Intraorbital optic nerve hemangioblastoma with von Hippel–Lindau disease. *Journal of Neurosurgery*, **56**, 426–9.

Seizinger, B. R., *et al.* (1988). Von Hippel–Lindau disease maps to the region of chromosome 3 associated with renal cell carcinoma. *Nature*, **332**, 268–9.

Seizinger, B. R., *et al.* (1991). Genetic flanking markers refine diagnostic criteria and provide insights into the genetics of von Hippel–Lindau disease. *Proceedings of the National Academy of Sciences USA*, **88**, 2864–8.

Smalley, S. R., *et al.* (1990). Radiotherapeutic considerations in the treatment of hemangioblastomas of the central nervous system. *International Journal of Radiation Oncology, Biology and Physiology*, **18**, 1165–71.

Solomon, D. and Schwartz, A. (1988). Renal pathology in von Hippel–Lindau disease. *Human Pathology*, **19**, 1072–9.

Spencer, W. F., Novick, A. C., Montie, J. E., Streem, S. B., and Levin, H. S. (1988). Surgical treatment of localized renal cell carcinoma in von Hippel–Lindau disease. *Journal of Urology*, **139**, 507–9.

Trimble, M., Caro, J., Talalla, A., and Brain, M. (1991). Secondary erythrocytosis due to a cerebellar hemangioblastoma: demonstration of erythropoietin mRNA in the tumor. *Blood*, **78**, 599–601.

Tory, K., *et al.* (1989). Specific genetic change in tumors associated with von Hippel–Lindau disease. *Journal of the National Cancer Institute*, **81**, 1097–101.

VHL News (1992). *Newsletter of the Hippel–Lindau Syndrome Foundation, Inc*, P. O. Box 733, Toms River, NJ 08754-0733, USA.

VHL Family Forum (1993). *Newsletter of the VHL Family Alliance*, No. 1, March. 171 Clinton Road, Brookline, MA 02146, USA.

Vogel, F. and Motulsky, A. G. (1979). Mutation. In *Human genetics: problems and approaches*, p. 296. Springer-Verlag, New York.

Wing, G. L., Weiter, J. J., Kelly, P. J., Albert, D. M., and Gonder, J. R. (1981). Von Hippel–Lindau disease: angiomatosis of the retina and central nervous system. *Opthalmology*, **88**, 1311–14.

Yimoyines, D. J., Topilow, H. W., Abedin, S., and McMeel, J. W. (1982). Bilateral peripapillary exophytic retinal hemangioblastomas. *Opthalmology*, **89**, 1388–92.

PART III

*Autosomal dominant polycystic kidney disease:
natural history and genetics*

13

Definition and natural history of autosomal dominant polycystic kidney disease

Patricia A. Gabow

This chapter serves to present in broad overview much of what will be discussed in detail in subsequent chapters. It is hoped that it will present a panoramic snapshot of the entire disorder while permitting subsequent chapters to take 'close-up' views.

Definition, genetics, and epidemiology

The term 'autosomal dominant polycystic kidney disease' (ADPKD) at once both represents and misrepresents the disorder. As the name implies, the disease is hereditary, being transmitted in an autosomal dominant pattern. Therefore, each offspring of an affected person has a 50 per cent chance of inheriting the parental chromosome which carries the abnormal gene and hence the disease. Since the disease is inherited on an autosome, there is no gender difference in the frequency of the disease in males and females. However, there are differences in the phenotypic manifestations of the disorder by gender (see below). Although the name portrays a renal cystic disorder, this is only, in part, correct. In fact, the disease is characterized by both renal and extrarenal manifestations as well as by both cystic and non-cystic abnormalities (Gabow 1990, 1993). Many of these aspects will be discussed in detail in subsequent chapters.

ADPKD displays considerable phenotypic variability both between and within families; there is variability in both the array of manifestations and in the severity of individual manifestations. Elucidation of the genetics of the disorder has begun to provide an explanation for some of this variability. The interfamily variability can be explained in part by the occurrence of genetic heterogeneity, that is, more than one gene can produce ADPKD (Reeders *et al*. 1985; Kimberling *et al*. 1988; Romeo *et al*. 1988). The first ADPKD gene located was found to be on the short arm of chromosome 16 (Reeders *et al*. 1985). This has been called ADPKD1 in the nephrology literature. ADPKD1 appears to account for 90 per cent of the disease among whites of European origin (Kimberling *et al*. 1991). A second gene which produces ADPKD has been labelled ADPKD2 by nephrologists and is located on chromosome 4 (Kimberling *et al*. 1993; Peters *et al*. 1993). Preliminary data suggest there may be ADPKD families in which the ADPKD gene is not located on either chromosome 16 or chromosome 4, suggesting that there may be even a third ADPKD gene (Daoust *et al.* 1993). The initial information on the location of the ADPKD genes permitted diagnosis to be made in at-risk individuals with gene linkage techniques (see below).

In 1994, the ADPKD1 gene itself was cloned (EPKDC 1994). Although we do not yet know the gene product of either the ADPKD1 or ADPKD2 gene, it is likely that they are different. This raises the question: 'Do the ADPKD1 and ADPKD2 gene cause a different clinical picture?' In fact, members of ADPKD1 families appear to have earlier disease onset with renal cyst development, hypertension, and renal failure at a younger age than do members of ADPKD2 families (see below).

Although the presence of different causative genes can explain interfamily variability, it cannot explain intrafamily variability since within a single family the same gene would be present in all affected members. Milutinovic *et al.* (1992) have demonstrated that 38 per cent of affected family members have non-comparable degrees of renal insufficiency and 53 per cent had non-comparable severity of renal structural involvement as assessed by renal size. The most dramatic manifestation of this intrafamily variability occurs in families with children who manifest the disease *in utero* or in the first year of life. In one study of 11 such children from 8 families, all of their affected parents had disease onset in adult life (Fick *et al.* 1993). In fact, 3 of the 8 parents were unaware they had ADPKD until the birth of the affected child prompted their own evaluation. Moreover, all the affected parents had normal renal function at time of study at a mean age of 34.4 years. Of note, all of the affected parents were mothers and 8 of the 11 offsprings were daughters. Moreover, early onset children tended to cluster in certain families; three families had more than one child with very early onset of ADPKD. The occurrence of congenital onset of disease in offspring of affected mothers is strikingly similar to a pattern observed in myotonic dystrophy, another autosomal dominant disease (Harper and Dyken 1972). In myotonic dystrophy this pattern has been called 'genetic anticipation', that is, earlier disease onset and greater disease severity in successive generations.

A recent study examined the pedigrees of 242 ADPKD families for such examples of genetic anticipation (Fick *et al.* 1994*b*). Anticipation was considered to have occurred in a family if there was a very early onset child (i.e. *in utero* or in the first year of life) or if ESRD occurred 10 years earlier in an offspring in comparison to his or her affected parent. Given the availability of better disease management with better antihypertensive therapy and better antibiotic treatment for cyst infection and the better understanding of the disease as well as diagnosis of milder cases with better imaging techniques, one would predict a better or at least a similar course of disease in the younger generation. However, 53 per cent of the informative ADPKD families demonstrated anticipation (Fick *et al.* 1994*b*). In examining 221 informative individual parent–offspring pairs, 39 per cent of the offspring had a worse course of disease than did their affected parent (Fick *et al.* 1994*b*). These results suggest anticipation in ADPKD. In disorders, such as myotonic dystrophy, which demonstrate clinical anticipation, the genetic mechanism is increased triplet repeats within the gene (Harley *et al.* 1992*a*). An increasing number of repeats relates to earlier onset and increased disease severity. An individual with a low number of repeats may have a pre-mutation and may not manifest clinical signs and symptoms. At the opposite end of the disease spectrum, children with congenital presentation of the disease have the largest numbers of repeats (Harper and Dyken 1972; Brook *et al.* 1992; Buxton *et al.* 1992; Fu *et al.* 1992; Harley *et al.* 1992*a*; *b*). At present, it is not known if this is the mechanism involved in the intrafamily variability seen in ADPKD. However, the cloning of the ADPKD1 gene will permit this question to be answered.

ADPKD is one of the most common hereditary diseases and certainly the most common hereditary renal disease. Estimates of the frequency of the disease based on autopsy series range from approximately 1/160 to 1/1000 individuals (Oppenheimer 1934). The frequency of clinical diagnosis is considerably less, reflecting the large number of people who never have the diagnosis made in life. In fact, in a study of Olmstead County, Minnesota, it was estimated that the annual incidence figure of 1.38/100 000 person-years would double if cases found at autopsy were included (Iglesias *et al.* 1983). The incidence figures based on autopsy information make the disease 15 times more common than cystic fibrosis and 10 times more common than sickle-cell disease.

ADPKD appears to occur throughout the world and among all ethnic populations. It has been suggested that it is less common in Africa (Seedat *et al.* 1984) and less common in blacks than in whites in the United States (Easterling 1977; Eggers *et al.* 1984). However, the studies have not been extensive. The overall percentage of end-stage renal disease (ESRD) due to ADPKD is smaller in blacks than in whites (Yium *et al.* 1994). This probably reflects the higher occurrence of other renal diseases among blacks with ESRD than among whites. In fact, in a recent study the frequency of ESRD due to ADPKD adjusted for the population revealed a similar frequency in blacks and whites (Yium *et al.* 1994). None the less this may not represent equal frequency of the gene in black and white populations; rather it may simply represent a more aggressive course of the disease in blacks leading to an equal occurrence of ADPKD-ESRD in blacks and whites (see below). Although ADPKD occurs in the Hispanic and Native American populations, there are little to no data regarding the frequency of the disorder in either of these two ethnic groups. The frequency of the ADPKD1 and ADPKD2 genes in different ethnic and racial groups is not known.

Methods of diagnosis

Patients present to the physician for consideration of diagnosis of ADPKD because of symptoms that suggest the diagnosis, a family history of the disease, and/or the renal abnormalities compatible with ADPKD found unexpectedly on a imaging study or during a surgical procedure. Each of these present somewhat different choices to the physician. The most frequent presenting symptoms of ADPKD are hypertension, acute or chronic flank or back pain, urinary tract infection, nephrolithiasis, gross haematuria, or a palpable abdominal mass

(Oppenheimer 1934; Higgins 1952; Dalgaard 1957; Milutinovic *et al.* 1984; Delaney *et al.* 1985; Zeier *et al.* 1988). Some patients do present initially with renal insufficiency or with extrarenal manifestations of the disease, including rupture of an intracranial aneurysm (Dalgaard 1957; Hatfield and Pfister 1972; Delaney *et al.* 1985). None of these symptoms is pathognomonic of ADPKD, but most of the renal signs and symptoms, with the possible exception of chronic pain and hypertension, would prompt a renal imaging study and hence permit the diagnosis to be established. Certainly, both hypertention and chronic flank or back pain in a person with a family history of ADPKD should prompt evaluation. Twenty-eight to 32 per cent of adults with ADPKD are in fact asymptomatic for the disease (Gabow *et al.* 1984; Milutinovic *et al.* 1984). In the circumstance in which a patient is asymptomatic but has a positive family history, the physician should counsel the patient prior to performing any diagnostic test regarding the implications of a positive diagnosis (Gabow *et al.* 1989*a*). Under the current health care system, a positive diagnosis carries with it difficulties in obtaining both health and life insurance (Fick *et al.* 1992). In preliminary data from one study 28 per cent of ADPKD patients had been denied health insurance at least once (Fick *et al.* 1992). Thirty-four per cent had not informed their employer that they had ADPKD and 17 per cent had not informed their insurer for fear of loss of insurance (Fick *et al.* 1992). Pre-symptomatic diagnosis in children raises the additional concerns of the psychological effects on both the child and the parent of a positive diagnosis and of the child's ability to participate fully in informed consent. For these reasons, non-clinically directed testing of asymptomatic children and adults is not advised (Gabow *et al.* 1989*a*). However, if an asymptomatic individual who has been appropriately counselled still wishes to know his or her status there are several diagnostic options.

Diagnosis of ADPKD relies either on renal imaging or genetic testing. Renal imaging is the easiest, least expensive, and most readily available method to diagnose the disease. Renal imaging requires only the person needing the diagnostic information to be tested and it supplies valuable information on the structural severity of the renal disease. The need for only the interested individual to be tested will eventually also be the case in ADPKD1 when direct gene testing becomes available. Gene linkage techniques requires at least two other affected family members to be tested (Kimberling *et al.* 1991). Moreover, currently the family testing for linkage analysis costs approximately US$1500 per family in commercial DNA laboratories.

Among the renal imaging modalities, ultrasonography (US) is the easiest and least expensive method. US does not require contrast exposure, does not involve exposure to radiation, can be performed easily even in young children, can be performed safely in pregnant women and fetuses, is generally available, and costs only about US$450 per examination. However, it is more operator-dependent than the other possible imaging modalities of computed tomography (CT) or magnetic resonance imaging (MRI). With any renal imaging technique, there are no number of renal cysts which absolutely equates to polycystic kidney disease.

However, a definition which is widely used is bilateral cysts totalling at least three in an adult in an ADPKD family (Bear *et al.* 1984; Churchill *et al.* 1984; Parfrey *et al.* 1990). Recently, there are data accumulating which compare the results of gene linkage studies of individuals in ADPKD1 families with US (Parfrey *et al.* 1990; Ravine *et al.* 1994; Gabow *et al.* 1994). An initial study estimated that US will detect the presence of renal cysts and permit a positive diagnosis of ADPKD in 68 per cent of gene carriers under age 30 and 89 per cent of gene carriers over age 30 (Bear *et al.* 1992). A recent study by Ravine *et al.* (1994) compared the results of gene linkage analysis with US in 204 individuals over age 15 years and at 50 per cent risk in ADPKD1 families. There was concordance of the DNA testing prediction and the US diagnosis in 97.6 per cent of the subjects; however, the sensitivity of US using the criteria stated above was 88.5 per cent in subjects between the ages of 15 and 29 and 100 per cent in individuals over age 30. The positive and negative predictive values by age groups for various number of cysts are shown in Table 13.1. From these data Ravine *et al.* (1994) suggest a modification of the diagnostic criteria for individuals known to be at 50 per cent risk for the disease based on the patient's age: two cysts either unilateral or bilateral in people less than 30 years of age, two cysts in each kidney in people age 30 to 59 years, and at least four cysts in each kidney in individuals over age 60. Although the authors agree that the criteria would be less stringent if other manifestations of ADPKD, such as liver cysts, were present this was not formally included in the analysis.

There are currently three studies which address the issue of the utility of US in children in ADPKD families. In one study with preliminary data 76 children in 31 ADPKD1 families were examined with both US and DNA-linkage techniques; a diagnosis of ADPKD was made if any cyst was detected with US. There was a 0 per cent false positive and a 4 per cent false negative rate in children greater than 10 years old and a 22 per cent false negative rate in children less than 10 years old (Gabow *et al.* 1994). Three of the 38 children with

Table 13.1 Positive (PPV) and negative (NPV) predictive values of various ultrasound diagnostic criteria

Criteria PPV(%)/NPV(%) at age (years):						
	20	30	40	50	60	70
**1 cyst	100/96.6	97.7/100	96.9/100	77.2/100	73.8/100	45.5/100
**2 cysts*	100/96.6	99.2/100	98.9/100	95.6/100	94.7/100	61.2/100
**2 cysts in one kidney, > 1 cyst in the other	100/90.5	99.2/100	98.9/100	98.2/100	97.9/100	85.2/100
**2 cysts in each kidney	100/87.7	100/100	100/100	100/100	100/100	90.7/100
**4 cysts in each kidney	100/85.1	100/89.9	100/100	100/100	100/100	96.9/100

*Unilateral or bilateral. Taken from Ravine *et al.* (1994)

detectable cysts who were predicted by gene linkage to be gene carriers had unilateral cysts only (Gabow *et al.* 1994).

Two additional studies provide longitudinal data on children in ADPKD families. In one study, 37 children who initially had no cysts detected by US were re-examined; seven of the children had detectable cysts on the second examination 11.2 years later (Sedman *et al.* 1987). In a subsequent study from the same institution, follow-up was available in 39 children 3.7 years after their first visit. No child who initially was without cysts had detectable cysts on the follow-up visit (Fick *et al.* 1994*a*). Moreover, three of the four children with a single cysts on the first study had progressed to have multiple renal cysts on follow-up (Fick *et al.* 1994*a*). Similarly, 13 of the 22 children classified as ADPKD initially on the basis of any renal cysts had an increase in cyst number on the second examination (Fick *et al.* 1994*a*). These studies underscore the variability with age in the utility of US in establishing the diagnosis. Fetuses require even different criteria for diagnosis of ADPKD. *In utero* the most common renal imaging abnormalities in affected fetuses are large kidneys and a hyperechoic appearance (Fellows *et al.* 1976; Loh *et al.* 1977; Chevalier *et al.* 1981; Garel *et al.* 1983; Main *et al.* 1983; Farrell *et al.* 1984; Hayden *et al.* 1984; Fryns *et al.* 1986; Pretorius *et al.* 1987; Ceccherini *et al.* 1989; Gal *et al.* 1989; Journel *et al.* 1989; Fick *et al.* 1993). In the study by Fick *et al.* (1993) cysts were detected in only 3 of 10 fetuses or children who were diagnosed in the first year of life on the basis of the other imaging characteristics and an affected parent. It is not known what percentage of fetuses who carry the gene will demonstrate any characteristic ultrasonographic abnormalities. One study have examined 13 fetuses at 50 per cent risk for ADPKD but with no early onset siblings in the family with US examination and found no fetuses who had phenotypic evidence of ADPKD (Fick *et al.* 1993). However, US screening was positive in three fetuses as early as 21 weeks of gestation who had a sibling with detectable disease *in utero* or in the first year of life (Fick *et al.* 1993). This suggests that in the general ADPKD population, fetal US is not a very sensitive diagnostic test and is best utilized in families in whom there is another early onset sibling.

Therefore, since renal US abnormalities are not universally present in individuals with the ADPKD1 gene, particularly before age 30, how and when does a clinician need to define gene carriers in this population? Computed tomography may demonstrate detectable cysts in a very few patients with completely normal US. More frequently, it simply permits the detection of additional small cysts. However, it cannot readily be used in children nor can it be employed for fetuses. In these circumstances one must utilize gene linkage or direct gene testing to establish the diagnosis. For those individuals in ADPKD1 families the presence of the gene mutation itself will be able to be determined in certain research laboratories. However, it is not yet readily available; until it is, individuals in ADPKD1 families and all ADPKD2 families will still need to rely on gene linkage. An example of this type of testing is shown in Fig. 13.1 (Gabow 1993). At least two affected family members in addition to the individual in question must be studied. This permits identification of the probe allele which is travel-

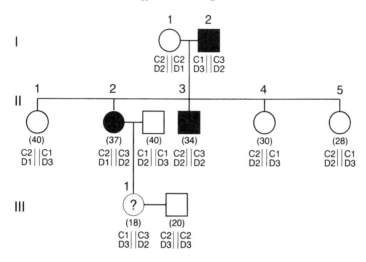

Fig. 13.1 Pedigree of a Kindred with ADPKD1. (○), female family members; (□), male family members; (●, ■) affected members; ages are shown in parentheses. Subject III-1 wished to know her status before her marriage. US was negative. Two types of chromosome 16p markers were used (C and D). The three possible alleles are indicated (1, 2, 3). Markers C and D are assumed to flank the ADPKD1 gene, each within 5 cM of the ADPKD1 gene locus. These types are depicted below each symbol. In this family the haplotype C3, D2 is transmitted with the ADPKD1 gene. Therefore, Subject III-1 has an approximately 99 per cent chance of being a gene carrier. (Taken from Gabow, P. A. (1993). Autosomal dominant polycystic kidney disease. *New England Journal of Medicine*, **329**, 332–42.)

ling with the ADPKD gene in a given family. In this setting, if DNA probes which flank the ADPKD1 gene are used in the testing, the gene status can be defined with 99 per cent reliability in most ADPKD1 families (Breuning *et al.* 1987). There are no data to define the precision yet in ADPKD2 families, but it is likely to be quite similar.

Differential diagnosis

The renal cystic disorders and their characteristics are shown in Table 13.2 (Fick and Gabow 1994). The need to consider any of these other disorders in addition to ADPKD is substantially influenced by the presence of other affected family members, the age of the subject, the size of the kidneys, the number of cysts and the presence of other non-renal manifestations. In a patient who has a strong family history of autosomal dominant inherited renal cystic disease, bilaterally enlarged polycystic kidneys and no extrarenal manifestations which are not seen in ADPKD, no other disorder need be considered. Similarly, a fetus or a new-born with large hyperechoic kidneys and a parent with classic ADPKD need not have other diagnostic possibilities evaluated.

Table 13.2 Comparison of various cystic renal disorders

Feature	ADPKD	TS	VHL	ARPKD	JN/MCD	MSK	ARCD	Simple cysts
Inheritance	AD, ≈ 10% new mutations	AD, ≈ 66% new mutations	AD, <10% new mutations	AR	AR/AD	None	None	None
Linkage to chromosome	16, 4 gene to chromosome 16 indentified	9, 16 gene to chromosome 16 indentified	3 gene indentified	6	2	NA	NA	NA
Prevalence	1/200–1/1000	1/10 000	1/36 000	Rare	Rare	Common	up to 90% of long-term (>10 years) dialysis patients	11.5% age 50–70 years
Age of clinical onset	Usually adults and adults	Children adults young adults	Usually rarely	Children, Adults	Children/ adults	Usually and adults	Children	Adults
Method of diagnosis	US, linkage	US, brain CT or MRI, linkage	US, brain CT or MRI, linkage	US, occasionally liver or renal biopsy	Non reliable	IVP	CT/US	US
Presenting symptom	Pain, haematuria, infection, family screening	Seizures, renal bleeding, cardiac arrhythmias, skin lesions, mental retardation	Retinal, brain or renal tumours. pheochromocytoma	Abdominal mass, HTN, ESRD, portal HTN	Polyuria, anaemia, ESRD	Renal calculi, infection	Haematuria, pain, malignancy, screening US	Incidental finding on US

Table 13.2 *Continued*

Feature	ADPKD	TS	VHL	ARPKD	JN/MCD	MSK	ARCD	Simple cysts
Hypertension	60–75% of adults	Occurs	Patients with phaeochromocytoma	Common	Late in the course	No	Dependent on underlying disease	No
Gross Haematuria	42% of adults	Occurs	Patients with renal carcinoma	Occurs	Rare	Common	Occurs	Rare
Nephrolithiasis	20–36% of adults	No	No	No	No	Common	No	No
Renal size	Normal early, later enlarged	Normal or enlarged	Enlarged tumorous	Enlarged	Reduced	Normal	Reduced, normal or enlarged	Normal
Extrarenal manifestations	Common[a]	Common[b]	Common[c]	Congenital hepatic fibrosis	Occur in JN	No	No	No
Renal malignancy	Rare	Occurs	Very common	Not reported	Rare	No	Common	Rare

ADPKD, autosomal dominant polycystic kidney disease; TS, Tuberous sclerosis; VHL, von Hippel–Lindau; ARPKD, autosomal recessive kidney disease; JN, juvenile nephronophthisis; MCD, medullary cystic disease; ARCD, acquired renal cystic disease.

AD, autosomal dominant; AR, autosomal recessive; NA, not applicable; US, ultrasound; CT, computed tomography; MRI, magnetic resonance imaging; IVP, intravenous pyelography; HTN, hypertension; ESRD, end-stage renal disease.
[a]e.g. liver cysts, heart valve abnormalities, intracranial aneurysms, diverticula; [b]skin, brain, heart, retina; [c]retina, brain, phaeochromocytoma.

In a fetus, infant, or a child with a negative family history for PKD who presents with large kidneys with increased echogenicity the other major diagnostic possibility to consider is autosomal recessive polycystic kidney disease (ARPKD). Although discrete cysts favour the diagnosis of ADPKD, the US appearance of the two diseases can be indistinguishable. The easiest and most readily available way to distinguish ADPKD and ARPKD is to have the parents undergo US. In this setting it is important to know that the lack of family history in the parents is not sufficient to exclude the diagnosis of ADPKD; 27–60 per cent of parents of children with very early onset disease did not know they had the disease until after the birth of an affected child (Pretorius *et al.* 1987; Fick *et al.* 1993). A negative US in the parents strongly favours the diagnosis of ARPKD particularly if the parents are over 30 years of age. It is possible in parents younger than 30 years of age that one of them has the ADPKD gene but has not yet demonstrated cysts. Also in this circumstance, one must always consider the possibility of non-paternity. The other diagnostic possibility to consider is tuberous sclerosis (TS), which can present early in life as polycystic disease (Wenzl *et al.* 1970; Cole *et al.* 1987). Although TS is a dominant disease, it appears to have a very high spontaneous mutation rate so that the parents could demonstrate no abnormalities (Fahsold *et al.* 1991; Osborne *et al.* 1991; Northrup 1992; Roach 1992). Simple cysts are not usually considered in the differential diagnosis of ADPKD in children, particularly the very young, since they are uncommon in children (Ahmed 1972; Gordon *et al.* 1979; Kramer *et al.* 1982; Mir *et al.* 1983). The difficulty in correctly diagnosing the disease in children is underscored by a study in which 48 children with PKD were diagnosed with the disease in the first year of life and survived for at least one month. Eighteen of these children could not be placed in a specific disease category; four of six children who were ultimately diagnosed as having ADPKD were initially misdiagnosed as ARPKD (Cole *et al.* 1987).

The circumstance of an affected child with no clear family history will be one in which direct gene testing for ADPKD1, the most common form of PKD, will be helpful when it is commercially available. Also in families with more than one affected child, gene linkage analysis for ARPKD will be helpful when it becomes commercially available (Zerres *et al.* 1994). In adults, the other diagnostic possibility most commonly considered is that of simple renal cysts. The widespread use of US and the frequency of simple cysts in the general population result in renal cysts often being detected unexpectedly. A recent study from Australia examined ultrasonograms from 729 individuals age 15 to more than 70 years old with normal renal function who were referred for symptoms unrelated to the urinary tract, in an attempt to determine the frequency and characteristics of simple cysts in the general population (Ravine *et al.* 1993). They confirmed that renal cysts increase in frequency with age occurring in zero per cent of those aged 15–29 years; 1.7 per cent of those aged 30–49 years; 11.5 per cent of those aged 50–70 years; and 22.1 per cent of those older than 70 years of age (Ravine *et al.* 1993). Bilateral renal cysts were uncommon in the general population occurring in only 1 per cent of those aged 30–49 years; 4 per cent of those aged 50–70 years; and 9 per cent of those older than 70 (Ravine *et al.* 1993).

Therefore, bilateral cysts very strongly favour one of the polycystic renal diseases rather than simple cysts especially in those under 50 years of age. Renal size is not particularly helpful in distinguishing simple renal cysts from ADPKD since 18 per cent of ADPKD patients early in the course of the disease when they have only a few cysts have normal sized kidneys (Gabow *et al.* 1984).

Tuberous sclerosis (TS) and von Hippel–Lindau (VHL) disease are also in the differential diagnosis of ADPKD in the adult; in fact, as in children, TS has been misdiagnosed as ADPKD in adults (Anderson and Tannen 1969; Durham 1987). Careful attention to both the extrarenal as well as the renal manifestations should help prevent this misdiagnosis. Acquired renal cystic disease (ARCD) also needs to be included in the differential diagnosis of ADPKD in the circumstance in which cysts are first noted in an adult or child who already has renal insufficiency. Acquired renal cystic disease rather than ADPKD becomes the likely diagnosis when the kidneys are normal in size or small and the cysts are few in number; by the time renal insufficiency occurs in ADPKD the kidneys are large and renal cysts are too numerous to count on an imaging procedure.

Natural history of ADPKD

Renal disease

The natural history of ADPKD to date has focused largely on the renal disease. The evolution of the renal disease includes the progressive development of renal cysts and the progression of renal functional changes including the occurrence of renal insufficiency in some patients. It is clear that cysts exist in fetal tissue and can be visualized by imaging procedures in fetuses (see above). It is unknown if all the cysts that will ever form are present in fetal life and only enlarge subsequently or if more tubules become cystic with time. The large hyperechoic kidneys that are seen in some affected fetuses become less echogenic over time and the kidneys do not appear to grow at the same rate as the infant and young child so that during this time the kidneys may appear less enlarged than they did at birth. As discussed above, children diagnosed after the first year of life often have few and small cysts and not infrequently only unilateral cysts. In fact only 18 per cent have relatively severe disease with greater than 10 cysts in both kidneys (Fick *et al.* 1994*a*). Also, as discussed above, the available longitudinal data in children demonstrated structural progression of the disease in terms of cyst number, cyst size and/or renal volume in 86 per cent of them (Fick *et al.* 1994*a*). Thus, by adulthood, only 18 per cent of those with cysts and normal renal function have normal sized kidneys (Gabow *et al.* 1984) and approximately the same percentage of adults over age 50 will have kidneys which although enlarged are less than 15 cm in length (Milutinovic *et al.* 1990). In adults, renal size correlates positively with age. There is less information on the structural disease progression in families with ADPKD2; however, it appears that individuals with this gene may develop cysts at an older age (Parfrey *et al.* 1990). In a study by Parfrey *et al.* (1990) 46.6 per cent of 125 individuals less than 30 years old in ADPKD1 families had detectable cysts with US compared to 11.1 per cent of 27 individuals of the same age in ADPKD2 families, suggesting a later age of onset of renal cysts in ADPKD2. These data also provide some information regarding the disease penetrance; 51.4 per cent of the 70 members of ADPKD1 families over the age of 30 had detectable, bilateral cysts (Parfrey *et al.* 1990). Since one would predict statistically that 50 per cent of at-risk individuals would have cysts, this suggests complete gene penetrance at over the age of 30 in ADPKD1. Formal estimates suggest 99 per cent penetrance as defined as renal cysts by the age of 55. (Dobin *et al.* 1993).

There appears to be a strong correlation between a number of the signs and symptoms of ADPKD, particularly pain and hypertension, and the severity of the structural abnormalities. Children with 10 or more renal cysts are more likely to have flank and/or back pain as well as hypertension (Fick *et al.* 1994*a*). Among adults, those with kidneys greater than 15 cm are more likely to have pain (Milutinovic *et al.* 1984). Moreover, among ADPKD adults renal size is significantly larger in those with hypertension compared to those who are normotensive (Gabow *et al.* 1990*a*). The relationship between these findings and the severity of the cystic disease is underscored by the alleviation of both the pain and the hypertension with cyst decompression procedures (Bennett *et al.* 1987; Frang *et al.* 1988; Elzinga *et al.* 1993).

The earliest renal functional abnormality appears to be a renal concentrating defect. Although the defect is mild and does not produce polyuria or polydipsia, it can be detected in children (Fick *et al.* 1994*a*). The maximum urinary concentrating ability in children with normal renal function but with severe structural involvement (>10 renal cysts) is significantly lower than in children with less renal involvement as well as unaffected siblings (823 ± 54, 940 ± 22, 945 ± 21 mm/kg, respectively) (Fick *et al.* 1994*a*). In adults with normal renal function maximum urinary osmolality is lower than it is in unaffected family members (680 ± 14 vs. 812 ± 23 mm/kg, $P<0.0001$) and declines with age (Gabow *et al.* 1989*b*). As in children, those adults with larger kidneys demonstrated the greatest impairment in concentrating ability (Gabow *et al.* 1989*b*). This suggests that the renal architectural disruption that occurs as a consequence of the cysts is in part responsible for the concentrating defect. This architectural disruption and consequent impaired renal concentrating ability and reduced medullary trapping of ammonia has also been suggested to be responsible for the decrease in ammonia excretion observed in ADPKD adults with normal renal function (Torres *et al.* 1994).

Of course, the most important renal functional abnormality in ADPKD is renal failure. Interestingly, the presence of the ADPKD gene alone does not necessarily eventuate in end-stage renal disease (ESRD). Approximately 50 per cent of all ADPKD patients are alive without ESRD at about 60 years of age (Churchill *et al.* 1984; Parfrey *et al.* 1990; Gabow *et al.* 1992*b*). Moreover, there is considerable variability in the age of ESRD from childhood to old age. This raises the question of what other factors besides the presence of the gene itself influence the development of ESRD in ADPKD. First, the type of gene appears to have considerable influence on the progression of ESRD (Parfrey *et al.* 1990; Gabow *et al.* 1992*b*). In one study the patients with ADPKD1 would have been expected to exceed a serum creatinine of 1.5 mg/dl at the age of 49 years whereas patients with the ADPKD2 gene would not have exceeded this level until over 70 (Gabow *et al.* 1992*b*). Although not found in all studies (Gonzalo *et al.* 1990; Bear *et al.* 1992), a number of studies have demonstrated that women have less rapid progression to ESRD than do men (Dalgaard 1957; Gretz *et al.* 1989; Gabow *et al.* 1992*b*). The data on the effect of the gender of the parent passing on the ADPKD gene on the course of the renal disease in the offspring have been inconsistent (Bear *et al.* 1992; Gabow *et al.* 1992*b*). However, the largest study of children with very early onset ADPKD demonstrated that these children were much more likely to have received the gene from an affected mother than from an affected father (Fick *et al.* 1993). Ethnicity may also influence the course of the disease. Black ADPKD patients have earlier onset of ESRD than do white ADPKD patients; in one study this represented a 12.2 year difference (Yium *et al.* 1994). This difference is even more pronounced among black patients with ADPKD who also have sickle haemoglobin. Black patients with AS haemoglobin have the onset of ESRD at 38.2 years in comparison to 48.1 years in black ADPKD patients with AA haemoglobin and 55.2 years in white patients with ADPKD (Yium *et al.* 1994).

An earlier age of diagnosis has also been shown to be associated with an earlier onset of ESRD (Gabow *et al.* 1992*b*). This is particularly dramatic in children who are diagnosed with the disease by US *in utero* or in the first year of life. In one study, 10 of 11 such children had hypertension and 3 of 11 impaired renal function or ESRD before the age of 5 years (Fick *et al.* 1993).

Hypertension appears to have a dramatic effect on renal function (Iglesias *et al.* 1983; Gabow *et al.* 1992*b*). Patients with hypertension exceed a serum creatinine concentration of 1.5 mg/dl at an average age of 47 years in comparison to 66 years in normotensive patients (Gabow *et al.* 1992*b*). Hypertensive males appear to have the worst progression of renal insufficiency and normotensive females the best course of the disease (Fig. 13.2). The effect of pregnancy on renal disease progression in ADPKD has been reported both to have no effect (Milutinovic *et al.* 1983) and to worsen the outcome (Gabow *et al.* 1992*b*; Chapman *et al.* 1994*a*). A study by Milutinovic *et al.* (1983) examined the occurrence of ESRD in relationship to pregnancy number and concluded that there was no adverse effect of pregnancy on renal function. Three of the eight women who had more than three pregnancies and were over 40 years of age were in ESRD and six of the eight women who had one, two, or three pregnancies and were over the age of 40 had ESRD. Another study utilizing longitudinal data analysis demonstrated that women who had three or more pregnancies had a more severe course of the renal disease than women who had fewer pregnancies; women with three or more pregnancies reached a serum creatinine of 1.5 mg/dl at the age of 51, compared with those aged 59 with ADPKD and fewer pregnancies (Gabow *et al.* 1992*b*). Subsequent studies demonstrated that the detrimental effect of pregnancy number on renal function appeared to be

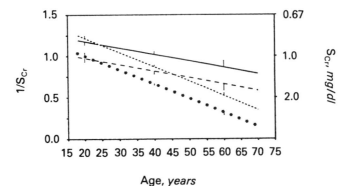

Fig. 13.2   The combined effects of gender and blood pressure on renal function. (——), mean for normotensive females; (– – –), normotensive males; (• • •), hypertensive females; (∗ ∗ ∗), hypertensive males. The *P*-value for gender in the presence of hypertension in the model is less than 0.001, as is the P-value for hypertension in the presence of gender in the model. (Taken from Gabow, P. A., *et al.* (1992*b*). Factors affecting the progression of renal disease in autosomal-dominant polycystic kidney disease. *Kidney International*, **41**, 1311–19.)

confined to hypertensive ADPKD women (Chapman *et al.* 1994*a*). The occurrence of both microscopic and gross haematuria also appear to be related to a worse renal outcome at any given age (Gabow *et al.* 1992*a,b*). In fact, in one study a greater number of episodes of gross haematuria was associated with a higher serum creatinine concentration (Gabow *et al.* 1992*a*). The amount of proteinuria also appears to relate directly to the severity of the renal dysfunction (Chapman *et al.* 1994*b*).

Structural severity also relates to the severity of the renal functional impairment. The larger the kidneys the worse the renal function for any given age (Gabow *et al.* 1992*b*). This is why the occurrence of renal insufficiency in a patient with normal or small sized kidneys and a few cysts should raise the question of another cystic disease, including acquired cystic disease.

Extrarenal disease

The most common extrarenal manifestation of ADPKD is hepatic cysts. Hepatic cysts are very rare in children and increase with age (Milutinovic *et al.* 1989; Gabow *et al.* 1990*b*; Fick *et al.* 1994*a*). However, unlike with renal cysts, the increasing severity of the structural disease with time is not associated with impairment of hepatic function. In some patients, mostly women, the hepatic cystic disease becomes severe creating morbidity in terms of discomfort, pain, and early satiety (Everson *et al.* 1987; Gabow *et al.* 1990*b*; Newman *et al.* 1990). (See also Chapter 21.)

Another gastrointestinal manifestation of ADPKD is colonic diverticuli. In a study by Scheff *et al.* (1980), 10 of 12 (83 per cent) ESRD–ADPKD patients had diverticular disease demonstrated with barium enema compared to 10 of 31 (32 per cent) patients with ESRD from other causes and 45 of 120 (38 per cent) age-matched people without renal failure. Although the natural history of this manifestation has not been well studied four of 10 ADPKD patients with diverticuli in the Scheff study developed a colonic perforation which occurred in no patient in the control group (Scheff *et al.* 1980). Moreover, in examining reported cases of diverticular complications in ESRD patients it appears that ADPKD patients are over-represented in the group, suggesting that the natural history of diverticular disease is more fraught with problems in ADPKD (Gabow 1990).

Cardiac manifestations, including valvular abnormalities, hypertrophy, and perhaps congenital heart disease, are other frequent extrarenal manifestations of ADPKD. Two studies demonstrate approximately a 25 per cent occurrence of mitral valve prolapse in ADPKD patients (Hossack *et al.* 1988; Timio *et al.* 1992). In addition, ADPKD patients have a higher frequency of the symptoms often associated with mitral prolapse than is present in a control group. In the two prospective studies 36–40 per cent of ADPKD patients complained of palpitations and 25–27 per cent had atypical chest pain compared to 9–17 per cent and 9–10 per cent, respectively of the random control population (Hossack *et al.* 1988; Timio *et al.* 1992). Aortic valvular abnormalities have also been reported in the disease (Leier *et al.* 1984; Hossack *et al.* 1988; Timio *et al.* 1992). In fact, in the retrospective study of Leier *et al.* (1984), dilatation of the aortic root and annulus with aortic regurgitation was the most common valvular abnormality noted. In the two prospective studies, aortic valvular incompetence was found in 9 and 19 per cent of the ADPKD patients compared to 1 and 5 per cent of the random controls (Hossack *et al.* 1988; Timio *et al.* 1992). Although the natural history of the valvular disease has not been extensively studied, some ADPKD patients have required aortic valve replacement (Leier *et al.* 1984; Zeier *et al.* 1988). Left ventricular hypertrophy is the other very common cardiac abnormality found in ADPKD patients. An increase in left ventricular mass begins in childhood (Zeier *et al.* 1993) and by adulthood 18–24 per cent of adult ADPKD patients have cardiac hypertrophy as measured by echocardiography criteria compared to 3 and 6 per cent of the control groups (Hossack *et al.* 1988; Timio *et al.* 1992). In an autopsy study, 54 of 61 patients demonstrated an increase in cardiac weight (Fick *et al.* 1995).

Timio *et al.* (1992) began to define the natural history of the valvular abnormalities and of the cardiac hypertrophy by echocardiographic measurements. There was only a 2–5 per cent increase in the frequency of valvular abnormalities over a 10-year follow-up period; there was no information on the change in severity of the symptoms or structural abnormality in individual patients. The frequency of left ventricular hypertrophy increased by 11 per cent over a 10-year period; however, again no information on the progression in individual patients is available (Timio *et al.* 1992).

A prospective study of cardiovascular abnormalities in 126 children from ADPKD families demonstrated a 12 per cent incidence of mitral valve prolapse in the affected children compared to 3 per cent in the unaffected children ($P < 0.08$) (Ivy *et al.* in press). In addition, there was a 5 per cent incidence of congenital heart disease in affected children compared to 3 per cent in the unaffected children (Ivy *et al.* 1995).

The other major vascular abnormality in ADPKD is intracranial aneurysms which occur in 5–10 per cent of all ADPKD patients (Torres *et al.* 1990; Chapman *et al.* 1992; Schievink *et al.* 1992; Huston *et al.* 1993). The natural history of aneurysms in ADPKD patients remains to be defined completely. None the less, it appears that ADPKD patients rupture intracranial aneurysms at a younger age and have a greater morbidity and mortality than patients in the general population who suffer ruptured intracranial aneurysms (Lozano and Leblanc 1992; Chapman *et al.* 1993). Moreover, it is now clear that ADPKD patients with aneurysms may have multiple aneurysms and that they may develop more over time (Chauveau *et al.* 1990, 1992; Chapman *et al.* 1992; Lozano and Leblanc 1992). (This subject is discussed in more detail in Chapter 22.)

Ultimately, the consequences of the renal and extrarenal manifestations interplay to define the overall natural history of the disease. Since the early 1900s there has been an apparent increase in survival of ADPKD patients (Iglesias *et al.* 1983; Roscoe *et al.* 1993; Fick *et al.* 1994*b*). In a study from the Mayo Clinic there was a significantly greater departure from expected survival in patients with the disease from 1956 to 1980 in comparison to patients from 1935 to 1955 (Iglesias *et al.* 1983). In Dalgaard's classic study of the disease (1957), the mean age of death was 51.5 years. A recent large study demonstrated an increase in age of death from 51 ± 1 years in patients who died before 1975 to 59 ± 2 years in patients who died after 1975 (Fick *et al.* 1994*b*). Of note, the increase in survival was noted only among patients who were in ESRD at the time of death (Fick *et al.* 1994*b*). Those patients with ESRD had a mean age of death of 49 ± 1 years before 1975 and 60 ± 2 years after 1975 reflecting the introduction of renal replacement therapy. ADPKD patients with ESRD may have somewhat better overall survival than patients with ESRD from other causes (Roscoe *et al.* 1993). The mean age of death among those who died before reaching ESRD was unchanged over the same time period being 55 ± 5 years before 1975 and 55 ± 4 years after 1975 (Fick *et al.* 1994*b*). Prior to 1975, the most frequent causes of death were infection and uraemia and after 1975 the most frequent causes were cardiac disease and infection (Fig. 13.3). Eleven to 12 per cent of ADPKD patients died of acute neurological events (Roscoe *et al.* 1993; Fick *et al.* 1994*b*). Among patients with ESRD, there was a greater frequency of death from infection and cerebral vascular accidents in ADPKD patients compared to patients with other causes of ESRD (Roscoe *et al.* 1993). Among ADPKD patients who died of infection, in 47 per cent the source of the infection was directly related to a manifestation of ADPKD, including renal and hepatic cyst infections, and ruptured colonic diverticuli (Fick *et al.* 1994*b*). Thus, it appears that greater attention to cardiovascular risk factors and more attention to sources of infection may even further improve the survival of ADPKD patients.

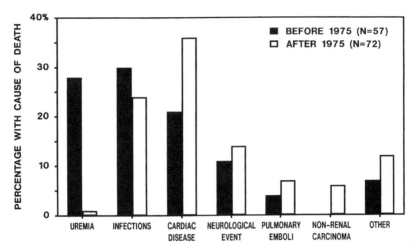

Fig. 13.3 Primary causes of death in individuals with ADPKD dying before or after 1975. (Taken from Fick, G. M., Johnson, A. M., Hammond, W. S., Gabow, P. A. (1995). Causes of death in autosomal dominant polycystic kidney disease. *Journal of the American Society of Nephrology*, **5**, 2048–56.)

Acknowledgements

This research was supported by Grant 5 POI DK34039, Human Polycystic Kidney Disease (PKD), awarded by the Department of Health and Human Services, Public Health Service, NIDDK, and the Clinical Research Center, Grant MORR-00051 from the General Clinical Research Centers Research Program of the Division of Research Resources, National Institutes of Health.

References

Ahmed, S. (1972). Simple renal cysts in childhood. *British Journal of Urology*, **44**, 71–5.

Anderson, D. and Tannen, R. L. (1969). Tuberous sclerosis and chronic renal failure. *American Journal of Medicine*, **47**, 163–168.

Bear, J. C., Parfrey, P. S., Morgan, J. M., Martin, C. J., and Cramer, B. C. (1992). Autosomal dominant polycystic kidney disease: New information for genetic counselling. *American Journal of Medical Genetics*, **43**, 548–53.

Bear, J. C., *et al.* (1984). Age at clinical onset and at ultrasonographic detection of adult polycystic kidney disease: Data for genetic counselling. *American Journal of Medical Genetics*, **18**, 45–53.

Bennett, W. M., Elzinga, L., Golper, T. A., and Barry, J. M. (1987). Reduction of cyst volume for symptomatic management of autosomal dominant polycystic kidney disease. *Journal of Urology*, **137**, 620–2.

Breuning, M. H., *et al.* (1987). Improved early diagnosis of adult polycystic kidney disease with flanking DNA markers. *Lancet*, **2**, 1359–61.

Brook, D., *et al.* (1992). Molecular basis of myotonic dystrophy: Expansion of a trinu-cleotide (CTG) repeat at the 3′ end of a transcript encoding a protein kinase family member. *Cell*, **68**, 799–808.

Buxton, J., *et al.* (1992). Detection of an unstable fragment of DNA specific to individuals with myotonic dystrophy. *Nature*, **355**, 547–8.

Ceccherini, I., *et al.* (1989). Autosomal dominant polycystic kidney disease: Prenatal diagnosis by DNA analysis and sonography at 14 weeks. *Prenatal Diagnosis*, **9**, 751–8.

Chapman, A. B., *et al.* (1992). Intracranial aneurysms in autosomal dominant polycystic kidney disease. *New England Journal of Medicine*, **327**, 916–20.

Chapman, A. B., Johnson, A. M., and Gabow, P. A. (1993). Intracranial aneurysms in patients with autosomal dominant polycystic kidney disease: How to diagnose and who to screen. *American Journal of Kidney Diseases*, **22**, 526–31.

Chapman, A. B., Johnson, A. M., and Gabow, P. A. (1994a). Pregnancy outcome and its relationship to progression of renal failure in autosomal dominant polycystic kidney disease. *Journal of the American Society of Nephrology*, **5**, 1178–85.

Chapman, A. B., Johnson, A. M., Gabow, P. A., and Schrier, R. W. (1994b). Overt proteinuria and microalbuminuria in autosomal dominant polycystic kidney disease. *Journal of the American Society of Nephrology*, **5**, 1349–54.

Chauveau D., Sirieix, M. E., Schillinger, F., Legendre, C., and Grunfeld, J. P. (1990). Recurrent rupture of intracranial aneurysms in autosomal dominant polycystic kidney disease. *British Medical Journal*, **301**, 966–7.

Chauveau, D., Pirson, Y., Verellen-Dumoulin, C., and Grünfeld, J-P. (1992). Ruptured intracranial aneurysms in autosomal dominant polycystic kidney disease. *Journal of the American Society of Nephrology*, **3**, 293.

Chevalier, R. L., Garland, T. A., and Buschi, A. J. (1981). The neonate with adult-type autosomal dominant polycystic kidney disease. *International Journal of Pediatric Nephrology*, **2**, 73–7.

Churchill, D. N., Bear, J. C., Morgan, J., Payne, R. H., McManamon, P. J., and Gault, M. H. (1984). Prognosis of adult onset polycystic kidney disease re-evaluated. *Kidney International*, **26**, 190–3.

Cole, B. R., Conley, S. B., and Stapleton, F. B. (1987). Polycystic kidney disease in the first year of life. *Journal of Pediatrics*, **111**, 693–9.

Dalgaard, O. Z. (1957). Bilateral polycystic disease of the kidneys: A follow-up of two hundred and eighty-four patients and their families. *Acta Medica Scandinavica (Suppl.)*, **328**, 1–255.

Daoust, M. C., Bichet, D. G., and Somlo, S. (1993). A French-Canadian family with autosomal dominant polycystic kidney disease unlinked to ADPKD1 and ADPKD2 (abstract). *Journal of the American Society of Nephrology*, **4**, 262.

Delaney, V. B., Adler, S., Bruns, F. J., Licinia, M., Segel, D. P., and Fraley, D. S. (1985). Autosomal dominant polycystic kidney disease: Presentation, complications, and prognosis. *American Journal of Kidney Diseases*, **5**, 104–11.

Dobin, A., Kimberling, W. J., Pettinger, W., Bailey-Wilson, J. E., Shugart, Y. Y., and Gabow, P. (1993). Segregation analysis of autosomal dominant polycystic kidney disease. *Genetic Epidemiology*, **10**, 189–200.

Durham, D. S. (1987). Tuberous sclerosis mimicking adult polycystic kidney disease. *Australian and New Zealand Journal of Medicine*, **17**, 71–3.

Easterling, R. E. (1977). Racial factors in the incidence and causation of end-stage renal disease. *Transactions of the American Society of Artificial Internal Organs*, **23**, 28–32.

Eggers, P. W., Connerton, R., and McMullen, M. (1984). The Medicare experience with end-stage renal disease: Trends in incidence, prevalence, and survival. *Health Care Financing Review*, **5**, 69–88.

Elzinga, L. W., Barry, J. M., and Bennett, W. M. (1993). Surgical management of painful polycystic kidneys. *American Journal of Kidney Diseases*, **22**, 532–7.

EPKDC (The European Polycystic Kidney Disease Consortium) (1994). The polycystic kidney disease 1 gene encodes a 14 kb transcript and lies within a duplicated region on chromosome 16. *Cell*, **77**, 881–94.

Everson, G. T., Scherzinger, A., Leff, N., Lee, E., Seibert, J., and Manco-Johnson, M. (1987). Liver cell, liver cyst and kidney volumes in subjects with autosomal dominant polycystic kidney disease with liver cysts (Abstract). *Hepatology*, **7**, 1100.

Fahsold, R., Rott, H-D., and Lorenz, P. (1991). A third gene locus for tuberous sclerosis is closely linked to the phenylalanine hydroxylase gene locus. *Human Genetics*, **88**, 85–90.

Farrell, T. P., Boal, D. K., Wood, B. P., Dagen, J. E., and Rabinowitz, R. (1984). Unilateral abdominal mass: An unusual presentation of autosomal dominant polycystic kidney disease in children. *Pediatric Radiology*, **14**, 349–52.

Fellows, R. A., Leonidas, J. C., and Beatty, E. C. Jr (1976). Radiologic features of 'adult type' polycystic kidney disease in the neonate. *Pediatric Radiology*, **4**, 87–92.

Fick, G., Johnson, A., and Gabow, P. (1992). Health insurance and life insurance in patients with autosomal dominant polycystic kidney disease (Abstract). *Journal of the American Society of Nephrology*, **3**, 295.

Fick, G. M., *et al.* (1993). Characteristics of very early onset autosomal dominant polycystic kidney disease. *Journal of the American Society of Nephrology*, **3**, 1863–70.

Fick, G. M. and Gabow, P. A. (1994). Hereditary and acquired cystic disease of the kidney. *Kidney International*, **46**, 951–64.

Fick, G. M., Duley I. T., Johnson A. M., Strain J. D., Manco-Johnson, M. L., and Gabow, P. A. (1994*a*). The spectrum of autosomal dominant polycystic kidney disease in children. *Journal of the American Society of Nephrology*, **4**, 1654–60.

Fick, G. M., Johnson A. M., and Gabow, P. A. (1994*b*). Is there evidence for anticipation in autosomal-dominant polycystic kidney disease? *Kidney International*, **45**, 1153–62.

Fick, G. M., Johnson, A. M., Hammond, W. S., and Gabow, P. A. (1995). Causes of death in autosomal dominant polycystic kidney disease. *Journal of the American Society of Nephrology*, **5**, 2048–56.

Frang, D., Czvalinga, I., and Polyak, L. (1988). A new approach to the treatment of polycystic kidneys. *International Urology and Nephrology*, **20**, 13–21.

Fryns, J. P., Vandenberghe, K., and Moerman, F. (1986). Mid-trimester ultrasonographic diagnosis of early manifesting 'adult' form of polycystic kidney disease (Letter). *Human Genetics*, **74**, 461.

Fu, Y-H., *et al.* (1992). An unstable triplet repeat in a gene related to myotonic muscular dystrophy. *Science*, **255**, 1256–8.

Gabow, P. A. (1990). Autosomal dominant polycystic kidney disease — More than a renal disease (review). *American Journal of Kidney Diseases*, **16**, 403–13.

Gabow P. A. (1993). Autosomal dominant polycystic kidney disease. *New England Journal of Medicine*, **329**, 332–42.

Gabow, P. A., Iklé, D. W., and Holmes, J. H. (1984). Polycystic kidney disease: Prospective analysis of nonazotemic patients and family members. *Annals of Internal Medicine*, **101**, 238–47.

Gabow, P. A., *et al.* (1989*a*). Gene testing in autosomal dominant polycystic kidney disease: Results of National Kidney Foundation Workshop. *American Journal of Kidney Diseases*, **13**, 85–7.

Gabow, P. A., *et al.* (1989*b*). The clinical utility of renal concentrating capacity in polycystic kidney disease. *Kidney International*, **35**, 675–80.

Gabow, P. A., *et al.* (1990*a*). Renal structure and hypertension in autosomal dominant polycystic kidney disease. *Kidney International*, **38**, 1177–80.

Gabow, P. A., Johnson, A. M., Kaehny, W. D., Manco-Johnson, M. L., Duley, I. T., and Everson, G. T. (1990*b*). Risk factors for the development of hepatic cysts in autosomal dominant polycystic kidney disease. *Hepatology*, **11**, 1033–7.

Gabow, P. A., Duley, I., and Johnson, A. M. (1992*a*). Clinical profiles of gross hematuria in autosomal dominant polycystic kidney disease. *American Journal of Kidney Diseases*, **20**, 140–3.

Gabow, P. A., *et al.* (1992*b*). Factors affecting the progression of renal disease in autosomal-dominant polycystic kidney disease. *Kidney International*, **41**, 1311–19.

Gabow, P., Johnson, A., Kimberling, W., Velidi, M., Fowler, T., and Strain, J. (1994). Utility of ultrasonography in children in families with chromosome 16 autosomal dominant polycystic kidney disease (ADPKD1). *Journal of the American Society of Nephrology*, **5**, 646.

Gal, A., *et al.* (1989). Childhood manifestation of autosomal dominant polycystic kidney disease: No evidence for genetic heterogeneity. *Clinical Genetics*, **35**, 13–19.

Garel, L., Sauvegrain, J., and Filiatrault, D. (1983). Dominant polycystic disease of the kidney in a newborn child: Report of one case. *Annals of Radiology*, **26**, 183–6.

Gonzalo, A., Rivera, M., Quereda, C., and Ortuno, J. (1990). Clinical features and prognosis of adult polycystic kidney disease. *American Journal of Nephrology*, **10**, 470–4.

Gordon, R. L., Pollack, H. M., Popky, G. L., and Duckett, J. W. Jr (1979). Simple serous cysts of the kidney in children. *Radiology*, **131**, 357–61.

Gretz, N., Zeier, M., Geberth, S., Strauch, M., and Ritz, E. (1989). Is gender a determinant for evolution of renal failure? A study in autosomal dominant polycystic kidney disease. *American Journal of Kidney Diseases*, **14**, 178–83.

Harley, H. G., *et al.* (1992*a*). Expansion of an unstable DNA region and phenotypic variation in myotonic dystrophy. *Nature*, **355**, 545–6.

Harley, H. G., *et al.* (1992*b*). Unstable DNA sequence in myotonic dystrophy. *Lancet*, **339**, 1125–8.

Harper, P. S. and Dyken, P. R. (1972). Early-onset dystrophia myotonica: Evidence supporting a maternal environmental factor. *Lancet*, **2**, 53–5.

Hatfield, P. M. and Pfister, R. C. (1972). Adult polycystic disease of the kidneys (Potter type 3). *JAMA*, **222**, 1527–31.

Hayden, C. K. Jr, Swischuk, L. E., Davis, M., and Brouhard, B. H. (1984). Puddling: A distinguishing feature of adult polycystic kidney disease in the neonate. *American Journal of Roentgenology*, **142**, 811–12.

Higgins, C. C. (1952). Bilateral polycystic kidney disease: Review of ninety-four cases. *Archives of Surgery*, **65**, 318–29.

Hossack, K. F., Leddy, C. L., Johnson, A. M., Schrier, R. W., and Gabow, P. A. (1988). Echocardiographic findings in autosomal dominant polycystic kidney disease. *New England Journal of Medicine*, **319**, 907–12.

Huston, J. III, Torres, V. E., Sulivan, P. P., Offord, K. P., and Wiebers, D. O. (1993). Value of magnetic resonance angiography for the detection of intracranial aneurysms in autosomal dominant polycystic kidney disease. *Journal of the American Society of Nephrology*, **3**, 1871–7.

Iglesias, C. G., Torres, V. E., Offord, K. P., Holley, K. E., Beard, C. M., and Kurland, L. T. (1983). Epidemiology of adult polycystic kidney disease, Olmstead County, Minnesota: 1935–1980. *American Journal of Kidney Diseases*, 2, 630–9.

Ivy, D. D., Shaffer, E. M., Johnson, A. M., Kimberling, W. J., and Gabow, P. A. (1995). Cardiovascular abnormalities in children with autosomal dominant polycystic kidney disease, *Journal of the American Society of Nephrology*, 5, 2032–6.

Journel, H., Guyot, C., Barc, R. M., Belbeoch, P., Quemener, A., and Jouan, H. (1989). Unexpected ultrasonographic prenatal diagnosis of autosomal dominant polycystic kidney disease. *Prenatal Diagnosis*, 9, 663–71.

Kimberling, W. J., Fain, P. R., Kenyon, J. B., Goldgar, D., Sujansky, E., and Gabow, P. A. (1988). Linkage heterogeneity of autosomal dominant polycystic kidney disease. *New England Journal of Medicine*, 319, 913–18.

Kimberling, W. J., Pieke-Dahl, S. A., and Kumar, S. (1991). The genetics of cystic diseases of the kidney. *Seminars in Nephrology*, 11, 596–606.

Kimberling, W. J., Kumar, S., Gabow, P. A., Kenyon, J. B., Connolly, C. J., and Somlo, S. (1993). Autosomal dominant polycystic kidney disease: Localization of the second gene to chromosome 4q13–q23. *Genomics*, 18, 467–72.

Kramer, S. A., Hoffman, A. D., Aydin, G., and Kelalis, P. P. (1982). Simple renal cysts in children. *Journal of Urology*, 128, 1259–61.

Leier, C. V., Baker, P. B., Kilman, J. W., and Wooley, C. F. (1984). Cardiovascular abnormalities associated with adult polycystic kidney disease. *Annals of Internal Medicine*, 100, 683–8.

Loh, J. P., Haller, J. O., Kassner, E. G., Aloni, A., and Glassberg, K. (1977). Dominantly-inherited polycystic kidneys in infants: Association with hypertrophic pyloric stenosis. *Pediatric Radiology*, 6, 27–31.

Lozano, A. M. and Leblanc, R. (1992). Cerebral aneurysms and polycystic kidney disease: A critical review. *Canadian Journal of Neurological Sciences*, 19, 222–7.

Main, D., Mennuti, M. T., Cornfeld, D., and Coleman, B. (1983). Prenatal diagnosis of adult polycystic kidney disease (Letter). *Lancet*, 2, 337–8.

Milutinovic, J., Fialkow, P. J., Agodoa, L. Y., Phillips, L. A., and Bryant, J. I. (1983). Fertility and pregnancy complications in women with autosomal dominant polycystic kidney disease. *Obstetrics and Gynecology*, 61, 566–70.

Milutinovic, J., Fialkow, P. J., Agodoa, L. Y., Phillips, L. A., Rudd, T. G., and Bryant, J. I. (1984). Autosomal dominant polycystic kidney disease: Symptoms and clinical findings. *Quarterly Journal of Medicine*, 53, 511–22.

Milutinovic, J., Schabel, S. I., and Ainsworth, S. K. (1989). Autosomal dominant polycystic kidney disease with liver and pancreatic involvement in early childhood. *American Journal of Kidney Diseases*, 13, 340–4.

Milutinovic, J., Fialkow, P. J., Agodoa, L. Y., Phillips, L. A., Rudd, T. G., and Sutherland, S. (1990). Clinical manifestations of autosomal dominant polycystic kidney disease in patients older than 50 years. *American Journal of Kidney Diseases*, 15, 237–43.

Milutinovic, J., et al. (1992). Intrafamilial phenotypic expression of autosomal dominant polycystic kidney disease. *American Journal of Kidney Diseases*, 19, 465–72.

Mir, S., Rapola, J., and Koskimies, O. (1983). Renal cysts in pediatric autopsy material. *Nephron*, 33, 189–95.

Newman, K. D., Torres, V. E., Rakela, J., and Nagorney, D. M. (1990). Treatment of highly symptomatic polycystic liver disease: Preliminary experience with a combined hepatic resection-fenestration procedure. *Annals of Surgery*, 212, 30–7.

Northrup, H. (1992). Tuberous sclerosis complex: Genetic aspects. *Journal of Dermatology*, **19**, 914–19.

Oppenheimer, G. D. (1934). Polycystic disease of the kidney. *Annals of Surgery*, **100**, 1136–58.

Osborne, J. P., Fryer, A., and Webb, D. (1991). Epidemiology of tuberous sclerosis. *Annals of the New York Academy of Sciences*, **615**, 125–7.

Parfrey, P. S., *et al.* (1990). The diagnosis and prognosis of autosomal dominant polycystic kidney disease. *New England Journal of Medicine*, **323**, 1085–90.

Peters, D. J. M., *et al.* (1993). Chromosome 4 localization of a second gene for autosomal dominant polycystic kidney disease. *Nature Genetics*, **5**, 359–62.

Pretorius, D. H., Lee, M. E., Manco-Johnson, M. L., Weingast, G. R., Sedman, A. B., and Gabow, P. A. (1987). Diagnosis of autosomal dominant polycystic disease in utero and in the young infant. *Journal of Ultrasound in Medicine*, **6**, 249–55.

Ravine, D., Gibson, R. N., Donlan, J., and Sheffield, L. J. (1993). An ultrasound renal cyst prevalence survey: Specificity data for inherited renal cystic diseases. *American Journal of Kidney Diseases*, **22**, 803–7.

Ravine, D., Gibson, R. N., Walker, R. G., Sheffield, L. J., Kincaid-Smith, P., and Danks, D. M. (1994). Evaluation of ultrasonographic diagnostic criteria for autosomal dominant polycystic kidney disease 1. *Lancet*, **343**, 824–7.

Reeders, S. T., *et al.* (1985). A highly polymorphic DNA marker linked to adult polycystic kidney disease on chromosome 16. *Nature*, **317**, 542–4.

Roach, E. S. (1992). Neurocutaneous syndromes. *Pediatric Clinics of North America*, **39**, 591–620.

Romeo, G., *et al.* (1988). A second genetic locus for autosomal dominant polycystic kidney disease. *Lancet*, **2**, 8–10.

Roscoe, J. M., Brissenden, J. E., Williams, E. A., Chery, A. L., and Silverman, M. (1993). Autosomal dominant polycystic kidney disease in Toronto. *Kidney International*, **44**, 1101–8.

Scheff, R. T., Zuckerman, G., Harter, H., Delmez, J., and Koehler, R. (1980). Diverticular disease in patients with chronic renal failure due to polycystic kidney disease. *Annals of Internal Medicine*, **92**, 202–4.

Schievink, W. I., Torres, V. E., Piepgras, D. G., and Wiebers, D. O. (1992). Saccular intracranial aneurysms in autosomal dominant polycystic kidney disease. *Journal of the American Society of Nephrology*, **3**, 88–95.

Sedman, A., *et al.* (1987). Autosomal dominant polycystic kidney disease in childhood: A longitudinal study. *Kidney International*, **31**, 1000–5.

Seedat, Y. K., Naicker, S., Rawat, R., and Parsoo, I. (1984). Racial differences in the causes of end-stage renal failure in Natal. *South African Medical Journal*, **65**, 956–8.

Timio, M., Monarca, C., Pede, S., Gentili, S., Verdura, C., and Lolli, S. (1992). The spectrum of cardiovascular abnormalities in autosomal dominant polycystic kidney disease: A 10-year follow-up in a five-generation kindred. *Clinical Nephrology*, **37**, 245–51.

Torres, V. E., Wiebers, D. O., and Forbes, G. S. (1990). Cranial computed tomography and magnetic resonance imaging in autosomal dominant polycystic kidney disease. *Journal of the American Society of Nephrology*, **1**, 84–90.

Torres, V. E., Keith, D. S., Offord, K. P., Kon, S. P., and Wilson, D. M. (1994). Renal ammonia in autosomal dominant polycystic kidney disease. *Kidney International*, **45**, 1745–53.

Wenzl, J. E., Lagos, J. C., and Albers, D. D. (1970). Tuberous sclerosis presenting as polycystic kidneys and seizures in an infant. *Journal of Pediatrics*, **77**, 673–5.

Yium, J., Gabow, P., Johnson, A., Kimberling, W., and Martinez-Maldonado, M. (1994). Autosomal dominant polycystic kidney disease in blacks: Clinical course and effects of sickle-cell hemoglobin. *Journal of the American Society of Nephrology*, **4**, 1670–4.

Zeier, M., Geberth, S., Ritz, E., Jaeger, T., and Waldherr, R. (1988). Adult dominant polycystic kidney disease — Clinical problems (Editorial). *Nephron*, **49**, 177–83.

Zeier, M., Geberth, S., Schmidt, K. G., Mandelbaum, A., and Ritz, R. (1993). Elevated blood pressure profile and left ventricular mass in children and young adults with autosomal dominant polycystic kidney disease. *Journal of the American Society of Nephrology*, **3**, 1451–7.

Zerres, K., *et al.* (1994). Mapping of the gene for autosomal recessive polycystic kidney disease (ARPKD) to chromosome 6p21-cen. *Natural Genetics*, **7**, 429–32.

14

Cloning strategies and genetics of type 1 autosomal dominant polycystic kidney disease

Gregory Germino

In the case of polycystic kidneys, we do not yet have a therapy which can hinder the manifestations of the disease, far less cure the patient. (O. Z. Dalgaard, 1957)

Introduction

It has been nearly 40 years since Dalgaard concluded his landmark study with this observation. Sadly, renal failure remains a common outcome for those inheriting the disease gene. Despite the development of diagnostic tools that now allow identification of such individuals long before they become symptomatic, our therapeutic armamentarium is limited to treatments for the associated complications (hypertension, infection, pain). Aggressive control of blood pressure has many laudatory benefits, possibly including the delay of renal failure in hypertensive individuals, but there are no data proving that it significantly affects the underlying disease process. Indeed, a significant number of normotensive individuals also develop renal failure. Dietary protein modification, similarly proposed as an effective retardant for most causes of renal failure, has recently been found to be ineffective in the treatment of autosomal dominant polycystic kidney disease (ADPKD) (Klahr *et al.* 1994), a result that would not have been very surprising to Dalgaard: 'It is still not known whether the prognosis can be improved by treatment of the chronic uraemia with the so-called low-protein diet. It seems unlikely that a low-protein diet should have any influence on the progression of the cyst formation, but in some cases the patients appear to feel better.' (Dalgaard 1957).

So why are we still in this unhappy state? It certainly is not for lack of effort! The studies of hundreds of investigators have greatly improved our understanding of this disease as summarized in the other chapters of this monograph. Its pathogenesis, however, has proven to be much more complicated than even Dalgaard could have imagine. It has been learned that there are innumerable ways to make a cystic kidney. Moreover, it has recently been discovered that ADPKD actually is comprised of three, clinically very similar diseases (Kimberling *et al.* 1988, 1993; Romeo *et al.* 1988; Peters *et al.* 1993; Daoust *et al.* 1993). Although a few features are shared by many of the naturally occurring and experimental forms of the disease, a common pathway treatable by a 'magic bullet' has not been defined.

The natural history of the disease offers cause for hope, however. Unlike the autosomal recessive form of polycystic disease in which many individuals are severely affected at birth and die soon thereafter, the slowly progressive course of the autosomal dominant form offers many opportunities for early diagnosis and intervention. This feature also presents a major challenge: the therapy may be required throughout the life of an individual and therefore its risks must be less than that of simply offering supportive care. At least 50 per cent of individuals inheriting the disease never develop renal failure, and many of the remainder have a relatively uncomplicated course until their fifth or sixth decade. Presently, we have no way of identifying the individuals most at risk to suffer a more severe course. It seems likely that therapies specifically targeted at the underlying pathophysiology of the disease, provided to individuals most at risk, offer the greatest promise.

Essential to this approach is the identification of the primary defect that initates cyst formation. Elusive since Steiner first concluded that polycystic kidney disease had 'an outstandingly hereditary character' almost 100 years ago (Steiner 1899), a recent breakthrough finally has led to the discovery of the gene mutated in the most common form of this disease, PKD1. This chapter reviews the molecular genetic analyses that culminated in this discovery and discusses the implications of what was found.

Positional cloning

Given the inherited nature of a disease like PKD1, the primary defect must be associated with an alteration of DNA. Theoretically, one could simply compare the entire genomic sequence of an individual suffering from the disease with that of unaffected individuals and identify the pathogenic difference. Determining the entire sequence of one individual is currently an impossible challenge for mere mortals. Although very large laboratories *may* be able to process up to 10^5 nucleotides (bases, b)/day, the standard laboratory is very unlikely to generate more than 10^3b/day of perfect sequence. The scale of the problem becomes much clearer when one considers that the size of the haploid genome (i.e. one copy of each of the autosomes and one sex chromosome) is 3×10^9 bases! Even if we could overcome this hurdle, we would likely discover hundreds of irrelevant sequence differences. Nonetheless, this approach would eventually lead to the gene's discovery given enough money and lifetimes.

Unfortunately, most of us lack the resources of 'heaven' or the life span of 'angels'. Thus, investigators have long sought alternative approaches that would hasten the process. It had been hoped that study of the physiology, biochemistry, and cell biology of the disease would provide clues. Although these approaches have provided some important insights, they have not been able to distinguish primary from secondary processes. Fortunately, developments in molecular biology over the past decade have yielded powerful tools that have been applied to genetic problems in a relatively new approach termed 'positional cloning' (Collins 1992; Germino and Somlo 1992). In this approach, disease genes are identified on the basis of their chromosomal position using genetic methods rather than on the basis of the complex phenotypes they produce. Molecular genetic techniques have reduced the complexity of the search for mutant DNA sequences by four to five orders of magnitude and have been successfully used to identify the genes mutated in an ever growing list of diseases. The principles underlying their use are very simple:

1. Scattered throughout the genome are thousands of short stretches of DNA that differ within the population in their length or sequence (genetic markers). Although some are clinically apparent, such as eye colour or blood type, the majority can only be detected using molecular techniques. The specific chromosomal address of each genetic marker is called its locus, and each of the variants at a particular locus is called an allele. The map location of several thousand, evenly spaced genetic markers has been defined over the past decade (Donis-Keller *et al.* 1987; Cohen *et al.* 1993; Weissenback *et al.* 1992; Orr *et al.* 1993; Beutow *et al.* 1994; Gyapay *et al.* 1994).

2. Meiotic recombination is an evolutionary engine that shuffles the alleles along a chromosome's length, producing novel haplotypes (a group of alleles at two or more separate loci close together on a chromosome that tend to be inherited together), but preserves the general chromosome structure (Fig. 14.1). The frequency with which this occurs is in part determined by the distance separating two loci. The alleles of genes or genetic markers that are situated adjacent to each other on the same chromosome segment almost always are inherited together and are said to be linked, whereas markers on different chromosomes segregate randomly during meiosis and are unlinked.

3. One can identify the chromosomal address of novel, unmapped genetic markers by comparing their inheritance pattern to that of a battery of previously mapped markers. This process has been used to construct highly detailed linkage maps spanning the entire human genome (Orr *et al.* 1993; Beutow *et al.* 1994; Gyapay *et al.* 1994).

4. Genetic disease develops as a consequence of an inherited sequence variation that disrupts the normal function of a gene product. Though one does not know the sequences of the different alleles at the disease locus, one can identify each by the phenotype it produces. Thus, a disease gene may be thought of as a genetic marker with a rare allele that causes a scoreable phenotype.

5. One can map the unknown gene responsible for causing an inherited disease by treating it like any other genetic marker. Inheritance of the disease phenotype is compared to that of an array of mapped genetic markers. Depending on the number of at-risk individuals available for analysis and the density of genetic markers that have been localized to the disease interval, one might be able to map the disease to a segment of $\leq 10^6$ base pairs in length (typically ≤ 1 per cent recombination).

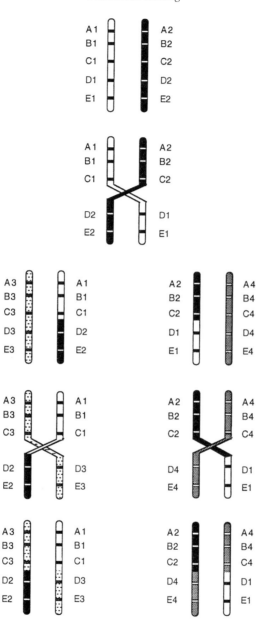

Fig. 14.1 *Meiotic recombination.* Each letter identifies a unique polymorphic locus on a chromosome and the numbers identify its alleles. The composite of alleles for each chromosome defines its haplotype. The 'cross-overs' that develop between homologous chromosome pairs during meiosis result in equal exchange of genetic material between the partners. The net effect is the generation of novel haplotypes.

6. A physical map that determines the actual length in nucleotides of the interval between the flanking genetic markers is then generated and used to guide cloning of the segment. The cloned interval is screened for candidate expressed sequences, and the latter are scanned for disease-specific variants. The sequences of the normal gene and its disease-producing variants are determined, and these are used to deduce the likely primary structures of their encoded proteins. The latter often provide clues to the gene product's function and the first insights into the pathogenesis of the disease.

The search for PKD1

Localization to a 500 kb segment of chromosome 16

The first negative linkage study was published over 40 years ago, back before the triple helical structure of DNA was known and when one could still report such things (Fergusson 1949)! Dalgaard subsequently attempted linkage analysis using a better defined clinical database. Although he failed to find linkage because of a paucity of available genetic markers, his detailed analysis of affected individuals and their families determined the natural course of the disease, its incidence within the Caucasian population, and the range of disease-associated manifestations. Based on his observations, he concluded that: 'A single gene causes the syndrome of malformations: polycystic kidneys–polycystic liver–congenital aneurysm of the basal arteries of the brain, with wide variation, particularly in the two last components. This hypothesis will be of importance for the understanding of the pathogenesis of the malformations' (Dalgaard 1957). Subsequent studies have confirmed most of his observations, and his work provided an essential foundation for later genetic studies.

In a pattern repeated in the final step of the gene's discovery, good fortune together with careful science ushered in the next phase of the project. A gene for autosomal dominant polycystic kidney disease was found to segregate with a hypervariable genetic marker that had previously been cloned from the alpha-globin region, localizing the gene to chromosome 16p13.3 (Reeders *et al.* 1985). This report was soon followed by another that erroneously concluded there was only one locus for ADPKD (Reeders *et al.* 1987). Although subsequent studies soon discovered additional disease gene loci (Kimberling *et al.* 1988, 1993; Romeo *et al.* 1988; Peters *et al.* 1993; Daoust *et al.* 1993), the chromosome 16-linked form of the disease (PKD1) was found to be the most common, accounting for ~ 79–91 per cent of all cases of ADPKD (Peters and Sandkuijl 1992). Detailed genetic maps were generated and used to define more precisely the genetic interval for PKD1 (Germino *et al.* 1990; Breuning *et al.* 1990; Somlo *et al.* 1992). A physical map established that the closest flanking genetic markers were less than 500 kb apart (Breuning *et al.* 1990; Somlo *et al.* 1992), and two sets of overlapping genomic clones spanning virtually the entire interval were isolated (Somlo *et al.* 1992).

Cloning candidate genes

An intensive search for candidate genes within the PKD1 interval rapidly identified over 20 unique sets of expressed sequences (cDNA clones) that detected a minimum of 60 kb of mRNA by Northern analysis (Germino *et al.* 1991, 1993). Most of the genes were found to be expressed in multiple tissues including normal and cystic kidney. A transcription map of the interval was generated by mapping the cDNA clones with respect to genomic landmarks (Fig. 14.2). The gaps between sets of mapped clones suggest that there are likely to be additional genes packed into this segment. At least partial sequences have been determined for each of the sets of cDNA clones and compared to the various gene and protein sequence databases (GenBank, Swissprot, and EMBL) and a number of important homologies have been identified (Somlo and Germino 1995).

Mutation detection

One of the more challenging problems in positional cloning is the final step of mutation detection. Technological advances have resulted in more rapid and sensitive methods for discovering linkage, cloning genomic segments, and identifying candidate genes; but few substantive changes have improved the efficiency of mutation analysis. Scanning cloned intervals for pathogenic mutations remains a very labour-intensive process. Hybridization studies of Southern blots of DNA of individuals affected with a disease is the most rapid assay for detecting

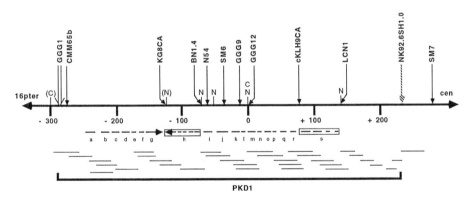

Fig. 14.2 *Map of the PKD1 region on chromosome 16.* The genetic markers GGG1 and NKG92.6SH1.0 define the genetic interval for PKD1. The segments at the bottom of the figure represent an overlapping set of cosmid and phage genomic clones whereas the lettered lines identify cDNA clones. The arrows identify the transcriptional orientation of TSC2 and PKD1 (g and h, respectively). Above the map are listed some important landmarks and genetic markers. The number immediately below the map define physical distance in kilobases (1000 bp). C and N identify restriction sites for *Cla*I (C) and *Not*I (N) (not all sites are shown).

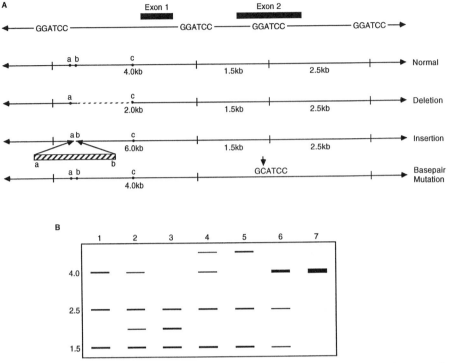

Fig. 14.3 *Mutation detection by Southern blot analysis.* (A) Restriction map of a genomic segment which encodes two exons of a candidate gene (exon 1 and exon 2). Sites for the restriction endonuclease *Bam*HI are listed (GGATCC). Digestion with this enzyme yields three fragments that can be detected by a radiolabelled probe complementary to exons 1 and 2: 4.0 kb, 1.5 kb, and 2.5 kb. In this example, three different types of mutation are illustrated: (a) a deletion that removes a 2.0 kb genomic fragment flanked by 'a' and 'c'; (b) an insertion of 2.0 kb between 'a' and 'b'; and (c) a single base pair mutation that changes a G to a C and thereby destroys the restriction site for *Bam*HI. (B) Schematic of an autorad of a Southern blot probed with exons 1 and 2. In this example, DNA samples described in (A) were digested with *Bam*HI, separated by size by gel electrophoresis, transferred to a nylon membrane, and probed with radiolabelled copies of exons 1 and 2. Fragment length is indicated on the left. Lane 1, a normal control; lane 2, heterozygous deletion; lane 3, homozygous deletion; lane 4, heterozygous insertion; lane 5, homozygous insertion; lane 6, heterozygous for a single base pair mutation; lane 6, homozygous for a single base pair mutation. Note that the respective band intensities vary depending on the number of loci that share identical restriction maps. The 4.0 kb band in lane 2 is one half of the intensity of that in lane 1 because a deletion altered only one of the two loci. The homozygous individual (lane 3) loses both 4.0 kb fragments and acquires a novel 2.0 kb band of an intensity ~ equal to that of the 4.0 kb. The loss of the *Bam*HI site due to a point mutation results in the generation of a novel 4.0 kb band that cannot be distinguished by size from that encoding exon 1. The respective band intensities change as illustrated, however (lanes 6, 7).

deletions, insertions, rearrangements, or oligo-sequence differences that alter a restriction site(s) (Fig. 14.3). While the power of the approach is in its ability to scan thousands of base pairs of multiple individuals simultaneously, its usefulness is limited by its poor sensitivity — fragment sizes must differ by at least 5 per cent in order to be resolved. Single or oligo-base pair differences are the most common pathogenic mutations and are usually missed by Southern blot screens unless the differences fortuitously alter a restriction site. One can improve the likelihood of success by increasing both the number of individuals and restriction enzymes used in generating the Southern blots since most diseases are caused by a number of unique mutations. The probability of this approach succeeding is highest for diseases with a moderately high *de novo* mutation rate. It is possible, however, that one may never find the right combination of enzymes/individuals. One could screen hundreds of individuals with cystic fibrosis with a battery of enzymes and still miss the most common CF mutation (the Δ508 deletion of 3 bp) for example.

At some poorly defined point, failure to find disease-specific variants with the Southern blot approach ultimately requires one to employ sequence-based techniques. Direct sequence analysis is the most sensitive but is the most labourious. Overlapping sets of oligonucleotide primers placed 300–400 bp apart are used to amplify short segments of the candidate gene by the polymerase chaing reaction using either the mRNA or DNA of normals and affected individuals as template. One compares the sequences and characterizes any differences. Anyone who has ever attempted DNA sequencing is painfully aware of the obstacles that prevent the attainment of perfect sequence. Several alternative sequence-based approaches have been developed that overcome this problem. Fragments are amplified as described above but then indirectly scanned for sequence differences using one of four techniques: (1) single strand conformation polymorphism analysis (SSCP) (Orita *et al.* 1989); (2) denaturing gradient gel electrophoresis (DGGE) (Myers *et al.* 1985); (3) RNAse protection (Myers *et al.* 1988); or (4) chemical cleavage (Cotton 1989). The advantages and limitations of each are beyond the scope of this review. SSCP is the method most commonly used and is illustrated in Fig. 14.4. Although the method is technically simple, it is most sensitive in detecting differences in fragments between 150- and 200 bp in length (Sheffield *et al.* 1993). Even so, it still can miss between 5 and 30 per cent mutations.

In the case of PKD1, Southern blot hybridization studies of the DNA of affected individuals failed to identify any disease-specific differences in their restriction maps (Somlo *et al.* 1992), and sequence-based approaches were reluctantly initiated. This task was greatly complicated by both the large number (> 20) of candidate genes as well as the cumulative length of their mRNA (> 60 000 bp). Complete (if not necessarily perfect) sequence is required in order to generate overlapping sets of primers spaced no more than 200 bp apart. Additional mapping and sequence information of exon–intron boundaries is required if genomic DNA is to be used as template. Further confounding the search was the extraordinarily complicated nature of the largest candidate, KG8.

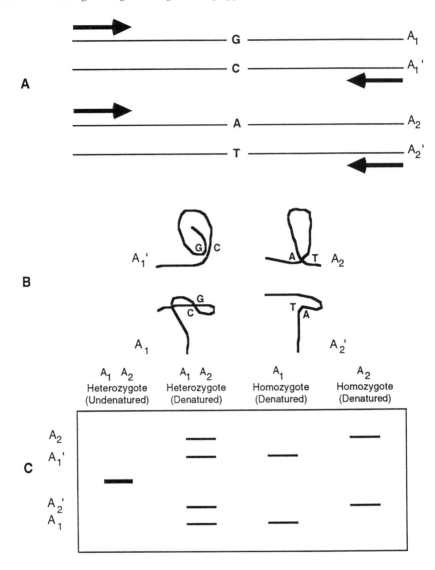

The mRNA encoded by this gene is > 12 kb, and two-thirds of its sequence is replicated in multiple copies elsewhere on chromosome 16 (discussed below). It was in this quicksand that the project quickly became mired.

Reducing the genetic interval approaches

Reducing the size of the genetic interval and thus the number of potential candidates became a high priority. One strategy had been to screen a large number of meioses for recombinations between the disease locus and the closest flanking markers (Fig. 14.5). Such recombinations could be further evaluated

◀ **Fig. 14.4** *Single-strand conformation polymorphism analysis (SSCP).* (A) Oligonucleotide primers (arrows) are used to amplify a 150–200 bp fragment. In this example, the individual has two alleles (A1, A2) of a gene that differ in sequence at a single base pair. Two sets of fragments of identical length are generated by PCR. (B) Each DNA fragment actually is comprised of two strands (sense, A1/A2, and antisense, A1′/A2′). They can be separated by heating in a strong denaturant that breaks the hydrogen bonds between them. Diluting the sample prevents the two strands from re-annealing, whereas reducing or removing the denaturant allows the sample to self-anneal between complementary sequences. The conformation of each strand is determined by its sequence. Sense and antisense strands often differ. Single or oligo-base pair changes also can alter the conformation of the molecule. (C) Schematic autoradiograph of an SSCP gel. DNA fragments are denatured as described in (B) and then electrophoresed through a nondenaturing gel. The latter serves to dilute the denaturant and allow separation of molecules based on size *and* conformation. The undenatured sample runs as a single band because the two alleles do not differ in length and have an identical conformation, whereas the mobility of the single stranded molecules greatly depends on the molecules' conformation.

with internal genetic markers. If recombination was still observed, the internal markers would have become the new closest flanking markers. Unfortunately, recombination events are rarely observed when the loci are as close as those flanking PKD1, and only a handful were observed out of the > 1000 meioses that were studied. No recombinant events were detected between PKD1 and any of the internal markers such as KG8CA, GGG9, and cKLH9CA (Fig. 14.2) (Somlo *et al.* 1992). Even the rare recombinations observed between GGG1 or 92.6SH1.0 and PKD1 that were used to define the limits of the interval had to be interpreted cautiously. An unusually late onset of disease, a misdiagnosis, laboratory error, or gene conversion event could account for an apparent recombination (pseudo-recombinant) between the disease and flanking markers (Fig. 14.5). The term 'pseudo-recombination' describes an apparent recombination between the disease locus and its flanking markers that is not due to crossing-over between homologous chromosomes during meiosis. The probability of detecting probable 'pseudo-recombinants' approaches that of discovering true combinant events when genetic markers are as closely linked as GGG1 and 92.6SH1.0. Failure to distinguish between the two can result in mislocalization of the disease locus and a significant prolongation of the search. The discordant genetic localization data involving proximal genetic markers for PKD1 likely were a result of a pseudo-recombination (Somlo *et al.* 1992).

Another approach used to refine the localization of PKD1 was to search for linkage dysequilibrium between alleles of the internal genetic markers and the disease phenotype (Fig. 14.6). This property is observed when a disease mutation has spontaneously arisen or been imported through a founder effect into a population on a single or small number of ancestral chromosomes. Immediately after introduction of a new mutation into a population, the haplotype of all affected individuals is identical. Over time, recombination events cause deviation from the ancestral haplotype. The rate of change depends on the genetic dis-

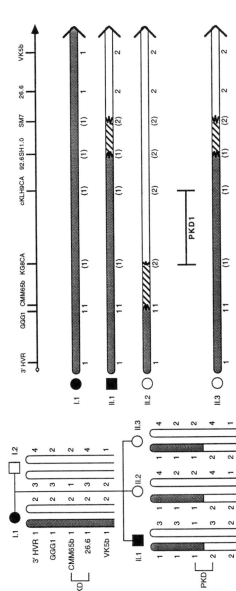

Fig. 14.5 *Narrowing the genetic interval with recombination mapping* On the left is the pedigree of a family with PKD1. The shaded chromosome represents the haplotype that segregates with the disease in this imaginary family. Recombination has occurred between the markers CMM65b and 26.6 in all three individuals in the second generation. II.1, II.2, and II.3 appear to share identical genotypes with the listed markers despite having different phenotypes. On the right is a genetic map that lists the genotype of key individuals with the previous set of flanking genetic markers as well as newer, internal ones. The additional markers are very useful for refining the genetic interval (alleles in parentheses). Individuals II.1 and II.3 share the same genotype yet one is clinically affected and the other is not. II.3 is an example of a 'pseudo-recombination'. This individual either has had a gene conversion event (the mutant allele has been replaced by the normal one) or a diagnostic error has been made (perhaps age-related). Clinically affected individuals are much more informative than those who are unaffected since false positives are much less likely than false negatives.

tance between loci, the rate of new mutations developing at either the disease or marker loci, and the time interval between introduction of the mutation and genetic testing. Alleles of polymorphic markers very close to a disease locus often maintain their association over long periods of time. Haplotype analysis evaluates the ancestral recombination history of a disease and nearby genetic loci within a population.

Linkage dysequilibrium is said to be present when one discovers an association of a specific *allele* with the disease phenotype in a population of unrelated affected individuals. It is important to emphasize the difference between this approach and testing for genetic linkage. In the latter, alleles at linked loci cosegregate with a disease phenotype within a family but not necessarily across families (Fig. 14.6). Genetic linkage is a more powerful technique since it is able to detect an association between loci and disease at a much greater genetic distance. It cannot be practically used to determine gene order, however, when genetic distance is less than < 1 per cent recombination because the number of meioses required becomes too large. Conversely, linkage dysequilibrium is much less likely to be observed when the genetic distance between markers is ≥ 1 per cent recombination but can be very useful in ordering genetic markers that are very close together (Lander and Botstein 1986; Ramsay *et al.* 1993; Hästbacka *et al.* 1990). Identification of a cluster of markers in linkage dysequilibrium with a disease may help define new boundaries that define a smaller genetic interval. This approach was extremely useful in narrowing the search for the Huntington disease gene to only one of the two multi-megabase intervals that had been previously implicated by discordant recombination mapping information (Snell *et al.* 1992; MacDonald *et al.* 1991). A Finnish group has recently used this approach to narrow the interval for the diastrophic dysplasia gene to less than 70 000 bp prior to its cloning (Hästbacka *et al.* 1990, 1994).

Testing for linkage dysequilibrium in PKD1 yielded interesting but non-definitive results. Linkage dysequilibrium was observed between the disease phenotype and alleles of genetic markers that map near the centromeric end of the interval in several European populations (Peral *et al.* 1994; Pound *et al.* 1992; Elles 1992; Wright *et al.* 1993; Snarey *et al.* 1994). Haplotype analysis was inconclusive but suggested KG8 and 92.6SH1.0 as possible boundaries (Peral *et al.* 1994). These data led to some investigators to favor a more centromeric location for PKD1 (Pound *et al.* 1992; Wright *et al.* 1993; Snarey *et al.* 1994). Data presented in later sections of this chapter illustrate why one must be very cautious in the interpretation of linkage dysequilibrium data.

A final genetic approach derives from the observation that PKD1 mutations often are variable in their expression. Allelic mutations are likely to account for at least some of the interfamilial variation but cannot explain the intrafamilial differences. A genetic model of pathogenesis must also explain why only a small fraction of the total number of nephrons become cystic despite all cells being derived from a common progenitor cell (the gamete) with the mutation. One simple explanation is that the mutation is not static within a family or an individual. A class of mutations with this property has been recently described

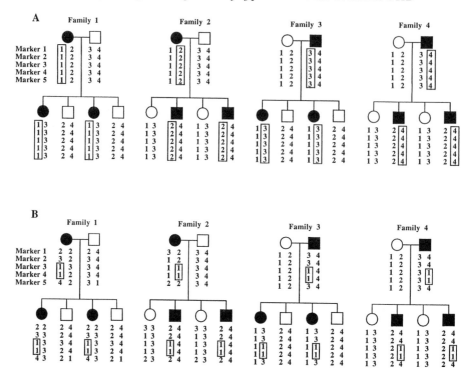

Fig. 14.6 *Linkage analysis vs. linkage dysequilibrium.* (A) The haplotypes for a series of markers from a chromosome segment of four families with an autosomal dominant disease are listed. There is clear segregation of one of the haplotypes with the disease (large box) within each family because the disease is genetically linked to these loci. Note that each family has a different *allele* segregating with the disease. (B) The haplotypes of four families with an autosomal dominant disease are presented (as above). In this example, segregation of a haplotype with the disease is again noted for each family. The alleles at two loci are identical in all affected families (small box) whereas the extended haplotypes are not similar. The original mutation within this population is likely to have arisen on an ancestral haplotype with the alleles '1–1' at markers 3 and 4. Alleles at the other markers are not in linkage dysequilibrium because they are further away from the disease locus, and recombination has shuffled the disease locus onto different genetic backgrounds.

(Kuhl and Caskey 1993; Warren and Nelson 1993; Caskey *et al.* 1992; Willems 1994). These unstable DNA elements comprise GC-rich trinucleotide repeats that frequently lengthen as a consequence of somatic and meiotic mutation, and their length directly correlates with the clinical severity of the disease (Andrew *et al.* 1993; Tsilfidis *et al.* 1992; O'Hoy *et al.* 1993). Unstable trinucleotide repeats have been implicated in the pathogenesis of 11 human diseases (Brook *et al.* 1992; La Spada *et al.* 1991; Huntington Disease Collaborative Research Group 1993; Orr *et al.* 1993; Knight *et al.* 1993; Koide *et al.* 1994; Burke *et al.*

1994; Nancarrow *et al.* 1994; Parrish *et al.* 1994; Kawaguchi *et al.* 1994; Verkerk *et al.* 1991). Several of the diseases are characterized by a progressive increase in the severity of the illness with successive generations, a phenomenon called 'anticipation'. A high apparent *de novo* mutation rate is another feature shared by many of these disorders.

Several editorials have proposed that unstable trinucleotide repeats may be the primary cause of the phenotypic variation observed in PKD1 (Caskey *et al.* 1992; Reeders 1992). This model could explain many of the clinical features of the disorder: (1) renal cysts arise only from nephron segments in which the repeats have undergone mitotic expansion; (2) phenotypic variation within a family correlates with the length of the repeats, with severely affected children having greatly expanded repeats (Kääriäinen 1987; Fick *et al.* 1993); (3) anticipation occurs as a result of successive intergenerational increases in repeat length (Fick *et al.* 1994); (4) apparent *de novo* mutations result from the expansion of a pre-mutation, an allele with an increased number of repeats that does not cause disease but is at very high risk of developing a pathogenic expansion in subsequent generations (Caskey *et al.* 1992; Andrew *et al.* 1993; Tsilfidis *et al.* 1992). Another appealing aspect of this model is that the genomic clones could be rapidly screened by hyridization studies for the presence of trinucleotide repeats. One group searching for the myotonic dystrophy gene used this approach to swiftly move from isolation of a yeast artificial chromosome to identification of the disease gene in less than six months (Fu *et al.* 1992). Unfortunately, a search of the PKD1 genomic clones for unstable trinucleotide repeats was negative (Somlo *et al.* 1992). These data do not exclude a role for unstable elements in the pathogenesis of PKD1, however, since it is possible they have been deleted by the bacterial host cells during propagation of the clones.

Reducing the interval functional approaches

It has been recently proposed that detailed transcription maps will greatly expedite disease gene identification. In this paradigm, one scans the list of genes that map to an interval of interest and selects for further analysis those whose protein products have functions most consistent with the pathophysiology of the disease. For example, a gene with homology to collagen chains would be a better candidate for a disease of the basement membrane than one with homology to alpha-globin. This approach was recently used by Shiang and co-workers to identify the fibroblast growth receptor gene as the gene mutated in the most common form of dwarfism, achondroplasia (Shiang *et al.* 1994). Given that we had a detailed transcription map of the PKD1 interval, we sought to prioritize the candidates on the basis of their predicted function.

Perhaps the most striking observation was that many of the candidates encoded proteins with functions consistent with current hypotheses of cystogenesis. For example, some investigators have proposed a defect in cell-sorting mechanisms as the primary cause of cyst formation in ADPKD based on the discovery of altered polarity for several membrane proteins (e.g. Na-K ATPase, EGF receptor) in cyst-lining epithelium (Wilson *et al.* 1991; Wilson 1991). One of the PKD1 candidate genes is likely to be a novel member of the rab family of proteins, a class of small GTP-binding proteins important in regulating intra-cellular membrane trafficking (Bourne 1988; Chavrier *et al.* 1990; Bucci *et al.* 1992; van der Sluijs *et al.* 1992; Simons and Zerial 1993).

An alternative hypothesis is that cysts arise as a consequence of a primary abnormality of cellular proliferation or cell fate determination (Wilson 1991; Calvet 1993). There are PKD1 candidates that may be important in these processes. The murine homologue of one is a transcription factor which is in its active, phosphorylated form (i.e. DNA-binding) in proliferating cells and is thought to repress expression of genes important in inhibiting the cell cyle. Another candidate is a member of the cyclin F family. Ankryin repeats, a feature of NIK9, is a motif common to a handful of transcription factors, cell cycle proteins, and receptors important in cell fate determination (Blank *et al.* 1992; Lux *et al.* 1990; Artavanis-Tsakonas 1988; Spence *et al.* 1990). One PKD1 candidate encodes a domain shared by a different class of transcription factors as well as repetitive region (WD-40 repeats) thought likely to mediate protein–protein interactions (Neer *et al.* 1994). Two additional genes in the region also have WD-40 repeats. Many members of the WD-40 repeat family function to regulate cell growth, cell fate determination and membrane trafficking (Neer *et al.* 1994). Lastly, the gene mutated in 30 per cent of all cases of tuber-ous sclerosis was discovered to be one of our candidates. Tuberin encodes a possible GTPase that functions as a tumour suppressor (EC16TSC 1993).

These data illustrate the limits of attempting to prioritize based upon putative function. First, the successful application of this approach requires an under-standing of the pathophysiology of the disorder. The biology of most diseases studied by a positional cloning approach is poorly understood, however. In the case of ADPKD, the mechanisms underlying cyst formation had been so broadly defined that members of many diverse families of proteins could be considered likely candidates, including virtually all of the genes mapping to the interval. Ironically, the two most clinically important genes in the region (TSC2 and PKD1) were among the handful without likely functions at the time of their initial discovery.

The PKD1 breakthrough

The agonal search was ended literally by a major breakthrough (EPKDC 1994)! The first clue was the discovery that a major form of tuberous sclerosis mapped to the PKD1 interval (Kandt *et al.* 1992). A second study used genetic markers from the PKD1 region and determined that renal angiomyolipomas, a common feature of tuberous sclerosis, had somatic deletions centred about the micro-satellite repeat, KG8 (Green *et al.* 1994). This strongly implied that TSC2 was a tumour suppressor gene. At about the same time, a Portuguese family was discovered in which there was a child with polycystic kidneys and tuberous sclerosis but whose mother and sibling only suffered from polycystic kidneys (EPKDC 1994). Cytogenetic analysis revealed that the mother and sister had balanced translocations between chromosome 16 and 22 [46XX t(16; 22)(p13.3; q11.21)], whereas the child with TSC and PKD had an unbalanced karyotype and was monosomic for 16p13.3-16pter as well as for 22q11.21-22pter [45XY/−16–22+der(16)(16qter-16p13.3::22q11.21-22qter)] (Fig. 14.7) (EPKDC 1994).

The authors reasoned that the translocation, common to all three, was likely responsible for causing the PKD by disrupting a gene at 16p13.3. They also suspected that the tuberous sclerosis gene was likely to be distal to the 16p13.3 breakpoint since the child with the deletion also had TSC. Further analysis of the family with polymorphic genetic markers localized the breakpoint to the interval bounded by GGG1 and SM6 (Figs 14.2, 14.7). The child with the un-

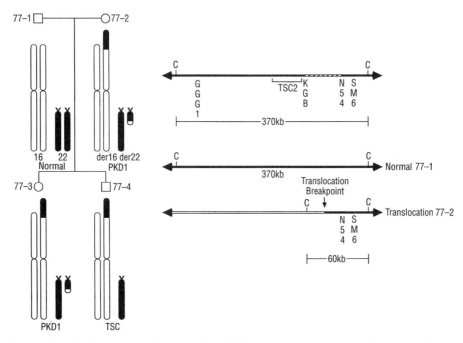

Fig. 14.7 *16p13.3 translocation identifies PKD1.* On the left is the pedigree of a family that had members with tuberous sclerosis and ADPKD (adapted from EPKDC 1994). A balanced translocation between 16p13.3 and 22q11.21 was common to all individuals with ADPKD. The single individual with tuberous sclerosis had an unbalanced translocation that resulted in loss of one copy of 16p13.3-16pter and 22q11.21-22pter. A long-range restriction map (similar to that in Fig 14.2) is on the right. The marker SM6 was discovered to be heterozygous in 77-4 whereas GGG1 was hemizygous. Pulsed field mapping determined that the SM6 marker detected a 60 kb *Cla*I (C) fragment in 77-2, 3, 4 but a 370 kb band in the unaffected parent, 77-1. This placed the breakpoint within 60 kb of the centromeric *Cla*I site.

balanced translocation was hemizygous for GGG1 but polymorphic for SM6. Pulsed field mapping determined that the breakpoint was within 60 kb of the marker SM6. The consortium then set out to identify both genes.

Pulsed field analysis of 260 individuals with tuberous sclerosis identified 10 with overlapping deletion involving the genomic region near KG8 (EC16TSC 1993). The smallest deletion mapped completely within a gene that was immediately to KG8 (Figs 14.2, 14.7), and this gene was ultimately identified as TSC2 (EC16TSC 1993). The 3′ end of TSC2 was discovered to be ~20 kb distal to the polycystic breakpoint, however. These results suggested that the cystic disease in individuals with the balanced translocation was due to a disruption of a separate gene just proximal to TSC2 and not a complication of tuberous sclerosis.

In their search for TSC2, the consortium had isolated an additional set of cDNA clones that detected a 14 kb transcript. It was determined that the orientation of this gene was opposite that of TSC2, with its 3′ end mapping very close to the 3′ end of TSC2. Genomic clones spanning the translocation breakpoint detected the 14 kb transcript on Northern blot (EPKDS 1994). Subsequent analyses confirmed that this gene was interrupted by the translocation, and a novel transcript was detected by Northern blot of fibroblast RNA isolated from the affected mother and daughter. Three additional mutations altering the normal gene transcript (called *PBP* for *P*olycystic *B*reak*P*oint) were also discovered (Fig. 14.7): two intragenic deletions (one a *de novo* event) and a splicing defect. Taken together, these studies confirmed that mutations within the *PBP* gene could result in the typical phenotype of ADPKD.

Characterization of the PKD1 gene, *PBP*

PKD1 is a unique member of a novel gene family

Perhaps the most notable and challenging feature of the gene is its bipartite structure. Sequence from the 3′ end of the gene is specific to the PKD1 region whereas 5′ sequences are found replicated in multiple copies elsewhere on the short arm of chromosome 16. This complicated feature had been first encountered during the generation of the genomic map of the region (Germino *et al.* 1992). Most attempts at chromosome walking towards the telomere from N54 (Fig. 14.2) landed elsewhere on chromosome 16. The end fragment of the cosmid cGGG1 hybridized to multiple other loci, and library screening with this sequence identified clones with similar but non-identical restriction maps (Fig. 14.8). Eventually two 16p13.3-specific cosmid clones, overlapping by less than 2 kb, were isolated that spanned the replicated segment of ~40–50 kb. The replicated segment was discovered to have a highly conserved CpG island very close to its centromeric border and thus thought likely to harbour a member of a gene family. A set of cDNA clones was soon isolated that mapped to the replicated segments. The most telomeric member of the set was ultimately linked to the PKD1-specific clone KG8 by the polymerase chain reaction using first stand cDNA as template. Studies were in progress to further characterize the sequence

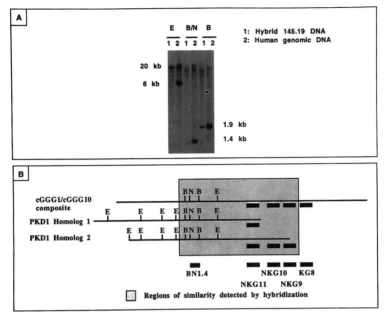

Fig. 14.8 *A set of clones from PKD1 region detects other homologous loci.* (A) The genomic fragment BN1.4 of the PKD1-specific cosmid cGGG10 hybridizes to a 20 kb *Eco*RI fragment in the cosmid and in the radiation hybrid cell line 145.19 that contains 16p13.3 as its only human DNA component (Ceccherini *et al.* 1992; Himmelbauer *et al.* 1991). Faint 20 kb and very prominent 6 kb bands are detected in total genomic human DNA. The relative intensity of the 20 kb and 6 kb fragments reflects the different copy number of each fragment (1 vs. 4-6, respectively). The 6 kb band is not present in 145.19 DNA, thereby proving that the homologous loci do not map to 16 p13.3. The identical hybridization pattern detected with BN1.4 of *Bam*HI/*Not*I and *Bam*HI digests of the 145.19 hybrid and total human genomic DNA indicates that all loci share several highly conserved restriction sites, suggesting very high sequence homology among the loci. (B) Multiple homologues were isolated by chromosome walking with BN1.4, and a comparison of the restriction maps for three loci are illustrated. Sequences common to all three loci extend from the *Bam*HI site towards the right through the length of the homologous cosmid clones. The cDNA clones NKG11, NKG10, NKG9 hybridize to both the PKD1-specific genomic clone and its homologues whereas KG8 is specific to the PKD1 region.

of the KG8 and its homologues when the European Consortium published its remarkable discovery.

The absolute number of *PBP* homologues has not yet been defined. The report of the European Consortium Group (ECG) described between 2 and 4 loci clustered together on 16p13.1. A precise number could not be determined by fluorescent *in situ* hybridization (FISH) analysis of metaphase chromosomes because of the proximity of the loci and the limited resolution of this technique (~ 1 million base pairs). FISH studies of interphase nuclei by A. Baldini suggest that between 3 and 6 loci are clustered together on 16p13.1 (Emory, unpublished results) (Fig. 14.9). The different results are at least partly due to the differences in technique — the latter allows far better resolution (< 100 000 base pairs) since the chromatin is not condensed. This may not be the entire explanation, however. Baldini also detected by FISH of metaphase chromosomes a third site of hybridization on 16p near the centromere. The apparent inconsistency may reflect true differences in the number of homologues per individual. Southern blot studies of panels of individuals both with and without PKD1 suggest variability in the number of homologues within the population (T. Watnick, unpublished results) (Fig. 14.10).

Both the published study and ours have determined that the PKD1 homologues are transcribed. In the *Cell* report (EPKDC 1994), the authors describe Northern results using fragments of the replicated 5′ end. They observed three additional mRNA species (21 kb, 17 kb, and 8.5 kb) in an astrocytoma cell line that were not detected using the PKD1-specific end fragment. A 3′ derived

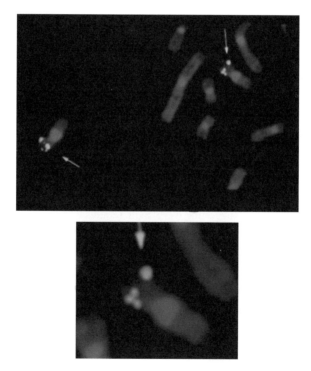

Fig. 14.9 *FISH analysis of PKD1 gene family.* A genomic cosmid of a PKD1-homologue has been hybridized to human chromosomes in metaphase under very stringent conditions after pre-blocking highly repetitive sequences (Alu elements). Several hybridization signals are visible on the short arm of chromosome 16 (16p13.3, 16p13.1). The stronger signal at 16p13.1 identifies the cluster of highly conserved loci. The photograph at the bottom is an enlargement of one of the chromosome 16s. (Photograph courtesy of A. Baldini, Baylor.)

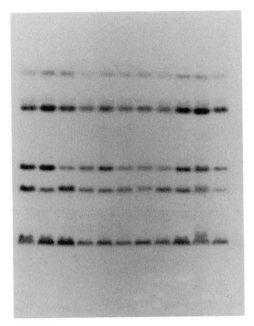

Fig. 14.10 *Variability in the copy number of PKD1 homologues?* An autorad of a Southern blot of genomic DNA digested with PstI and probed with a radiolabelled fragment of *PBP*. Five bands are detected. The relative intensity of bands within a lane varies among the individuals. A similar difference is seen with other enzymes. Variability in the number of homologues is likely to be a partial explanation for the different hybridization patterns. (Photograph courtesy of T. Watnick, Johns Hopkins.)

fragment, specific to the family of homologues and not found within PKD1, also hybridized to the 21 kb, 17 kb, and 8.5 kb mRNAs but did not detect the 14 kb PKD1 transcript. These studies confirmed that the other transcripts were derived from loci other than PKD1. It is unknown whether the homologues give rise to protein products or are transcribed pseudogenes. The observation that the number of homologues appears to be variable implies a non-essential role for at least some of them. These data further suggest though do not prove that some if not all of the homologues are pseudogenes. The biological significance of the homologues with respect to PKD is also unknown. Studies in my laboratory have failed to detect the 21 kb and 17 kb transcripts in mRNA derived from either fetal or cystic kidney (see below).

Southern blot hybridization data using cDNA clones that map to the replicated segment suggest that the PKD1 gene and its homologues have a very high level of sequence identity. The clones cross-hybridize at maximal stringency and restriction maps of the loci are virtually identical for many enzymes. Sequence analysis of partial length cDNA clones derived from the PKD1 locus as well as several homologues confirm these initial impressions. Very long stretches of sequence are identical with differences comprising ~1 per cent of the total.

Additional study will be required to determine whether this level of homology extends through the full length of the replicated portion.

Comparison of the restriction maps and sequences of the PKD1 gene to its homologues has determined that the homologues more closely resemble each other than they do PKD1 These data imply that PKD1 gene may have been the ancestral gene. After an initial duplication, the sequences of the two may have gradually diverged with the homologue subsequently undergoing additional rounds of replication. The mechanism underlying the original duplication and subsequent replications is not yet known. The observation that the number of homologues per individual appears to vary within the population implies a dynamic process.

The high degree of sequence conservation shared by the family has a number of important implications. As discussed briefly in a preceding paragraph, the shared segment spans much of the coding region of the gene and may include many of its most important functional domains. The protein products of homologues that are not pseudogenes (if such exist) may be functionally related to PKD1 and may be involved in modulating the severity of the disease. We had hypothesized (prior to the discovery of linkage of PKD2 to chromosome 4) that mutations altering one of the homologues might be involved in the unlinked forms of the disease. This theory was quickly refuted for PKD2 when linkage analysis of several large families excluded linkage to genetic markers mapping near the homologues (S. Somlo, unpublished results). Studies of non-PKD1 and non-PKD2 families are currently underway. It is also possible that allelic variants at homologous loci may account for intrafamilial differences in disease expression (see below).

On a more practical level, the extremely high level of similarity will make it difficult to generate reagents for the 5' region specific for each member of the family. Detecting mutations specific to the PKD1 locus will be especially challenging given its replicated nature since most methods screen short PCR-amplified fragments of only several hundred bases in length. It is quite likely that the sequence of many fragments will be identical among the family. Primers designed to common sequences will amplify alleles of all loci. Given that there may be as many as six loci, each with two alleles (unless there is variation in the number of homologues/chromosome, in which the case there may be only one allele present for a locus), such a PCR reaction may yield a population of molecules derived from as many as 12 original segment. Distinguishing a single abnormal product out of a mix containing the other 11 identical alleles may be impossible. Discriminating normal variants (polymorphisms) from pathogenic mutations also will be difficult. This problem may not be simply overcome by designing primers to the flanking intronic sequences. It appears that the very high degree of sequence conservation amongst the loci may involve both exonic and intronic sequences. Detailed sequence analysis of intronic sequences of both the PKD1 gene and at least two of its homologues may be required to resolve this issue.

Characterization of the PKD1 gene

Sequence analysis

So what insights have thus far resulted from discovery of the gene? Far fewer than one would have envisaged when first setting out on such an adventure. Comparison of the published sequence to the publicly available databases (GenBank, EMBL) yielded few clues. The hydropathy plot of the deduced protein revealed several possible membrane-spanning segments, but no unambiguous motifs or functional domains were identified. The gene was thought likely to encode a large protein given its relatively short 3′ untranslated portion (~1000 bp). Preliminary studies in my laboratory have suggested a minimum coding size of at least 3000 amino acids. It is extremely likely that complete sequence analysis will soon yield important clues as to the function of the normal gene product.

Mutation studies

Mutation analyses often yield important clues concerning structure–function relationships of the normal gene product. Unfortunately, little can be concluded from the published results. Only a handful of mutations altering the 3′ end have been discovered despite intensive analysis (Fig. 14.11). Each of the mutations has been unique and resulted in the generation of a novel transcript. The translocation that was discovered to disrupt *PBP* in the Portuguese family produced a novel mRNA that was overexpressed in the fibrobalsts of affected individuals. A second family was discovered to have a 5.5 kb genomic deletion that removed approximately 3 kb of the mRNA. A third individual was discovered to have a *de novo* 2 kb genomic deletion that resulted in a frameshift deletion of 446 bp. Lastly, a fourth individual was identified with a single base pair change at +1 of the splice

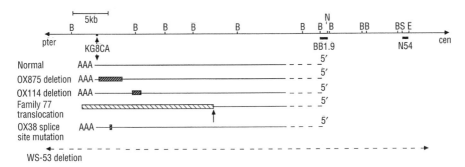

Fig. 14.11 *Summary of mutations disrupting PBP transcript.* Five mutations have been reported to date by the EPKDC (1994). Three were deletions, one was a mutation altering a donor splice site that resulted in the deletion of an exon, and the last was the original translocation described in Fig. 14.7. The largest deletion (WS-53) resulted in loss of TSC2, PKD2, and neighbouring genes and was associated with massive renal cystic disease. All of the mutations (except for the last) result in the generation of an abnormal transcript.

donor site. This mutation produced a splicing defect that resulted in an in-frame deletion of a 135 bp exon. The only feature common to the mutant proteins, if stably produced, is that each lacks the peptide sequence defined by the aforementioned splicing defect. Though this might imply an important regulatory role for this segment, it has no significant homologies and includes no obvious motifs.

The apparent clustering of mutations likely reflects ascertainment bias since this portion of the gene is most easily analysed. Indeed, failure to find more out of the > 100 individuals that have been screened both by the ECG as well as ourselves suggests a probable clustering of mutations within the 5′ replicated region of the gene. The studies of linkage dysequilibrium that found evidence of common haplotypes suggest that a set of common mutations will be identified, consistent with this hypothesis. The large number of haplotypes, however, implies either the existence of multiple mutations and/or the *de novo* development of the same mutation on different genetic backgrounds. Further evidence is provided by the observation that *de novo* mutations do not appear to be rare events in this disease. Two out of the four mutations reported by the ECG were *de novo*. These issues will be resolved by the characterization of more mutations.

Molecular mechanisms of disease

Understanding the process whereby mutations cause disease often provides additional insights into the pathophysiology of a disease. Dominant disorders like PKD can arise through a number of mechanisms: (1) from mutations that result in the production of an abnormal protein with a new function or an increase in its normal activity (a 'gain of function mutation'); (2) from mutations that result in the production of an abnormal protein that interferes with the function of the product of the other allele (a 'dominant negative mutation'); or (3) from mutations that reduce or eliminate the activity of the protein (Hodgkin 1993). In the last case, the loss may only involve the inherited mutant allele and thereby cause disease as a consequence of haploinsufficiency. Alternatively, a dominant disorder can be recessive on a cellular level with the second 'hit' arising through somatic mutation.

The mutations reported to date are consistent with each of the proposed mechanisms. Loss of the 3′ end of the protein might cause a loss of negative regulatory sequences, thereby resulting in a new activity. The loss may instead remove peptide or RNA sequences that normally enhance its degradation. This could result in increased quantities of active protein and cause disease through increased activity. A dominant negative effect may result from the protein product of the 5′ replicated sequence if it binds to the normal product or the normal product's binding partners within a multicomponent structure, thereby inactivating the normal product's function. Alternatively, the mutations may result in an unstable or less functional RNA or protein product. Supporting evidence for haploinsufficiency is provided by the discovery of an individual with massive cystic disease and deletion of both *PBP* and TSC2 (EPKDC 1994). Lastly, it is possible that multiple mechanisms underly the development of disease. Either too much or too little of the normal product may be problematic. Additional data will be required to resolve this issue.

It has been previously proposed that PKD1 might develop as a consequence of a 'two-hit' process (Reeders 1992). An appealing aspect of this model is that it can simply explain the intrafamilial variation in expression of ADPKD. It also can explain why only a fraction of nephrons become cystic despite all inheriting an identical mutation. According to this model, the germ line mutation of PKD1 is necessary but insufficient for cysts to form. Sporadic mitotic mutations must inactivate the second allele and thereby result in a growth advantage, polarity differences, etc. Variability in the frequency with which the second alleles are lost determines the severity of disease.

There is a common clinical feature that argues against this hypothesis. Though only a small percentage of nephrons become cystic, the number of renal cysts is still very large. This suggests a much higher rate of mutation involving the other allele than has been observed for most other tumour suppressor genes. Somatic mutations typically accumulate in rapidly or continuously proliferating organs like the colon or skin. One would expect relatively few 'second hits' in the mature kidney given its relatively low rate of mitosis. It might be argued that somatic mutations arise during renal development when the organ is more proliferative. Consistent with this view is the observation that at least some renal cysts can be found *in utero* (Reeders *et al.* 1986; Waldherr *et al.* 1989; Michaud *et al.* 1994). The large number of renal cysts detected in the ADPKD kidney (100–1000) is orders of magnitude greater than that discovered in hereditary disorders involving other tumour suppressors such as familial Wilms' tumour or retinoblastoma, however. This would imply the presence of an unstable DNA element within the PKD1 gene (either a trinucleotide repeat or a mutation hotspot) that frequently mutates during the development of the kidney when there is a high mitotic rate. To date, no such elements have been found.

Expression studies in human organs

As was previously mentioned, the ECG detected expression of *PBP* in human cell lines derived from multiple tissues (Wilms' tumour, hepatoma, fibroblast, lymphoblast, and astrocytoma) using a probe derived from the 3′ locus-specific portion of the gene. The authors have suggested that this pattern of expression is consistent with the systemic nature of ADPKD. Unfortunately, the authors did not analyse RNA prepared from tissue samples. Study of the expression pattern of a gene in fetal tissues as well organs that manifest the disease phenotype often yield important additional insights. Our preliminary studies of fetal and adult human tissues performed in collaboration with Dr Patricia Wilson suggest that the level of expression of *PBP* may be greater in fetal and cystic kidney and liver than in normal adult kidney or liver. Curiously, we do not detect expression of the 17 or 21 kb homologues in normal fetal kidney and liver, normal adult liver, nor cystic kidneys and liver using a cDNA clone derived from the replicated region of *PBP*. Study of adult kidneys are inconclusive. The 8.5 kb transcript is observed, however, and its level of expression roughly correlates with that of the 14 kb *PBP* mRNA.

These data suggest that expression of the PKD1 gene may be developmentally regulated and imply an important role for the normal gene product in renal and hepatic development. In contrast, the Northern blot data suggest that the 21 kb and 17 kb homologues may play little role in the normal formation of either the kidney or liver or in the pathogenesis of cyst formation. The significance of the 8.5 kb transcript is currently unknown. The correlation of its expression to that of *PBP* implies co-ordinate expression. One explanation for this may be that the homologue encoding this transcript is more similar to *PBP* than the others, sharing similar regulatory sequences. An alternative interpretation is that the *PBP* locus also generates an 8.5 kb transcript through alternative splicing. Thus, the 8.5 kb mRNA band detected by 5' end probes may represent more than one set of transcripts: at least one from a homologous locus and another from PKD1. The latter would be likely to share 5' regulatory sequences and thus exhibit similar patterns of expression.

The increased level of expression of *PBP* in cystic epithelium compared to normal adult tubules would seem at first glance to be inconsistent with haplo-insufficiency as the molecular mechanism whereby mutations result in disease. One would expect that increased expression of both the disease and normal alleles would compensate for the decreased functionality of a mutated copy if haplo-insufficiency were the sole explanation. The apparent 'up-regulation' of the expression of *PBP* would suggest one of a number of other dominantly acting mechanisms: (1) mutations altering regulatory sequences; (2) mutations resulting in enhanced stability of the mRNA of the disease transcript; and (3) gain of function or dominant negative mutations that increase expression through a direct or indirect effect of their mutant gene products. None of the models, however, can easily explain why only a fraction of the nephron segments become cystic without invoking somatic mutations (due to either an unstable DNA element or a 'second hit').

An alternative explanation for the observed phenomena is that there are two mechanisms underlying the increased expression of *PBP*. The normal down-regulation that occurs in the development of the kidney may not occur in cystic epithelia. The gene may be somehow involved in transducing signals, perhaps from the extracellular matrix, tubular lumen, or cell–cell contact, that result in 'flipping' a developmental switch. One of the normal consequences of flipping the switch is a down-regulation of *PBP* expression. Failure to pass through this stage results in persistent expression of *PBP* and perhaps some of the other developmental defects that have been observed in cystic epithelia. This hypothesis is consistent with the haplo-insufficiency model because the expression of *PBP* has not been up-regulated to compensate for loss of functional protein. The variable clinical expression of the disease can also be explained by this proposal. A critical minimal quantity of functional protein may be required for the switch to occur. The absolute amount may vary between nephron segments or even cells. Cells or segments falling below this critical level may fail to flip the switch and thus continue proliferating, retaining expression of other fetal genes, and exhibiting polarity patterns more consistent with fetal than adult kidney. Later increases in *PBP* gene expression in cystic epithelia may be regulated by other transcription factors.

This model, if proven true, would imply a critical role for PKD1 in the final differentiation pathway of tubules. Overexpression of the normal gene product (via transfection in cell culture systems or gene therapy *in vivo*) might be predicted to correct the quantitative defect and thereby lead to normalization of affected epithelia. It is also possible, however, that there is a critical temporal window for the activity of the normal gene product that is defined by other developmentally regulated co-factors. Cells with levels of functional *PBP* protein falling below the threshold may become commited to the cyst fate, and subsequent overexpression may not be able to correct the developmental block. This obviously is an important issue since it has therapeutic implications.

Clinical significance and future directions

Gene testing

A primary aim of studying the pathogenesis of ADPKD is to gain insights that might lead to effective and safe therapies. Although the identification of the gene was an important milestone, it is clear that much remains to be done before we realize our goal. The complicated bipartite nature of the gene, its large size and the large number of mutations that are likely to alter it will make direct gene testing for mutations a tedious chore. Population-based studies may ultimately identify subsets of common mutations that can be used in rapid assays. Nonetheless, the complexity of the gene will delay the development of a clinical test for use in pre-symptomatic testing (especially important in the evaluation of living related donors for renal transplantation), and linkage analysis is likely to remain useful. The certainty of a linkage-based diagnosis is determined by the genetic distance between the markers that flank the disease gene, their informativeness within the family being tested and the number of individuals in the family available for testing. The identification of KG8 as the PKD1 gene should improve the accuracy of linkage testing since lying within its 3′ untranslated region is the a highly polymorphic marker, KG8-CA, that is a microsatellite that can be rapidly evaluated using PCR (Germino *et al.* 1993; Snarey *et al.* 1994). Recombination between this marker and the disease should be an extremely rare event. Indeed, screening with KG8 is an excellent method for identifying families likely to have either PKD2 or PKD3. Several additional PCR-typeable markers discovered near the 5′ end of the gene also will be useful (Peral *et al.* 1994; Snarey *et al.* 1994).

Determining the pathobiology of renal cyst formation

Understanding the biology of the gene and the mechanism of its mutations will require multiple complementary approaches. The tools necessary to develop these approaches are rapidly being generated now that the gene has been identified. Complete sequence of the primary protein structure will soon be available. A number of laboratories have already generated antibodies that are currently being characterized. Numerous cell culture and organ culture systems have previously been developed that will be useful for characterizing the biochemistry of the gene, manipulating its expression, and studying the effect of mutations on a host of cellular properties (matrix formation, polarity, gene expression, signal transduction). Partial length cDNAs for the murine form of PKD1 have been cloned and are currently being used to determine its complete expression pattern during development. Preliminary studies done in collaboration with my laboratory have determined that the murine gene encodes a > 13 kb transcript that also is widely expressed (Konrad Trauth and Feng Qian). Mouse models of ADPKD with mutations of the murine form of PKD1 currently are under development. These will be useful for determining the effects of PKD1 mutations on renal development and for testing the efficacy of therapies.

Gene therapy

Gene therapy often is heralded as the ultimate answer to inherited diseases, and many patients often enquire as to when it will be available for PKD1. There are formidable challenges that must first be overcome before we can seriously consider this for ADPKD. Getting very large genes into the 'correct' cells and expressing them in a regulated manner are difficult technical problems that are likely to be at least partially resolved over the next few years by the many groups working on gene therapy for other diseases. Getting transgenes into cystic structures may prove to be an extra challange. Better understanding of the functional components of *PBP* may allow design a of minigene that is capable of correcting the defect. The minigene may be more compatible with current gene vector delivery systems.

It is essential, however, that we understand the mechanism whereby mutations result in dysfunction before we consider treating PKD1 with either *PBP* mini- or maxigenes. Dominantly acting mutations (either gain of function or dominant negative) are not treatable with standard gene therapy approaches. Rather, one would have to seek ways to inactivate expression of the disease allele or increase instability of its mRNA using methods that are less robust and less developed for clinical applications (antisense oligonucleotides, ribozymes). Haplo-insufficiency may be ideally suited for genetic therapeutic correction if the cells have not become committed to the cyst epithelial cell type.

Manipulating other steps in the pathway to cyst formation

It seems likely that a number of other factors besides mutations altering *PBP* may influence the clinical manifesation of the disease. There may be other genetic loci that encode products that modify the severity of the disease expression. It is well recognized in animal models of cystic disease that breeding the mutant gene into another genetic background significantly alters expression of the disease. The study of twin pairs, being co-ordinated by the European Concerted Action Group, and the evaluation of large carefully characterized clinical databases such as that collected at University of Colorado may be very useful for comparing the genotype and phenotype of affected siblings, using candidate genes as markers (the other PKD1 allele, tuberous sclerosis 1 and 2, von Hippel–Lindau, PKD2, ARPKD, downstream effectors, hypertension genes, etc.). Lastly, studies of animal models suggest that epigenetic and environmental influences also may play an important role in affecting disease progression. Identification of these factors and understanding their role in the pathophysiology of this disorder may yield therapies effective at retarding or preventing cyst growth and end-stage renal disease.

Note added in proof

The complete genomic and cDNA sequence of PKD1 has been determined since submission of this manuscript (Burn *et al.* 1995; International Consortium 1995; Hughes *et al.* 1995). The gene extends ~53 kb, yields a 14.2 kb mRNA distributed over 46 exons and encodes a protein 4302 amino acids in length whose structure is presented in Fig. 14.12. The coding region begins with a 23 amino acid hydrophobic signal sequence which is then followed by a series of extracellular domains. The most striking feature is the presence of two leucine-rich repeats (LRR) flanked on their amino- and carboxy-ends by conserved cysteine-rich clusters. This motif is thought to be involved in protein–protein interactions and has been found in >40 proteins of diverse function (Kobe and Deisenhofer 1994). The specific combination of LRRs with both flanking clusters has been found in only three sets of proteins to date: Toll, slit, and the Trk proto-oncogene family. Toll and slit are *Drosophila* developmental proteins that are essential for determining ventral–dorsal polarity and neurogenesis, respectively. The Trk family of proteins are tyrosine kinase receptors for the family of nerve growth factors (Hashimoto *et al.* 1988; Rothberg *et al.* 1990) (NGF) and are important in signal transduction.

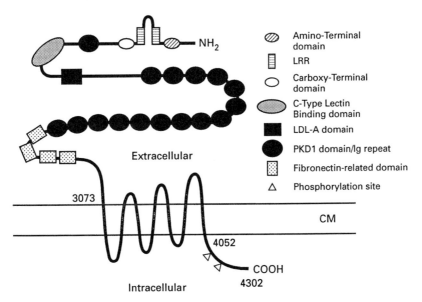

Figure 14.12 Structure of polycystin, the PKDI gene product.

The second most important characteristic of polycystin is that it is very likely to be a membrane protein with very large extracellular region. In our study, we used two complementary protein structure prediction programs to analyse the sequence and determined that a set of 7 transmembrane (TM) segments were identified by both algorithms. In our model (Figure 13), the amino- and carboxy-ends of the protein lie on opposite ends of the membrane, with the carboxy terminus lying within the cytoplasm. The later study by Hughes *et al.* (1995) used a different program and concluded that there were likely to be 11 TM segments. Both models clearly differ from that proposed by the International Consortium (1995) which identified one potential TM element but left the issue unresolved.

Other important features of polycystin include:

a) a region of homology to the LDL-A module of the LDL receptor;

b) a tandemly repeated ~80 amino acid module with structural similarity to the I set of immunoglobulin domains (Ig). One study identified a cluster of 15 repeats whereas another defined 13 (Hughes *et al.* 1995). An isolated Ig repeat is also found just after the flank-LRR-flank module near the amino end of the protein. This module is similar to those found in cell-adhesion molecules and cell-surface receptors.

c) 4 tandemly repeated elements with similarity to fibronectin Type III repeats are adjacent to the Ig repeat cluster. Similar modules are found in matrix proteins, cell-surface receptors and cell-adhesion molecules.

d) The cytoplasmic carboxy terminus includes a tyrosine kinase phosphorylation site as well as a consensus sequence for cyclic nucleotide phosphorylation.

There are two additional aspects of the genomic sequence that are noteworthy (Burn *et al.* 1995). First, we have determined that the original sequence of *PBP* had three sequencing errors. The most important of these was an error due to a GC compression that resulted in a deletion of two Cs near the carboxy terminus. Inclusion of the additional nucleotides in the corrected sequence changes the reading frame and results in the replacement of the original 92 residues with 12 novel amino acids. This has important implications with respect to the immunolocalization study by Van Adelsberg and Frank (1995) that used antibodies generated to the originally published *PBP* carboxy terminus. Readers are urged to use caution in interpreting the results of this report as there are presently no data to suggest that the peptide is part of the PKD1 protein (Harris *et al.* 1995). The second interesting and possibly important observation is that in the middle of the gene within an intron is the largest polypyrimidine tract yet identified. This element has been reported to be important in regulating the transcription of other genes (Young *et al.* 1991; Glaser *et al.* 1990; Hoffman *et al.* 1990; Boran *et al.* 1991). It also poses special challenges to DNA polymerases for replication since it is likely to form triple helical structures. Preliminary studies in my laboratory have determined that it is polymorphic in length in both affected and unaffected individuals. What role if any it may play in the pathogenesis of the disease awaits further analysis.

In sum, polycystin is likely to be a membrane glycoprotein that is involved in cell–cell and/or cell–matrix interactions with a cytoplasmic carboxy terminus that may participate in cellular signalling. Given our expression studies (expression of *PKD1* mRNA and protein is normally developmentally regulated but is increased in cystic epithelia), one downstream effect of its activity may be to down-regulate its own expression. Polycystic has a novel mix of cell recognition domains and is likely to bind a number of other extra- and intracellular proteins. The genes encoding binding partners for polycystin are obvious candidate genes for other forms of PKD if mutated. Likewise, these genes may be important modifiers of *PKD1* disease expression. Finally, identification and characterization of these partners and the pathways whereby mutations in *PKD1* result in cystogenesis may yield new therapeutic agents.

Concluding remarks

Identification of the PKD1 gene using molecular genetic techniques has ushered in a new era for PKD research and has again proven the invaluable contribution of positional cloning to the study of disease. Analysis of the gene and its protein product will likely yield important insights into the normal development of the kidney (and liver). Determining the pathway between the inherited mutation of *PBP* and disease may identify likely candidate genes for PKD2 and PKD3. Understanding the molecular mechanism whereby mutations result in disease may result in effective gene-based therapies. Alternatively, steps along the cysto-genic pathway may be more easily and effectively blocked by therapeutic interventions than genetic manipulation of *PBP*.

Perhaps, even by the 40th anniversary of its publication, the ADPKD community will soon complete the long-awaited epilogue of Dalgaard's seminal work.

Acknowledgements

Many thanks to the families and clinicians who have enthusiastically participated in studies on ADPKD. Special thanks to the former members of the laboratories of Dr Reeders and Dr Frischauf who have contributed to many of the studies described in this chapter. I am especially indebted to my collaborators, the members of my laboratory, and our Research Administrator, Ms Sidney McGaughey. The author is the Irving Blum Scholar of the Johns Hopkins University School of Medicine. This work was funded by the following sources: NIH DK01423, NIH DK48006, the Marion Merrell Dow/PKRF Research Merit Award, and the National Kidney Foundation.

References

Andrew, S. E., *et al.* (1993). The relationship between trinucleotide (CAG) repeat length and clinical features of Huntington's disease. *Nature Genetics*, **4**, 398–403.

Artavanis-Tsakonas, S. (1988). The molecular biology of the Notch locus and the fine tuning of differentiation in Drosophila. *Trends in Genetics*, **4**, 95–100.

Baran, N., Lapidot, A., and Manor, H. (1991). Formation of DNA triplexes accounts for arrests of DNA synthesis at d(TC)n and d(GA)n tracts. *Proc. Natl. Acad. Sci. USA.*, **88**, 506–11.

Beutow, K. H., *et al.* (1994). Integrated human genome-wide maps constructed using the CEPH reference panel. *Nature Genetics*, **6**, 391–3.

Blank, V., Kourilsky, P., and Israel, A. (1992). NF-κB and related proteins: Rel/dorsal homologies meet ankyrin-like repeats. *Trend in Biochemical Sciences*, **17**, 135–40.

Bourne, H. R. (1988). Do GTPases direct membrane traffic in secretion? *Cell*, **56**, 669–71.

Breuning, M. H., *et al.* (1990). Map of 16 polymorphic loci on the short arm of chromosome 16 close to the polycystic kidney disease gene (PKD1). *Journal of Medical Genetic*, **27**, 603–13.

Brook, J. D., *et al.* (1992). Molecular basis of myotonic dystrophy: expansion of a trinucleotide (CTG) repeat at the 3′ end of a transcript encoding a protein kinase family member. *Cell*, **68**, 799–808.

Bucci, C., *et al.* (1992). The small GTPase rab5 functions as a regulatory factor in the early endocytic pathway. *Cell*, **70**, 715–28.

Burke, J. R., *et al.* (1994). The Haw River syndrome: dentatorubropallidoluysian atrophy (DRPLA) in an African-American family. *Nature Genetics*, **7**, 521–4.

Burn, T. J., Connors, T. D., Dackowski, W. R., Petry, L. R., Van Raay, T. J., Millholland, J. M., Venet, M., Miller, G., Hakim, R. H., Landes, G. M., Klinger, K. W., Qian, F., Onuchic, L. F., Watnick, T., Germino, G. G. and Doggett, N. (1995). The American PKD1 Consortium. Analysis of the genomic sequence for the autosomal dominant polycystic kidney disease (PKD1) gene predicts the presence of a leucine-rich repeat. *Hum. Molec. Genet.* **4**, 575–82.

Calvet, J. P. (1993). Polycystic kidney disease: primary extracellular matrix abnormality or defective cellular differentiation? *Kidney International*, **43**, 101–18.

Caskey, C. T., Puzzuti, A., Fu, Y. H., Fenwick, R. G. Jr, and Nelson, D. L. (1992). Triplet repeat mutations in human disease. *Science*, **256**, 784–9.

Chavrier, P., Vingron, M., Sander, C., Simons, K., and Zerial, M. (1990). Molecular cloning of YPTa/SEC4-related cDNAs from an epithelial cell line. *Molecular and Cell Biology*, **10**, 6578–85.

Ceccherini, I., *et al.* (1992). Construction of a fine structure map of chromosome 16 by using radiation hybrids. *Proceedings of the National Academy of Sciences USA*, **89**, 104–8.

Cohen, D., Chumakov, I., and Weissenbach, J. (1993). A first-generation physical map of the human genome. *Nature*, **366**, 698–701.

Collins, F. S. (1992). Positional cloning: let's not call it reverse anymore. *Nature Genetics*, **1**, 3–6.

Cotton, R. G. (1989). Detection of single base pair changes in nucleic acids. *Biochemistry Journal*, **263**, 1–10.

Dalgaard, O. Z. (1957). Bilateral polycystic disease of the kidneys: a follow-up of two hundred and eighty-four patients and their families. *Acta Medica Scandinavica* (Suppl.), **328**, 1–251.

Daoust, M. C., Bichet, D. G., and Somlo, S. (1993). A French-Canadian family with autosomal dominant polycystic kidney disease (ADPKD) unlinked to ADPKD1 or ADPKD2. *Journal of the American Society of Nephrology*, **4**, 262.

Donis-Keller, H., *et al.* (1987). A genetic linkage map of the human genome. *Cell*, **51**, 319–37.

Elles, R. G. (1992). Linkage disequilibrium between D16S94 and the locus for adult polycystic kidney disease (PKD1). *Journal of Medical Genetics*, **29**, 758.

EC1I6TSC (European Chromosome 16 Tuberous Sclerosis Consortium) (1993). Identification and characterization of the tuberous sclerosis gene on chromosome 16. *Cell*, **75**, 1305–15.

EPKDC (European Polycystic Kidney Disease Consortium) (1994). The polycystic kidney disease 1 gene encodes a 14 kb transcript and lies within a duplicated region on chromosome 16. *Cell*, **77**, 881–94.

Fergusson, J. D. (1949). Observations on familial polycystic disease of the kidney. *Proceedings of the Royal Society of Medicine*, **42**, 806–14.

Fick, G. M., *et al.* (1993). Characteristics of very early onset autosomal dominant polycystic kidney disease. *Journal of the American Society of Nephrology*, **3**, 1863–70.

Fick, G. M., Johnson, A. M., and Gabow, P. A. (1994). Is there evidence for anticipation in autosomal-dominant polycystic kidney disease? *Kidney International*, **45**, 1153–62.

Fu, Y. J., *et al.* (1992). An unstable triplet repeat in a gene related to myotonic muscular dystrophy. *Science*, **255**, 1256–8.

Germino, G. G. and Somlo, S. (1992). A positional cloning approach to inherited renal disease. *Seminars in Nephrology*, **12**, 541–53.

Germino, G. G., *et al.* (1990). Identification of a locus which shows no genetic recombination with the autosomal dominant polycystic kidney disease gene on chromosome 16. *American Journal of Human Genetics*, **46**, 925–33.

Germino G., *et al.* (1991). The isolation and characterization of candidate genes for the chromosome 16-linked form of autosomal dominant polycystic kidney disease. *Journal of the American Society of Nephrology*, **2**, 253.

Germino, G. G., *et al.* (1992). The gene for autosomal dominant polycystic kidney disease lies in a 750-kb CpG-rich region. *Genomics*, **13**, 144–51.

Germino, G. G., Somlo, S., Weinstat-Saslow, D., and Reeders, S. T. (1993). Positional cloning approach to the dominant polycystic kidney disease gene, PKD1. *Kidney International Supplement*, **39**, S20–5.

Glaser, R. L., Thomas, G. H., Siegfried, E., Elgin, S. C., and Lis, J. T. (1990). Optimal heat-induced expression of the *Drosophila* hsp26 gene requires a promoter sequence containing (CT)n. (GA)n repeats. *J. Mol. Biol.*, **211**, 751–61.

Green, A. J., Smith, M., and Yates, J. R. (1994). Loss of heterozygosity on chromosome 16p13.3 in hamartomas from tuberous sclerosis patients. *Nature Genetics*, **6**, 193–6.

Gyapay, G., *et al.* (1994). The 1993–94 Genethon human genetic linkage map. *Nature Genetics*, **7**, 246–9.

Harris, P., Germino, G. G., Klinger, K., Landes, G., and Van Adelsberg, J. (1995). The PKD1 gene product. *Nature Med.*, **1**, 493.

Hashimoto, C., Hudson, K. L., and Anderson, K. V. (1988). The Toll gene of *Drosophila*, required for dorsal–ventral embryonic polarity, appears to encode a transmembrane protein. *Cell*, **52**, 269–79.

Hästbacka, J., Kaitila, I., Sistonen, P., and de la Chapelle A. (1990). Diastrophic dysplasia gene maps to the distal long arm of chromosome 5. *Proceedings of the National Academy of Sciences USA*, **87**, 8056–9.

Hästbacka, J., *et al.* (1994). The diastrophic dysplasia gene encodes a novel sulfate transporter: positional cloning by fine-structure linkage disequilibrium mapping. *Cell*, **78**, 1073–87.

Himmelbauer, H., Germino, G. G., Ceccherini, I., Romeo, G., Reeders, S. T., and Frischauf, A. -M. (1991). Saturating the region of the polycystic kidney disease gene with NotI linking clones. *American Journal of Human Genetics*, **48**, 325–34.

Hodgkin, J. (1993). Fluxes, doses and poisons: molecular perspectives on dominance. *Trends in Genetics*, **9**, 1–2.

Hoffman, E. K., Trusko, S. P., Murphy, M., and George, D. L. (1990). An S1 nuclease-sensitive homopurine/homopyrimidine domain in the c-Ki-ras promoter interacts with a nuclear factor. *Proc. Natl. Acad. Sci. USA.*, **87**, 2705–9.

Hughes, J., Ward, C. J., Peral, B., Aspinwall, R., Clark, K., San Millán, J. L., Gamble, V., and Harris, P. C. (1995). The polycystic kidney disease 1 (PKD1) gene encodes a novel protein with multiple cell recognition domains. *Nature Genet.*, **10**, 151–60.

Huntington Disease Collaborative Research Group (1993). A novel gene containing a trinucleotide repeat that is expanded and unstable on Huntington's disease chromosomes. *Cell*, **72**, 971–83.

The International Polycystic Kidney Disease Consortium (1995). Polycystic kidney disease: the complete structure of the *PKD1* gene and its protein. *Cell*, **81**, 289–98.

Kääriäinen, H. (1987). Polycystic kidney disease in children: a genetic and epidemiological study of 82 finnish patients. *Journal of Medical Genetics*, **24**, 474–81.

Kandt, R. S., *et al.* (1992). Linkage of an important gene locus for tuberous sclerosis to a chromosome 16 marker for polycystic kidney disease. *Nature Genetics*, **2**, 37–41.

Kawaguchi, Y., *et al.* (1994). CAG expansions in a novel gene for Machado–Joseph disease at chromosome 14q32.1. *Nature Genetics*, **8**, 221–8.

Kimberling, W. J., Fain, P. R., Kenyon, J. B., Goldgar, D., Sujansky, E., and Gabow, P. A. (1988). Linkage heterogeneity of autosomal dominant polycystic kidney disease. *New England Journal of Medicine*, **319**, 913–18.

Kimberling, W. J., Kumar, S., Gabow, P. A., Kenyon, J. B., Connolly, C. J., and Somlo, S. (1993). Autosomal dominant polycystic kidney disease: localization of the second gene to chromosome 4q13-q23. *Genomics*, **18**, 467–72.

Klahr, S., *et al.* (1994). The effects of dietary protein restriction and blood-pressure control on the progression of chronic renal disease. Modification of Diet in Renal Disease Study Group. *New England Journal of Medicine*, **330**, 877–84.

Knight, S. J. L., *et al.* (1993). Trinucleotide repeat amplification and hypermethylation of a CpG island in FRAXE mental retardation. *Cell*, **74**, 127–34.

Kobe, B., and Deisenhofer, J. (1994). The leucine-rich repeat: a versatile binding motif. *Trends biochem. Sci.*, **19**, 415–21.

Koide, R., *et al.* (1994). Unstable expansion of CAG repeat in hereditary dentatorubral-pallidoluysian atrophy (DRPLA). *Nature Genetics*, **6**, 9–13.

Kuhl, D. P. and Caskey, C. T. (1993). Trinucleotide repeats and genome variation. *Current Opinion in Genetics and Development*, **3**, 404–7.

Lander, E. S. and Botstein, D. (1986). Mapping complex genetic traits in humans: new methods using a complete RFLP linkage map. *Cold Spring Harbor Symposium on Quantitative Biology*, **51**, 49–62.

La Spada, A. R., Wilson, E. M., Lubahn, D. B., Harding, A. E., and Fischbeck, K. H. (1991). Androgen receptor gene mutations in X-linked spinal and bulbar muscular atrophy. *Nature*, **352**, 77–9.

Lux, S. E., John, K. M., and Bennett, V. (1990). Analysis of cDNA for human erythrocyte control proteins. *Nature*, **344**, 36–42.

MacDonald, M. E., *et al.* (1991). Complex patterns of linkage disequilibrium in the Huntington disease region. *American Journal of Human Genetics*, **49**, 723–34.

Michaud, J., *et al.* (1994). Autosomal dominant polycystic kidney disease in the fetus. *American Journal of Medical Genetics*, **51**, 240–6.

Myers, R. M., *et al.* (1985). Detection of single base substitutions in total genomic DNA. *Nature*, **313**, 495–8.

Myers, R. M., Larin, Z., and Maniatis, T. (1988). Detection of single base substitutions by ribonuclease cleavage of mismatches in RNA:DNA duplexes. *Science*, **230**, 1242–6.

Nancarrow, J. K., *et al.* (1994). Implications of FRA16A structure for the mechanism of chromosomal fragile site genesis. *Science*, **264**, 1938–41.

Neer, E. J., Schmidt, C. J., Nambudripad, R., and Smith, T. F. (1994). The ancient regulatory-protein family of WD-repeat proteins. *Nature*, **371**, 297–300.

O'Hoy, K. L., *et al.* (1993). Reduction in size of the myotonic dystrophy trinucleotide repeat mutation during transmission. *Science*, **259**, 809–12.

Orita, M., *et al.* (1989). Detection of polymorphisms of human DNA by gel electrophoresis as single-strand conformation polymorphisms. *Proceedings of the National Academy of Sciences USA*, **86**, 2766–70.

Orr, H. T., *et al.* (1993). Expansion of an unstable trinucleotide CAG repeat in spinocerebellar ataxia type 1. *Nature Genetics*, **4**, 221–6.

Parrish, J. E., *et al.* (1994). Isolation of a GCC repeat showing expansion in FRAXF, a fragile site distal to FRAXA and FRAXE. *Nature Genetics*, **8**, 236–42.

Peral, B., *et al.* (1994). Evidence of linkage disequilibrium in the Spanish polycystic kidney disease 1 population. *American Journal of Human Genetics*, **54**, 899–908.

Peters, D. J. M., and Sandkuijl, L. A. (1992). Genetic heterogeneity of polycystic kidney disease in Europe. *Contributions in Nephrology*, **97**, 128–39.

Peters, D. J. M., *et al.* (1993). Chromosome 4 localization of a second gene for autosomal dominant polycystic kidney disease. *Nature Genetics*, **5**, 359–62.

Pound, S. E., Carothers, A. D., Pignatelli, P. M., MacNicol, A. M., Watson, M. L., and Wright, A. F. (1992). Evidence for linkage disequilibrium between D16S94 and the adult onset polycystic kidney disease (PKD1) gene. *Journal of Medical Genetics*, **39**, 247–8.

Ramsay, M., *et al.* (1993). Haplotype analysis to determine the position of a mutation among closely linked DNA markers. *Human Molecular Genetics*, **2**, 1007–14.

Reeders, S. T. (1992). Multilocus polycystic disease. *Nature Genetics*, **1**, 235–7.

Reeders, S. T., Breuning, M. H., Davies, K. E., *et al.* (1985). A highly polymorphic DNA marker linked to adult polycystic kidney disease on chromosome 16, *Nature*, **317**, 542–4.

Reeders, S. T., Zerres, K., Gal, A., Hogenkamp, T., Propping, P., Schmidt, W., *et al.* (1986). Prenatal diagnosis of autosomal dominant polycystic kidney disease with a DNA probe. *Lancet*, **2**, 6–8.

Reeders, S. T., Breuning, M. H., Ryynanen, M. A., *et al.* (1987). A study of genetic linkage heterogeneity in adult polycystic kidney disease. *Human Genetics*, **76**, 348–51.

Romeo, G., Costa, G., Catizone, L., Germino, G. G., Weatherall, D. J., Devoto, M., *et al.* (1988). A second genetic locus for autosomal dominant polycystic kidney disease. *Lancet*, **ii**, 8–10.

Rothberg, J. M., Jacobs, J. R., and Goodman, C. S., Artavanis-Tsakonas (1990). *slit*: an extracellular protein necessary for development of midline glia and commissural axon pathways contains both EGF and LRR domains. *Genes and Dev.*, **4**, 2169–87.

Sheffield, V. C., Beck, J. S., Kwiteck, A. E., Sandstrom, D. W., and Stone, E. M. (1993). The sensitivity of single-strand conformation polymorphism analysis for the detection of single base substitutions. *Genomics*, **16**, 325–32.

Shiang, R., Thompson, L. M., Zhu, Y. Z., Church, D. M., Fielder, T. J., Bocian, M., *et al.* (1994). Mutations in the transmembrane domain of FGFR3 cause the most common genetic form of dwarfism, achondroplasia. *Cell*, **78**, 335–42.

Simons, K. and Zerial, M. (1993). Rab proteins and the road maps for intracellular transport. *Neuron*, **11**, 789–99.

Snarey, A., *et al.* (1994). Linkage disequilibrium in the region of the autosomal dominant polycystic kidney disease gene (PKD1). *American Journal of Human Genetics*, **55**, 365–71.

Snell, R. G., *et al.* (1992). A recombination event that redefines the Huntington disease region. *American Journal of Human Genetics*, **51**, 357–62.

Somlo, S. and Germino, G. G. (1995). Adult polycystic kidney disease. In *Molecular biology in health and disease*, (ed. D. Schlondorff and J. Bonventre). Marcel Dekker, New York.

Somlo, S., *et al.* (1992). Fine genetic localization of the gene for autosomal dominant polycystic kidney disease (PKD1) with respect to physically mapped markers. *Genomics*, **13**, 152–8.

Somlo, S., *et al.* (1992). Is autosomal dominant polycystic kidney disease (ADPKD) the result of heritable unstable DNA sequences? *Journal of the American Society of Nephrology*, **3**, 302.

Spence, A. M., Coulson, A., and Hodgkin, J. (1990). The product of fem-1, a nematode sex-determining gene, contains a motif found in cell cycle control proteins and receptors for cell-cell interactions. *Cell*, **60**, 981–90.

Steiner (1899). *Deutsche medizinische Wochenschrift*, **25**, 677.

Tsilfidis, C., MacKenzie, A. E., Mettler, G., Barcelo, J., and Korneluk, R. G. (1992). Correlation between CTG trinucleotide repeat length and frequency of severe congenital myotonic dystrophy. *Nature Genetics*, **1**, 192–5.

Van Adelsberg, J. S. and Frank, D. (1995). The PKD1 gene produces a developmentally regulated protein in mesenchyme and vasculature. *Nature Medicine*, **1**, 359–64.

van der Sluijs, P., Hull, M., Webster, P., Male, P., Goud, B., and Mellman, I. (1992). The small GTP-binding protein rab4 controls an early sorting event on the endocytic pathway. *Cell*, **70**, 729–40.

Verkerk, A. J. M. H., *et al.* (1991). Identification of a gene (FMR-1) containing a CGG repeat coincident with a breakpoint cluster region exhibing length variation in fragile X syndrome. *Cell*, **65**, 905–14.

Waldherr, R., Zerres, K., Gal, A., and Enders, H. (1989). Polycystic kidney disease in the fetus. *Lancet*, 274–5.

Warren, S. T. and Nelson, D. L. (1993). Trinucleotide repeat expansions in neurological disease. *Current Opinion in Neurobiology*, **3**, 752–9.

Weissenbach, J., *et al.* (1992). A second-generation linkage map of the human genome. *Nature*, **359**, 794–801.

Willems, P. J. (1994). Dynamic mutations hit double figures. *Nature Genetics*, **8**, 213–15.

Wilson, P. D. (1991). Cell biology of human autosomal dominant polycystic kidney disease. *Seminars in Nephrology*, **11**, 607–16.

Wilson, P., Sherwood, A. C., Palla, K., Du, J., Watson, R., and Norman, J. T. (1991). Reversed polarity of Na^+-K^+-ATPase: mislocalization to apical plasma membranes in polycystic kidney disease epithelia. *American Journal of Physiology*, **260**, F420–30.

Wright, G. D., Hughes, A. E., Larkin, K. A., Doherty, C. C., and Nevin, N. C. (1993). Linkage disequilibrium between the CA microsatellite D16S83 and PKD1. *Journal of the American Society of Nephrology*, **4**, 827.

Young, S. L., Krawczyk, S. H., Matteucci, M. D., and Toole, J. J. (1991). Triple helix formation inhibits transcription elongation *in vitro*. *Proc. Natl. Acad. Sci. USA.*, **88**, 10023–6.

15

Genetic heterogeneity of autosomal dominant polycystic kidney disease

M. H. Breuning and D. J. M. Peters

Introduction

Quite often one and the same hereditary disease can be caused by mutations at several distinct genes. ADPKD is a good example. At least two genes are involved, PKD1 on chromosome 16, and PKD2 on chromosome 4.

Cysts in the kidney are common and non-specific. Polycystic kidneys can be found in the fetus, or at birth as a congenital malformation, as a manifestation of autosomal recessive disease, or as a feature of a more complex malformation syndrome (for a review see Chapter 7).

By far the most common form of polycystic kidney disease (PKD) is inherited as an autosomal dominant trait. The clinical course of this disease is highly variable and differs both between different affected members of the same family, as well as between different families. In addition to the landmark study by Dalgaard (1957) many authors have described clinical aspects of the disease. Although family studies had been performed previously, the investigation of PKD only became feasible after ultrasonography (US) was developed, as this was a simple, non-invasive technique for the detection of kidney cysts (Hogewind *et al.* 1980; Bear *et al.* 1984). Because not all individuals affected with PKD in a pedigree could be reliably identified by US, especially at younger ages, and because the technique could not be used for prenatal diagnosis, several groups began to search for a genetic marker linked to the mutation causing PKD. Within a year, Steve Reeders and colleagues found that a highly polymorphic marker on chromosome 16, 3´HVR was closely linked to PKD in a set of large families (Reeders *et al.* 1985) (Fig. 15.1). This genetic locus, mutations at which were causing cystic kidneys, was called PKD1. However, despite extremely rapid progress in the development of techniques for DNA analysis it took nine years until the PKD1 gene was identified (EPKDC 1994).

Linkage analysis in PKD families

A large number of highly polymorphic loci is now known on the short arm of chromosome 16, near the PKD1 gene (see Fig. 15.1). In a given family or set of families with dominantly inherited PKD, linkage to polymorphic genetic markers

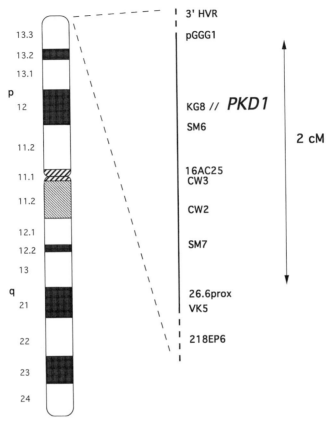

Fig. 15.1 *Map of the short arm of chromosome 16, around PKD1.* KG8, SM6, CW2, CW3 (Peral *et al.* 1994), SM7 (Harris *et al.* 1991), and 16AC2.5 (Thompson *et al.* 1992) are microsatellite markers. pGGG1 (Germino *et al.* 1990), 26-6 (Breuning *et al.* 1990*b*; Saris *et al.* 1990), VK5 (Hyland *et al.* 1990), 218EP6 (Snijdewint *et al.* 1990) are restriction fragment length polymorphisms (RFLP), 3'HVR (Jarman and Higgs, 1988) is a variable number of tandem repeat (VNTR). KG8 is located in the 3'HVR (Jarman and Higgs, 1988) is a variable number of tandem repeats (VNTR). KG8 is located in the 3'untranslated region of the PKD1 gene (EPKDC 1994).

is analysed using the lod score method (Ott 1985). The lod score is the logarithm of the odds for linkage, the likelihood that the results obtained by marker typing are due to linkage to the disease gene at a given recombination fraction divided by the likelihood that the results are due to chance (Ott 1985).

In general, when a disease gene has already been mapped, a lod score of > +2 is considered convincing evidence for linkage; and means that the results of the family study are more than a hundred times more likely to be due to linkage of the disease gene and the marker than due to chance. A lod score of below –2 is considered as evidence against linkage; the results are more than a hundred times less likely to be due to linkage to the markers used. In other words, when a lod score of < -2 is found in a PKD family using chromosome 16 markers, the mutation causing the disease is very likely *not* to have taken place in the PKD1 gene, but in some other gene.

Unfortunately, such decisive lod scores can only be obtained in very large families where sufficient adult family members have consented to donate blood for DNA typing and to undergo US scanning to look for cysts. Such large families have been investigated for research purposes (Reeders *et al.* 1985; Breuning *et al.* 1989*a*,*b*, 1990). In clinical practice, however, most families are small and incomplete due to early death of affected family members.

Applications of linked DNA markers in PKD families

The polymorphic DNA markers linked to the PKD1 gene have been used for presymptomatic and prenatal diagnosis of the disease (Reeders *et al.* 1986, 1989; Turco *et al.* 1991). In some cases, DNA studies have been used to select suitable donors for kidney transplantation among the siblings of patients with PKD (Hannig *et al.* 1992). When linked markers are used for such purposes two crucial points have to be addressed.

First, one has to realize that the risk assessment is not based on direct mutation analysis. In a family study, polymorphic DNA markers are used to follow the inheritance of a disease causing mutation. As a consequence, one has to establish reliably in each family under study which alleles of the polymorpic markers are linked to the mutation. This is called the linkage phase. Therefore, in families with only one single individual available for DNA analysis, linkage studies are impossible. Preferably, one should have DNA from several affected and unaffected family members in at least two generations. If in a family the affected parent has died, but the unaffected spouse is still among the living, DNA from this individual is of great value to establish the linkage phase of the DNA markers in the children. Secondly, evidence is needed to show that in the family under study PKD is indeed caused by a mutation in the short arm of chromosome 16, at the PKD1 gene.

Just after linkage between PKD and chromosome 16 markers had been established, the disease seemed genetically homogeneous. In all families studied, linkage with the chromosome 16 markers was found (Reeders *et al.* 1987). However, very soon after these reports appeared, several families were reported in which linkage between chromosome 16 markers and the mutation causing PKD was confidently excluded (Romeo *et al.* 1988; Kimberling *et al.* 1988; Norby *et al.* 1989; Norby and Schwartz 1990).

Mutations at two distinct genes can cause PKD

The fact that not all families with autosomal dominant PKD inherit the mutation in close linkage with DNA markers on chromosome 16 means that cysts are not always caused by mutations at PKD1 gene and that at least one, possibly more, genes can be involved in ADPKD.

Exclusion of the mutation causing PKD from chromosome 16 is most easily proven using informative flanking markers — markers on either side of the PKD1 gene (Fig. 15.2). If affected children from a patient inherit different alleles of two closely linked polymorphic markers flanking the gene as shown in Fig. 15.2, this can either be explained by recombination on both sides of the mutated gene, which is a very rare event, or by non-linkage of the mutation and the markers.

Among our first PKD families we had a sibship of nine, at first only informative for 3´HVR (Fig. 15.3). Either 4 or 5 recombinants were found, giving a lod score of −2.4. Flanking markers, such as 24-1 (D16S80) (Breuning *et al.* 1987) and CRI-090 (D16S45) (Keith *et al.* 1990), were uninformative at the time. Later, VK5 (D16S96) (Hyland *et al.* 1990) was found to be informative in this sibship, showing apparent double recombinants, or, more likely, independent segregation of the mutation causing PKD and the 3´HVR-VK5 haplotypes, giving a three-point score of −6.6 (Fig. 15.3).

The family described by Romeo (Romeo *et al.* 1988) was informative for 3´HVR (D16S85) and CRI-090 (D16S45). The family described by Kimberling *et al.* (1988) was very large, giving a sufficiently low lod score of −6.266 using only the affected family members, and 3´HVR as a single genetic marker. Many 'unlinked' families have been described subsequently (Mandich *et al.* 1990; Brissenden *et al.* 1991; A. F. Wright *et al.* 1993; Fossdal *et al.* 1993; G. D. Wright *et al.* 1993; Peral *et al.* 1993; Jeffery *et al.* 1993).

At present, several highly informative microsatellite markers are being used to analyse the PKD1 gene (Fig. 15.1) (Harris *et al.* 1991; Peral *et al.* 1994), facilitating the construction of haplotypes around the PKD1 locus which makes the detection or exclusion of linkage easier, even in small families.

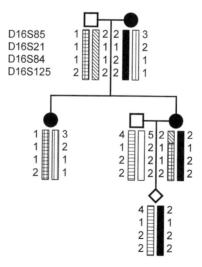

Fig. 15.2 *Small PKD family tested with markers flanking PKD1.* The affected sisters inherit different haplotypes around PKD1 from the affected parent. The mutation causing PKD is most likely not at PKD1.

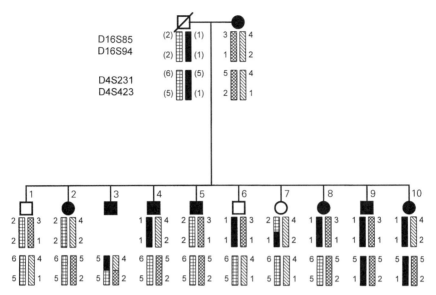

Fig. 15.3 *Sibship of ten with at least 4 recombinants between PKD and D16S85 (3'HVR).* The flanking marker D16S94 (VK5) gives decisive information that the mutation causing PKD is not in the short arm of chromosome 16, at PKD1. Linkage with chromosome 4 markers D4S231 and D4S423, haplotype 5,2. Person 3 was added later.

The search for the PKD2 gene

With genetic heterogeneity of autosomal dominant PKD firmly established, the question arose, of course, on which chromosome the second gene for PKD was located. Since the 'unlinked' form of PKD is relatively rare, the search for a linked marker could only be carried out by the few groups who had access to large families. Kimberling's group used a large family from Italian origin (Kimberling *et al.* 1988), at first with restriction fragment length polymorphisms and polymorphic protein markers (Kumar *et al.* 1990, 1991).

We used the large Australian family (Ravine *et al.* 1992), the Danish family (Norby and Schwartz 1990), and several other families from Cyprus (C. Deltas *et al.* 1995), Iceland (Fossdal *et al.* 1993), and the Netherlands. Both Kimberling's group and our own mainly used the highly polymorphic CA-repeat 'microsatellite' markers spread over all chromosomes which had been described by J. Weber (Weber and May 1989). Unfortunately, the PKD2 gene turned out not to be very close to any of the approximately 300 most widely used markers. After these markers had been tested, and more then 60 per cent of the genome had been excluded, both groups simultaneously 'struck gold' in one of the larger gaps in the exclusion map, on chromosome 4 (Kimberling *et al.* 1993; Peters *et al.* 1993).

Thus, the PKD2 gene was mapped to chromosome 4, between the markers D4S231 and D4S414/D4S423 (Fig. 15.4). The map of this particular region of the chromosome has since been refined, and cloning in overlapping yeast

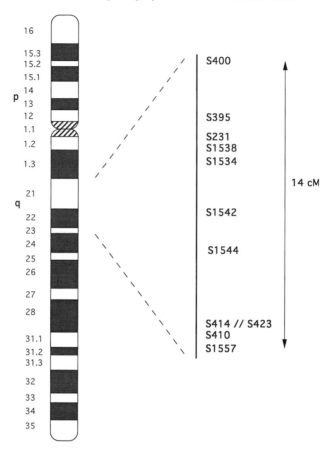

Fig. 15.4 *Map of the long arm of chromosome 4, around PKD2.* All markers are microsatellites. D4S231 is obtained from Milles *et al.* (1993), the other markers from Weissenbach *et al.* (1992).

artificial chromosomes (YACs) is almost complete. However, the physical distance between the two closest flanking markers is at least 8 megabases, which means that the interval has to be reduced considerably, using recombination events in informative families as was done for the PKD1 gene by Somlo and co-workers (Somlo *et al.* 1992) before a meaningful search for the PKD2 gene can begin.

The PKD2 gene is not on chromosome 2

Norby and Schwartz (1990) reported a lod score of +2.11 at a recombination frequency of 10 per cent using the marker YNH24 (D2S44) in the large Danish family, indicating possible localization of the mutation on chromosome 2. Subsequent studies using more polymorphic DNA markers from the relevant

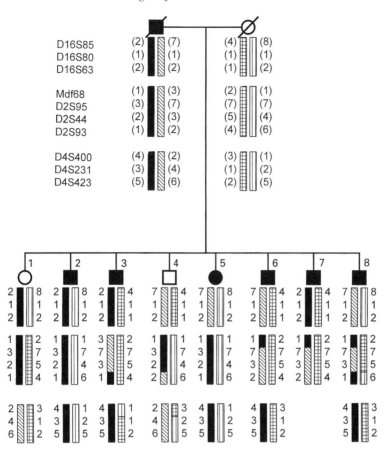

Fig. 15.5 *Analysis of the Danish PKD family with markers on chromosome 16, 2, and 4.* Part of the Danish PKD family showing non-linkage to chromosome 16 markers, apparent double recombinants with chromosome 2 markers (II-3, vs II-2 and II-5) and linkage to chromosome 4 markers, haplotype 4, 3, 5.

region of chromosome 2 revealed conflicting recombinants, confidently excluding the mutation from this chromosome (Fig. 15.5). Moreover, the Danish family gave a multipoint lod score of +4.26 with markers flanking PKD2 (Peters *et al.* 1993) localizing the mutation to chromosome 4 instead of to chromosome 2.

Is there a third gene for autosomal dominant PKD?

Now that two distinct genes, one on chromosome 16 (PKD1) and one on chromosome 4 (PKD2) have been well defined as the location of mutations responsible for autosomal dominant PKD, one can ask whether even more loci are involved in this disease. Indeed, two groups have reported families which appear not to show linkage with either chromosome 16 or 4 markers. One family is of

French-Canadian origin and was described by Somlo and co-workers (Daoust *et al.* 1994), the other is from Portugal and was recently reported by de Almeida *et al.* (1995).

Thus, the existence of a third form of ADPKD seems likely. Unfortunately, both families are of sufficient size to exclude well-defined areas of the genome, but are as yet too small to be useful for a genome-wide search in order to localize the mutation causing PKD.

PKD2 shows slower progression of the disease

It has been known for a long time that the clinical course of ADPKD is highly variable between different families as well as between different members of the same family. Little is known about the factors influencing progression of the disease toward kidney failure. However, when affected members from families with a mutation at the PKD1 locus are compared to those from families with a mutation at PKD2, the latter develop hypertension, end-stage renal failure, and lethal complications at a later age (Parfrey *et al.* 1990; Ravine *et al.* 1992). Although affected members with slow progression of the disease have also been described among the families PKD1 (Ryynanen *et al.* 1987), there is a general tendency to develop end-stage renal failure at an earlier age in PKD1 families than PKD2 families (Parfrey *et al.* 1990; Ravine *et al.* 1992; unpublished observations in several Dutch families). One should realize that these data come from the comparison of small numbers of large families, representing a relatively small set of mutations at the PKD1 and PKD2 genes. It is therefore questionable whether the data are relevant to all PKD families.

In any case, one should be careful not to use this clinical distinction in isolated cases of PKD. When a person with PKD over the age of 75 has no kidney failure, one cannot conclude from this finding alone that the causative mutation must be located at the PKD2 locus. Such a conclusion can only be reached by performing linkage studies with informative DNA markers on a sufficient number of members of the family, or, by the time it is technically possible, by direct mutation detection.

Frequency of the different forms of ADPKD

Genetic heterogeneity of the disease leads to the question: 'how often is PKD caused by mutations in chromosome 16 as opposed to chromosome 4?' This can be calculated with computer programs, such as HOMOG (Ott 1985), which use the admixture test. Adjusted lod scores from all families are summed assuming different proportions of linked families. This proportion is called 'alpha'. The highest lod score obtained, corresponds to the most likely value of alpha. When all families show linkage to the marker, alpha is 1; when none of the families shows linkage, alpha is 0.

At first, alpha was found to be 1, or almost 1, in all families showing linkage to chromosome 16 markers (Reeders *et al.* 1987). After 'unlinked' families had been described, alpha decreased a little, indicating that the vast majority of families showed linkage to PKD1, and that the 'unlinked' form of PKD was rare (Pieke *et al.* 1989). By far the most extensive set of families has been studied by Peters and Sandkuijl (1992) who found an alpha of 0.86 with 95 per cent confidence limits of 0.79–0.89 in a set of 328 families from eight European countries. A similar value for alpha was found in Spanish families (Peral *et al.* 1993), and families from Scotland (Wright *et al.* 1993), but the confidence limits of alpha were wide due to the small number of families tested.

It is intriguing that in the first sets of families, 'unlinked' families were rarely or never detected, then subsequently, one-fifth to one-tenth of the total number of ADPKD families tested. Probably some sort of selection has occurred in each of these studies. Initially, research groups focused on large families that would give interpretable lod scores. If mutations at PKD1 indeed lead to a more rapidly progressive disease, such patients are more likely to be detected at haemodialysis units or transplantation clinics. Since PKD leads to more morbidity and mortality in the extended family, distantly related family members may be more willing to collaborate with pre-symptomatic US and DNA studies.

The families in the European study (Peters and Sandkuijl 1992) were collected in order to identify recombinants between PKD1 and flanking markers with the aim of refining the mapping of the gene (Breuning 1994). It is likely that during these investigations families containing apparent recombinants may have been studied more thoroughly, leading to the detection of more 'unlinked' families.

An unbiased assessment of alpha — the proportion of families with a mutation at the PKD1 gene, or PKD2 — appears to be very difficult, if not impossible with current approaches to PKD patients and families.

Risk calculation under heterogeneity

Only a few mutations have been identified in the PKD1 gene to date (EPKDC 1994). Routine procedures for direct mutation detection are not available, and the search for the PKD2 gene is just beginning. Therefore, prenatal and pre-symptomatic diagnosis of PKD will have to rely on linked genetic markers for some time to come.

As mentioned above, such studies are straightforward in large families where the linkage phase of the markers can be reliably determined. In small or incomplete families, however, the linkage phase can be uncertain, precluding assignment of the mutation to either chromosome 4 or 16, and thus a reliable assessment of risk becomes impossible. In practice, such small families should be typed with both chromosome 4 and 16 markers. Subsequently, one should try to make haplotypes by hand and draw an 'old-fashioned' pedigree showing these haplotypes. Several computer programs are now available for storage and drawing of pedigrees (Fenton and Sandkuijl 1992) (Cyrillic[R]). Any inconsistencies in the data will become immediately apparent during this procedure. This is necessary because computer programs used for lod score calculations do not always detect linkages and show errors in the dataset.

If haplotypes cannot be ascertained by inspection of the pedigree, and many different explanations of the data remain likely, one cannot expect the programs (e.g. MLINK) to give decisive lod scores. However, the calculation should be carried out because linkage programs compute likelihoods for all possible combinations of markers for all individuals in the pedigree, typed or untyped. Thus, the analysis gives an objective assessment of the amount of linkage information in the pedigree. Therefore it is a good check on manual haplotyping.

Most computer programs would require separate calculations for the two different PKD loci. A practical and quick approach was designed by Janssen *et al.* (1990) who combined the two loci for tuberous sclerosis on a single 'imaginary chromosome'. In the same way, the polymorphic markers around PKD1 and PKD2 (Figs 15.1 and 15.5) can be connected on a 'PKD chromosome' and, subsequently, likelihoods can be calculated for all possible locations of the mutation at the same time. By comparing the likelihoods obtained for different intervals it can be determined how much more likely a certain location of the PKD mutation is, relative to the other possibilities. Of course, the a priori chances of the mutation mapping to PKD1 or to PKD2 of 85 per cent and 15 per cent, respectively, should also be taken in account.

Conclusion

The genetic heterogeneity of PKD does not preclude pre-sympromatic or prenatal diagnosis of PKD and it does make the diagnosis with linked markers more complex. Prenatal diagnosis, in particular, requires thorough preparation, preferably before the start of pregnancy.

References

Bear, J. C., *et al.* (1984). Age at clinical onset and at ultrasonographic detection of adult polycystic kidney disease — data for genetic counselling. *American Journal of Medical Genetics*, **18**, 45–53.

Breuning, M. H. (1994). Towards prevention of renal failure caused by inherited polycystic kidney disease. In *Advances in medical biology*, (ed. C. Baya), pp. 3–12. IOS Press. Amsterdam.

Breuning, M. H., *et al.* (1987). Improved early diagnosis of adult polycystic kidney disease with flanking DNA markers *Lancet*, **2**, 1359–61.

Breuning, M. H., *et al.* (1989*a*). Characterization of DNA probes for diagnosis of Huntington's chorea and adult polycystic kidney disease. In *Molecular probes, technology and medical applications*, (ed. A. Albertini, P. Paoletti, and L. Cavalli-Sforza). Raven, New York.

Breuning, M. H. *et al.* (1989*b*). *Characterization of new probes for diagnosis of polycystic kidney disease (PKD1)*, pp. 65–75. Liss, New York.

Breuning, M. H. *et al.* (1990*a*). Map of 16 polymorphic loci on the short arm of chromosome 16 close to the polycystic kidney disease gene (PKD1). *Journal of Medical Genetics*, **27**, 603–13.

Breuning, M. H., Snijdewint, F. G. M., Smits, J. R., Dauwerse, J. G., Saris, J. J., and Van Ommen, G.-J. B. (1990*b*). A TaqI polymorphism identified by 26-6 (D16S125) proximal to the locus affecting adult polycystic kidney disease (PKD1) on chromosome 16. *Nucleic Acids Research*, **18**, 3106.

Brissenden, J. E., Roscoe, J. M., Simpson, N. E., and Silverman, M. (1991). Linkage exclusion between the autosomal dominant polycystic kidney disease locus and chromosome 16 markers in a new family. *Journal of the American Society of Nephrology*, **2**, 913–19.

Constantinou-Deltas, C. D. *et al.* (1995). Genetic heterogeneity in adult dominant polycystic kidney disease in Cypriot families. *Human Genetics*, **95**, 416–23.

Dalgaard, O. Z. (1957). Bilateral polycystic disease of the kidneys: a follow-up of two hundred and eighty four patients and their families. *Acta Medica Scandinavica*, **328**, 1–255.

Daoust, M. C., Reynolds, D. M., Bichet, D. G., and Somlo, S. (1994). Evidence for a third genetic locus for autosomal dominant polycystic kidney disease. *Genomics*,

de Almeida, S. *et al.* (1995). Autosomal dominant polycystic kidney disease: evidence for a third locus in a Portuguese family. *Human Genetics*, **96**, 83–8.

EPKDC (European Polycystic Kidney Disease Consortium) (1994). The polycystic kidney disease 1 gene encodes a 14 kb transcript and lies within a duplicated region on chromosome 16. *Cell*, **77**, 881–94.

Fenton, I. and Sandkuijl, L. A. (1992). Megabase/PKD: A genetic database for polycystic kidney disease. In *Contributions to nephrology 97: Polycystic kidney disease*, (ed. M. H. Breuning, M. Devoto, and G. Romeo), pp. 118–27. Karger, Basel.

Fossdal, R., *et al.* (1993). Icelandic families with autosomal dominant polycystic kidney disease: families unlinked to chromosome 16p13.3 revealed by linkage analysis. *Human Genetics*, **91**, 609–13.

Germino, G. G., *et al.* (1992). The gene for autosomal dominant polycystic kidney disease lies in a 750 kb CpG-rich region. *Genomics*, **13**, 144–51.

Hannig, V. L., Erickson, S. M., and Phillips, J. A. (1992). Utilization and evaluation of living-related donors for patients with adult polycystic kidney disease. *American Journal of Medical Genetics*, **44**, 409–12.

Harris, P. C., Thomas, S., Ratcliffe, P. J., Breuning, M. H., Coto, E., and Lopez-Larrea, C. (1991). Rapid genetic analysis of polycystic kidney disease 1 by means of a microsatellite marker. *Lancet*, **II**, 1484–7.

Hogewind, B. L., Veltkamp, J. J., Koch, C. W., and de Graeff, J. (1980). Genetic counseling for adult polycystic kidney disease. Ultrasound a useful tool in pre-symptomatic diagnosis? *Clinical Genetics*, **18**, 168–72.

Hyland, V. J., *et al.* (1990). Probe, VK5B, is located in the same interval as the autosomal dominant adult polycystic kidney disease locus, PKD1. *Human Genetics*, **840**, 286–8.

Janssen, L. A. J., *et al.* (1990). Genetic heterogeneity in tuberous sclerosis. *Genomics*, **8**, 237–42.

Jarman, A. P., and Higgs, D. R. (1988). A new hypervariable marker for the human alpha globin gene cluster. *American Journal of Human Genetics*, **43**, 249–56.

Jeffery, S., Saggar-Malik, J. S., Morgan, S., and MacGregor, G. A. (1993). A family with autosomal dominant polycystic kidney disease not linked to chromosome 16p13.3. *Clinical Genetics*, **44**, 173–6.

Keith, T. P., *et al.* (1990). Genetic linkage map of 46 DNA markers on human chromosome 16. *Proceedings of the National Academy of Sciences USA*, **87**, 5754–8.

Kimberling, W. J., Fain, P. R., Kenyon, J. B., Goldgar, D., Sujansky, E., and Gabow, P. A. (1988). Linkage heterogeneity of autosomal dominant polycystic kidney disease. *New England Journal of Medicine*, **319**, 913–17.

Kimberling, W. J., Kumar, S., Gabow, P. A., Kenyon, J. B., Connolly, C. J., and Somlo, S. (1993). Autosomal dominant polycystic kidney disease: localization of the second gene to chromosome 4q13-q23. *Genomics* **18**, 467–72.

Kumar, S., Kimberling, W. J., Gabow, P. A., Shugart, Y. Y., and Pieke-Dahl, S. (1990). Exclusion of autosomal dominant polycystic kidney disease type II (ADPKD2) from 160 cM of chromosome 1. *Journal of Medical Genetics*, **27**, 697–700.

Kumar, S., Kimberling, W. J., Gabow, P., and Kenyon, J. B. (1991) Genetic linkage studies of autosomal dominant polycystic kidney disease: search for the second gene in a large Sicilian family. *Human Genetics*. **87**, 129–33.

Mandich, P., *et al*. (1990). Autosomal dominant polycystic kidney disease: A linkage evaluation of heterogeneity in Italy. *American Journal of Medical Genetics*. **35**, 579–81.

Mills, K. A., *et al*. (1993). Genetic and physical maps of human chromosome 4 based on dinucleotide repeats. *Genomics*, **14**, 209–19.

Norby, S. and Schwartz, M. (1990). Possible locus for polycystic kidney disease on chromosome 2. *Lancet*, **1**, 323–4.

Norby, S., Sorensen, A. W. S., and Boesen, P. (1989). Non-allelic heterogeneity of autosomal dominant polycystic kidney disease. In *Progress in clinical and biological research. Genetics of kidney disorders*, (ed. C. S. Bartsocas), pp. 83–8. Liss, New York.

Ott, J. (1985). *Analysis of human linkage*. Johns Hopkins, Baltimore.

Parfrey, P. S., *et al* (1990). The diagnosis and prognosis of autosomal dominant polycystic kidney disease. *New England Journal of Medicine*, **323**, 1085–90.

Peral, B., *et al*. (1993). Estimating locus heterogeneity in autosomal dominant polycystic kidney disease (ADPKD) in the Spanish population. *Journal of Medical Genetics*, **30**, 910–13.

Peral, B., *et al*. (1994). Evidence for linkage disequilibrium in the Spanish Polycystic Kidney Disease I population *American Journal of Human Genetics*, **54**, 899–908.

Peters, D. J. M. and Sandkuijl, L. A. (1992). Genetic heterogeneity of polycystic kidney disease in Europe. In *Contributions to nephrology. Polycystic kidney disease*, (ed. M. H. Breuning, M. Devoto, and G. Romeo), Vol. 97, pp. 128–39. Karger, Basel.

Peters, D. J. M., *et al*. (1993). Localization of the second gene for autosomal dominant polycystic kidney disease on chromosome 4. *Nature Genetics*, **5**, 359–62.

Pieke, S. A., Kimberling, W. J., Kenyon, J. B., and Gabow, P. (1989). Genetic heterogeneity of polycystic kidney disease: An estimate of the proportion of families unlinked to chromosome 16 *American Journal of Human Genetics*, **45**, A58.

Ravine, D., *et al*. (1992). Phenotype and genotype heterogeneity in autosomal dominant polycystic kidney disease. *Lancet*, **340**, 1330–3.

Reeders, S. T., *et al*. (1985). A highly polymorphic DNA marker linked to adult polycystic kidney disease on chromosome 16. *Nature*, **317**, 542–4.

Reeders, S. T., *et al*. (1986). Prenatal diagnosis of autosomal dominant polycystic kidney disease using a DNA probe. *Lancet*, **2**, 7–9.

Reeders, S. T., *et al*. (1987). A study of genetic linkage heterogeneity in adult polycystic kidney disease. *Human Genetics*, **76**, 348–51.

Reeders, S. T., Germino, G. G., and Gillespie, G. A. J. (1989). Mapping the locus of autosomal dominant polycystic kidney disease: diagnostic application. *Clinical Chemistry*, **35**, B13–16.

Romeo, G., *et al.* (1988). A second genetic locus for autosomal dominant polycystic kidney disease. *Lancet*, **2**, 8–10.

Ryynanen, M. A., Dolata, M. M., Lamainen, E., and Reeders, S. T. (1987). Localisation of a mutation producing autosomal dominant polycystic kidney disease without renal failure. *Journal of Medical Genetics*, **24**, 462–5.

Saris, J. J., *et al.* (1990). Rapid detection of a new polymorphism near the gene for adult polycystic kidney disease. *Lancet*, **I**, 1102–3.

Snijdewint, F. G. M., Saris, J. J., Dauwerse, J. G., Breuning, M. H., and Van Ommen, G.-J. B. (1990). Probe 218EP6 (D16S246) detects RFLP's close to the locus affecting adult polycystic kidney disease (PKD1) on chromosome 16. *Nucleic Acids Research*, **18**, 3108.

Somlo, S. *et al.* (1992). Fine genetic localization of the gene for autosomal dominant polycystic kidney disease (PKD1) with respect to physically mapped markers. *Genomics*, **13**, 152–8.

Thompson, A. D., Shen, Y., Holman, K., Sutherland, G. R., Callen, D. F., and Richards, R. I. (1992). Isolation and characterization of (AC)n microsatellite genetic markers from human chromosome 16. *Genomics*, **13**, 402–8.

Turco, A., Peissel, B., Gammaro, L., Maschio, G., Pignatti, P. F. (1991). Linkage analysis for the diagnosis of autosomal dominant polycystic kidney disease, and for the determination of genetic heterogeneity in Italian families. *Clinical Genetics*, **40**, 287–97.

Weber, J. L. and May, P. E. (1989). Abundant class of human DNA polymorphisms which can be typed using the polymerase chain reaction. *American Journal of Human Genetics*, **44**, 388–96.

Weissenbach, J., *et al.* (1992). A second-generation linkage map of the human genome. *Nature*, **359**, 794–801.

Wright, A. F., *et al.* (1993). A study of genetic linkage heterogeneity in 35 adult-onset polycystic kidney disease families. *Human Genetics*, **90**, 569–71.

Wright, G. D., *et al.* (1993). Genetic linkage analysis, clinical features and prognosis of autosomal dominant polycystic kidney disease in Northern Ireland. *Quarterly Journal of Medicine*, **86**, 459–63.

PART IV

*Autosomal dominant polycystic kidney disease:
clinical features*

16
Hypertension in polycystic disease
Michael L. Watson

Introduction

Reports of hypertension in association with polycystic kidney disease (PKD) began to appear in the literature in the early part of the twentieth century (Braasch 1916; Schacht 1931). Most of these reports related to patients who had chronic renal failure as a consequence of cystic kidney disease (Braasch and Schacht 1933; Rall and Odell 1949; Higgins 1952), and it was noted that in these patients the incidence of hypertension was very much higher than in age- and sex-matched controls with end-stage renal disease secondary to pyelonephritis (Schacht 1931). More recently, it has become clear that blood pressure increases well before the onset of detectable renal impairment in up to 75 per cent of patients (Hansson *et al.* 1974; Milutinovic *et al.* 1984; Watson *et al.* 1986; Gabow 1990) and increases progressively with age (Fig. 16.1). Whether there is a significant difference between the sexes remains unclear; Gabow *et al.* (1990) reported more severe hypertension at an earlier age in males whereas others have not observed the same differences, at least in the rate of deterioration in renal function (Bear *et al.* 1992).

Because of the need to delay development of end-stage renal failure and prevent the rupture of cerebral aneurysms, detection and effective treatment of raised blood pressure has become one of the most important aspects of patient management. This chapter will discuss the assessment of hypertension, review the pathophysiology, and then examine the significance of hypertension in the management of patients of different ages.

Assessment of blood pressure

The primary value of treating hypertension is to prevent target organ damage; most particularly damage to the kidneys. The aim is, therefore, the early detection and treatment of mild hypertension and subsequent monitoring to ensure continuing control. The detection of more severe levels of hypertension is straightforward but milder increases are more difficult to assess. Not only are the increases above the 'normal range' small, but there are a number of confounding influences, the most important of which is the significance of the 'white coat phenomenon' (Pickering *et al.* 1988). Blood pressure (BP) recorded in a clinic

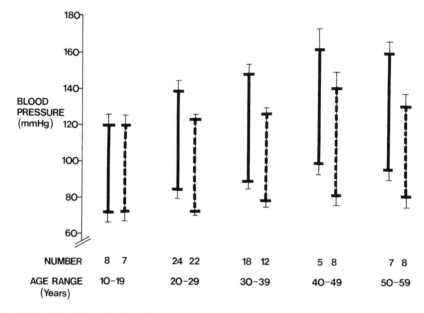

Fig. 16.1 Systolic and diastolic BP of patients affected by polycystic kidney disease compared with the BP of their unaffected relatives. (——), affected; (– – – –), unaffected. (From Watson *et al.* 1986.)

environment may be disproportionately high compared with results when the patient is in an 'unstressed state'. The recording of multiple readings on separate occasions assists in this assessment, but the measurement of BP outside the clinic environment by portable equipment provides useful further data and a better indication of actual BP. Ambulatory BP monitoring systems permit frequent measurement of BP over periods of 24–48 hours; the consistency of hypertension can therefore be assessed. Using this technique in essential hypertension, good correlations have been obtained between the development of target organ damage such as left ventricular hypertrophy and the level of BP (Devereux *et al.* 1983; Drayer *et al.* 1987). This is probably achieved at least in part by eliminating the higher BP associated with the 'white coat effect' (Gosse *et al.* 1993).

Results of ambulatory BP measurements have not been widely reported in autosomal dominant PKD (ADPKD). In a recent study, we compared clinic BP readings obtained using a Hawksley random zero sphygmomanometer after patients rested for 15 minutes with results of mean daytime BP readings obtained using an ambulatory system (SpaceLabs 90207 SpaceLabs Inc., Redmond, WA, USA). The results suggest a reasonable correlation between the two, but the random zero tends to overestimate diastolic pressure. With the ambulatory systems, BP can also be recorded during the night and an assessment made of the diurnal variation in pressure. The BP often drops significantly at night, and therefore the 24-hour mean BP is even lower than readings obtained during the day at the clinic.

The variability of diurnal variation in BP in individual ADPKD patients is interesting. The usual picture is of substantial hypertension during the day, and subsequent fall in pressure at night (Fig. 16.2). In others, there may be a complete loss of this nocturnal decline in pressure (Fig. 16.3). The integrated level of BP over a 24-hour period is thus significantly higher in the latter case compared with an individual who has the usual night-time decline. Other studies have also provided evidence that secondary hypertension as a consequence of renal disease is associated with significant attenuation of the day/night variability (Portaluppi *et al.* 1991; Morduchowicz *et al.* 1993). Many patients do not fit into such a clear category of showing either diurnal variation in pressure, or no such change. BP during the day may show marked lability, but overall ambulatory BPs do provide useful additional information over and above the usual clinic BP. Further detailed studies are awaited to establish the long-term value of such measurements in relation to improvement of BP control and prediction of target organ damage.

Pathophysiology

The cause of the early rise in BP remains controversial. Detailed information on the genetic background of ADPKD is only now becoming available, but there is no data as yet to suggest a direct role for the genetic defect in the genesis of hypertension, and no co-segregation of the mutated gene with other genes known to be associated with development of hypertension.

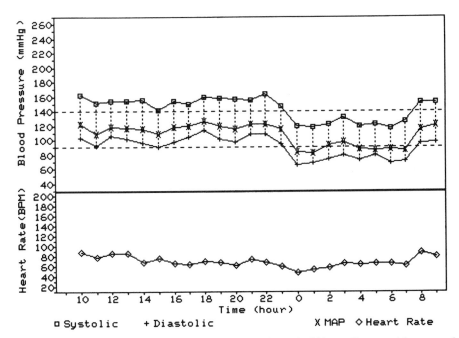

Fig. 16.2 Average hourly BP of patient with polycystic kidney disease without renal failure: normal diurnal variations. □, systolic; x, mean; +, diastolic.

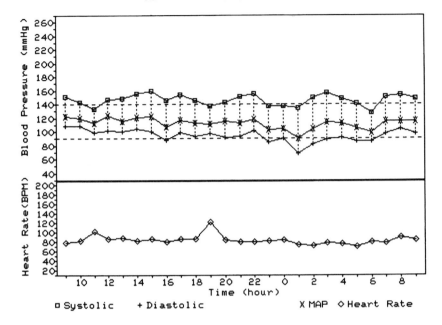

Fig. 16.3   Average hourly BP of patient with polycystic kidney disease without renal failure: no diurnal variation. □, systolic; x, mean; +, diastolic.

It is much more likely that the rise in BP is secondary to renal damage. Indeed, there is a direct relationship between the volume of the kidneys and the severity of hypertension (Gabow *et al.* 1992), but how this relates to the underlying pathogenesis is less certain. A number of factors may be important, and these are described below.

Sodium balance

The extracellular fluid and/or plasma volume is clearly expanded in patients with ADPKD well before the onset of renal failure (Nash 1977; Valvo *et al.* 1985; Danielsen *et al.* 1986*b*; Harrap *et al* 1991), although some of the earlier studies concentrated on patients with renal impairment (Leenen *et al.* 1975). Harrap and co-workers studied a group of affected patients with good renal function and minimal renal impairment and compared them with unaffected matched relatives (Harrap *et al.* 1991). The total exchangeable sodium was significantly elevated in affected compared to unaffected offspring (Table 16.1). Average total body water and plasma volume were also greater in affected offspring, but the confidence interval for the differences was relatively wide. Calculation of the expanded total body water coincided well with the predicted increase in extracellular fluid volume based on the increase in exchangeable sodium, suggesting that expansion that occurred was in the extracellular fluid

Table 16.1 Renal haemodynamics and fluid volume characteristics of ADPKD families

	Unaffected	Affected	95% CI
Glomerular filtration rate ml/min/1.73 m2	100 (23)	97 (19)	−18–10
Effective renal plasma flow ml/min/1.73 m2	605 (118)	532 (86)*	−140– −05
Exchangeable sodium mmol/kg	38.0 (3.5)	40.8 (2.3)*	0.9–4.8
Total body water ml/kg	573 (71)	594 (64)	−22–62
Plasma volume ml/kg	39.6 (8.5)	41.7 (4.6	−2.4–6.6

Results are mean (50). The approximate 95 per cent confidence interval (CI) is for the difference between means. * $P < 0.0005$ compared to unaffected. (From Harrap *et al.* 1991.)

space. Demonstration of a difference in extracellular fluid space between normotensive and hypertensive patients is less clear. Danielsen reported no difference in the extracellular fluid volume between control subjects and affected patients with mild hypertension and renal insufficiency (Danielsen *et al.* 1986*b*). Bell found no difference in the plasma volume between normotensive and hypertensive ADPKD patients (Bell *et al.* 1988) — a direct contrast to Valvo, who found a significant increase in plasma volume in the hypertensives compared with the normotensive patients (Valvo *et al.* 1985).

Sodium retention contributes significantly to the hypertension of chronic renal failure (Dathan *et al.* 1973). However, renal salt wasting is a well-described feature of ADPKD and in these circumstances severe sodium restriction may exacerbate the renal failure (Leenen *et al.* 1975) — indeed an inverse relationship between decreasing creatinine clearance and extracellular fluid volume has been reported (Danielsen *et al* 1986*b*).

The critical importance of sodium balance increases with decreasing glomerular filtration rate. Inulin clearance increased in affected patients when dietary sodium was increased from 20 mmol/day to 200 mmol/day, and the increase was greatest in those patients with the lowest baseline glomerular filtration rate (Schmid *et al.* 1990). Conflicting results are reported on the effects of dietary sodium restriction on BP. Although Nash reported a fall in BP on severe sodium restriction (10 mmol/day, Nash 1977), there was no change of pressure in another group of patients (Bell *et al.* 1988), although the dietary sodium intake (20 mmol/day) was slightly higher in the latter. In another study, systolic BP increased but diastolic was unchanged when affected subjects were changed from a dietary sodium intake of 20 mmol/day to 200 mmol/day (Schmid *et al.* 1990).

The demonstrable expansion of the extracellular fluid volume in ADPKD patients before the onset of renal failure implies a mechanism of sodium retention additional to the effects of renal damage, and indeed there is evidence in favour of enhanced renal tubular sodium and water reabsorption in ADPKD (D'Angelo *et al.* 1975). In contrast, other studies (Danielsen *et al.* 1986*a*; Torres *et al.* 1989) suggested that ADPKD patients excrete an intravenous sodium and water load more rapidly than control subjects. The latter study also demonstrated a shift in the pressure–natriuresis curve in the hypertensive patients which is corrected by the administration of an angiotensin converting enzyme inhibitor (Torres *et al.* 1991). The wide variability of the data, and limited numbers in each group add to the difficulties in comparing and contrasting the results in these different studies.

In association with expansion of the extracellular fluid volume, changes in cardiac function would be expected. Valvo *et al.* (1985) reported that cardiac index was increased with a good correlation between plasma volume and cardiac output, whereas Brod and co-workers found the cardiac indices to be normal (Brod *et al.* 1982). Baseline cardiac index was similar in another group of normotensive and hypertensive ADPKD patients but cardiac index increased more during exercise whilst on a high sodium diet in the hypertensives compared with the normotensive group (Bell *et al.* 1988). A greater increase in atrial natriuretic factor in hypertensives on high sodium intake and with exercise compared with normotensives, in conjunction with the observation on cardiac index, pointed towards enhanced venoconstriction in hypertensive ADPKD patients.

Renal vascular resistance

There are many reports of increased renal vascular resistance in essential hypertension (Uneda *et al.* 1984; Ruilope *et al.* 1994). Indeed, there appears to be a familial component to the increased renal vascular resistance (Van Hooft *et al.* 1991), suggesting a primary pathogenetic role in essential hypertension (Bianchi *et al.* 1979). Renal vascular resistance is also increased early in the course of ADPKD (Watson *et al.* 1992), but in all these patients significant cyst formation has occurred and it is therefore uncertain whether there has been a primary increase in renal vascular resistance or whether the change is secondary to the presence of cysts. In favour of the latter proposition, Hollenberg and co-workers demonstrated that in ADPKD, as with advanced nephrosclerosis, but in contra-distinction to essential hypertension, there was loss of the renal vasodilator response to a variety of renal vasodilators (Hollenberg *et al.* 1975). This loss of vasodilatory capacity may contribute to sodium retention.

Renin angiotensin system

Inevitably, questions arise as to the role of the renin angiotensin system in contributing to raised renal vascular resistance. A number of studies have reported increases in plasma renin activity (PRA) in ADPKD (Nash 1977; Chapman *et al.* 1990). Harrap and co-worker reported PRA measurements in patients with good renal function and demonstrated a significantly higher level in affected compared to unaffected patients (Harrap *et al.* 1991). Since the extracellular fluid volume was significantly expanded in the same group, the clear implication is that renin is inappropriately elevated for the degree of extracellular fluid volume expansion in affected patients. The same group reported smaller but significant increases in plasma aldosterone, but other hormones with mineralocorticoid activity were not increased (Table 16.2). In another study, PRA was not found to be significantly increased in ADPKD patients with minimal renal impairment. However, although the patients were matched in terms of urinary sodium excretion, there were no measurements of extracellular fluid volume although plasma volume was significantly increased (Nash 1977). Renin might therefore still have been inappropriately high in relation to the state of the extracellular fluid volume (Nash 1977; Chapman *et al.* 1990; Harrap *et al.* 1991). More convincing evidence for lack of a significant role of the renin angiotensin system was the absence of a significant vasodepressor response to saralasin (an angiotensin II antagonist) (Anderson *et al.* 1979). However, this compound does have some partial agonist activity which may have been significant. An alternative approach has been to use the acute response to angiotensin-converting enzyme inhibitors to probe the renal effects of the renin angiotensin system. The marked renal vasodilation that follows administration of antiotensin-converting enzyme inhibitors, without change in glomerular filtration rate (GFR) (Fig. 16.4) indicates a marked vasospastic effect of angiotensin in the renal vasculature (Chapman *et al.* 1990; Torres *et al.* 1991; Watson *et al.* 1992). The alternative explanation of an increase in levels of bradykinin or prostaglandins in response to the inhibitor is unlikely (Watson *et al.* 1992), but will only definitely be excluded by observing the renal vascular response to angiotensin II antagonists such as losartan.

Further evidence of increased renin activation is a study comparing matched populations of ADPKD and essential hypertensives (Chapman *et al.* 1990). The ADPKD patients had higher supine and erect PRA, as well as a higher level 60 minutes after captopril; a similar result to that reported by Bell *et al.* (1988).

There are, at present, no data on extra renal synthesis of renin in ADPKD. The most likely explanation of increased renal synthesis relates to cyst expansion. Expanding cysts may either cause direct pressure on the juxtaglomerular apparatus or alternatively compress arterioles within the kidney leading to lower glomerular perfusion and a baroreceptor-mediated increase in renin release. Direct visualization of this process has been obtained by renal angiography (Cornell 1970; Ettinger *et al.* 1969), with the demonstration of attenuation of blood vessels around cysts. There are other lines of evidence to support the enhanced activity of the renin angiotensin system. Immunocytochemical studies of tissue slices from polycystic kidneys demonstrated marked variability of the number of renin granules in the juxtaglomerular apparatus of normal sections of kidney. In the normal sections, some showed only a few renin-positive cells, whereas others showed marked hyperplasia of renin-containing cells. The renin-containing cells also extended along the afferent arteriole and were identifiable in the walls of some efferent arterioles (Graham and Lindop 1988). In scarred areas and in fibrous tissue the same distribution as in the normal sections was observed, but additional renin-containing cells were often present in the vascular poles of sclerosed glomeruli, and in the walls of small arterioles closely related to the cyst wall. Others have demonstrated increased renin granules in the juxtaglomerular apparatus of those kidneys and also in renal tubules (Torres

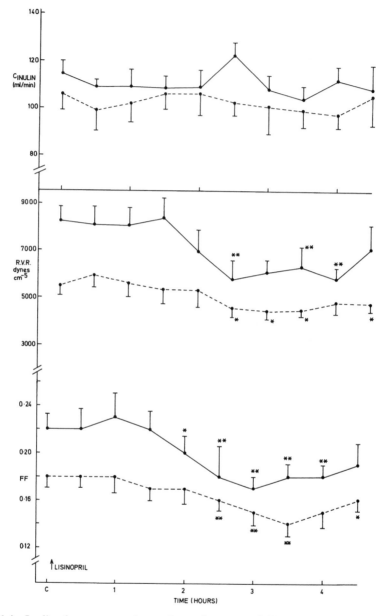

Fig. 16.4 Inulin clearance, renal vascular resistance, and filtration fraction before and after lisinopril (10 mg). (– – –), affected patients; (——), unaffected relatives. $^{*}P < 0.05$; $^{**}P < 0.01$ from control values in the same group.

et al. 1992). Their finding of detectable concentrations of renin in cyst fluid and the demonstration of the capacity of tubulo-cystic epithelium to synthesize renin, further supports the notion of enhanced activity.

There is, therefore, a substantial body of evidence supporting the presence of increased activity of the renin angiotensin system in the affected kidneys. Although this may contribute to the development and maintenance of hypertension, it may also have a role in accelerating the rate of renal damage by causing focal areas of ischaemia within the kidneys.

Atrial natriuretic peptide (APN)

Comparison of ANP levels in normotensive and hypertensive patients suggests that there is no difference. However, on a high sodium diet the levels increased significantly more in the hypertensive patients compared to the normotensive group (Bell *et al.* 1988). Confirmation of these findings has been interpreted to indicate that central venoconstriction is a contributory factor to the genesis of hypertension. In one study of patients without renal failure the levels of ANP in affected patients were not significantly higher than in unaffected patients (Harrap *et al.* 1991) (Table 16.2), whereas in another study patients had a lower GFR but the ANP was significantly increased compared to normal controls, and the same further increase on a high sodium diet was observed (Schmid *et al.* 1990). It seems most likely that any increase in ANP levels is a phenomenon secondary to extracellular fluid volume expansion rather than having any primary pathogenetic role.

Sympathetic nervous system

Bell and co-workers found no evidence of enhanced sympathetic nervous activity in hypertensives compared to the normotensive group either on the basis of baseline level of norepinephrine or in the response of the two groups to suppression with clonidine or phentolamine (Bell *et al.* 1988).

Table 16.2 Humoral characteristics of families with ADPKD

	Unaffected	Affected	95% CI
Plasma renin activity μU/ml	14.0 (11.0,26.5)	26.2 (14.5, 36.5)*	−2.0–22.0
Atrial natriuretic peptide pg/ml	29.5 (22.0, 40.5)	34.0 (26.5, 50.0)	−7.0–17.0
Aldosterone μg/100 ml	2.0 (1.5,2.0)	2.5 (2.0, 3.0)*	0.0–1.0
Cortisol μg/100 ml	5.5 (4.5,7.0)	4.5 (3.5,6.0)	−2.0–1.0
11-Deoxycotisol ng/100 ml	10.5 (6.5,16.0)	13.0 (8.0,26.0)	−4.0–7.0
Corticosterone ng/100 ml	255 (139,357)	250 (134,393)	−126–143
18-Hydroxycorticosterone ng/100 ml	23.8 (17.0,38.0)	36.0(16.0,44.5)	−8.0–23.0
Deoxycortisone ng/100 ml	8.5 (5.0,12.0)	8.5 (4.5,12.0)	−4.0–4.0

All values are expressed as median with the approximate 95% confidence interval (CI) of the median in parentheses. The 95 per cent CI is the approximate 95 per cent CI for the difference in medians. *$P < 0.05$ (one-tailed test) compared to unaffected. (From Harrap *et al.* 1991.)

Deficient renal vasodilator systems

The two most likely deficient vasodilator systems are the bradykinin/kinin system and the vasodilator prostaglandins such as PGE_2 and PGI_2. Again, there is no evidence to suggest that these systems are deficient in the kidneys of patients with ADPKD (Bell *et al.* 1988; Watson *et al.* 1992). More recently, data have been published on the renal vasodilator response to nitric oxide, and the renal vasoconstrictor effect of low doses of the nitric oxide inhibitor L-NAME (Lahera *et al.* 1992). The extent to which these changes may be important in modulating renal vascular resistance and sodium retention in either essential hypertension or ADPKD (Romero *et al.* 1992) remains unclear.

Sodium potassium ATPase

A defect in Na-K ATPase might explain both the occurrence of cysts in the kidneys and conceivably, if present systemically, account for vascular changes that might elevate BP (Rosskopf *et al.* 1993). In the study by Harrap *et al.* (1991) of matched affected and unaffected patients, measurements of erythrocyte sodium and potassium and transmembrane sodium efflux showed that although intracellular electrolyte levels were similar, total efflux rate constants for sodium were greater in unaffected offspring, and this appeared to result from lower rates of oubain-sensitive efflux in red cells of affected offspring (Table 16.3). There was also a negative correlation between total exchangeable sodium and oubain-sensitive sodium efflux rate constant in both affected and unaffected groups. Whether the change in efflux rate constant relates to cause or effect is uncertain, but given the correlation in both affected and unaffected patients, it most likely relates to a more general physiological relationship between sodium and circulating inhibitors of Na-K ATPase (De Wardener and Clarkson 1985). Isolation of the protein defect(s) related to the underlying genetic mutation associated with ADPKD will permit better investigation of such a hypothesis, but at present there is no good supportive evidence. Studies that have been published suggest that changes in the red cell Na-K ATPase activity are more

Table 16.3 Erythocyte electrolyte characteristics of ADPKD families

	Unaffected	Affected	95% CI
Red cell Na conc. mmol/litre	5.7 (1.7)	5.2 (0.9)	−1.3–0.4
Red cell K conc. mmol/litre	105(5)	100(7)	−7–1
$ERC_t h^{-1}$	0.447(0.062)	0.412(0.065)	−0.076–0.006
$ERC_{os} h^{-1}$	0.2888(0.042)	0.258(0.040)*	−0.056– −0.002
$ERC_{fs} h^{-1}$	0.019(0.009)	0.020(0.011)	−0.008–0.006

Results are mean (standard deviation). ERC_t, ERC_{os}, and ERC_{fs} are the total, oubain-sensitive and frusemide-sensitive components of the erythrocytic sodium efflux rate constant. The 95 per cent confidence interval (CI) is for the difference between means. $*P < 0.05$ compared to unaffected. (From Harrap *et al.* 1991.)

likely to correlate with changes in sodium balance rather than constitute part of an underlying pathogenic system.

Coincidental causes

There are case reports of hyperaldosteronism in association with ADPKD, but these are sporadic and unlikely to be part of an underlying pathogenetic mechanism (Bobrie *et al.* 1992; Saeki *et al.* 1986). Although many cases have not been reported in the literature, it is surprising that more have not been published, given the high incidence of ADPKD. The same can be said of renal artery stenosis. Stenosis of the renal arteries may occur as a consequence of cyst expansion, but other pathologies, such as fibromuscular dysplasia and atherosclerotic vascular disease, may occur in conjunction with ADPKD (Messerli *et al.* 1978). Correction of such reversible causes of hypertension could have substantial benefit for individual patients.

Genetic factors

The nature of the underlying genetic defect has some influence on the development of hypertension — patients with ADPKD unlinked to chromosome 16 appear to have a lower incidence of hypertension — but this may merely relate to less severe renal damage from cyst formation (Ravine *et al.* 1992).

It is possible, however, that an individual might not only inherit cystic kidney disease, but in addition also inherit a predisposition to essential hypertension. Simultaneous elevation of BP a consequence of the latter, whatever the mechanism, may, in combination with ADPKD, result in rapid acceleration of the rate of BP increase. Indeed hypertension in unaffected parents seems to be associated with accelerated renal damage in affected offspring (see Chapter 17).

Hypertension and end-organ damage in ADPKD

Death from cardiovascular causes is very common in ADPKD. Dalgaard, in an extensive post-mortem study reported that 64 per cent of patients died from cardiovascular disease (Dalgaard 1957). Hypertension is a major contributor to these causes. Retrospective data from the Mayo Clinic confirms the serious prognosis attached to hypertensive ADPKD patients, both for kidney and patient survival compared with normotensive patients (Fig. 16.5) (Iglesias *et al.* 1983). Systems of particular relevance to consider are the kidney, heart and circulation, and, because of the high incidence of aneurysms, the brain.

Kidney

In a longitudinal study of the effects of ageing there was a significant negative correlation between mean BP and the rate of decline of creatinine clearance with time in years in a population of 'normal subjects' (Lindeman *et al.* 1984).

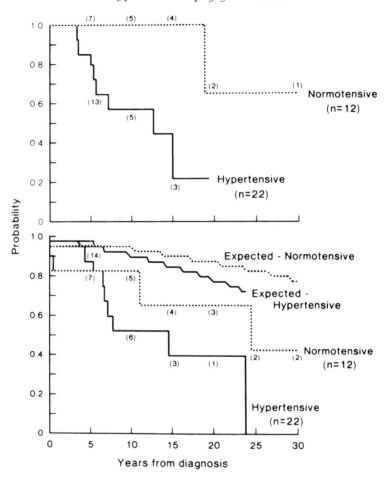

Fig. 16.5 Actuarial kidney (top) and patient (bottom) survival among symptomatic cases of ADPKD by status at diagnosis (1935–80). Hypertensive = diastolic BP ≥ 90 mmHg at diagnosis; normotensive = diastolic BP < 90 mmHg at diagnosis. From Iglesias *et al.* (1983).

The mechanism of this effect is unclear but hypertension is a potent cause of sclerosis of the afferent arterioles in the kidney (Williams and Harrison 1937). In ADPKD, studies of these processes in the earlier phases are by necessity limited, but those undertaken later in the natural history do suggest that significant vessel sclerosis occurs (Zeier *et al.* 1988). The extent to which this in turn accelerates renal failure or results in further elevation of BP is unclear. Recent data leave little doubt that accelerated deterioration of renal function is associated with hypertension (Gabow *et al.* 1992). Confidence of this correlation was further increased by an association in the same study between left ventricular mass and deterioration of renal function. That this association was not merely a consequence of renal damage was indicated by the independence of the relationships of hypertension to deterioration of renal function and that of renal volume to the deterioration of renal function.

This, despite the fact that there is a very clear relationship between hypertension and renal size. Moreover there is a clear relationship between the presence of proteinuria and microalbuminuria and elevation of mean arterial pressure and more severe renal cystic involvement (Chapman *et al.* 1994). These issues are explored in more detail in Chapter 17.

It seems unlikely that hypertension *per se* accelerates the rate of cyst formation, however, haematuria is slightly more common in hypertensives and this may have an effect on progression of renal impairment (Gabow *et al.* 1992).

Heart and circulation

Left ventricular hypertrophy has been recognized as an important complication of hypertension for many years. It is recognized that left ventricular hypertrophy is a poor prognostic factor in essential hypertension with a significant relationship between left ventricular mass and both the incidence and mortality from cardiovascular disease (Levy *et al.* 1990). The extent of elevation of BP appears to be the most important determinant. Moreover, left ventricular hypertrophy appears to occur early in the course of ADPKD (Zeier *et al.* 1993) and may be related to the relatively high nocturnal BPs that have been recorded in young ADPKD patients. Preventing the development of left ventricular hypertrophy is clearly an important part of the strategy for improving blood pressure control in ADPKD.

Valvular lesions of the heart are more common in ADPKD, the mitral valve being most commonly affected (Hossack *et al.* 1988) and may account for some of the high incidence of left ventricular hypertrophy. Changes in the aortic root might have been a consequence of hypertension, but is more likely a consequence of a connective tissue abnormality (Leier *et al.* 1984).

Coronary vascular disease appears to be more common in ADPKD than in the general population, with ADPKD patients on dialysis having a high mortality from cardiovascular disease. It seems likely that long-standing modest elevations of BP will result in accelerated atherogenesis.

Cerebral aneurysms

Hypertension is a risk factor for rupture of cerebral aneurysms (Chauveau *et al.* 1994). In ADPKD, rupture of cerebral aneurysms in young patients appears to be associated with hypertension, although overall there is not a particularly strong relationship between increased BP and rupture of aneurysms. Good control of BP is an important component of long-term management of patients who have already suffered from one rupture, particularly because they may be at increased risk of developing further aneurysms.

The significance of hypertension in different age groups

Childhood involvement

Childhood forms of PKD have usually been regarded as having a particularly poor prognosis. This is primarily because only very severely affected individuals presented with symptoms or complications in early life. The worst affected may present in the neonatal period, whereas others may have massive kidneys within a few months of birth (Blyth and Ockenden 1971; Kääriäinen *et al.* 1988). Most of these patients were thought to have the autosomal recessive disease. Out of 10 children with ADPKD who were studied, 9 developed hypertension. Four of these developed hypertension in the first year of life and three had severe hypertension controlled by multiple drug therapy (Fick *et al.* 1993). In another series only 4 of the 14 patients in the age range 2–29 years with ADPKD required antihypertensive medication (Kääriäinen *et al.* 1988). In comparison, in the same study, 11 of the 14 patients with autosomal recessive disease in the age range 2–23 years required antihypertensive medication. As screening becomes more widespread it is only to be expected that more affected infants will be identified, many of whom will not have the poor prognosis associated with the more severe form. Sedman *et al.* (1987) in a study of children of ADPKD families reported that only 5 per cent of children who had negative US examinations had hypertension (> 150/90 or 95 per cent for age). Seven per cent of the children who were considered to be potentially affected, whereas, 22 per cent of those definitely affected had hypertension. Few of the children in the latter group had renal failure.

Others have not found the same high incidence of hypertension in affected children. In one study, 6 of 22 offspring were diagnosed as affected (age range 1–14 years) but none at that time had hypertension (Taitz *et al.* 1987). In the same study four children presented very early in life with massively enlarged kidneys, but in one at least hypertension in the first year was controlled with drug therapy and subsequently resolved (Kaye and Leny 1974). Corroborating these findings, Zeier and co-workers found none of 12 children under the age of 15 had hypertension; however, 12 young adults (age 15–25 years) had significantly higher daytime and nocturnal BPs (Zeier *et al.* 1993). Clearly, early detection and treatment of hypertension is important. It is probably unrealistic, however, to think in terms of significantly delaying the rate of renal progression by such control in the very early severely affected cases, in whom the rate of progression is determined by massive renal structural damage.

Adolescence

There is no doubt that BP significantly increases in many adolescents with ADPKD (Zeier *et al.* 1993). The increase may at first only be a small increase in nocturnal pressure or even as a more labile pressure than usual. Left ventricular hypertrophy does appear at this age, however, and although there is no supporting evidence, it is possible that vascular change and accelerated renal damage is also taking place. Differentiation of those with raised BP depends on the measurement of multiple BP readings with or without the use of ambulatory measurement. Early intervention with treatment may have significant long-term benefits but at present these are difficult to quantify.

The subgroup most at risk in this age group are those with cerebral aneurysms in whom hypertension is often an associated feature (Chauveau *et al.* 1994). Confirmation of the presence of an aneurysms in such individuals will emphasize the need for good BP control.

Adults

The consistent feature of ADPKD is that hypertension usually develops well before the onset of renal failure, and this remains true in adult life. The data on natural history do not yet permit the prediction of onset of measurable renal impairment, but in some individuals it may be as much as 10 years after the detection of hypertension. In others (a minority) hypertension is not a feature at all, despite the onset of renal impairment. Many of the latter will have significant salt wasting. In a study of patients over the age of 50, 69 per cent had hypertension, and even in subjects with good renal function (creatinine < 133 µmol/l, 60 per cent had significant hypertension. Only two of the 32 patients were asymptomatic and only one of these had significant hypertension (Milutinovic *et al.* 1990). With more widespread screening this will almost certainly prove to be an underestimate of asymptomatic individuals with hypertension.

Some patients undergo uninephrectomy for various clinical reasons. Although this in itself does not accelerate renal failure, uninephrectomized patients with fast progression to renal failure did have higher BP (Zeier, *et al.* 1992).

The severity of renal involvement, as assessed by measurement of kidney size, suggests a direct correlation between the severity and the extent of BP elevation (Milutinovic *et al.* 1990; Gabow, *et al.* 1992), in the same way that there appears to be a correlation between kidney size and deterioration of renal function. Target organ damage is often well established in early adult life and the emphasis must remain on good BP control to prevent its progression. Racial differences in incidence and progression of ADPKD are very poorly documented, although a recent study comparing blacks and whites in US centres suggests that hypertension, at least late in the disease, is not significantly different in the two groups (Yium *et al.* 1994). The same may well not be true in the early stages of the disease.

Pregnancy

Pregnancy in affected individuals does not appear to be associated with a decline in renal function. Many affected mothers will not have significant renal impairment at the time of pregnancy and there appears to be no significant complications in this group, although there are very little data in the literature on BP.

Patients with renal impairment are clearly more at risk, and data from the litera-ture, although limited, suggest that these patients with three or more preg-nancies suffer from a subsequent more rapid deterioration of renal function (Gabow *et al.* 1992).

Transplantation

Hypertension remains common after renal transplantation in ADPKD patients (Fitzpatrick *et al.* 1990). Eight of 12 patients transplanted without bilateral nephrectomy (67 per cent), required antihypertensive medication compared with 20 of 42 (48 per cent) of the patients who had previous bilateral nephrectomy. Other data support this observation (Coles *et al.* 1972; Cohen 1973; McHugh *et al.* 1980) and emphasizes the continuing pressor effect of the residual cystic kidney.

Target blood pressure

Confirmatory evidence for the value of good BP control in ADPKD is less readily available, and indeed some is contradictory (Franz and Reubi 1983). Much of the information in ADPKD can only be derived from studies examin-ing renal function in a variety of different renal diseases (Alvestrand *et al.* 1988; Williams *et al.* 1988; Roseman *et al.* 1989; Brazy *et al.* 1989) in which ADPKD contributed a subset of the patients. Part of the difficulty may reside in the complex nature of the relationships; data suggest that there is not a linear rela-tionship between BP and renal function, but a sigmoid relationship, best de-scribed by a polynomial regression (Gonzalo *et al.* 1992). This study also highlights the importance of average mean arterial pressure as the best predictor of progression, as opposed to systolic and diastolic pressures.

Epidemiological data suggest that normotensive ADPKD patients have better survival than hypertensives; normotension being designated as a diastolic BP < 90 mmHg (Iglesias *et al.* 1983). The target figure to achieve for 'controlled blood pressure' remains arbitrary. It is easier to extrapolate from data in other forms of hypertension. The most acceptable target pressure on this basis is 130/85, although achieving this target may not be appropriate in the elderly with impaired cardiovascular function (Fifth report of the Joint National Commitee on Detection, Evaluation and Treatment of High Blood Pressure 1993). The advantage of reducing systolic and diastolic pressure below 140 and 90 mmHg, respectively, is marginal, control at this level having been reported to induce a 50 per cent reduction in the rate of decline of reciprocal plasma creatinine (Bergstrom *et al.* 1985). However, in the recent study of diet and BP in chronic renal disease, in which patients with ADPKD constituted 24 per cent of the study population, there was no discernible benefit in reducing mean BP to less than 92 mmHg (equivalent to 125/75) compared with less than 107 mmHg (equivalent to 140/90) in those in the 18- to 60-year-old age group, or in those aged greater than 61 from less than 113 mmHg (equivalent to 160/90) to less than 98 mmHg (equivalent to 145/75) (Klahr *et al.* 1994). 'Supercontrol' did not therefore appear to confer added benefit, although all patients had a creatinine clearance of less than 70 ml/min/1.73 m^2 body surface area. Moreover, as a group the ADPKD patients appeared to have a more rapid decline in renal function than patients with other forms of renal disease (Klahr *et al.* 1994). More optimistic results have been reported on delaying the progression of hypertensive nephrosclerosis by good BP control (Lee *et al.* 1993).

Choice of therapy

Pharmacological agents

The mechanism of progression of renal damage in ADPKD is multifactorial, but extrapolation of data from other conditions such as diabetes mellitus suggest that glomerular hypertension may be important (Anderson *et al.* 1990). Ideally, drugs should therefore be selected which, in addition to lowering systemic BP, also reduce glomerular hypertension (Bakris 1993; Campanacci *et al.* 1993). Antihypertensive drugs differ in their effects on glomerular hypertension depending on their pharmacological action (Ruilope *et al.* 1994). In acute studies in man, metoprolol and nifedipine induced glomerular hyperfiltration in comparison with captopril and celiprolol (Bohler *et al.* 1993). In other studies, there appears to be a distinct advantage in using either angiotensin-converting enzyme inhibitors or certain calcium antagonists, since in animal models these drugs not only lower BP, but also lower glomerular capillary pressure and slow progression of glomerulosclerosis (Bakris, 1991). Extrapolating from data in diabetic patients is of limited value, but there is evidence to support the contention that angiotensin-converting enzyme inhibitors and calcium antagonists preferentially slow the decline of glomerular filtration rate in diabetes mellitus (Slataper *et al.* 1993).

Comparison of the renal haemodynamic effects of lisinopril, verapamil, and amlodipine in a group of patients with chronic renal failure from a variety of causes including ADPKD failed to show any real difference in the action of one drug type vs. another at least in respect of the effects of lowering BP and renal haemodynamics (August *et al.* 1993).

More detailed assessment of the effects of angiotensin-converting enzyme inhibitors on renal haemodynamics in ADPKD supports this data (Chapman *et al.* 1990; Watson *et al.* 1992) and suggests that, both on the basis of hypotensive action and benefit as regards interfering with potential mechanisms of renal damage, these drugs are the treatment of choice. The inclusion of angiotensin-converting enzyme inhibitors in any therapeutic regimen is therefore attractive. Indeed, there is also the potential benefit, although yet to be proven, that angiotensin-converting enzyme inhibitors may slow the process of atherogenesis (Schuh *et al.* 1993). Unfortunately, some patients that have more advanced disease have also been reported to develop an acute reversible deterioration of renal function as a consequence of angiotensin-converting enzyme inhibition (Chapman *et al.* 1991). This may in part be a consequence of the salt wasting that may become more important when renal impairment is more advanced

(Leenen *et al.* 1975). The same may well not apply in patients much earlier in the course of their disease and, at present, there is probably reasonable justification for widespread use of angiotensin-converting enzyme inhibitors. There appears little hard information to influence the choice of diuretic. The choice of drug is therefore wide, with some advantage in using angiotensin-converting enzyme inhibitors in the earlier stages of the disease.

Special attention should, however, be payed to monitoring of renal function in elderly patients since they may well be more sensitive to the effects of sodium depletion and sympathetic inhibition.

Other methods

Renal cyst decompression is undertaken for a number of reasons, mostly for the relief of pain. There are also reports that decompression of cysts results in alleviation of hypertension (Bennett *et al.* 1987; Frang *et al.* 1988). If the effects were predictable this would be an attractive therapeutic option, but it is true to say that the main indication for cyst puncture remains alleviation of pain, with benefit on BP control being a potential but unpredictable additional benefit.

Conclusion

Successful control of blood pressure is one of the main challenges for clinicians caring for patients with ADPKD. With the use of modern drugs, good control can be achieved in the vast majority of cases. Further developments in anti-hypertensive therapy are likely to facilitate this in the future.

The critical question is to what extent good blood pressure control delays the progression of renal impairment, and particularly, whether there is value in achieving good blood pressure control early in the course of the disease. Further long-term data will be required before a definitive answer can be given.

References

Alvestrand, A., Gutierrez, A., Bucht, H., and Bergstrom, J. (1988). Reduction of blood pressure retards the progression of chronic renal failure in man. *Nephrology, Dialysis and Transplantation*, 3, 624–31.

Anderson, R. J., Miller, P. D., and Linas, S. L. (1979). Role of the renin-angiotensin system in hypertension of polycystic kidney disease. *Mineral and Electrolyte Metabolism*, 2, 137–41.

Anderson, S., Brenner, B. M., Laragh, J., and Brenner, B. (ed.) (1990). The critical role of nephron mass and intraglomerular pressure for initiation and progression of experimental hypertensive renal disorders. In *Hypertension: pathophysiology diagnosis and management*. pp. 1163–76. Raven, New York.

August, P., Lenz, T., and Laragh, J. H. (1993). Comparative renal hemodynamic effects of lisinopril, verapamil and amlodipine in patients with chronic renal failure. *American Journal of Hypertension*, 6, S148–54.

Bakris, G. L. (1991). The effects of calcium antagonists on renal hemodynamics, urinary protein excretion, and glomerular morphology in diabetic states. *Journal of the American Society of Nephrology*, 2 (Suppl.), 21–9.

Bakris, G. L. (1993). Hypertension in diabetic patients. *American Journal of Hypertension*, 6, S140–7.

Bear, J. C., Parfrey, P. S., Morgan, J. M., Martin, C. J., and Cramer, B. C. (1992). Autosomal dominant polycystic kidney disease: new information for genetic counselling. *American Journal of Medical Genetics*, 43, 548–53.

Bell, P. E., Hossack, K. F., Gabow, P. A., Durr, J. A., Johnson, A. M., and Schrier, R. W. (1988). Hypertension in autosomal dominant polycystic kidney disease. *Kidney International*, 34, 683–90.

Bennett, W. M., Elzinga, L., Golper, T. A., and Barry, J. M. (1987). Reduction of cyst volume for symptomatic management of autosomal dominant polycystic kidney disease. *Journal of Urology*, 137, 622–4.

Bergstrom, J., Alverstrand, A., Bucht, H., and Gutierrel, A. (1985). Progression of chronic renal failure in man is retarded with more frequent clinical follow-up and better blood pressure control. *Clinical Nephrology*, 25, 1–6.

Bianchi, G. *et al.* (1979). A renal abnormality as a possible cause of 'essential' hypertension'. *Lancet*, 1, 173–7.

Blyth, H. and Ockenden, B. G. (1971). Polycystic disease of kidneys and liver presenting in childhood. *Journal of Medical Genetics*, 8, 257–84.

Bobrie, G., Sirieix, M., Day, M., Landais, P., Lacombe, M., and Grunfeld, J. F. (1992). Autosomal dominant polycystic kidney disease with primary hyperaldosteronism. *Nephrology, Dialysis and Transplantation*, 7, 647–50.

Bohler, J., Becker, A., Reetze-Bonorden, P., Woitas, R., Keller, E., and Schollmeyer, P. (1993). Effect of anti hypertensive drugs on glomerular hyperfiltration and renal haemodynamics. *European Journal of Clinical Pharmacology*, 44 (Suppl.), S55–6.

Braasch, W. F. (1916). Clinical data of polycystic kidney. *Surgery, Gynaecology and Obstetrics*, 23, 697–702.

Braasch, W. F. and Schacht, F. W. (1933). Pathological and clinical data concerning polycystic kidney. *Surgery, Gynaecology and Obstetrics*, 57, 467–75.

Brazy, P. C., Stead, W. W., and Fitzwilliam, F. (1989). Progression of renal insufficiency: Role of blood pressure. *Kidney International*, 45, 670–4.

Brod, F., Bahlmann, J., Cachovan, M., Hubrich, W., and Pretschner, P. D. (1982). Mechanisms for the elevation of blood pressure in human renal disease. *Hypertension*, 4, 839–44.

Campanacci, L., Fabris, B., Fischetti, F., Bardelli, M., Uran, F., and Carretta, R. (1993). ACE inhibition in renal disease: Risks and benefits. *Clinical and Experimental Hypertension*, 15, 173–86.

Chapman, A. B., Gabow, P. A., Johnson, A., and Schrier, R. W. (1990). The renin-angiotensin-aldosterone system and autosomal dominant polycystic kidney disease. *New England Journal of Medicine*, 323, 1091–6.

Chapman, A. B., Gabow, P. A. and Schrier, R. W. (1991). Reversible renal failure associated with angiotensin converting enzyme inhibitors in polycystic kidney disease. *Archives of Internal Medicine*, 115, 769–73.

Chapman, A. B., Johnson, A. M., Gabow, P. A., and Schrier, R. W. (1994). Overt proteinuria and microalbuminuria in autosomal dominant polycystic kidney disease. *Journal of the American Society of Nephrology*, 5, 1349–54.

Chauveau, D., Pirson, Y., Verellen-Dumoulin, C., Macnicol, A. M., Gonzalo, A., and Grunfeld, J. P. (1994). Intracranial aneurysms in autosomal dominant polycystic kidney disease. *Kidney International*, **45**, 1140–6.

Cohen, S. L. (1973). Hypertension in renal transplant recipients: Role of bilateral nephrectomy. *British Medical Journal*, **3**, 78–81.

Coles, G. A., Crosby, D. L., and Jones, G. R. (1972). Hypertension following cadaveric renal transplantation. *Postgraduate Medical Journal*, **48**, 399–404.

Cornell, S. H. (1970). Angiography in polycystic disease of the kidneys. *Journal of Urology*, **103**, 24–6.

D'Angelo, A., Mioni, G., Ossi, E., Lupo, A., Valvo, E., and Maschio, G. (1975). Alterations in renal tubular sodium and water transport in polycystic kidney disease. *Clinical Nephrology*, **3**, 99–105.

Dalgaard, O. Z. (1957). Bilateral polycystic disease of the kidneys: A follow-up study of 284 patients and their families. *Acta Medica Scandinavica*, **158** (Suppl.), 328.

Danielsen, H., Nielsen, A. H., Pedersen, E. B., Herlvesen, P., Kornerup, H. J., and Posborg, V. (1986*a*). Exagerated natriuresis in adult polycystic kidney disease. *Acta Medica Scandinavica*, **219**, 59–66.

Danielsen, H., Pedersen, E. B., Nielsen, A. H., Herlevsen, P., Kornerup, H. J., and Posborg, V. (1986*b*). Expansion of extracellular volume in early polycystic kidney disease. *Acta Medica Scandinavica*, **219**, 399–405.

Dathan, J. R., Johnson, D. B., and Goodwin, F. J. (1973). The relationship between fluid compartment volumes, renin activity and blood pressure in chronic renal failure. *Clinical Science Molecular Medicine*, **280**, 978–81.

De Wardener, H. E. and Clarkson, E. M. (1985). Concept of natriuretic hormone. *Physiological Reviews*, **65**, 658–9.

Devereux, R. B. *et al.*, (1983). Left ventricular hypertrophy in patients with hypertension: importance of blood pressure response to regularly recurring stress. *Circulation*, **68**, 470–6.

Drayer, J. M., Weber, M. A., and De Young, J. L. (1987). Blood pressure as a determinant of cardiac left ventricular muscle mass. *Archives of Internal Medicine*, **143**, 90–2.

Ettinger, A., Kahn, P. C., and Wise, H. M. (1969). The importance of selective renal angiography in the diagnosis of polycystic kidney disease. *Journal of Urology*, **102**, 156–61.

Fick, G. M., *et al.* (1993). Characteristics of very early onset autosomal dominant polycystic kidney disease. *Journal of the American Society of Nephrology*, **3**, 1863–70.

Fifth report of the Joint National Committee on Detection, Evaluation and Treatment of High Blood Pressure, 1993, *Archives of Internal Medicine*, **153**, 154–83.

Fitzpatrick, P. M., Torres, V., Charboneau, J. W., Offord, K. P., Holley, K. E., and Zincke, H. (1990). Long-term outcome of renal transplantation in autosomal-dominant polycystic kidney disease. *American Journal of Kidney Disease*, **15**, 535–43.

Frang, D., Czalinga, I., and Polyak, L. (1988). A new approach to the treatment of polycystic kidneys. *International Journal of Urology and Nephrology*, **20**, 13–21.

Franz, K. A. and Reubi, F. C. (1983). Rate of functional deterioration in polycystic kidney disease. *Kidney International*, **23**, 526–9.

Gabow, P. A., Ikle, D. W., and Holmes, J. H. (1984). Polycystic kidney disease: Prospective analysis of non azotaemic patients and family members. *Annals of Internal Medicine*, **101**, 238–47.

Gabow, P. A., Chapman, A. B., Johnson, A. M., Tangel, D. J., Duley, I. T., Kaehny, W. D., Manco-Johnson, M., and Schrier, R. W. (1990). Renal structure and hypertension in autosomal dominant polycystic kidney disease. *Kidney International*, **38**, 117–80.

Gabow, P. A., Johnson, A. M., and Kaehny, W. D. (1992). Factors affecting the progression of renal disease in autosomal dominant polycystic kidney disease. *Kidney International*, **41**, 1311–19.

Gonzalo, A., Gallego, A., Rivera, M., Orte, L., and Ortuno, J. (1992). Shape of the relationship between hypertension and the rate of progression of renal failure in autosomal dominant polycystic kidney disease. *Nephron*, **62**, 52–7.

Gosse, P., Promax, H., Durandet, P., and Clementy, J. (1993). 'White Coat' hypertension: No harm for the heart. *Hypertension*, **22**, 766–70.

Graham, P. C. and Lindop, G. B. (1988). The anatomy of the renin-secreting cell in adult polycystic kidney disease. *Kidney International*, **33**, 1084–90.

Hansson, L., Karlander, L. E., Lundgren, W., and Peterson, L. E. (1974). Hypertension in polycystic kidney disease. *Scandinavian Journal of Urology*, **8**, 203–5.

Harrap, S. B., *et al.* (1991). Phenotypic characteristics of young adults with contrasting genetic predisposition to adult polycystic kidney disease. *Kidney International*, **40**, 501–8.

Higgins, C. C. (1952). Bilateral polycystic kidney disease. *Archives of Surgery*, **65**, 318–29.

Hollenberg, N. K., *et al.* (1975). Renal vascular tone in essential and secondary hypertension: hemodynamics and angiographic responses to vasodilators. *Medicine*, **54**, 29–44.

Hossack, K. F., Leddy, C. L., Johnson, A. M., Gabow, P. A., and Schrier, R. W. (1988). Echocardiographic findings in autosomal dominant polycystic kidney disease. *New England Journal of Medicine*, **319**, 907–12.

Iglesias, C. G., Torres, V., Offord, K. P., Holley, K. E., Beard, C. M., and Kurland, L. T. (1983). Epidemology of adult polycystic kidney disease. Olmsted County, Minnesota: 1935–1980. *American Journal of Kidney Disease*, **2**, 630–9.

Kääriainen, H., Koskimies, O., and Norio, R. (1988). Dominant and recessive polycystic kidney disease in children: Evaluation of clinical features and laboratory data. *Padiatric Nephrology*, **2**, 296–302.

Kaye, C. and Lewy, P. R. (1974). Congenital appearance of adult-type (autosomal dominant) polycystic kidney disease: report of a case. *Journal of Pediatrics*, **85**, 807–10.

Klahr, S., *et al.* (1994). The effects of dietary protein restriction and blood pressure control on the progression of chronic renal disease. *New England Journal of Medicine*, **330**, 877–84.

Lahera, V., Salazar, J., Salom, M. G., and Romero, J. C. (1992). Deficient production of nitric oxide induces volume-dependent hypertension. *Journal of Hypertension*, **10**, S173–7.

Lee, H. C., Mitchell, H. C., Van Dreal, P., and Pettinger, W. A. (1993). Hyperfiltration and conservation of renal function in hypertensive nephrosclerosis patients. *American Journal of Kidney Disease*, **21** (Suppl. 1), 68–74.

Leenen, F. H., Galla, S. J., Redmond, D. P., Vagnucci, A. H., McDonald, R. H. and Shapiro, A. P. (1975). Relationship of the renin-angiotensin-aldosterone system and sodium balance to blood pressure regulation in chronic renal failure of polycystic kidney disease. *Metabolism*, **24**, 589–603.

Leier, C. V., Baker, P. B., Kilman, J. W., and Wooley, C. F. (1984). Cardiovascular abnormalities associated with adult polycystic kidney disease. *Annals of Internal Medicine*, **100**, 683–8.

Levy, D., Garrison, R. J., Savage, D. D., Kannell, W. B., and Castelli, W. P. (1990). Prognostic implications of echocardiographically determined left ventricular mass in the Framingham study. *New England Journal of Medicine*, **322**, 1561–6.

Lindeman, R. D., Tobin, J. D., and Shock, N. W. (1984). Association between blood pressure and the rate of decline in renal function with age. *Kidney International*, **26**, 861–8.

McHugh, M. I., Tanboga, H., and Marcen, R. (1980). Hypertension following renal transplantation: The role of the hosts kidneys. *Quarterly Journal of Medicine*, **49**, 395–403.

Messerli, F. H., De Carvalho, J. G., Mills, N. L., and Frohlich, E. D. (1978). Renal artery stenosis and polycystic kidney disease. *Journal of Urology*, **8**, 279–80.

Milutinovic, J., Fialkow, P. J., Agadoa, L. Y., Phillips, L. A., Rudd, T. D., and Bryant, J. I. (1984). Autosomal dominant polycystic kidney disease: Symptoms and clinical findings. *Quarterly Journal of Medicine*, **53**, 511–22.

Milutinovic, J., Fialkow, P. J., Agadoa, L. Y., Phillips, L. A., Rudd, T. G., and Sutherland, S. (1990). Clinical manifestations of autosomal dominant polycystic kidney disease in patients older than 50 years. *American Journal of Kidney Disease*, **15**, 237–43.

Morduchowicz, G., Zabludowski, J., Wittenberg, C., Winkler, J., and Boner, G. (1993). Ambulatory blood pressure monitoring assessment of blood pressure control in hypertension associated with chronic renal failure. *Nephrology, Dialysis and Transplantation*, **8**, 1169–71.

Nash, D. A. (1977). Hypertension in polycystic kidney disease without renal failure. *Archives of Internal Medicine*, **137**, 1571–5.

Pickering, T. G., James, J. D., and Boddie, C. (1988). How common is white coat hypertension? *Journal of the American Medical Association*, **259**, 225–8.

Portaluppi, F., Montanari, L., Massari, M., Di Chiara, V., and Capanna, M. (1991). Loss of nocturnal decline of blood pressure in hypertension due to chronic renal failure. *American Journal of Hypertension*, **4**, 20–6.

Rall, J. E. and Odel, H. M. (1949). Congenital polycystic disease of the kidney review of the literature and data on 207 cases. *American Journal of Medical Science*, **218**, 399–407.

Ravine, D., *et al.* (1992). Phenotype and genotype heterogeneity in autosomal dominant polycystic kidney disease. *Lancet*, **340**, 1330–3.

Romero, J. C., Lahera, V., Salom, M. G., and Biondi, M. L. (1992). Role of endothelium-dependent releasing factor nitric oxide on renal function. *Journal of the American Society of Nephrology*, **2**, 1371–87.

Rosman, J. B., *et al.* (1989). Protein restricted diet in chronic renal failure: A four year follow up shows limited indication. *Kidney International*, **36** (Suppl. 27), S96–102.

Rosskopf, D., Dusing, R., and Siffert, W. (1993). Membrane sodium-proton exchange and primary hypertension. *Hypertension*, **21**, 607–17.

Ruilope, L. M., Lahera, V., Rodicio, J. L., and Romero, J. C. (1994). Are renal hemodynamics a key factor in the development and maintenance of arterial hypertension in humans. *Hypertension*, **23**, 3–9.

Saeki, S., Ogihara, T., and Masugi, F. (1986). A case of primary aldosteronism with polycystic kidney disease. *Nippon Naika Gakkai Zasshi*, **1**, 28–32.

Schacht, F. W. (1931). Hypertension in cases of cogenital polycystic kidney. *Archives of Internal Medicine*, **47**, 500–9.

Schmid, M., *et al.* (1990). Natriuresis-pressure relationship in polycystic kidney disease. *Journal of Hypertension*, **8**, 277–83.

Schuh, J. R., Blehm, D. J., Friedrich, G. E., McMahon, E. G., and Blaine, E. H. (1993). Differential effects of renin-angiotensin system blockade on atherogenesis in cholesterol-fed rabbits. *Journal of Clinical Investigation*, **91**, 1453–8.

Sedman, A., *et al.* (1987). Autosomal dominant polycystic kidney disease in childhood: A longitudinal study. *Kidney International*, **31**, 1000–5.

Slataper, R., Vicknair, N., Sadler, R., and Bakris, G. L. (1993). Comparative effects of different antihypertensive treatments on progression of diabetic renal disease. *Archives of Internal Medicine*, **153**, 973–80.

Taitz, L. S., Brown, C. B., Blank, C. E., and Steiner, G. M. (1987). Screening for polycystic kidney disease: Importance of clinical presentation in the new born. *Archives of Diseases of Childhood*, **62**, 45–9.

Torres, V., Wilson, D. M., Offord, K. P., Burnett, J. C., and Romero, J. C. (1989). Natriuretic response to volume expansion in polycystic kidney disease. *Mayo Clinic Proceedings*, **64**, 509–15.

Torres, V., Wilson, D. M., Burnett, J. C., Johnson, C. M., and Offord, K. P. (1991). Effect of inhibition of converting enzyme on renal hemodynamics and sodium management in polycystic kidney disease. *Mayo Clinic Proceedings*, **66**, 1010–17.

Torres, V., *et al.* (1992). Synthesis of renin by tubulocystic epithelium in autosomal dominant polycystic kidney disease. *Kidney International*, **42**, 364–73.

Uneda, S., *et al.* (1984). Renal hemodynamics and renin-angiotensin system in adolescents genetically predisposed to essential hypertension. *Journal of Hypertension*, **2**, (Suppl. 3), S437–9.

Valvo, E., *et al.* (1985). Hypertension of polycystic kidney disease: Mechanisms and hemodynamic alterations. *American Journal of Nephrology*, **5**, 176–81.

Van Hooft, I., Grobbee, D. E., Derky, F. H., de Leeuw, P. Schalekamp, M. A., and Hofman, A. (1991). Renal hemodynamics and the renin-angiotensin-aldosterone system in normotensive subjects with hypertensive and normotensive parents. *New England Journal of Medicine*, **324**, 1305–11.

Watson, M. L., Macnicol, A. M., and Allan, P. L. (1986). Genetic markers for polycystic kidney disease and their implications for detection of hypertension. *Journal of Hypertension*, **4** (Suppl. 6), 40–1.

Watson, M. L., Macnicol, A. M., Allan, P. L., and Wright, A. F. (1992). Effects of angiotensin converting enzyme inhibitor in adult polycystic kidney disease. *Kidney International*, **41**, 206–10.

Williams, P. S., Fass, G., Bone, J. M. (1988). Renal pathology and proteinuria determine progression in untreated mild/moderate chronic renal failure. *Quarterly Journal of Medicine*, **67**, 343–5.

Williams, R. H., and Harrison, T. R. (1937). A study of the renal arteries in relation to age and to hypertension. *American Heart Journal*, **14**, 645–58.

Yium, J., Gabow, P. A., Johnson, A., Kimberling, W., Martinez, and Maldonado, M. (1994). Autosomal dominant polycystic kidney disease in Blacks: Clinical cause and effects of sickle-cell hemoglobin. *Journal of the American Society of Nephrology*, **4**, 1670–4.

Zeier, M., Geberth, S., Ritz, E., Jaeger, T., and Waldherr, R. (1988). Autosomal dominant polycystic kidney disease — clinical problems. *Nephron*, **49**, 177–83.

Zeier, M., Geberth, S., Gonzalo, A., Chauveau, D., Grunfeld, J. P., and Ritz, E. (1992). The effect of uninephrectomy on progression of renal failure in autosomal dominant polycystic kidney disease. *Journal of the American Society of Nephrology*, **3**, 1119–23.

Zeier, M., Geberth, S., Schmidt, K. G., Mandelbaum, A., and Ritz, E. (1993). Elevated blood pressure profile and left ventricular mass in children and young adults with autosomal dominant polycystic kidney disease. *Journal of the American Society of Nephrology*, **3**, 1451–7.

17

Progression to renal insufficiency

Eberhard Ritz, Martin Zeier, and Rüdiger Waldherr

Introduction

Since the reputed first description of polycystic kidney disease post-mortem by Eustachio Fine in 1986, the disease was viewed, until recently, as leading inexorably to end-stage renal failure. This view may have to be modified, however, in the light of recent observations that indicate that previous estimates have been too negative as a result of ascertainment bias (Churchill *et al.* 1984). In the seminal paper of Dalgaard (Dalgaard 1957) all the 173 patients who had come to autopsy had suffered from uraemia unless they had died as a result of subarachnoid haemorrhage or urological complications. Churchill (1984) was the first to note, however, that a substantial proportion of autosomal dominant poly-cystic kidney disease (ADPKD) patients do not reach end-stage renal failure (ESRF). In an inception cohort study on 140 subjects from 17 kindreds in Newfoundland, Churchill documented that some subjects were carriers of the trait, but failed to develop endstage renal disease. The probability of one of the following: developing end-stage renal disease (ESRD); requiring dialysis/transplantation; or dying, was estimated using a time-to-event analysis. The probability of being alive and not having ESRD was 77 per cent by the age of 50, 57 per cent by the age of 58, and 52 per cent by the age of 73 years. These results have subsequently been confirmed by several other investigators (Gabow *et al.* 1984; Simon *et al.* 1989).

In one of our own series (Zeier 1993) covering 64 affected individuals the median age at ESRF was 52.5 years in males ($n = 34$), and 58 years in females ($n = 30$). By the age of 50, 45 per cent of the patients required dialysis or trans-plantation, and at the age of 60 the proportion was 80 per cent. Table 17.1 shows the age at the time of renal death according to gender in 29,319 individuals with ADPKD as reported by the EDTA registry (Ritz *et al.* submitted). In the past, it had been assumed that in ADPKD, ESRF occurs only beyond the third decade. It has become apparent, however, that children may reach ESRF after birth or in the first years of their lives (Gal *et al.* 1989). Although pre-viously such children were thought to represent misdiagnosed cases of recessive PKD, there is now consensus that perinatal renal failure is also a rare, but proven outcome in ADPKD. It appears that the pathogenesis of this outcome differs from the more common delayed development of ESRF and may perhaps have a distinct molecular basis.

Table 17.1 Autosomal dominant polycystic kidney disease: age at start of renal replacement therapy

Age (yrs)	Males (%)	Females (%)
< 15	0.13	0.17
15–24	0.39	0.50
25–34	3.1	2.35
35–44	19.7	14.9
45–54	38.1	37.1
55–64	26.8	30.3
65–74	9.94	12.5
> 75	1.89	2.21
Total (*n*)	17 692	11 627

There is obviously large variability of the age at renal death and the question arises whether this is due to: (1) variability of the rate of progression; (2) variability of the age of onset of renal failure; or (3) both (1) and (2). This will be discussed more fully below. The extent to which variability is due to genetic factors or environmental influences is currently unresolved. However, recent studies have clearly indicated genetic heterogeneity of ADPKD, the majority being coded on chromosome 16p13.3 (PKD1) (Reeders *et al.* 1985), but a sizeable proportion, perhaps 20 per cent or more, being coded on chromosome 4 (PKD 2) (Romeo *et al.* 1988). Possibly, even more subtypes may exist (Daoust *et al.* 1994). Renal prognosis is different in the two subtypes (see below). Interestingly, age at onset of ESRD is more homogenous within families than between families (Zeier *et al.* 1994a; Torra *et al.* 1994). The coefficient of variation of age at renal death between individuals was 20 per cent between families and 11 per cent within families in a series collected by our group, and smaller within-family variance was also reported from Barcelona (Torra *et al.* 1994). As indicated in Fig. 17.1, although age of onset of ESRF is more homogenous within families, the dispersion is such that the clinical value in predicting onset of ESRF is limited. The extent to which intrafamilial homogeneity is due to genetic factors (disease heterogeneity, e.g. PKD1 vs. PKD2; different intragenic mutations; non-allelic genetic determinants), or environmental factors remains unresolved. In this context, it is of particular interest that in preliminary studies no significant difference of age at renal death is noted between monozygotic and dizygotic twins (Grünfeld, personal communication). This observation, if confirmed, would cast doubt on the notion that the genetic background plays a major role in determining progression of ADPKD. Our case material also shows that the rate of progression becomes progressively smaller with advancing age. It is unclear, however, whether this is due to a greater proportional contribution of PKD2 in the higher age brackets.

The interesting issue has recently been raised as to whether a trend exists for renal death to occur at progressively higher ages. The discussion was based on

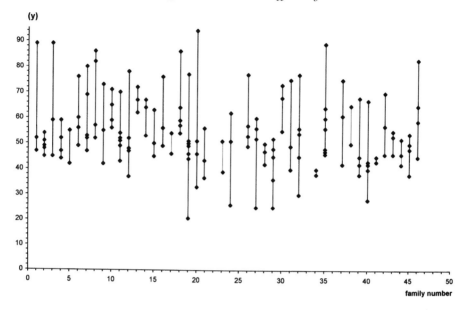

Fig. 17.1   Age at renal death in different families. Age at renal death (ordinate) in 46 different families (abscissa). Each symbol denotes age at renal death in one family member.

observations from Toronto (Roscoe *et al.* 1993), indicating that the age of onset of ESRF has increased in recent decades, possibly as a result of better medical management of such patients. These data, although encouraging, have not been consistently confirmed by other investigators. Table 17.2 shows our own observations; age at renal death has recently been higher. It is possible that the somewhat younger age in the post-mortem series (1950–70) compared to the higher age for individuals accepted for dialysis/transplantation is the result of ascertainment bias (i.e. acceptance of patients for renal replacement therapy at a somewhat earlier age). On the other hand, it is possible that in recent decades some individuals, as a result of antihypertensive treatment, never had ESRF, thus biasing the statistics based on ESRF estimates in an unfavourable direction.

Table 17.2   Age at renal death (autopsy for uraemia or start of renal replacement therapy) over four decades

Percentile	Age at renal death (1950–60)	Age at renal death (1980–90)
75th	71 yrs	74 yrs
Median	62 yrs	59 yrs
25th	44 yrs	52 yrs
No. of patients	21	23

Rate of progression of ADPKD

Until the mid-1980s, textbook wisdom held that the rate of progression in ADPKD was considerably lower compared to glomerular diseases (e.g. glomerulonephritis, Dalgaard 1971). We were struck by the observation (Gretz *et al.* 1989) that the rate of progression of renal failure in ADPKD was on average very rapid, the median interval between elevation of serum creatinine to 3 mg/dl and acceptance for renal replacement therapy being approximately 30 months (Fig. 17.2). This observation has been confirmed in several studies, for example, the observations in the Hopital Necker, Paris (Hannedouche *et al.* 1989) with an average rate of progression of 0.49 ml/min/month and the MDRD trial (MDRD in press), with 6.4 ml/min/year in males and 5.1 ml/min/year in females with moderate renal failure and a glomerular filtration rate (GFR) of 25–50 ml/min/1.73 m². Similarly, from the data of Gabow *et al.* (1992), an average rate of progression of approximately 5.0 ml/min/year can be estimated.

Effect of gender on progression of ADPKD

As shown in Fig. 17.3, median age at renal death was significantly lower in males than in females (Gretz *et al.* 1989). In individuals with serum creatinine levels above 3 mg/dl, this study showed a similar average rate of progression in the two genders. A gender difference was not noted in prepubertal subjects with renal disease (e.g. cystinosis or nephronophthisis). A factor predisposing male individuals to more adverse renal prognosis may be higher prevalence and severity of hypertension, at least early in the course of the disease. Theoretically, increased transcription of the renin gene under the influence of androgens could

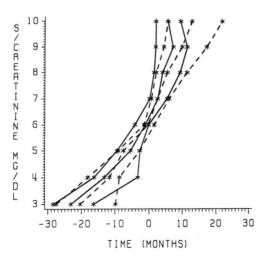

Fig. 17.2 Time interval between moderate renal failure (S-creatinine 3 mg/dl) and ESRF (S-creatinine 10 mg/dl) in male (——) and female (– – – –) patients with ADPKD. The lines represent 25th, 50th, and 75th percentiles. From Gretz *et al.* (1989).

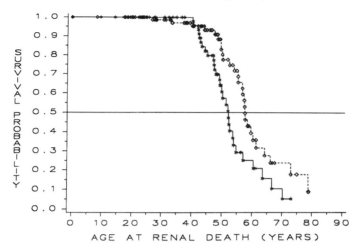

AGE AT RENAL DEATH (YEARS)

Fig. 17.3 Survival analysis of the age at renal death according to gender in 158 ADPKD patients. (*), men; (◇) women. From Gretz *et al.* (1989).

also play a role (Wagner *et al.* 1990). It is of interest that in the Han: SPRD model of cystic renal disease renal prognosis is also worse in male animal models, and that orchidectomy favourably affects evolution of renal failure (Zeier *et al.* in press). However, there have been some reports to the contrary (Gonzalo *et al.* 1990; Simon *et al.* 1991). The more benign course in female ADPKD patients has now been confirmed in a number of studies (Gabow *et al.* 1992). In contrast to the above estimates (Gretz *et al.* 1989), based on measurements of S-creatinine, the preliminary results of the recent MDRD trial (MDRD in press) show a more attenuated rate of progression in females compared to males; this finding was based on direct measurements of GFR.

Effect of urological complications on progression

ADPKD is known to be associated with a great number of urological problems (Zeier *et al.* 1988; Higashihara *et al.* 1992), urinary tract infection (UTI), urolithiasis, and particularly episodes of macrohaematuria. Previously, such urological complications often led to uninephrectomy (Zeier *et al.* 1991*b*; Bennett *et al.* 1985), but this has recently become rare because of better patient management, for example, use of antibiotics with good tissue-penetration characteristics (Bennett *et al.* 1985), use of lithotripsy, and non-invasive management of renal haemorrhage. In our own experience (Zeier *et al.* 1988), symptomatic UTI was the presenting symptom in 23 per cent. Thirty per cent of patients entering ESRF had experienced at least one symptomatic episode. Gross haematuria was the presenting feature of ADPKD in 23 per cent and had been present in 42 per cent of patients by the time ESRF had occurred. The corresponding figures for nephrolithiasis were 15 per cent and 20 per cent, respectively.

The issue of whether such urological complications adversely affect renal outcome has remained somewhat controversial. We found no relation between the presence of symptomatic UTI and risk of ESRF. However, in a larger cohort, Gabow *et al.* (1984) found that, at least in males, symptomatic UTI was associated with more adverse renal prognosis; the absence of an effect in females may be due to the frequent occurrence of lower UTI (i.e. infection), without invasion of renal tissue. Time will show whether the above findings are still relevant today with the availability of better antibiotic treatment.

There is no convincing evidence as to whether the presence of nephrolithiasis (Torres *et al.* 1993) has an impact on renal prognosis. Historical observation are again obsolete in view of modern treatment modalities (e.g. extracorporeal shock wave, lithotripsy, and percutaneous nephrostolithotomy).

Of particular interest with respect to the potential mechanisms that are involved in progression of renal failure of ADPKD is the observation of Gabow (Gabow *et al.* 1984; Gabow 1990) that a history of one or more episodes of gross haematuria is associated with worse renal outcome. An adverse effect on renal prognosis was found even in patients with microscopic haematuria. This observation has been confirmed by others, but is in conflict with our own observations (unpublished).

Heterogeneity of ADPKD (PKD1 vs. PKD2 vs. PKD3)

The variant of PKD coded on chromosome 4 is called PKD2 (Bear *et al.* 1992; Kimberling *et al.* 1993). The observation of Bear *et al.* (1992), who documented a more benign renal prognosis in families with PKD2 has been confirmed by at least three other groups (Gabow *et al.* 1992; Kimberling *et al.* 1993; Ceccherini *et al.* 1992). Bear and co-workers' observation was that average age of renal death was 56.3 years in PKD1, and 68.7 years in PKD2 families. In a paper on the hypothetical PKD3 variety (Daoust *et al.* 1994), the age of death of the uraemic patient was 50–60 years.

Anticipation or imprinting and progression

In several monogenic disorders (e.g. myodystrophy and Huntington's chorea), onset of the disease tends to occur at progressively younger ages in successive generations. This is thought to reflect accumulation of repetitive sequences of unstable DNA (i.e. repetitive short nucleotide sequences). This model of genetic transmission of disease has also been considered for ADPKD. There has been considerable interest whether onset of renal failure was lower in successive generations of ADPKD individuals. Fick *et al.* (1994) noted that anticipation of ESRD is found in 49 per cent of informative families, when early onset children are included: 53 per cent of informative families have at least one parent–offspring pair with anticipation. This observation, if confirmed, would have quite important implications with respect to the genetic mechanisms involved. The type of mutations identified so far provides no strong evidence for unstable

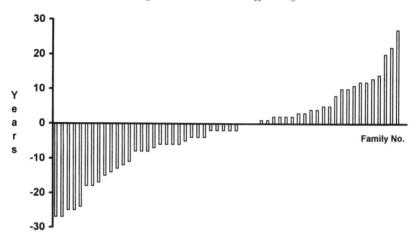

Fig. 17.4   Difference in age at renal death between parent and offspring in 54 families
with ADPKD. Negative values denote earlier age of onset of ESRF in offspring

DNA in ADPKD (EPKDC 1994). Furthermore, several groups, including ours,
failed to find evidence of anticipation (Torra *et al.* 1994; Geberth *et al.* 1994).
The difference of age at renal death (i.e. parent vs. offspring) in 46 patients
ranged from –26.3 years to +27.2 years, with a median of 1.05 years (Fig. 17.4).
Dispersion around the mean followed a Gaussian distribution according to the
Shapiro–Wilk test for normality (Geberth *et al.* 1994). Several authors noted
early onset of terminal renal failure in individuals who had inherited the
ADPKD trait from their mothers compared to those who had inherited
ADPKD from their fathers (Bear *et al.* 1992). This effect was interpreted as
evidence for imprinting. Imprinting refers to early partially irreversible
inactivation of DNA by methylation so that the transcriptional activities of
paternally and maternally transmitted DNA may differ, leading to unequal
expression of genes inherited from the two parents. Such an effect (i.e. earlier
onset of age at renal death in mother to son transmission) cannot be excluded on
the basis of our own findings (Geberth *et al.* submitted), but any such difference
is certainly minor and less than the 12-year difference in the original report
(Bear *et al.* 1992). The same may be true for the rate of progression (Grünfeld,
personal communication). Clearly, this issue requires further investigation.

Blood pressure and progression of ADPKD

Before antihypertensive treatment had become available, Hanson *et al.* (1974)
found established hypertension (i.e. blood pressure of 160/100 mmHg in 75 per
cent of patients with serum creatinine below 1.2 mg/dl and in 87 per cent of
patients with elevated serum creatinine). Table 17.3 shows the prevalence of
hypertension according to age and renal function, in ADPKD patients attending
the Heidelberg outpatient clinic. The prevalence of hypertension defined as

Table 17.3 Prevalence of hypertension (BP > 140/90, or antihypertensive treatment) in autosomal dominant polycystic kidney disease patients according to age and renal function

Age (yrs)	Normal renal function S-Cr < 1.2 mg/dl (n = 92)	Impaired renal functio S-Cr > 1.2 mg/dl (n = 125)
20–29	24/37 (65%)	6/7 (86%)
30–39	20/27 (74%)	15/16 (94%)
40–49	10/13 (77%)	52/60 (87%)
50–59	9/11 (82%)	27/31 (88%)
60–69	3/4 (75%)	9/11 (82%)

casual BP equal to or greater than 140/90 mmHg (or antihypertensive treatment) was considerably higher than in the age-matched general population even at serum creatinine levels below 1.2 mg/dl. Virtually all males with impaired renal function were hypertensive. The apparent decrease of prevalence with age may be a biostatistical artefact reflecting better survival of some normotensive patients. The higher BP in ADPKD patients compared to their non-affected siblings is shown in Fig. 17.5 (Watson *et al.* 1986). It is of note that in our cohort the prevalence of hypertension was similar in male and female patients (in contrast to that in the general population). Hypertension is also more common in smokers (again in contrast to the general population). (An interesting proposition is that this may be related to sympathetically mediated renal vasoconstriction under the influence of nicotine, but no direct data are available to support this hypothesis).

Several lines of evidence argue for a role of hypertension in progression of ADPKD. Vascular lesions are a prominent finding in the kidneys of ADPKD patients who have ESRF (Zeier, *et al.* 1991*a*), as discussed below. Sclerosis of renal arterioles (Fig. 17.6) was much more marked than sclerosis of the arterioles of other viscera. Sclerosis of intrarenal vessels, the hallmark of ADPKD, presumably reflects a particular susceptibility of renal vessels to BP-induced injury.

Hypertension is more frequent in ADPKD patients with impaired renal function (Zeier *et al.* 1994*b*), but such association does not provide evidence as to whether hypertension is the cause or the consequence of renal failure. Some authors attempted to solve this problem by comparing age at renal death (as an index of progression) in current and historical series (Roscoe *et al.* 1993). In the original series of Dalgaard (1957), age at patient death in 1957 was 41.5 years, whereas in a recent series ESRF occurred at an average age of 54.4 years (Roscoe *et al.* 1993). With some optimism, this finding was interpreted as indicating a more delayed onset of renal failure in recent decades as a result of antihypertensive treatment. Similar data were reported by others (Hannedouche *et al.* 1993). However, as indicated above, our own data are less reassuring in this respect (Table 17.2). In addition, a recent trial failed to show an effect of intensified antihypertensive treatment on the rate of progression in ADPKD (MDRD in press).

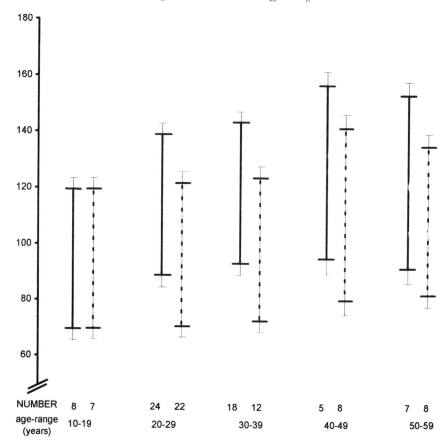

Fig. 17.5 Systolic and diastolic BP of patients affected by ADPKD (——); compared with the BP of their unaffected relatives (– – – –). From Watson *et al.* (1986).

It is of relevance to examine whether the presence of hypertension, or the level of BP, are related: (1) to the rate of progression; and (2) to age at onset of ESRD. A tendency for BP to rise is noted in carriers of the ADPKD trait as early as the second decade of life and this is particularly true for nocturnal BP (Zeier *et al.* 1993). We noted significantly higher BP, albeit within the range of normotension according to the World Health Organization, in patients with ADPKD after puberty, compared to matched controls. Even before puberty, however, left ventricular mass index (LVMI) (presumably an even more sensitive index of time-averaged BP exposure) was significantly higher in individuals with ADPKD compared to the matched controls (see Fig. 17.7). At a very early stage, BP is sodium-sensitive (Schmid *et al.* 1990; Harrap *et al.* 1991), and evidence for increased sensitivity of renal vasculature to ANG II (Watson *et al.* 1992) and inappropriately high ANG II-receptors (Schmid *et al.* 1990) is found. A constellation of a vasoconstricted, that is, ischaemic, sodium-retaining kidney with increased expression of renin both orthotopically in the juxtaglomerular

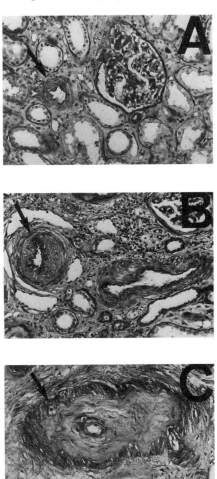

Fig. 17.6 Vascular lesions of various degrees in kidneys of patients with ADPKD and onset of ESRF (×190). (A) Arteriolar hyalinosis and mild intimal arterial thickening. (B) Moderate intimal fibrosis and medial thickening in interlobular and arcuate arteries. (C) Severe concentric sclerosis of interlobular and arcuate arteries. From Zeier *et al.* (1991*a*).

apparatus (Harrap *et al.* 1991) and ectopically in non-glomerular vessels (Zeier *et al.* 1991*a*; Graham and Lindop 1988; Torres *et al.* 1992), would be an ideal scenario for induction of vascular damage and renal interstitial fibrosis. This point is discussed in Chapter 16). Although there are good theoretical arguments to assume that a relation exists between BP and ADPKD progression, there are little data to prove it. Fig. 17.8 compares 1/S-creatinine and S-creatinine in normotensive and hypertensive ADPKD patients in the study of Gabow *et al.*

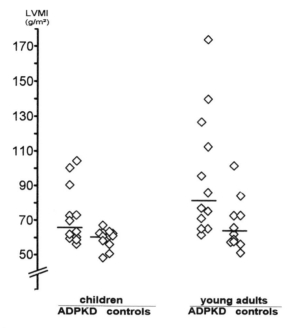

Fig. 17.7 Left ventricular mass index (LVMI) in children and young adults with ADPKD. The carriers of the ADPKD trait were compared to their age- and sex-matched controls. From Zeier *et al.* (1993).

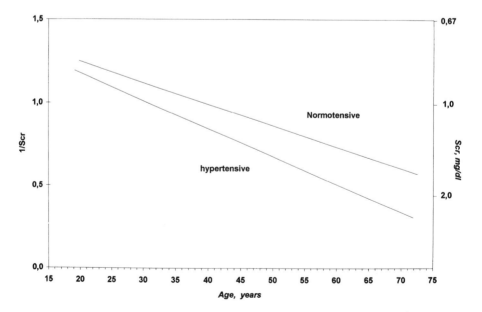

Fig. 17.8 The effect of BP on the progression of renal failure in 84 normotensive and 197 hypertensive ADPKD patients: 1/S-Cr and S-Cr one shown at different ages. From Gabow *et al.* (1984).

Table 17.4 Standardized graph 1/S-creatinine as a function of diastolic BP

Diastolic BP (mm Hg)	Slope
78	−5
87	−8
95	−13

Data courtesy of A. Gonzalo.

(1984). As shown in Table 17.4, a significant difference is found with respect to the slope 1/S-creatinine vs. time between normotensive and hypertensive ADPKD patients. However, this does not agree with observations in our own outpatient clinic. Recently, Grünfeld *et al.* (personal communication) found a modest correlation, at best, between achieved BP (during antihypertensive treatment) on the one hand, and progression of renal failure, assessed as loss of GFR according to the Cockroft formula, on the other.

A considerable lack of precise information continues to exist on this topic, and it is hoped that this will be resolved by appropriate prospective trials in the near future. However, we have recently tried to address this question using an entirely different approach. We reasoned that if hypertension were deleterious for renal function, superimposition of primary hypertension on ADPKD should cause more rapid deterioration of renal function and earlier onset of ESRF (Geberth *et al.* submitted). We examined 57 families where precise information was available concerning the BP of the parent who was not a carrier of the ADPKD trait (as verified by post-mortem or ultrasonography). As shown in Table 17.5, age at onset of ESRF was significantly lower in the offspring in families with primary hypertension (i.e. hypertension of the non-affected parent), than in offspring of families without primary hypertension. Since all offspring of patients with primary hypertension would not yet have developed hypertension by the third or fourth decade (i.e. when ESRF had occurred in ADPKD), the above difference is a minimum estimate. Nevertheless, the data strongly suggest that hypertension is deleterious for renal prognosis in ADPKD — as it is in other renal diseases, for example, in glomerulonephritis or diabetic nephropathy (Ritz *et al.* 1994).

Table 17.5 Age (years) at onset of ESRF in the offspring of 57 families with ADPKD, according to presence or absence of primary hypertension in the non-affected parent

BP in the non-affected parent	Age at renal death (trans. from mother)	Age at renal death (trans. from father)	Age at renal death (all patients combined)
Hypertension	47 (26–54) $n = 10$	51 (42–64) $n = 13$	49 (26–64) $n = 23$
Normotension	55 (28–82) $n = 18$	53 (42–69) $n = 16$	54 (28–69) $n = 34$
	n.s.	n.s.	P = 0.03

Diet and progression of ADPKD

Several uncontrolled retrospective trials suggested a benefit of protein-restricted diets on the rate of progression in ADPKD (Oldrizzi *et al.* 1985; Gretz *et al.* 1992). Oldrizzi *et al.* (1985) followed-up 17 patients with PKD having a mean serum creatinine of 2.4 mg/dl and substantial hypertension (mean arterial pressure (MAP) 114 mmHg) over an average of months providing a diet with 700 mg/day of phosphate and 0.6 g/kg protein/day. These patients were compared with a group of patients suffering from glomerulonephritis or PKD without dietary restriction. The authors concluded that in the intervention group a substantial proportion of patients (i.e. 68%) showed no progression. One has to be aware, however, of some methodological problems of this study, particularly its retrospective nature and the absence of matched controls.

In a group of patients with somewhat more advanced renal failure, the MDRD trial failed to note an effect of a diet with restricted protein and phosphorus intake on the rate of progression in patients with ADPKD (MDRD in press). Multivariate *post-hoc* analysis showed that in ADPKD patients (in contrast to patients with proteinuric glomerular disease) the rate of progression was completely unaffected by dietary intervention. This result is not unexpected in view of the fact that the kidney in ADPKD is already vasoconstricted (Harrap *et al.* 1991; Zeier *et al.* 1992). One would not anticipate a major benefit with respect to progression from protein restriction, an intervention which is thought to act, at least to a major extent, via reduction of renal perfusion and increase of preglomerular resistance.

Mechanisms of progression of ADPKD

In the past, it had been assumed on theoretical grounds that renal failure in ADPKD resulted from compression of residual normal renal parenchyma by expanding cysts, since renal tissue is trapped within the poorly distensible renal capsule (Franz and Reubi 1983; Zeier *et al.* 1992). Confirmation of this hypothesis by histological examination of renal tissue has not yet occurred, however. More recently, hyperfiltration and elevated glomerular pressure were thought to be the mechanisms underlying progression in a great number of renal diseases (Brenner *et al.* 1982). We tried to address this issue using two different approaches. First, according to the hyperfiltration theory, uninephrectomy should accelerate the rate of progression as demonstrated in various animal models of renal damage. We were able to collect a total of 47 patients with ADPKD from various European countries who had undergone uninephrectomy for urological emergencies. Median age at uninephrectomy was 41 years and median serum creatinine concentration 2.1 mg/dl. Progression to ESRF was noted in 28 of the 47 uninephrectomized patients. As shown in Fig. 17.9, the cumulative interval for the increase of serum creatinine from 4 to 8 mg/dl did not show accelerated progression in uninephrectomized patients (Zeier *et al.* 1991*b*). This observation provides an indirect argument against a potential role of hyperfiltration in progression of renal failure in ADPKD, at least in humans.

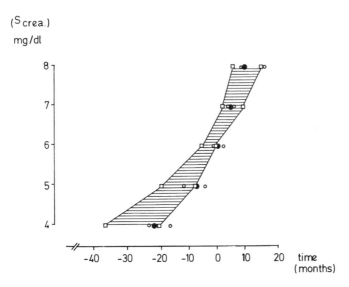

Fig. 17.9 Comparison of progression in uninephrectomized ADPKD patients and matched controls. The cumulative time interval for the increase of S-creatinine from 4 to 8 µg/dl in uninephrectomized ADPKD patients (○) and controls (●). The 25th, 50th, and 75th percentiles are shown. From Zeier *et al.* (1991b).

Interestingly in the Han: SPRD rat, (i.e. the male heterozygous polycystic rat), uninephrectomy accelerates progression, pointing to potential differences between human and rodent PKD (Zeier *et al.* in press). In a more direct approach, we recently compared (Zeier *et al.* 1991*a*) renal specimens obtained at surgery or post-mortem from ADPKD patients who had normal (or only borderline impairment of) renal function on the one hand, and patients with ESRF, on the other. Segmental glomerulosclerosis, the putative hallmark of hyperfiltration, was not a feature of ADPKD kidneys with ESRF (Fig. 17.10). However, global glomerulosclerosis, suggestive of renal ischaemia, was prevalent in the kidneys of ADPKD patients with terminal renal failure. The two features that were uniquely associated with ESRF were: (1) advanced vascular sclerosis of intrarenal arterioles (Fig. 17.6); and (2) marked interstitial fibrosis (Fig. 17.11). Semiquantitative scoring is given in Fig. 17.12. It is of note that sclerosis of afferent arterioles and interlobular arteries was present even in normotensive patients and was more severe in ADPKD patients than in patients with comparable renal dysfunction who suffered from glomerular disease. The vascular changes were vastly more marked in the kidney than in other organs, pointing to the particular susceptibility of renal vessels to a (hypothetical) insult, possibly related to elevated blood pressure, pressor agents (e.g. ANG II, growth factor, etc.). A second feature was severe interstitial fibrosis associated with scarce infiltrates of lymphocytes and macrophages and no evidence of extravasa-

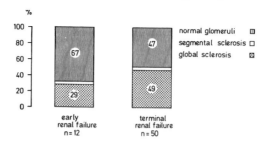

Fig. 17.10 Glomerular pathology in ADPKD patients in early and terminal renal failure. Symbols show percentage glomeruli with segmental sclerosis (□) or global sclerosis (▦); normal glomeruli (▥). Note low prevalence of segmental glomerulosclerosis. From Zeier *et al.* (1991a).

tion of tubular fluid; the latter was indicated by the absence of deposits of Tamm–Horsfall glycoprotein in the renal interstitium.

With respect to the possibility of compression of renal parenchyma by expanding cysts (Gretz *et al.* 1992), it is of note that in the ESRF kidneys intense tubular atrophy was found only in close vicinity to renal cysts, but not as a major generalized feature. A further argument against compression atrophy would be the observation that surgical decompression of cysts, which should relieve interstitial pressure, fails to improve GFR (Elzinga *et al.* 1992). We admit, however, that it is difficult to distinguish compression atrophy from atrophy as a result of interstitial fibrosis.

If a mechanical effect of cysts was involved in causing impairment of renal function, one would anticipate that a close relation existed between the number and the volume of cysts and the rate of progression. Such a relation is certainly not convincing. Gabow *et al.* (1984) found a highly significant ($P < 0.001$) relation between renal volume and adverse renal prognosis. Larger renal cysts (and also hepatic cysts) were associated with a more unfavourable renal outcome. Our limited experience suggests that this may well be the case in younger patients with ADPKD. A substantial number of elderly individuals, however, have normal or slightly impaired renal function despite the presence of huge renal cysts. Consequently, we do not find, overall, a relation between progression and the estimated number of cysts (by ultrasonography), or the diameter of the largest cysts (by ultrasonography) in our own patient material (unpublished observations). Whether the issue is confounded by a mixture of patients with PKD2, an intrisically more benign renal course, and a tendency to develop large cysts at an advanced age, is currently unresolved.

It emerges from the above that the mechanisms that cause progression of renal failure are poorly understood. Although convincing hypotheses have been advanced to explain the development of cysts (Ritz *et al.* 1993; Ye and Grantham 1993), the mechanisms leading to delayed loss of renal function in cyst-bearing kidneys are less well understood.

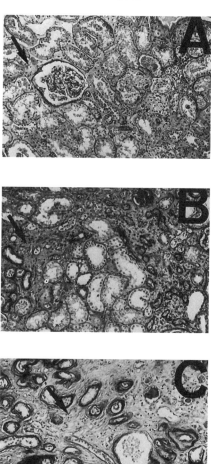

Fig. 17.11 Interstitial fibrosis and various degrees of tubular atrophy in kidneys of ADPKD patients with onset of ESRF (×125). (A) Small foci of mild interstitial fibrosis and occasional atrophic tubules. (B) Moderate focal interstitial fibrosis and tubular atrophy. (C) Diffuse severe interstitial fibrosis and widespread tubular atrophy. From Zeier *et al.* (1991*a*).

Conclusions

End-stage renal failure is the most dreaded complication of autosomal dominant polycystic kidney disease (ADPKD). However, recent observations show that progression is not universal. Factors that influence the rate of progression and the time of onset of terminal renal failure include the following: gender; type of disease (heterogeneity, i.e. PKD1 vs. PKD2); blood pressure; possibly cyst size;

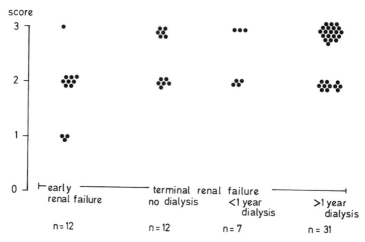

Fig. 17.12   Interstitial fibrosis scores in patients with ADPKD in early and terminal renal failure. From Zeier *et al.* (1991*a*).

number of episodes of macrohaematuria; and urinary tract infection. Interventions, for example, antihypertensive treatment and dietary restriction (i.e. restriction of protein and phosphate intake), are disappointingly ineffective in advanced renal failure. Based on theoretical consideration, antihypertensive treatment, particularly with ACE inhibitors, may be more effective if initiated early on. There is uncertainty concerning the mechanisms of progression, but glomerular hyperfiltration does not appear to play a role.

References

Bear, J. C., Parfrey, P. S., Morgan, J. M., Martin, C. J., and Cramer, B. C. (1992). Autosomal dominant polycystic kidney disease: new information for genetic counselling: *Am. J. Med. Genet.*, **43**, 548–53.

Bennett, W. M., Elzinga, L., Pulliam, J. P., Rashad, A. L., and Barry, J. M. (1985). Cyst fluid antibiotic concentrations in autosomal-dominant polycystic kidney disease. *Am. J. Kidney Dis.*, **6**, 400–4.

Brenner, B. M., Meyer, T. W., and Hostetter, T. H. (1982). Dietary protein intake and the progressive nature of kidney disease: the role of haemodynamically mediated glomerular injury in the pathogenesis of progressive glomerular sclerosis in ageing, renal ablation and and intrinsic renal disease. *New Engl. J. Med.*, **307**, 652–9.

Ceccherini, I., Matera, I., Sbrana, M., Di Donato, A., Yin, L., and Romeo, G. (1992). Radiation hybrids for mapping and cloning DNA sequences of distal 16p. *Somat. Cell. Mol. Genet.*, **18**, 319–24.

Churchill, D. N., Bear, J. C., Morgan, J., Payne, R. H., and McManamon, P. J. (1984). Prognosis of adult onset polycystic kidney disease re-evaluated. *Kidney Int.*, **26**, 190–3.

Dalgaard, O. Z. (1957). Bilateral polycystic kidney disease of the kidneys: a follow-up of two-hundred and eighty-four patients and their families. *Acta Med. Scand.*, **158**, 326–47.

Dalgaard, O. Z. (1971). Polycystic disease of the kidneys. In *Diseases of the kidney*, (2nd edn), (ed. by B. M. Strauss and L. G. Welt). Kluwer, Boston.

Daoust, M. C., Bichet, D. G., and Somlo, S. (1994). A French-Canadian family with autosomal dominant polycystic kidney disease (ADPKD) unlinked to ADPKD1 and ADPKD2 (Abstract). *J. Am. Soc., Nephrol.*, **4**, 262.

Elzinga, L. W., *et al.* (1992). Cyst decompression surgery for autosomal dominant polycystic kidney disease. (see Comments). *J. Am. Soc. Nephrol.*, **2**, 1219–26.

EPDKC (European Polycystic Kidney Disease Consortium) (1994). The polycystic kidney disease 1 gene encodes a 14 kb transcript and lies within a duplicated region on chromosome 16. *Cell* **77**, 6–20.

Fick, G. M., Johnson, A. M., and Gabow, B. A. (1994). Is there evidence for anticipation in autosomal-dominant polycystic kidney disease? *Kidney Int.*, **45**, 1153–62.

Fine, I. G. (1986). Eustachio's discovery of the renal tubule. *Am. J. Nephrol.*, **6**, 47–50.

Franz, K. A. and Reubi, E. C. (1983). Rate of functional deterioration in polycystic kidney disease. *Kidney Int.*, **23**, 526–9.

Gabow, P. A. (1990). Autosomal dominant polycystic kidney disease — more than a renal disease. *Am. J. Kidney Dis.*, **16**, 403–13.

Gabow, P. A., Ikle, D. W., and Holmes, J. H. (1984). Polycystic kidney disease: Prospective analysis of nonazotemic patients and family members. *Ann. Int. Med.*, **101**, 238–47.

Gabow, P. A., *et al.* (1992). Factors affecting the progression of renal disease in autosomal dominant polycystic kidney disease. *Kidney Int.*, **41**, 1311–19.

Gal, A., *et al.* (1989). Childhood manifestation of autosomal dominant polycystic kidney disease: no evidence for genetic heterogeneity. *Clin. Genet.*, **35**, 13–19.

Geberth, S., Zeier, M., Stier, E., and Ritz, E. (1994). No evidence for anticipation of age at renal death in autosomal dominant polycystic kidney disease (ADPKD). *J. Am. Soc. Nephrol.*, **5**, 646.

Geberth, S., Stier, E., Zeier, M., Mayer, G., and Ritz, E. (Submitted). More adverse renal prognosis of autosomal dominant polycystic kidney disease (ADPKD) in families with primary hypertension.

Gonzalo, A., Rivera, M., Quereda, C., and Ortuno, J. (1990). Clinical features and prognosis of adult polycystic kidney disease. *Am. J. Nephrol.*, **10**, 470–4.

Graham, P. C. and Lindop, G. B. (1988). The anatomy of the renin-secreting cell in adult polycystic Kidney Disease. *Kidney Int.*, **33**, 1084–90.

Gretz, N. and Strauch, M. (1992). Effect of a low-protein diet on the rate of progression of chronic renal failure in patients with polycystic kidney disease. *Contrib. Nephrol.*, **97**, 93–100.

Gretz, N., Zeier, M., Geberth, S., Strauch, M., and Ritz, E. (1989). Is gender a determinant for evolution of renal failure? A study in autosomal dominant polycystic kidney disease. *Am. J. Kidney Dis.*, **14**, 178–83.

Hannedouche, T., Chauveau, P., Fehrat, A., Albouze, G., and Jungers, P. (1989). Effect of moderate protein restriction on the rate of progression of chronic renal failure. *Kidney Int.*, (Suppl.), **27**, S91–5.

Hannedouche, T., Albouze, G., Chauveau, P., Lacour, B., and Jungers, P. (1993). Effects of blood pressure and antihypertensive treatment on progression of advanced chronic renal failure. *Am. J. Kidney Dis.*, **21**, 131–7.

Hansson, L., Karlander, L. E., Lundgren, W., and Peterson, L. E. (1974). Hypertension in polycystic kidney disease. *Scand. J. Urol. Nephrol.*, **8**, 203–205.

Harrap, S. B., *et al.* (1991). Renal, cardiovascular and hormonal characteristics of young adults with autosomal dominant polycystic kidney disease. *Kidney Int.*, **40**, 501–8.

Higashihara, E., Aso, Y., Shimazaki, J., Ito, H., Koiso, K., and Sakai, O. (1992). Clinical aspects of polycystic kidney disease. *J. Urol.*, **147**, 329–32.

Kimberling, W. J., Kumar, S., Gabow, P. A., Kenyon, J. B., Connolly, C. J., and Somlo, S. (1993). Autosomal dominant polycystic kidney disease: localization of the second gene to chromosome 4q13-q23. *Genomics*, **18**, 467–72.

MDRD (Modification in Diet in Renal Disease — Study Group) (in press). *JAMA*,

Oldrizzi, L., *et al.* (1985). Progression of renal failure in patients with renal disease of diverse etiology on protein-restricted diet. *Kidney Int.*, **27**, 553–7.

Reeders, S. T., *et al.* (1985). A highly polymorphic DNA marker linked to adult polycystic kidney disease on chromosome 16. *Nature*, **317**, 542–4.

Ritz, E., Fliser, D., Wiecek, A., and Siebels, M. (1994). Hypertension and renal disorders. In *Metabolic aspects of hypertension*, (ed. N. M. Kaplan) Dallas.

Ritz, E., Zeier, M., Geberth, S., and Waldherr, R. (1993). Autosomal dominant polycystic kidney disease (ADPKD) — mechanisms of cyst formation and renal failure. *Aust. N. Z. J. Med.*, **23**, 35–41.

Ritz, E., Jones, E., Waldherr, R., and Zeier, M. The patient with ADPKD on maintenance haemodialysis. *Nephron*, (submitted).

Romeo, G., Devoto, M., Costa, G., Roncuzzi, L., and Catizone, L. (1988). A second genetic locus for autosomal dominant polycystic kidney disease. Lancet **2**, 8–11.

Roscoe, J. M., Brissenden, J. E., Williams, E. A., Chery, A. L., and Silverman, M. (1993). Autosomal dominant polycystic kidney disease in Toronto. *Kidney Int.*, **44**, 1101–8.

Schmid, M., *et al.* (1990). Natriuresis-pressure relationship in polycystic kidney disease. *J. Hypertens.*, **8**, 277–3.

Simon, P. and Thebaud, H. E. (1989). Prognosis of adult polycystic kidney disease re-evaluated: Results of an investigation in 1112 patients from 369 kindreds (Abstract). *J. Am. Soc. Nephrol.*, **38**,

Simon, P., Thebaud, H. E., and Albouze, G. (1991). Comparative clinical study of early and late forms of kidney polycystic disease in adults. *Rev. Med. Intern.*, **12**, S345.

Torra, R., Darnell, A., Botey, A., Estivill, X., and Revert, L. (1994). Interfamilial and intrafamilial variability of clinical expression in autosomal dominant polycystic kidney disease. *Vimercate, abstract meeting on ADPKD*

Torres, V. E., *et al.* (1992). Synthesis of renin by tubulocystic epithelium in autosomal-dominant polycystic kidney disease. *Kidney Int.*, **42**, 364–73.

Torres, V. E., Wilson, D. M., Hattery, R. R., and Segura, J. W. (1993). Renal stone disease in autosomal dominant polycystic kidney disease. *Am. J. Kidney Dis.*, **22**, 513–19.

Wagner, D., *et al.* (1990). Androgen dependence and tissue specificity of renin messenger RNA expression in mice. *J. Hypertens.*, **8**, 45–52.

Watson, M. L., Macnicol, A. M., Allan, P. L., Clayton, J. E., Reeders, S. T., and Wright, A. F. (1986). Genetic markers for polycystic kidney disease and their implications for detection of hypertension. *J. Hypertens.*, **4**, (Suppl. 6), s40–1.

Watson, M. L., Macnicol, A. M., Allan, P. L., and Wright, A. F. (1992). Effects of angiotensin converting enzyme inhibition in adult polycystic kidney disease. *Kidney Int.*, **41**, 206–10.

Ye, M. and Grantham, J. J. (1993). The secretion of fluid by renal cysts from patients with autosomal dominant polycystic kidney disease. *N. Engl. J. Med.*, **329**, 310–13.

Zeier, M. (1993). Die autosomal dominante polycystische Nierenkrankheit (Zystennieren)-klinische, morphologische, molekularbiologische und tierexperimentelle Untersuchungen. Doctoral thesis. University of Heidelberg, Heidelberg.

Zeier, M., Geberth, S., Ritz, E., Jaeger, T., and Waldherr, R. (1988). Adult dominant polycystic kidney disease — clinical problems. *Nephron*, **49**, 177–83.

Zeier, M., Fehrenbach, P., Geberth, S., Möhring, K., Waldherr, R., and Ritz, E. (1991*a*). Renal histology in polycystic kidney disease with incipient and advanced renal failure. *Kidney Int.*, **42**, 1259–65.

Zeier, M., Geberth, S., Gonzalo, A., Chauveau, D., Grünfeld, J. P., and Ritz, E. (1991*b*). Effect of uninephrectomy and progression of renal failure in autosomal dominant polycystic kidney disease. *J. Am. Soc. Nephrol.*, **3**, 1119–23.

Zeier, M., Schmid, M., Nowack, R., Zacharewics, S., Hasslacher, C., and Ritz, E. (1992). The response of GFR to amino acids differs between autosomal dominant polycystic kidney disease (ADPKD) and glomerular disease (see Comments). *Nephrol. Dial. Transplant.*, **7**, 501–6.

Zeier, M., Geberth, S., Schmidt, K. G., Mandelbaum, A., and Ritz, E. (1993). Elevated blood pressure profile and left ventricular mass in children and young adults with autosomal dominant polycystic kidney disease. *J. Am. Soc. Nephrol.*, **3**, 1451–7.

Zeier, M., Geberth, S., Stier, E., and Ritz, E. (1994*a*). Evolution of renal failure in autosomal dominant polycystic kidney disease (ADPKD) is more homogenous within families. *Int. Congress in Nephrology. Jerusalem. 1993*, p 610.

Zeier, M., Ritz, E., Geberth, S., and Gonzalo, A. (1994*b*). Genesis and significance of hypertension in autosomal dominant polycystic kidney disease. *Nephron*, **68**, 155–8.

Zeier, M., Pohlmeier, G., Deerberg, F., Schönherr, R., and Ritz, E. (1994). Progression of renal failure in the HAN: SPRD polycystic kidney model. *Nephrol. Dial. Transplant.*, **9**, 1734–39.

18

Management of end–stage renal failure and problems of transplantation in autosomal dominant polycystic kidney disease

Bruce Culleton and Patrick S. Parfrey

Introduction

Autosomal dominant polycystic kidney disease is the most common renal cystic disease which causes end-stage renal disease (ESRD) in adults. In Canada, the prevalence of polycystic kidney disease (PKD) among registered ESRD patients was 6.3 per cent ($n = 1205$) at the end of 1991 (Canadian Organ Replacement Registry; CORR 1993). PKD occurred in 5.3 per cent ($n = 135$) of new patients starting ESRD therapy during 1991, an incidence virtually unchanged since the previous decade (CORR 1993). Prevalence rates are similar throughout the world, although it has been reported that the disease is rare in Africa (Habte and Abraha 1983), and may be less common in American blacks than whites (Torres *et al.* 1985).

Age of onset of end–stage renal disease (ESRD)

Symptomatic clinical presentation usually occurs between the second and sixth decades, with about half the patients having ESRD by the age of 60 years. (Parfrey *et al.* 1990; Gabow *et al.* 1992; Churchill *et al.* 1984). However, the age of onset has a considerable range, from 2 to 80 years being reported. Figure 18.1 shows the natural history of autosomal dominant polycystic kidney disease type I (Parfrey 1993). Cysts are nearly always present before the age of 30 years. On average, renal impairment has occured by the end of the fifth decade and end-stage disease occurs within the next 10 years. Those who do not develop ESRD usually maintain good renal function with serum creatinine less than 140 µmol/1 (Churchill *et al.* 1984), and have a life expectancy similar to the general population (Hatfield and Pfister 1972).

ESRD Therapy and ADPKD

Figure 18.2 shows the relatively good prognosis for patients with PKD disease who develop ESRD compared with other causes of ESRD (i.e. 70 per cent survival at five years; CORR 1993). Renal replacement therapy consists of

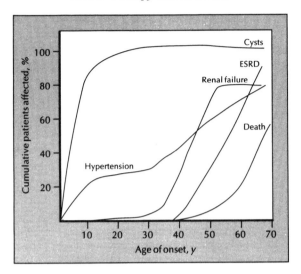

Fig. 18.1 The clinical course of autosomal dominant polycystic kidney disease. (From *Current Opinion in Nephrology and Hypertension* (1993), **2**, 192–200, with permission.)

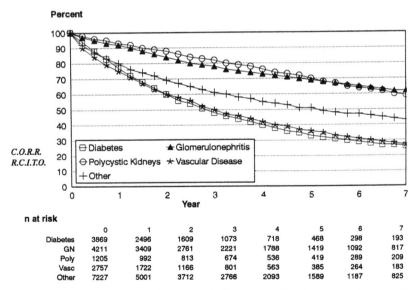

Fig. 18.2 Patient survival by primary renal disease in all registered patients in Canada from 1981 to 1991. (From the Canadian Organ Replacement Registry 1993, with permission.)

peritoneal or haemodialysis, or transplantation. The choice of therapy is highly dependent on individual patient factors, but is not significantly different from non-polycystic patients. The three existing modalities of treatment for end-stage renal failure are complementary and not mutually exclusive. In our patients who developed ESRD, dialysis and/or transplantation prolonged life by an average of 14 years (Barrett and Parfrey 1991).

Dialysis

The survival of patients with ADPKD appears to be as good as, if not better, than other non-diabetics on dialysis. Singh and Hanriharan (1991) reported survival for ESRD patients with ADPKD to be similar to that for the general ESRD population, excluding diabetics. Mendelssohn *et al.* (1988) reported 1- and 5-year actuarial survival rates of 93 and 77 per cent, respectively for ADPKD patients on haemodialysis, although there was no control comparison. Recent data from the EDTA registry confirmed actuarial survival was better for patients with ADPKD than for patients with other standard primary chronic renal disease, excluding diabetes mellitus (Ritz *et al.* 1994). In Canada, dialysis patients with PKD had a significant, beneficial hazard ratio for survival of 0.84, after adjustment for age, type of dialysis, primary diagnosis, calender period of starting ESRD therapy, and centre size (CORR 1993).

There is very little literature available concerning the treatment of patients with ADPKD by peritoneal dialysis. However, it is generally accepted that the large mass of the kidneys does not interfere with this form of dialysis (Ito *et al.* 1985; Barrett and Parfrey 1991; Singh and Hariharan 1991; Bennett and Elzinga 1993). Mendelssohn *et al.* (1988) reported that none of their patients needed to be transferred from peritoneal to haemodialysis for simple mechanical reasons. Minimal data exist concerning the efficacy of continuous ambulatory peritoneal dialysis (CAPD) in the treatment of uraemia in ADPKD patients, although there appears to be no reason why it should be different from the general non-polycystic population.

Clinical problems

In the ADPKD population on ESRD therapy, problems frequently encountered include those associated with the type of dialysis, and those associated with ADPKD itself — both renal and extrarenal problems. Other problems inherent with end-stage renal failure will not be discussed here.

The most common causes of death are related to infections and coronary artery disease (Singh and Hariharan 1991; Barrett and Parfrey 1991). It has recently been suggested that mortality from coronary artery disease is significantly less than that associated with other primary chronic renal diseases (Ritz *et al.* 1994). It has been postulated that the protective effect from a cardiac death appears to be related to less severe anaemia seen in ADPKD, a finding which has been previously documented (Vaughan 1990). This effect appears to be independent of left ventricular hypertrophy or lipoprotein parameters. In addition, cerebrovascular deaths are somewhat more frequent in ADPKD patients on dialysis, possibly because of aneurysmal bleeding (Ritz *et al.* 1994). Once dialysis is instituted, there is less difficulty in blood pressure control (Lazarus *et al.* 1971), and in fact, may be lower than average, with usual fluid removal, in the ADPKD population (Chester *et al.* 1978).

Comparative data on the frequency, duration, and reason for hospitalization in ADPKD patients of ESRD therapy are not available. Singh and Hanriharan (1991) reported a total hospital stay that amounted to 3 per cent of the total time at risk, which is not different from that in the non-ADPKD patients on ESRD therapy (Ito *et al.* 1985).

Problems associated with dialysis procedure

Problems associated with the dialysis procedure itself include vascular access problems in the haemodialysis group and peritonitis–catheter related infections in peritoneal dialysis patients. There is no literature to support a difference in vascular access problems in ADPKD patients compared with non-polycystic patients. With respect to recurrent or complicated peritonitis, the US National CAPD Registry found no difference in median number of months to first, second, or third episodes of peritonitis from the time CAPD was started in ADPKD patients compared to the patients with ESRD due to other cause (Nolph *et al.* 1985). This is also supported in other series (Singh and Hariharan 1991). However, there appears to be an increased incidence of peritonitis secondary to intestinal perforation which is felt to be due to colonic diverticula (Scheff *et al.* 1980). Subsequent reports have supported diverticula as a cause, but have also implicated ischaemic intestinal necrosis (Singh and Hariharan 1991; Graham *et al.* 1986).

Renal problems

Renal problems associated with ADPKD and ESRD include hypertension, pain, haemorrhage, urinary tract infections, renal masses (including malignancy), and nephrolithiasis. These problems are discussed in detail in other chapters and only points particular to the treatment of ESRD will be considered here.

Renal bleeding may take the form of haematuria, intracystic haemorrhage, or perirenal haemorrhage. The differential diagnosis includes neoplasms, calculi, and infections. Haemorrhage into cysts or perirenally is usually well seen by computed tomography (CT) (Levine and Grantham 1985). Cystoscopy, angiography, or CT imaging may be required to investigate the possibility of a neoplasm causing the haematuria. Dialysis with heparin does not necessarily increase the risk of bleeding (Delaney *et al.* 1985), but if major bleeding occurs, heparin should be avoided or closely controlled. Uraemia-associated coagulation defects may also predispose to bleeding. Bleeding is usually best managed with conservative measures including bed rest, analgesia, and transfusion as needed. Severe, persistent bleeding may require surgical intervention such as arterial embolization (Harley *et al.* 1980), or nephrectomy.

ESRD patients with cyst infections create major diagnostic and therapeutic difficulties. They may have new areas of renal tenderness and positive blood cultures, while their urine (if produced) may be sterile. Other sources of infection must be excluded. This includes infected liver cysts, diverticulitis, vascular access infection, or endocarditis — given the increased incidence of valvular abnormalities in the ADPKD population (Hossack *et al.* 1988). If a cyst or a complicated urinary tract infection is suspected in an ESRD patient, renal imaging is required. Plain films may show stones, obscuring of the psoas shadow, and gas collections. Ultrasound (US) or CT scanning may further delineate abscess collections (Gerzof and Gale 1982). [111I]-labelled leucocytes may be of some value in identifying the source of infection (Fortner *et al.* 1986; Bretan *et al.* 1988). Planar gallium scanning is of questionable benefit, with a sensitivity as low as 50 per cent (Schwab *et al.* 1987). The choice of antibiotics to treat renal cyst infections is discussed elsewhere in this text. In patients with ESRD, antibiotics often need adjustment by increasing dosing interval and supplementing after dialysis.

There are a number of case reports of renal malignancy coexisting with ADPKD (Ng and Suki 1980; Keith *et al.* 1994; Gatalica *et al.* 1994). There is also a high incidence of hyperplastic renal polyps (90 per cent) and micro-adenomas (24 per cent) (Zeier *et al.* 1988; Gregoire *et al.* 1987). It has been stated that the incidence of renal malignancy is higher than expected by chance, but the calculations are based on figures subject to selection bias (Bernstein *et al.* 1987). Also, autopsy studies have failed to demonstrate an increased risk of renal cell carcinoma in patients with ADPKD. On the other hand, the risk of renal cell carcinoma in dialysis patients with acquired renal cystic disease is unquestionably, approximately 0.5–1 per cent per year of observation (Lafayette *et al.* 1994). By the time a patient with ADPKD reaches ESRD the kidneys are usually very large and easily palpable. This makes differentiation of discrete, solid, renal masses difficult even with the best of imaging procedures. Symptoms, such as flank pain and haematuria, are common presenting symptoms for neoplasia, but are frequent symptoms in ADPKD anyway. For these reasons the diagnosis of kidney carcinoma in patients with ADPKD is often very difficult. In these instances CT, magnetic resonance imaging (MRI) (Hilpert *et al.* 1986; Keith *et al.* 1994), angiogram, or possibly nephrectomy may be required (Zeier *et al.* 1988).

Non-renal problems

Non-renal problems associated with ADPKD and ESRD include hepatic cysts, intracranial aneurysms, subdural haematomas, cardiac abnormalities, colonic diverticula, and pulmonary emboli.

Autopsy studies report liver cysts in 15–75 per cent of cases of ADPKD (Milutinovic *et al.* 1980). Cyst prevalence increases with age (Thomsen and Thaysen 1988), and is more frequently seen in females (Kaehny *et al.* 1988). In patients on dialysis, hepatic complications including liver cyst infection or carcinoma, may be responsible for death. Grunfeld (1985) reported 10.5 per cent of patients with ADPKD, undergoing haemodialysis, who died as a result of these hepatic complications. CT and radionuclide studies may be useful in determining infection in liver cysts (London *et al.* 1988). Gladziwa *et al.* (1993) has reported successful non-operative CT-guided percutaneous catheter drainage of infected liver cysts.

The management of cerebral aneurysms in ADPKD patients is similar for patients with normal renal function and for those with ESRD. This is discussed in detail elsewhere in this monograph (Chapter 22).

Subdural haematoma is an occasional complication in patients on dialysis. ADPKD was the underlying renal disease in 4 of 12 cases of subdural haematoma associated with haemodialysis. It is very uncommon in patients on CAPD, but two cases have been reported in patients with ADPKD (Wheeler 1987). This susceptibility may be related to poor vascular support by connective tissue.

The prevalence of mitral, aortic, and tricuspid valve disease is also increased in ADPKD and should always be considered in the ADPKD patient with bacteraemia, or fever with no obvious clinical source. Emboli from affected valves should always be considered in the patient who presents with a cerebrovascular accident.

The principal involvement of the gastrointestinal tract is colonic diverticula. The largest study to date has reported an 82 per cent frequency in 12 patients with ADPKD who were receiving dialysis (Scheff *et al.* 1980). Diverticular disease should always be considered when patients develop polymicrobial peritonitis while on peritoneal dialysis.

Pulmonary diseases, including infections, also cause significant morbidity in ADPKD patients on renal replacement therapy. Pulmonary embolism was reported to occur in 7 of 54 patients in one series (Singh and Hariharan 1991). The reason for this complication is not clear, and has not been reported elsewhere.

Transplantation

Renal transplantation was once thought to be too high a risk for most patients who develop end-stage renal disease secondary to ADPKD because of their relatively advanced age. With improvements in immunosuppressive therapy, and emphasis on quality of life, transplantation is now the treatment of choice for patients less than 65 years of age with end-stage renal disease and ADPKD. Of course, individual patient factors, such as extent of cardiovascular disease, presence of active infection, and suitability for immunosuppresive therapy, must also be considered.

Survival

Patient and graft survival appears to be similar to that of other non-diabetic controls (Figs 18.3 and 18.4) (CORR 1993, Fitzpatrick *et al.* 1990). The 5-year patient survival after transplantation is over 80 per cent, and the 5-year graft survival is about 70 per cent. Graft and patient survival of polycystic patients after renal transplantation is no different from those with glomerulonephritis, after adjustment for age, calendar period, centre size and donor source. ADPKD does not recur in grafts (Tzardis *et al.* 1989).

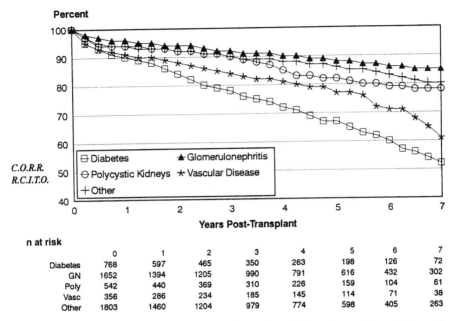

n at risk

	0	1	2	3	4	5	6	7
Diabetes	768	597	465	350	263	198	126	72
GN	1652	1394	1205	990	791	616	432	302
Poly	542	440	369	310	226	159	104	61
Vasc	356	286	234	185	145	114	71	38
Other	1803	1460	1204	979	774	598	405	263

Fig. 18.3   Patient survival after first cadaveric renal graft by primary diagnosis in registered patients in Canada, 1981–91 (From the Canadian Organ Replacement Registry 1993, with permission.)

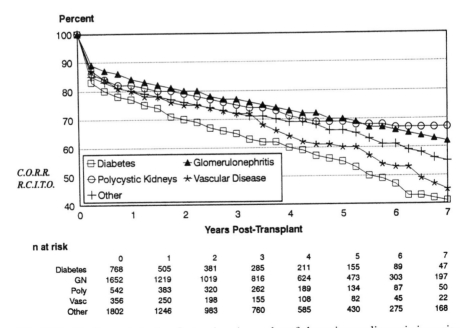

n at risk

	0	1	2	3	4	5	6	7
Diabetes	768	505	381	285	211	155	89	47
GN	1652	1219	1019	816	624	473	303	197
Poly	542	383	320	262	189	134	87	50
Vasc	356	250	198	155	108	82	45	22
Other	1802	1246	983	760	585	430	275	168

Fig. 18.4   Graft survival after first cadaveric renal graft by primary diagnosis in registered patients in Canada, 1981–91 (From the Canadian Organ Replacement Registry 1993, with permission.)

Though the question is often raised, there has not been a large prospective study comparing survival in haemodialysis patients with transplant patients. From retrospective analyses and small prospective studies there appears to be equivalent survival in both groups. Mendelssohn *et al.* (1988), in a small prospective series of 35 patients (mean age 50 years, range 28–65), showed no difference in 5-year survival of patients on haemodialysis vs. those receiving transplantation (77 and 73 per cent, respectively). Beyond five years a trend towards increased survival in the transplant group was seen.

Transplantation considerations

The majority of kidneys being transplanted are of cadaveric origin, mainly because of the hereditary nature of ADPKD. In an ADPKD population, Hannig *et al.* (1992) reported only 7 per cent of the transplants utilized a living related donor compared to the 20 per cent reported for all renal transplants. It has been accepted that related donors should be considered if they have a negative US or CT of kidney when aged over 30 years of age (Parfrey *et al.* 1990). However, in informative families, the use of gene linkage studies should allow the use of more living related donors. This approach has been limited by the necessity to have relatively large families. The recent discovery of a portion of the abnormal PKD1 gene brings closer the ability to detect the abnormal gene with a blood test from the potential donor.

ADPKD frequently leads to ESRD at an advanced age, which often increases the chances of clinically important cardiac disease being present prior to transplantation. This often requires an echocardiogram to assess left ventricular function as well as presence or absence of mitral valve disease. Aorto-iliac angiography is frequently performed as well because pelvic arteriosclerosis is commonly present. Some series report fewer than one-third of patients receive the standard end-to-end renal artery to internal iliac artery anastomosis because of this problem (Bennett and Elzinga 1993). In preventing post-transplant urinary retention, older men may require assessment of their prostate prior to surgery. Transurethral resection is the easiest way to manage significant prostatic hypertrophy. The management of diverticular disease prior to transplant remains controversial. Some centres advise routine screening in the form of a barium enema before elective transplant (Novick and Ho-Hseih 1985). However, prophylactic surgery is not widely accepted.

One of the major problems confronting transplant surgeons is whether or not to remove native polycystic kidneys. Routine, pre-transplant, bilateral nephrectomy was performed in many centres in the past. Papers continue to be published supporting the practice of ADPKD recipient bilateral nephrectomy (Rayner *et al.* 1990). However, a large body of evidence exists showing that patients transplanted with native kidneys *in situ* do not present major problems related to these kidneys (Sanfilippo *et al.* 1983; Mendelssohn *et al.* 1988; Ho-Hseih *et al.* 1987; Tzardis *et al.* 1989; Fitzpatrick *et al.* 1990).

But there have been no prospective trials to confirm these data. Certainly, the advantage of leaving native kidneys *in situ* leaves fewer problems with fluid balance, in particular if transplant rejection necessitates a return to peritoneal or haemodialysis, or if transplantation is delayed and the interval between nephrectomy and transplant is prolonged. The advent of erythropoietin has dramatically decreased the problem of anaemia in patients who have had bilateral nephrectomy. Our only indications for pre-transplant nephrectomy include those patients with frequent renal infections, neoplasia, or major bleeding. Occasionally, the sheer bulk of the kidneys may make surgery necessary to make room for a transplant.

Clinical problems

The risks and problems inherent with immunosuppression are no different in the ADPKD transplant patients than other transplant recipients. Causes of graft loss in patients with ADPKD are no different than from other patients with non-polycystic renal disease. Acute or chronic rejection, patient death with a functioning graft, and sepsis are the major reasons for graft loss (Delaney *et al.* 1991).

Hypertension following transplant remains a significant problem. This is felt to be mainly secondary to cyclosporin and its direct toxic effect at the level of the peripheral vasculature (Bennett and Porter 1988). Dose reduction may be of some benefit (Calabrese *et al.* 1982).

Not unexpectedly, death from cardiovascular events remain the primary cause of mortality in this patient group. There is no significant difference when compared to other age-matched transplant groups in previously reported series (Tzardis *et al.* 1989; Fitzpatrick *et al.* 1990; Singh and Hariharan 1991). However, Florijn *et al.* (1994) reported that the use of azathioprine in post-transplant ADPKD patients was associated with enhanced risk of cardiovascular death when compared with non-polycystic controls, and matched for age and cardiovascular risk factors. This has yet to be confirmed in other reports.

Conclusions

The prognosis of polycystic kidney disease during end-stage renal disease therapy is good compared to other causes of ESRD. Patients with ESRD appear to do quite well on haemodialysis and achieve an improvement in quality of life. Therefore, Transplantation should be offered to all patients who fulfil the usual criteria. The post-transplant management of these patients is not significantly different from that of non-polycystic transplant recipients.

References

Barrett, B. J. and Parfrey, P. S. (1991). Autosomal dominant polycystic kidney disease and end-stage renal disease. *Seminars in Dialysis*, **4**, 26–32.
Bennett, W. M. and Elzinga, L. W. (1993). Clinical management of autosomal dominant polycystic kidney disease. *Kidney International*, **44**, (Suppl. 42), S74–9.

Bennett, W. M. and Porter, G. A. (1988). Cyclosporin-associated hypertension. *American Journal of Medicine*, **85**, 131–3.

Bernstein, J., Evan, A. P., and Gardner, K. D. (1987). Epithelial hyperplasia in human polycystic kidney diseases. *American Journal of Pathology*, **129**, 92–101.

Bretan, P. N., Price, D. C., and McClure, R. D. (1988). Localization of abscess in adult polycystic kidney by indium-111 leukocyte scan. *Urology*, **32**, 169–71.

Calabrese, G., Vagelli, G., Cristofano, C., and Barsotti, G. (1982). Behaviour of arterial pressure in different stages of polycystic kidney disease. *Nephron*, **32**, 207–8.

CORR (Canadian Organ Replacement Registry) (1993, April). *1991 Annual Report*, Hospital Medical Records Institute, Don Mills, Ontario, Canada.

Chester, A. C., Argy, W. P., Rakowski, T. A., and Schreiner, G. E. (1978). Polycystic kidney disease and chronic haemodialysis. *Clinical Nephrology*, **10**, 129–33

Churchill, D. N., Bear, J. C., Morgan, J., Payne, R. H., McManamon, P. J., and Gault, M. H. (1984). Prognosis of adult onset polycystic kidney disease re-evaluated. *Kidney International*, **26**, 190–3.

Delaney, V. B., Adler, S., Bruns, F. J., Licinia, M., Segel, D. P., and Fraley, D. S. (1985). Autosomal dominant polycystic kidney disease: Presentation, complications, and prognosis. *American Journal of Kidney Disease*, **5**, 104–11.

Delaney, V., Sumrani, N., Butt, K. M. H., and Hong, J. H. (1991). The impact of cyclosporin in patients with adult polycystic kidney disease following transplantation. *Nephron*, **59**, 537–42.

Fitzpatrick, P. M., Torres, V. E., Charboneau, J. W., Offord, K. P., Holby, K. E., and Zincke, H. (1990). Long term outcome of renal transplantation in autosomal dominant polycystic kidney disease. *American Journal of Kidney Disease*, **15**, 535–43.

Florijn, K. W., Chang, P. C., van Der Woude, F. J., van Bockel, H., and van Saase, J. (1994). Long-term cardiovascular morbidity and mortality in autosomal dominant polycystic kidney disease patients after renal transplantation. *Transplantation*, **57**, 73–81.

Fortner, A., Taylor, A., and Datz, F. L. (1986). Advantage of Indium 111 leukocytes over ultrasound in imaging an infected renal cyst. *Journal of Nuclear Medicine*, **27**, 1147–9.

Gabow, P. A., *et al.* (1992). Factors affecting the progression of renal disease in autosomal dominant polycystic kidney disease. *Kidney International*, **41**, 1311–19.

Gatalica, Z., Schwarting, R., and Petersen, R. O. (1994). Renal cell carcinoma in the presence of adult polycystic kidney disease. *Urology*, **43**, 102–5.

Gerzof, S. G. and Gale, M. E. (1982). Computed tomography and ultrasonography for diagnosis and treatment of renal and retroperitoneal abscesses. *Urology Clinics of North America*, **9**, 185–93.

Gladziwa, U., Bohm, R., Malms, J., Keulers, P., Haasa, G., and Sieberth, H. G. (1993). Diagnosis and treatment of a solitary infected hepatic cyst in two patients with adult polycystic kidney disease. *Clinical Nephrology*, **40**, 205–7.

Graham, A. N., Neale, T. J., and Hatfield, P. J. (1986). End-stage renal failure due to polycystic kidney disease managed by continuous ambulatory peritoneal dialysis. *New Zealand Medical Journal*, **99**, 491–3.

Gregoire, J. R., Torres, V. E., Holley, K. E., and Farrow, G. M. (1987). Renal epithelial hyperplastic and neoplastic proliferation in autosomal dominant polycystic kidney disease. *American Journal of Kidney Disease*, **9**, 27–38.

Grunfeld, J. P., *et al.* (1985). Liver changes and complications in autosomal dominant polycystic kidney disease. *Advances in Nephrology*, **14**, 1–20.

Habte, B. and Abraha, A. (1983). Adult polycystic kidney disease in Ethiopians. *Ethiopian Medical Journal*, **21**, 193–6.

Hannig, V. L., Erickson, S. M., and Phillips, J. A. (1992). Utilization and evaluation of living-related donors for patients with adult polycystic kidney disease. *American Journal of Medical Genetics*, **44**, 409–12.

Harley, J. D., Shen, F. H., and Carter, S. J. (1980). Transcatheter infarction of a polycystic kidney for control of recurrent hemorrhage. *A. J. R.* **134**, 818–20.

Hatfield, P. M. and Pfister, R. C. (1972). Adult polycystic disease of the kidneys (Potter type 3). *Journal of the American Medical Association*, **222**, 1527–31.

Hilpert, P. L., *et al.* (1986). MRI of hemorrhagic renal cysts in polycystic kidney disease. *American Journal of Radiology*, **146**, 1167–72.

Ho-Hseih, H., Streem, S. B., Novick, A. C., Buszta, C., Steinmuller, D., and Goormastic, M. (1987). Renal transplantation for end-stage polycystic kidney disease. *Urology*, **30**, 322–6.

Ito, Y., Singh, S., and, Pollack V. E. (1985). Efficacy of dialysis treatment. In *Proceedings of the First International Workshop on Polycystic Kidney Disease*, (ed. J. J. Grantham and K. D. Gardner), pp. 160–8. Polycystic Kidney Research Foundation, Kansas City.

Kaehny, W. D., Manco-Johnson, M., Johnson, A. M., Tangel, D. J., and Gabow, P. A. (1988). Influence of sex on liver manifestations of autosomal dominant polycystic kidney disease. *Kidney International*, **33**, 196.

Keith, D. S., Torres, V. E., King, B. F., Zincke, H., and Farrow, G. M. (1994). Renal cell carcinoma in autosomal dominant polycystic kidney disease. *Journal of the American Society of Nephrology*, **4**, 1661–9.

Lafayette, R. A., Meyer, K. B., and, Levey A. S. (1994). Acquired cystic kidney disease. In *Principles and practice of dialysis*, (ed. W. L. Heurich), pp. 333–4. Williams & Wilkins, Baltimore.

Lazarus, J. M., Bailey, G. L., Hampers, C. L., and Merrill, J. P. (1971). Haemodialysis and transplantation in adults with polycystic renal disease. *Journal of the American Medical Association*, **217**, 1821–4.

Levine, E. and Grantham, J. J. (1985). High density renal cysts in autosomal dominant polycystic kidney disease demonstrated by CT. *Radiology*, **154**, 477–82.

London, R. D., Malik, A. A., and Train, J. S. (1988). Infection in a patient with polycystic kidney and liver disease: Noninvasive localization and treatment. *American Journal of Medicine*, **84**, 1082–5.

Mendelssohn, D. C., Harding, M. E., Cardella, C. J., Cook, G. T., and Uldall, P. R. (1988). Management of end-stage autosomal dominant polycystic kidney disease with haemodialysis and transplantation. *Clinical Nephrology*, **30**, 315–19.

Milutinovic, J., Fialkow, P. J., Rudd, T. G., Agodoa, L. Y., Phillips L. A., and Bryant, J. I. (1980). Liver cysts in patients with autosomal dominant polycystic kidney disease. *American Journal of Medicine*, **68**, 741–4.

Ng, R. C. K. and Suki, W. N. (1980). Renal cell carcinoma occurring in a polycystic kidney of a transplant recipient. *Journal of Urology*, **124**, 710–12.

Nolph, K. D., Cutler, S. J., and Seinberg, S. M. (1985). Continuous ambulatory peritoneal dialysis in the United States: A three year study. *Kidney International*, **28**, 198–205.

Novick, A. C. and Ho-Hseih, H. (1985). Renal transplantation. In *Problems in diagnosis and management of polycystic kidney disease*, (ed. J. J. Grantham and K. D. Gardner), pp. 172–9. Intercollegiate Press, Kansas City.

Parfrey, P. S. (1993). Hereditary renal disease. *Current Opinion in Nephrology and Hypertension*, **2**, 192–200.

Parfrey, P. S., *et al.* (1990). The diagnosis and prognosis of autosomal dominant polycystic kidney disease. *New England Journal of Medicine*, **323**, 1085–90.

Rayner, B. L., Cassidy, M. J. D., Jacobsen, J. E., Pascoe, M. D., Pontin, A. R., and van Zyl Smit, R. (1990). Is preliminary binephrectomy necessary in patients with autosomal polycystic kidney disease undergoing renal transplantation? *Clinical Nephrology*, **34**, 122–4.

Ritz, E., Zeier, M., Schneider, P., and Jones, E. (1994). Cardiovascular mortality of patients with polycystic kidney disease on dialysis: is there a lesson to learn? *Nephron*, **66**, 125–8.

Sanfilippo, F. P., Vaughn, W. K., Peters, T. G., Bollinger, R. R., and Spees, E. K. (1983). Transplantation for polycystic kidney disease. *Transplantation*, **36**, 54–9.

Scheff, R. T., Zuckerman, G., Harter, H., Delmez, J., and Koehler, R. (1980). Diverticular disease in patients with chronic renal failure due to polycystic kidney disease. *Annals of Internal Medicine*, **92**, 202–4.

Schwab, S. J., Bander, S. J., and Klahr, S. (1987). Renal infection in autosomal dominant polycystic kidney disease. *American Journal of Medicine*, **82**, 714–18.

Singh, S. and Hariharan, S. (1991). Renal replacement therapy in autosomal dominant polycystic kidney disease. *Nephron*, **57**, 40.

Thomsen, H. S. and Thaysen, J. H. (1988). Frequency of hepatic cysts in adult polycystic kidney disease. *Acta Medica Scandinavica*, **224**, 381–4.

Torres, V. E., Holley, K. E., and Offord, K. P. (1985). General features of autosomal dominant polycystic kidney disease: Epidemiology. In *Problems in diagnosis and management of polycystic kidney disease*, (ed. J. J. Grantham and K. D. Gardner), pp. 49–69. Intercollegiate Press, Kansas City.

Tzardis, P. J., *et al.* (1989). Renal transplantation in patients with polycystic kidney disease: A single centre experience. *Clinical Transplantation*, **3**, 325–30.

Vaughan, E. D. (1990). Erythropoietin in polycystic kidneys. (Editorial comment). *Journal of Urology*, **144**, 814.

Wheeler, R. P. (1987). Case report: Subdural hematoma in a patient on continuous ambulatory peritoneal dialysis. *American Journal of Medical Sciences*, **294**, 448–50.

Zeier, M., Geberth, S., Ritz, E., Jaeger, T., and Waldherr R. (1988). Autosomal dominant polycystic kidney disease — clinical problems. *Nephron*, **49**, 177–83.

19

Chronic pain and its medical and surgical management in renal cystic diseases

Joseph W. Segura, Bernard F. King, Sheila G. Jowsey, Patricia Martin, and Horst Zincke

Introduction

Pain, located in the abdomen, flank, or back is the most common initial complaint in autosomal dominant polycystic kidney disease (ADPKD) and, at some point in the course of the disease, affects the majority of patients (Dalgaard 1957; Iglesias *et al.* 1983, Gabow *et al.* 1984). The pain can be caused by cyst enlargement; bleeding (either confined to inside a cyst or leading to gross haematuria with passage of clots, or to a perinephric haematoma); urinary tract infection (acute pyelonephritis, infected cyst, perinephric abscess); nephrolithiasis and renal colic; rarely a coincidental renal cell carcinoma. Patients with ADPKD may also have abdominal pain related to definitely or presumably associated conditions. A large polycystic liver may cause dull aching and an uncomfortable sensation of heaviness. Hepatic cysts may become infected, especially after renal transplantation. Abdominal pain can result from diverticulitis which has been reported to occur with increased frequency in patients with ADPKD treated by chronic dialysis. ADPKD patients may be at higher risk of developing aortic abdominal aneurysms. Finally, these patients may develop pain for reasons unrelated to their underlying disease. Obviously, abdominal pain in ADPKD may be a diagnostic challenge. Renal and extrarenal sources of pain not directly caused by the cystic disease need to be aggressively sought out and treated accordingly. The purpose of this chapter is to discuss the management of chronic pain caused directly by the cystic disease. Patients with ADPKD often have a sensation of flank or abdominal fullness or heaviness, but this sensation is not usually painful and does not require special treatment. In a small subset of patients, however, the renal enlargement and distortion is accompanied by chronic, intermittent or unremitting, pain that may range from moderate discomfort to severe and disabling. The pain is usually exacerbated by physical activity. Data derived from clinical studies indicate that renal and cyst size correlate with the presence of pain (Hatfield and Pfister 1972), but exceptions to this rule are common. Why some patients remain asymptomatic while others with similar or less renal enlargement experience severe pain remains a mystery (Grantham 1992).

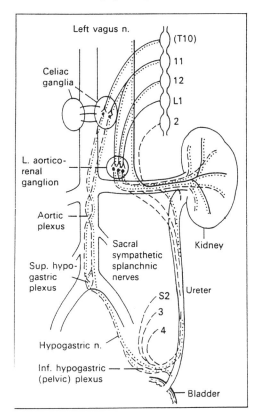

Fig. 19.1 Schematic illustration of the autonomic and sensory nerve pathways supplying the kidney and ureters. (Reproduced by permission from Ansell, J., *et al.* (1990). Diseases of the kidney and ureter. In *The management of pain*, (2nd edn), (ed. J. Bonica), pp. 1232–49. Lea & Febiger, Philadelphia PA.

Pathophysiology of pain

The pathophysiology of pain originating from the kidney is complex and depends on input from the sympathetic, parasympathetic, and sensory nervous system (Ansell *et al.* 1990) (Fig. 19.1). The sympathetic component includes preganglionic fibers from the T_{10}, T_{11}, and T_{12} spinal cord segments travelling via the lesser and least splanchnic nerves and synapsing in the coeliac or aorticorenal ganglion. Occasionally, the least (T_{12}) and 1st and 2nd lumbar splanchnic nerves may pass directly to, and synapse in the renal plexus located around the renal artery. The parasympathetic nerve supply includes preganglionic fibres from the vagus nerve. These traverse (without synapsing) the coeliac plexus before synapsing near the renal pelvis. Afferent (sensory) fibres whose neurones lie in the dorsal root ganglions of T_{10}, T_{11}, and T_{12} travel with the autonomic nerves.

The exact mechanism of pain is unknown but may be secondary to cyst expansion stretching the renal capsule, displacing renal parenchyma, or placing traction on the renal pedicle. It may be a well-localized visceral pain or it may cause a localized or referred somatic pain. Areas that have been described include the costovertebral angle, abdominal pain and spasm of the lateral rectus sheath and paraspinal muscles, pain in the inguinal and thigh area, and referred pain from diaphragmatic irritation.

Afferent sensory fibres travelling with the vagus nerve may explain the nausea that sometimes accompanies this pain. An increasing or changing quality of pain may indicate renal calculi, bleeding into a cyst or rupture, obstruction, infection, or a malignancy.

Management of pain by conservative measures

After reversible or self-limiting causes of pain have been excluded, an initial conservative approach is warranted. Treatment with non-opioid analgesics is preferable (Rummans 1994) with care taken when prescribing drugs which may have nephrotoxic properties, such as combination analgesic mixtures and non-steroidal anti-inflammatory drugs.

Adjunctive treatment with tricyclic antidepressants has been shown to be helpful. Antidepressants can have a dual role in patients with chronic pain. They can effectively treat depression, but they also are beneficial as adjuvant analgesics (Butler 1984). This effect is believed to be separate from the effect of the anti-depressants on mood disorders (Watson *et al.* 1982). Amitriptyline, imipramine, desipramine, doxepin, and clomipramine have all been found to be effective, usually in dosage ranges similar to those used for depression (Portenoy 1993). Amitriptyline is most commonly used in low doses (less than 75 mg at bedtime) and can be continued on a long-term basis with usually only minor side-effects secondary to its anticholinergic effects (i.e. sedation, dry mouth). Occasionally, difficulties with urinary obstruction, orthostatic hypotension, or dysrhythmias warrant discontinuation of the medication. Their exact mechanism in the relief of chronic pain is not known but is felt to involve the central descending sero-tonin pathways. These inhibitory pathways modulate both first- and second-order neurones in the dorsal horn of the spinal cord. They may also alleviate pain via their antidepressant properties and decrease the perception of pain. The newer antidepressants, including the selective serotonin re-uptake inhibitors, have not been as well studied as adjuvant agents for pain, and currently, are not widely used for analgesia.

Use of antispasmodics and trigger point injections may be useful for intermittent episodes of accompanying spasm or pain involving the paravertebral or abdominal musculature. A supporting garment (corset) may decrease some of the discomfort associated with tension on the renal pedicles.

Patients with severe pain may require narcotic analgesics. Traditionally, opiate analgesia has been viewed as problematic for chronic non-malignant pain because of the risk of developing tolerance and requiring escalating doses of opiates leading to the development of physical and psychological dependence. Portenoy (1993), in his comprehensive review of chronic pain management, argues that the current medical literature does not support these concerns and that the risk for addiction in chronic pain patients who have no history of substance abuse is small. However, controlled prospective studies have not been performed to validate this approach to chronic non-malignant pain. It is estimated that substance abuse is found in up to one-third of patients presenting to general hospitals (Swift 1993). Thus, a thorough review of the chronic pain patients past history of drug and alcohol use needs to be obtained and other non-opiate approaches to pain control considered before proceeding with opiate medications for chronic pain management. Acute episodes of pain usually can be managed well with opiate analgesia and pose less of a threat of physiological and psychological dependence. It has not been established whether long-acting opiates, such as methadone or sustained release oral morphine, are safer and more efficacious than shorter-acting forms of opiate analgesia for chronic pain. Other authors have argued that chronic pain patients are susceptible to negative behavioural consequences of long-term opiate analgesia. One study (Turner *et al.* 1982) found that patients with chronic pain who used narcotics and sedatives spent more money on medication per month, reported greater physical impairment, and had higher Minnesota Multiphasic Personality Inventory scores for hypochondriasis and hysteria when compared to chronic pain patients not using narcotics. This research reinforces the need for a careful psychological assessment of chronic pain patients who are being considered for opiate analgesia.

Splanchnic nerve blockade with local anaesthetic and steroid should be considered as a worthwhile alternative to the use of narcotic analgesics. By interrupting the transmission of pain via the splanchnic nerves, the pain may decrease beyond the duration of the local anaesthetic during acute exacerbations. Although only anecdotal, some patients have received prolonged relief following this procedure in the treatment of pain associated with polycystic kidney disease. More experience has been gained in the treatment of chronic pancreatitis with splanchnic nerve blockade utilizing a combination of local anaesthetic and steroid. Occasionally, patients may have several months of diminished pain with a need for intermittent series of injections every three to four months. The role of neurolytic blockade in chronic non-malignant pain is controversial and in general not recommended because of the concern of regeneration and problems associated with this.

Options when conservative measures fail

Once attempts at conservative management have been exhausted and the patients quality of life is diminishing, the physician has three choices in dealing with cysts causing chronic pain: (1) needle aspiration with or without injection of sclerosing agents; (2) open surgical decompression; and (3) laparoscopic fenestration of renal cysts. The selection of the best option in a particular case is a function of the severity of the symptoms, the morbidity of the procedure, the number, size, and location of the cysts, the level of renal function, and the presence of co-morbid conditions. In patients with moderate symptoms the pain secondary to surgical incisions, particularly a flank or a midline incision, may well be out of proportion to the symptoms justifying the intervention. Patients with advanced chronic renal insufficiency may be best treated by conservative measures and eventually bilateral nephrectomy. A further caveat reflects the issue of the location of the cysts responsible for the pain. In the absence of an obvious complicated cyst, it is generally assumed that larger cysts are the root of the patients problem, and the treatment is directed toward these cysts.

Cyst aspiration and sclerosis

Aspiration of renal cysts for diagnostic purposes has been standard procedure in many hospitals since 1939 (Göthlin 1987). Almost invariably re-accumulation of fluid causes a recurrence of the cyst of the same or larger size within weeks after the aspiration. To prevent these recurrences, a number of sclerosing agents since the 1950s have been injected into benign simple cysts at the time of the aspirations. Of these, 95 per cent ethanol, acidic solutions of tetracyclines (e.g. minocyclin hydrochloride) and bismuth phosphate are the most commonly used (Bean 1981; Holmberg 1992; Uemasu *et al.* 1993). The best results are obtained with ethanol sclerosis. The success rate of ethanol sclerosis for benign renal cysts exceeds 90 per cent (Bean 1981). The risk of recurrence may increase with the size of the cyst. Minor complications, such as microhaematuria, localized pain, transient fever, and systemic absorption of the alcohol can occur, but more serious complications, such as perirenal haemorrhage, pneumothorax, arteriovenous fistula, urinomas, and infections, are more rare. Complications from aspiration and the sclerosis of centrally located cysts are more common than when these procedures are performed for peripheral cysts. Aspiration of multiple cysts may provide transient pain relief in patients with ADPKD (Bennett *et al.* 1987). Unfortunately, the effect is short lived and most individuals experience recurrence of their pain within three to six months. Very limited information has been published on treatment of renal cysts by sclerosing agents in patients with ADPKD (Uemasu *et al.* 1993). The effectiveness and safety of these procedures in patients with ADPKD may be limited by the fact that the morbidity of the procedure is proportional to the number of cysts treated.

Technique

The patient is placed on a fluoroscopic X-ray table and an ultrasound (US) examination of the kidneys is performed. Under US guidance a 5 French pigtail Teflon catheter with side holes is inserted percutaneously into the cyst. The cyst is then completely aspirated and the volume of cyst fluid is recorded. Contrast material is injected into the cyst to exclude significant leakage or communication with the collecting system. The amount of contrast material varies but generally is about 25 per cent of the original cyst volume. The patient should be placed in multiple different positions (supine, oblique, lateral, etc.) and viewed under fluoroscopy to exclude leakage. After excluding leakage and completely removing the contrast medium, 15–25 per cent of the cyst volume is replaced with 95 per cent ethanol and the patient is placed in multiple positions (supine, oblique, lateral, etc.) to assure contact of the ethanol with the entire cyst wall. After 20 to 30 minutes the ethanol is completely aspirated and the catheter removed. The epithelial cells lining the cyst become fixed and non-viable within 1 to 3 minutes after contact with 95 per cent ethanol. It is claimed that ethanol does not result in significant damage to the renal parenchyma because it takes 4–12 hours for the ethanol to penetrate the cyst capsule and diffuse into the surrounding tissue (Bean and Rodan 1985).

Surgical cyst decompression

Surgical decompression of polycystic kidneys was pioneered in 1911 by Rovsing in Copenhagen. He described an open surgical procedure with puncture of multiple cysts and reported a marked and sustained reduction in renal size in three patients treated by this procedure. Over the next 40 years, multiple reports confirmed several beneficial effects of surgical cyst decompression, including pain relief (reviewed by Bennett *et al.* 1990). Surgical cyst decompression fell out of favour in the 1960s following the influential report by Bricker and Patton in two patients with renal insufficiency who experienced a deterioration of glomerular infiltration rate following the procedure (Bricker and Patton 1957). The concerns raised by this report were supported by subsequent studies of nine patients who underwent differential renal function studies before and after unilateral decompression of a polycystic kidney (Prat and Kocvara 1961; Milam *et al.* 1963). In most instances, the functional capacity of the decompressed kidney was impaired by the operation. This conclusion has been challenged because surgical decompressions and ureteral catheterizations for split renal function studies were often complicated by infection and because the rate of renal function decline before surgery was not considered. In 1980, Shangzhi and co-workers reported their experience with surgical cyst decompression in ADPKD. This study, which was later expanded to 96 cases, indicated that this surgery was effective in relieving pain and that the pain relief was maintained in 90 per cent of the patients after six months and 77 per cent after five years (Ye *et al.* 1986).

Between 1986 and 1990, 30 patients with ADPKD underwent surgical cystic compression at the University of Oregon and at the Mayo Clinic. Twenty-six of these patients had chronic pain. In these patients the probability of being free of pain post-operatively was 80 per cent at one year and 62 per cent at two years (Elzinga *et al.* 1992). In those patients who experienced relapse of their pain during the period of observation, the pain was often of less intensity than that present pre-operatively and narcotic analgesics were less often needed. Nineteen of the 30 patients underwent unilateral and the remaining 11 had bilateral cyst decompression surgery. One year after surgery the serum creatinine levels remained unchanged in patients with normal pre-operative renal function, whereas those with pre-operative progressive renal insufficiency had no difference in the mean slope of reciprocal serum creatinine plots preceding and after surgery. In patients who underwent unilateral surgery, a split function isotope scan showed no change in function of the operated kidney when compared with the non-operated kidney. The results indicated that surgical cystic decompression provides effective relief of chronic pain without compromising renal function, but did not support the use of this procedure to slow the progression of renal insufficiency. Surgical complications were limited and included upper urinary collecting system injury in two patients, urinary tract infection in two patients, bleeding requiring transfusion of two or three units of blood in three patients, incisional hernias in two patients and small bowel obstruction in one patient.

Technique

The approach for the surgical decompression of polycystic kidneys depends on whether one or both kidneys are treated, as well as on the size of the kidneys and number, size, and location of the cysts. The procedures are done preferably through a lumbar approach, since it is the least painful approach and allows the surgeon to insert the hand and mobilize the kidney progressively as the cysts are decompressed (Fig. 19.2). The patient is placed in the lateral decubitus position at an angle of 50° from prone with the table flexed at least at 15–20° angle in order to increase the distance between the 12th rib and extended inferiorly and slightly laterally from the proximal incision down toward the iliac crest. After incising the lumbodorsalis fascia, the sacrospinalis muscle and subsequently the quadratus lumborum are identified and held back by a Richardson retractor medially. Similarly, the anterior abdominal wall muscles are being held inferiorly to provide access to the muscle-free area where incision of the transversalis fascia in a vertical fashion will provide access to the Gerotas fascia surrounding the targeted kidney. Since there is only a small amount of fat within the Gerotas fascia over the expanding cysts, these can be easily identified, although a lumbotomy incision provides a relatively small field. Visualization of the entire kidney is eventually possible since, after decompression of several larger cysts, the kidney will be easily movable. The ureter will be identified and looped in order to prevent injury. Subsequently, using the cautery at a 40 watt setting, cysts are incised, and bleeding bridging areas of parenchyma are fulgurated to

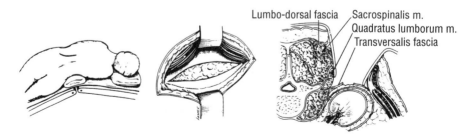

Lumbo-dorsal fascia   Sacrospinalis m.
                      Quadratus lumborum m.
                      Transversalis fascia

Fig. 19.2 Posterior surgical approach to the kidney. (Reproduced by permission from Novick, A. C. (1980). Posterior surgical approach to the kidney and ureter. *Journal of Urology*, **124**, 192–5.)

prevent bleeding. The use of intra-operative US facilitates the identification of cysts within the depth of the kidney. The cysts can be entered through the floor of more superficial previously unroofed cysts. Care should be taken not to enter the collecting system, which, however, is typically compressed by the large cysts and has not been a problem in our experience. US used throughout the procedure facilitates the decompression of most of the large cysts as shown by comparison of computed tomography (CT) scans obtained before and after the surgery (Fig. 19.3). The area is irrigated with 0.5 per cent neomycin solution at the end of the procedure. A medium size haemovac drain is placed and brought out through a separate stab wound and the facial layers closed with running 1-0 PDS suture. A subcutaneous haemovac is placed and the skin edges approximated with subcuticular 4-0 Vicryl. Patients treated by a lumbotomy approach

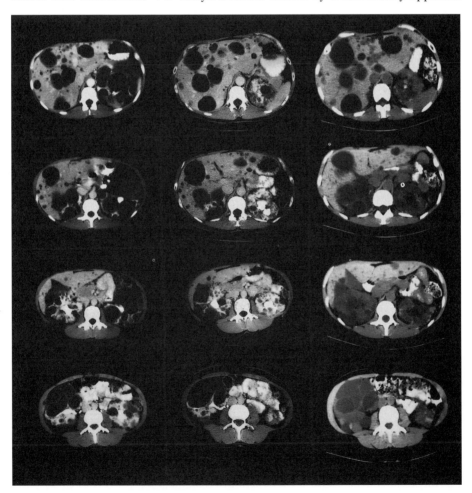

Fig. 19.3 CT scans of the abdomen before (left panels), three months after (middle panels), and one year after (right panels) surgical decompression of the left polycycstic kidney.

can usually be dismissed from the hospital within four or five days, after the in-dwelling haemovacs have been removed.

In certain instances where the patients body habitus does not allow an adequate approach through a lumbotomy incision or when the size of the kidney and number and distribution of the cysts on the pre-operative CT scan suggest that a lumbotomy approach will result in suboptimal results, consideration might be given to provide access through a subcostal incision, using a transperitoneal approach to the kidney. This is accomplished by mobilizing the right colon and kockerizing the duodenum, which provides easy access on the right. On the left, the splenic flexure of the colon is mobilized medially. The ureter is identified and isolated and looped for protection. This approach provides a better and more global visualization of the entire kidney but is not necessary in the vast majority of patients since the procedure can usually be easily accomplished through the above described lumbotomy incision.

In the case where both kidneys are to be explored, bilateral lumbotomy incisions can be used. In this case the patient is placed in the prone flexed position with a simultaneous approach being performed on each side. Alternatively, both kidneys can be operated simultaneously via transperitoneal midline approach.

Laparoscopic cyst decompression

Laparoscopy has been a standard part of the gynaecological armamentarium for many years. Over the last few years, laparoscopy has found a role in various urological applications, particularly pelvic lymph node dissection, renal surgery, and certain applications in paediatric urology (Sosa 1993). Its minimally invasive nature has appeal in the treatment of those patients whose problems require surgical treatment, yet can be managed without the precision and control of a standard open operation. Most of the tools and techniques which form the basis of urological laparoscopy were developed for gynaecological purposes which primarily involved the management of structures located in the peritoneal cavity. For this reason, most urological laparoscopic procedures are performed using a transperitoneal approach, although recently, techniques have been developed whereby laparoscopy can be performed using the retroperitoneum alone.

Solitary benign renal cysts have been fenestrated using laparoscopic techniques for several years (Morgan and Rader 1992; Stoller *et al.* 1993; Austoni *et al.* 1992; Nieh and Bihrle 1993; Rubenstein *et al.* 1993; Gelet *et al.* 1990). In most instances, these patients had failed previous needle aspiration with efforts to sclerose the cysts and in most cases the procedures were successful. Elzinga *et al.* (1993) used laparoscopy to decompress cysts in three ADPKD patients with complete pain relief in two and partial relief in one patient.

The only absolute contraindications to laparoscopy are an uncontrolled bleeding diathesis and an acute intra-abdominal inflammatory process such as peritonitis. Other more common relative contraindications may mean that some other approach is preferable in a specific situation. Previous abdominal surgery will result in adhesions making access difficult and exposure of the area of interest tedious. This is particularly true if previous colon surgery has included the area of the kidney which must be exposed. In our experience so far, we have not yet encountered a candidate for fenestration whose kidneys were so large as to preclude laparoscopy, although these patients clearly exist. As in all areas of surgery, those patients who are morbidly obese or misshapen owing to scoliosis or other anatomical abnormality may present technical challenges such that laparoscopy may be difficult to the point of impossibility.

That patients treated by laparoscopic surgery have shorter, smoother recovery periods than after an open operation for the same condition is beyond question. The real issue is whether the results are comparable to those achievable using open surgery and whether the results are durable. We have treated 11 patients with polycystic disease using transperitoneal laparoscopy with post-operative pain relief on short-term follow-up in the majority. In one patient, pain recurred several months later and CT scan showed that one cyst had reformed. This was successfully managed by percutaneous removal of the cyst wall. The reason for failure is unknown but presumably is because a large enough window of cyst wall was not removed. Laparoscopy at best will eliminate all important cysts and at worst will leave symptomatic cysts behind. Reduction in numbers of cysts may make cyst aspiration with injection of sclerosing agents more practical and the use of cyst aspiration to 'clean up' after laparoscopy (or open surgery) should be considered. Laparoscopic management of missed, recurrent, or new cysts in the previously operated field will be difficult, and this may limit the benefits from this procedure. While the long-term results of laparoscopic marsupialization remain unknown, in the short term it is clearly safe, practical, and effective. In the appropriately selected patient with ADPKD or with multiple renal cysts, laparoscopy should be the procedure of first consideration for removal of targeted cysts.

The main risk of laparoscopy for this indication is the risk that a significant cyst will be missed. However, it is hoped that regular use of intra-operative US will minimize this problem. A post-operative urinary leak occurred in one of our patients with a solitary cyst who was treated by percutaneous means. A drain was placed and the leak spontaneously resolved after a few days. Injury to the parenchyma in a left kidney generated some brisk bleeding which stopped after pressure and after thrombin-soaked gelfoam was placed in the parenchyma. Ready availability of the Argon-bean Coagulator should make this sort of problem easier to manage. Elzinga *et al.* (1993) reported a series of patients with cysts who were managed laparoscopically. Residual upper pole cysts were present in three patients and residual posterior cysts in two.

Technique

The patient is anaesthetized and prepared with the side of the kidney which must be approached elevated with sandbags to an angle of 30° (Fig. 19.4). The table is then rotated so that the patient is supine. We prefer that the anaesthesiologist not use nitrous oxide, if possible, because of the possibility of bowel distention. A nasogastric tube is used and a Foley catheter placed. If there has been no previous intra-abdominal surgery, a Veress needle is placed through an infra-umbilical incision and the pneumoperitoneum achieved. A 10–12 mm trocar is placed through this site and the telescope inserted. Assuming that inspection of the abdominal cavity reveals no complication or other factor which might mean that the procedure should be terminated, the table is rotated such that the flank is oriented at an angle of about 60° (Fig. 19.4). Three more 10–12 mm trocars are then inserted (Fig. 19.5), giving a total of four ports which are adequate for many situations. A fifth port is often necessary, but its placement should be delayed as its optimum location will depend on how the case develops. How the surgeon proceeds at this point depends on the pathology and the goals of treatment. Large cysts, especially those located anteriorly, inferiorly, and laterally are often readily visible and easily approached, frequently without having to reflect the colon. More commonly, however, the colon must be reflected in order to access the target cysts, particularly when these cysts are located medially, posteriorly, or superiorly. As a practical matter, nearly complete exposure of the kidney may be required (Fig. 19.6) (Hulbert 1992*a,b*). Intrarenal cysts present particular problems because their location can only be estimated and not determined precisely. These cysts are exposed by fenestrating other cysts which overlay the deeper intrarenal cysts. This problem is not limited to laparoscopy, as the same difficulty applies when the kidney is approached by open surgery. Cysts are opened by using the Endoshears as scissors or with cautery. As the cyst fluid escapes, the cyst wall is grasped with forceps and excised. It is very important to remove as much of the cyst wall as possible in order to minimize

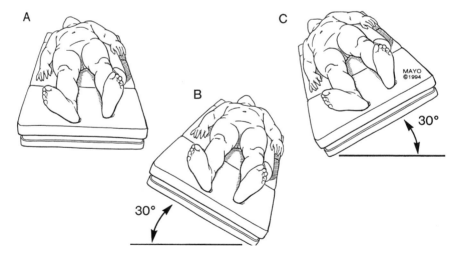

Fig. 19.4 After the patient has been anaesthetized and the flank supported in the approximate angle of 30° with sand bags (A), the patient is rotated supine and pneumoperitoneum achieved with the patient in this position (B). The table is then rotated fully to the opposite side so that the patient's flank is approximately at the 60° angle. It is this angle at which a left-sided cyst would be treated (C).

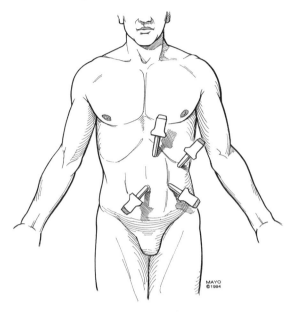

Fig. 19.5 Four 10–12 mm ports are used with an occasional fifth port. Two ports are placed under the rib cage, the third in the left lower quadrant, approximately lateral and slightly superior to the umbilicus near the anterior axillary line.

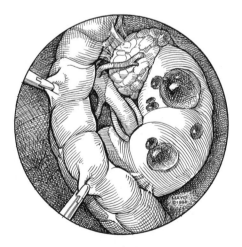

Fig. 19.6 The colon is reflected medially and retracted to reveal the kidney with the associated cysts. Anterior, lateral, and inferior cysts are obviously the easiest to treat.

the chances of the cyst reforming. Indeed, the main advantage of laparoscopy and open surgery over cyst aspiration is the fact that removal of the cyst wall is possible. As a matter of principle, the lining of the cyst is directly inspected, although incidental tumours are rare. Fulguration of the cyst lining is not usually done at open surgery and probably is not indicated as a routine measure laparoscopically. It can be tedious and one always risks inadvertent perforation into the collecting system, as happened to us on one occasion. One should have a clear idea of which cysts will be treated, as there is seemingly limitless number of small cysts whose treatment may bog down the operator in their management while larger, perhaps more 'important' cysts are missed. One should try to correlate each fenestrated cyst with its location on the CT scan in order to go through the kidney in an orderly manner (Fig. 19.7). When no further cysts can be identified via the laparoscope, it has become our practice to use intra-operative US in order to determine if we have missed a cyst. The radiologist places an external US probe on the patients flank, pushing the intra-abdominal side of the flank against the kidney. This is monitored laparoscopically to be certain which area of the kidney is being examined. Any residual cyst is then treated and the procedure terminated. A drain should be brought out of one of the ports. The typical patient leaves the hospital the next day or the day after, returning to average, sedentary activity after a few days.

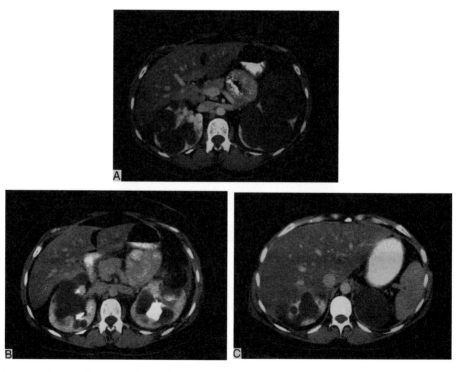

Fig. 19.7 (A) Pre-operative CT scan revealing large left renal cyst in a patient with ADPKD (B) Post-operative CT scan showing removal of the largest cysts. Note the crater-like fenestrated cyst on the anterior surface of the kidney. (C) A superior large renal cyst was missed intra-operatively.

Retroperitoneal laparoscopy

Gaur and co-workers described a technique whereby a space could be developed in the retroperitoneum after which standard laparoscopic techniques could be used for surgery on the kidney and ureter (Gaur *et al.* 1993). The patient is positioned in the flank position and after a short incision is made, a finger is placed in the retroperitoneum. A dilating balloon is placed in the retroperitoneum and the balloon filled with a litre of saline solution. This separates the peritoneum and immediately exposes the kidney, especially its posterior surface. This approach undoubtedly saves time and avoids some potential complications of the intraperitoneal approach. Shortcomings include a limited work space in the retroperitoneum compared to the transperitoneal approach and the risk that a tear in the peritoneal surface will result in loss of distension of the working space. We have not used this system, but some urologists regard it as preferable for renal laparoscopy (Kavoussi *et al.* 1991).

Percutaneous cyst resection

This approach may be regarded as a variant of the retroperitoneal approach. In this technique, the same methods which are standard practice for the management of renal stones are used in the retroperitoneal access to the kidney. Instead of the nephroscope being placed into the collecting system of the kidney, the nephroscope is placed outside the kidney adjacent to the cyst (Martinez-Sagarra and Sesmepo 1991). Under direct vision, the cyst is ruptured, the cyst wall removed, and the lining inspected. A drain is left indwelling. Because irrigating fluid must be used in order to see clearly, there is a risk of significant retroperitoneal extravasation; and so there is a limit as to how long the procedure might last. As a result, a percutaneous approach is not suited for the multiple cysts present in patients with ADPKD. Sironvalle *et al.* (1990) reported six cases performed without complication. Symptoms resolved in four of the six with a mean follow-up of over eight months. We have performed one case: a 47-year-old man underwent laparoscopic fenestration of several cysts with resolution of his pain. After six months the pain returned and CT scan revealed that one of the cysts had recurred. This was successfully fenestrated percutaneously, although the post-operative course was complicated by a urinary leak for a few days afterward. This resolved spontaneously.

Psychological aspects

The approach to the patient with chronic pain secondary to ADPKD must include a careful assessment of the patients psychological adaptation to his/her pain and also must address risk factors for the development of opiate dependence in patients exposed to opiate analgesia. Clinicians should consider psychiatric input on patients for whom pain complaints are resulting in family dysfunction, impaired job performance, or escalating demands for medication.

Some of these patients will benefit from a multidisciplinary behaviourally oriented approach to their pain, whereas others will need adjunctive treatment strategies, such as the use of tricyclic antidepressants or chemical dependence treatment.

The psychological sequalae of chronic pain in patients with ADPKD can manifest itself in concurrent depression, physiological and psychological dependence on opiate analgesics, and the development of social isolation and functional disability. Although surgical procedures and anaesthetic interventions may be of benefit in alleviating pain in these patients, treating depression and addressing psychological factors associated with pain is also beneficial in optimizing the patients adaptation to the illness and maintaining the best possible quality of life.

Psychiatrists can best address these complex issues by initially obtaining a thorough history of the nature and progression of the pain and how the pain has affected the patients ability to work, his/her relationships with family members, and how the patients mood has been affected by the pain. Careful attention to pre-morbid psychiatric conditions, such as depressive disorders, anxiety disorders, and chemical dependency, will yield valuable information about the patients risk for further psychiatric complications as the illness progresses. Of equal importance is the communication between the psychiatrist and nephrologist about the current medical and psychological findings and the timing of psychiatric interventions in the context of the patients current medical state. Often, the psychological profile of the patient and possible past chemical dependence will be important information in determining an approach to chronic pain.

The pain that patients experience from polycystic kidney disease can vary from mild discomfort to extreme pain (Grantham 1992). Psychological factors likely exacerbate pain in up to 40 per cent of pain cases (Stoudemire and Sandhu 1987). For these patients, their pain may become an agent with which they can meet certain psychological needs, including avoiding work responsibilities, being absolved of family expectations, or obtaining emotional nurturing that they might have lacked earlier in life.

The *Diagnostic and Statistical Manual of Mental Disorders* (APA, 1994) delineates several categories of psychiatric disorders that could present with a patient who complains of pain and also has autosomal dominant polycystic kidney disease (ADPKD). These include: pain disorder, somatization disorder, factitious disorder, and malingering. Pain disorders are diagnosed in patients who are significantly distressed by pain, have impairments in social, occupational, or other areas of function. Psychological factors are judged to be significant in the onset and severity of pain, and the pain is not intentionally feigned or produced. The pain becomes the major focus of the patients life. Iatrogenic opiate and benzodiazepine dependence or abuse often occurs in this setting. Somatization disorder is another psychiatric condition for which pain can be a complaint, however, these patients also complain of multiple other significant somatic complaints resulting in medical treatment or functional impairment. These symptoms are in excess of the medical condition that the patient has. The onset of the symptoms typically occurs before the age of 30 and the symptoms are not intentionally produced or feigned. These patients are at risk for illness produced because of iatrogenic interventions. These patients often visit multiple physicians and experience multiple medical procedures. Two other conditions exist for which an individual may actually feign physical symptoms and complain of pain. These conditions, factitious disorder and malingering, are differentiated by the individuals motivation for producing the symptoms. The factitious disorder patient produces symptoms in order to assume a sick role and continue to be engaged with care providers. Malingering patients produce symptoms in order to receive specific external incentives, such as obtaining compensation, obtaining drugs, or avoiding work or other responsibilities.

A careful psychiatric history focusing on the patient's adaptation to the pain and the pattern of pain in relation to the progression of symptoms may help in the diagnosis of a psychiatric disorder complicating the presentation of pain symptoms in a patient with ADPKD. Patients for whom psychological factors are prominent and have pain disorder or somatization disorder may benefit from a multidisciplinary approach to their pain (Turk *et al.* 1983) which includes: (1) psychological counselling, (2) physical and occupational therapy; and (3) psychological modalities of relaxation training, distraction techniques, and biofeedback (Fordyce *et al.* 1986). In the context of a comprehensive multidisciplinary programme, other factors contributing to the patients dysfunction may be identified, such as marital and family discord, the presence of affective disturbances, and the presence of chemical dependency. Further referral for marital counselling, treatment for chemical dependence, or the initiation of treatment for depression and anxiety may substantially improve the patients adaptation to chronic pain.

Depression does coexist with medical illness (Cohen-Cole *et al.* 1993) and can further impair a patients adaptation to pain. Depression has been associated with increased morbidity, length of hospital stay, and disability (Wells *et al.* 1989). The diagnosis of depression can be difficult in patients experiencing pain because pain can cause the neurovegetative symptoms seen in depression such as insomnia, decreased appetite, decreased concentration, and decreased energy. However, if a patient also complains of loss of interest in activities and has pervasive feelings of depression, a trial of antidepressants should be considered. Psychotherapy in combination with antidepressants often yields the best results in managing depression. Psychotherapeutic issues which need to be addressed in these patients include the losses experienced because of illness, role changes within the family, financial stressors due to illness, and concern over transmitting the illness to another generation.

Clinicians need to identify patients who have had substance abuse problems in the past and are at high risk for addiction if given opiate analgesia. Often, patients will deny or minimize past chemical dependence problems. Defensiveness in answering questions about past substance abuse can sometimes help identify potential at-risk patients. The CAGE questionnaire (Ewing 1984) is a well-studied, easily performed screening instrument for alcoholism which consists of the following four questions: (1) Have you ever felt the need to cut down on drinking? (2) Have you felt annoyed by criticisms of your drinking? (3) Have you had guilt feelings about drinking? (4) Have your ever taken an 'eye opener'? These questions, in addition to further history from the patients family members, will sometimes help identify previous behavioural patterns suggestive of chemical dependence.

Prescription drug dependence can sometimes be identified by evidence of escalating dosage requirements in the absence of any acute organic disease process, frequent visits to many doctors or different emergency rooms with demands for drugs, and repeated attempts to obtain more medication between visits. If these patterns are present, further history from family members should be obtained and further evaluation by a psychiatrist should be performed. Often, a past history of illicit drug use will become apparent in these patients. Such patients may require chemical dependence treatment combined with non-pharmacological pain management strategies to help them with future episodes of pain resulting from their polycystic kidney disease.

Future research will need to address the best ways of predicting which patients will benefit from behavioural measures and which will benefit from anaesthetic or surgical interventions. A recently published report on the importance of placebo effects in pain treatment (Turner *et al.* 1994) highlights the importance of factors such as the regression of the pain symptoms to the mean, the role of the physician and the physicians concern about the patient, and the patients and physicians expectations of treatment effects in the alleviation of pain. These factors can have an impact in the service of treating pain and avoiding more intrusive measures, such as opiate analgesia and invasive procedures.

References

APA (American Psychiatric Association) (1994). *Diagnostic and statistical manual of mental disorders*. (4th edn). American Psychiatric Association, Washington, DC.

Ansell, J., Gee, W., and Bonica, J. (ed.) (1990). Diseases of the kidney and ureter. In *The management of pain*, (2nd edn), (ed. J. Bonica), Vol. 2, pp. 1232–49. Lea & Febiger, Philadephia, PA.

Austoni, E., *et al.* (1993). Resezione di cisti renale. *Arch. It. Urol.*, **65**, 235–7.

Bean, W. J. (1981). Renal cysts: Treatment with alcohol. *Radiology*, **138**, 329–31.

Bean, W. J. and Rodan, B. A. (1985). Hepatic cysts: Treatment with alcohol. *Am. J. Roentgenol.*, **144**, 237–41.

Bennett, W. M., Elzinga, L., Golper, T. A., and Barry, J. M. (1987). Reduction of cyst volume for symptomatic management of autosomal dominant polycystic kidney disease. *J. Urol.*, **137**, 620–2.

Bennett, W. M., Elzinga, L. W., and Barry, J. M. (1990). Management of cystic kidney disease. In *The cystic kidney*, (ed. K.D. Gardner Jr and J. Bernstein), pp. 247–75. Kluwer, Boston.

Bricker, N. S. and Patton, J. F. (1957). Renal function studies in polycystic disease of the kidneys with observations on the effects of surgical decompression. *N. Engl. J. Med.*, **256**, 212–14.

Butler, S. (1984). Present status of tricyclic antidepressants in chronic pain. In *Advances in pain research and therapy: Recent advances in the management of pain*, (ed. C. R. Benedetti, C. R. Chapman, and G. Moricca) pp. 173–98. Raven, New York.

Cohen-Cole, S. A., Brown, F. W., and McDaniel, J. S. (1993). Assessment of depression and grief reactions in the medically ill. In *Psychiatric care of the medical patient*, (ed. A. Stoudemire and B. S. Fogel), pp. 53–69. Oxford University Press.

Dalgaard, O. Z. (1957). Bilateral polycystic disease of the kidneys: A follow-up of 285 patients and their families. *Acta Med. Scand. Suppl.*, **328**, 1–255.

Elzinga, L. W. *et al.* (1992). Cyst decompression surgery for autosomal dominant polycystic kidney disease. *J. Am. Soc. Nephrol.*, **2**, 219–26.

Elzinga, L. W., Barry, J. M., Lowe, B., and Bennett, W. M. (1993). Laparoscopic and retroperitoneoscopic cyst decompression in painful polycystic kidney disease (Abstract). *J. Am. Soc. Nephrol.*, **4**, 262.

Ewing, J. A. (1984). Detecting alcoholism: The CAGE questionnaire. *JAMA*, **252**, 1905–7.

Fordyce, W. E., Brockway, J., Bergman, J., and Spengler, D. (1986). A control group comparison of behavioural versus traditional management methods of acute back pain. *J. Behav. Med.*, **9**, 127–40.

Gabow, P. A., Ikle, D. W., and Holmes, J. H. (1984). Polycystic kidney disease: Prospective analysis of nonazotemic patients and family members. *Ann. Intern. Med.* **101**, 238–47.

Gaur, D. D., Agarwal, D. K., and Purohit, K. C. (1993). Retroperitoneal laparoscopic nephrectomy: Initial case report. *J. Urol.*, **149**, 103–5.

Gelet, A., Sanseverino, R., Martin, X., Leveque, J. M., and Dubernard, J. M. (1990). Percutaneous treatment of benign renal cysts. *Eur. Urol.*, **18**, 248–52.

Göthlin, J. H. (1987). Kidney puncture revisited. *Eur. J. Radiol.*, **7**, 76–82.

Grantham, J. J. (1992). Renal pain in polycystic kidney disease: When the hurt wont stop. *J. Am. Soc. Nephrol.*, **2**, 1161–2.

Hatfield, P. M. and Pfister, R. C. (1972). Adult polycystic disease of the kidneys (Potter type 3). *JAMA*, **222**, 1527–31.

Holmberg, G. (1992). Diagnostic aspects, functional significance and therapy of simple renal cysts. A clinical, radiologic and experimental study. *Scand. J. Urol. Nephrol. Suppl.*, **145**, 1–48.

Hulbert, J. C. (1992*a*). Laparoscopic approach to the retroperitoneum. *Semin. Urol.*, **10**, 227–31.

Hulbert, J. C. (1992*b*). Laparoscopic management of renal cystic disease. *Semin. Urol.*, **10**, 239–41.

Iglesias, G. C., Torres, V. E., Offord, K. P., Holley, K. E., Beard, C. M., Kurland, L. T. (1983). Epidemiology of adult polycystic kidney disease, Omsted County, Minnesota: 1935–1980. *Am. J. Kidney. Dis.*, **2**, 630–9.

Kavoussi, L. R., Clayman, R. V., Mikkelsen, D. J., and Meretyk, S. (1991). Ureteronephroscopic marsupialization of obstructing peripelvic renal cyst. *J. Urol.*, **146**, 411–14.

Martinez-Sagarra, J. M. and Sesmero, J. H. A. (1991). Quistes serosos renales: Resección percutánea translumbar. *Arch. Esp. Urol.*, **44**, 523–7.

Milam, J. H., Magee, J. H., and Bunts, R. C. (1963). Evaluation of surgical decompression of polycystic kidneys by differential renal clearance. *J. Urol.*, **90**, 144–9.

Morgan, C. Jr and Rader, D. (1992). Laparoscopic unroofing of a renal cyst. *J. Urol.*, **148**, 1835–6.

Nieh, P. T. and Bihrle, W. III (1993). Laparoscopic marsupialization of massive renal cyst. *J. Urol.*, **150**, 171–3.

Novick, A. C. (1980). Posterior surgical approach to the kidney and ureter. *J. Urol.*, **124**, 192–5.

Portenoy, R. K. (1993). Chronic pain management. In *Psychiatric care of the medical patient*, (ed. A. Stoudemire and B. S. Fogel), pp. 341–63. Oxford University Press.

Prat, V. and Kocvara, S. (1961). Evaluation of results after surgical treatment of polycystic kidneys by separate glomerular filtration tests. *Rozh. Chir.*, **40**, 383–9.

Rovsing, T. (1911). Treatment of multilocular renal cysts with multiple punctures. *Hospitalstid*, **4**, 105–16.

Rubenstein, S. C., Hulbert, J. C., Pharand, D., Schuessler, W. W., Vancaillie, T. G., and Kavoussi, L. R. (1993). Laparoscopic ablation of symptomatic renal cysts. *J. Urol.*, **150**, 1103–6.

Rummans, T. (1994). Nonopioid agents for treatment of acute and subacute pain. *Mayo Clin. Proc.*, **69**, 481–90.

Shangzhi, H., Shiyuan, A., Henning, J., Rong, Y., and Yufeng, C. (1980). Cyst decapitating decompression operation in polycystic kidneys. *Chinese Med. J.*, **93**, 773–8.

Sironvalle, M. S., *et al.* (1990). Reseccion percutanea de los quistes renales benignos. *Actas Urol. Esp.*, **14**, 349–51.

Sosa, R. E. (1993). Laparoscopy (Editorial) (1987). *J. Urol.*, **150**, 1110–11.

Stoudemire, A., and Sandhu, J. (1987). Psychogenic/idiopathic pain syndromes. *Gen. Hosp. Psychiatry*, **9**, 79–86.

Stoller, M. L., Irby, P. B. III, Osman, M., and Carroll, P. R. (1993). Laparoscopic marsupialization of a simple renal cyst. *J. Urol.*, **150**, 1486–8.

Swift, R. M. (1993). Alcohol and drug abuse in the medical setting. In *Psychiatric care of the medical patient*, (ed. A. Stoudemire and B.S. Fogel), pp. 139–53. Oxford University Press.

Turk, D. C., Meichenbaum, D., and Genest, M. (1983). Pain behavior medicine: A cognitive-behavioral perspective. Guilford Press, New York.

Turner, J. A., Calsyn, D. A., Fordyce, W. E., and Ready, L. B. (1982). Drug utilization patterns in chronic pain patients. *Pain*, **12**, 357–63.

Turner, J. A., Deyo, R. A., Loeser, J. D., Von Korff, M., and Fordyce, W. E. (1994). The importance of placebo effects in pain treatment and research. *JAMA*, **271**, 1609–14.

Uemasu, J., Fujiwara, M., Munemura, C., Tokumoto, A., and Kawasaki, H. (1993). Effects of topical instillation of minocycline hydrochloride on cyst size and renal function in polycystic kidney disease. *Clin. Nephrol.*, **39**, 140–4.

Watson, C. P. N., Evans, R. J., Reed, K., Merskey, H., Goldsmith, L., and Warsh, J. (1982). Amitriptyline versus placebo in post-herpetic neuralgia. *Neurology*, **32**, 671–3.

Wells, K. B., *et al.* (1989). The functioning and well-being of depressed patients: Results from the medical outcomes study. *JAMA*, **262**, 914–19.

Ye, M., An, S., Jiang, H., Sheng, S., and He, S. (1986). Clinical analysis of 141 cases of adult polycystic kidney disease. *Chin. J. Surg.*, **24**, 73–6.

PART V

Autosomal dominant polycystic kidney disease: complications

20

Miscellaneous renal and systemic complications of autosomal dominant polycystic kidney disease including infection

Lawrence W. Elzinga and William M. Bennett

As a multiorgan genetic disease, autosomal dominant polycystic kidney disease (ADPKD) has protean manifestations. Many of the more common and better understood complications and issues are covered separately in this monograph, including hypertension, renal failure, cystic liver disease, and cerebral aneurysms. This chapter addresses miscellaneous additional topics, including the very important subject of renal and hepatic infection.

Renal and urinary tract infection

General considerations

Infection of the urinary tract is a frequent complication in patients with ADPKD. In various clinical series, symptomatic urinary tract infection (UTI) was the presenting clinical finding in approximately 20 per cent of patients. Fifty to seventy-five per cent of all patients with ADPKD experience at least one clinical UTI during the course of their disease (Simon and Thompson 1955; Dalgaard 1957; De Bono and Evans 1977; Multinovic *et al.* 1984; Delaney *et al.* 1985). A vast majority occur in women, analagous to UTI in the general population. Urinary tract instrumentation with a bladder catheter or cystoscope is a frequent precipitating factor (Delaney *et al.* 1985; Schwab *et al.* 1987).

The incidence of upper tract infection involving the renal parenchyma or the cysts themselves is unknown. When it occurs, eradication of the infection is often unsuccessful despite prolonged antibiotic therapy, leading to the development of septicaemia and perinephric abscess necessitating surgical drainage or nephrectomy in a high percentage of cases. Over a 42-month observation period, Sweet and Keane (1979) discovered eight symptomatic UTI in 24 ADPKD patients undergoing chronic haemodialysis. Despite prompt and prolonged treatment with appropriate antibiotics, five patients subsequently developed perinephric abscess. Three of these patients died. Similarly, antibiotic therapy failed in four of five patients with infected polycystic kidneys reported by

Waters *et al.* (1979). These reports underscore the therapeutic difficulties and serious consequences of infection in polycystic kidneys.

Animal models

Studies in animal models of cystic disease suggest an enhanced susceptibility of the cystic kidney to infection. Following an intravenous inoculation of *Escherichia coli*, rats with cystic disease readily developed pyelonephritis when compared to non-cystic control animals who were remarkably resistant to renal infection (Kime *et al.* 1962). Other studies suggest that ambient environmental exposure to bacteria and endotoxin may enhance cyst formation and accelerate the deterioration of renal function (Gardner and Evan 1984*a*; Werder *et al.* 1984). However, there are no definitive clinical data supporting a role for uncomplicated UTI on the progression of renal dysfunction in ADPKD (Mitcheson *et al.* 1977; Franz and Reubi 1983).

Clinical and laboratory characteristics

Cystitis in the patient with ADPKD presents with the usual dysuria, pyuria, urgency, and suprapubic pain. Renal involvement with infection should be considered in a patient with persistent fever and flank pain, even in the absence of bacteriuria, since infected cysts may not communicate with the urinary space. Distinguishing between renal parenchymal and cyst infection often poses a difficult diagnostic problem. The experience of Schwab *et al.* (1987) with 26 episodes of renal infection in patients with ADPKD suggests that the presence of positive urine cultures and white blood cell casts favours a parenchymal infection, whereas positive blood cultures and development of a discrete new palpable area of tenderness in the involved kidney is indicative of a cyst infection. In fact, all 15 of their patients with cyst infection demonstrated a new discrete area of palpable renal tenderness. Nevertheless, in a bacteraemic patient with negative urine cultures, the source of infection may be uncertain and the clinical differentiation of renal infection from other septic processes, including hepatic cyst infection, may prove to be a diagnostic dilemma.

Pyonephrosis, with purulent infection confined to the upper renal collecting system, may develop in a kidney with partial or complete ureteral obstruction (Sklar *et al.* 1987). Obstruction may be due to purulent debris, calculus, blood clot or, less commonly, extrinsic ureteropelvic junction compression by a contiguous cyst.

Diagnostic imaging techniques

Renal imaging should be undertaken whenever a complicated UTI is suspected in a patient with ADPKD. Unfortunately, the gross structural deformation of the cystic kidney often reduces the diagnostic accuracy of imaging procedures that are otherwise quite reliable with anatomically normal kidneys. Plain films may show the presence of renal or ureteric calculi. Nephrolithiasis, which occurs in approximately 20 per cent of ADPKD subjects (Torres *et al.* 1988), is a well-recognized cause of renal infections recalcitrant to antibiotic therapy in the general population. The plain radiograph of the abdomen should also be examined for indefinite psoas muscle shadows, renal or perirenal gas collections which suggest parenchymal abscess formation. Perinephric abscess is probably best detected by computed tomography (CT) (Hoddick *et al.* 1983). In patients with normal renal function, intravenous pyelography can be used to search for ureteral obstruction. It is desirable, if possible, to avoid retrograde pyelography because of the increased risk of sepsis following instrumentation, particularly in an already infected urinary tract.

The diagnosis of renal cyst infection is hampered by the lack of reliable imaging techniques to identify the infected cyst (Rothermel *et al.* 1977; Betan *et al.* 1988). A wide variety of imaging modalities have been used but no systematic evaluation of the relative value of each modality has been performed. Renal sonography, which is extremely useful in the initial diagnosis of polycystic kidney disease, often cannot distinguish between complex septated patterns in multiple cysts from abscesses. Similarly, CT may fail to demonstrate any cysts with CT density clearly suggestive of abscess. Furthermore, CT findings compatible with cyst infection (i.e. thickened, indistinct cyst walls and increased CT density of the cyst contents), may be produced by previous haemorrhage into a cyst (Levine and Grantham 1981). Although nuclear scintigraphic studies may assist in localizing cyst infection, diagnostic accuracy is poorly quantified. Gallium-67 scanning, which is highly sensitive in localizing other abscesses, is less useful in the evaluation of the abdomen and pelvis because of interference from the 10 per cent of isotope excretion entering the bowel over the 48 hours after injection. In one study, planar [^{67}Ga] scanning had a sensitivity of only 50 per cent for detecting cyst infection (Schwab *et al.* 1987). Sensivity may be improved with gallium SPECT imaging (Amesur *et al.* 1988). Other authors have advocated the use of indium-labelled leucocyte imaging (Betan *et al.* 1988). In patients with renal failure, indium white cell scanning has the additional advantage since there is no bowel isotope-excretion and thus renal function is not a factor in isotope transport to a site of renal inflammation.

Microbiology

While difficult to document by controlled prospective studies in the literature, small patient series, and case reports support the belief that the pathogenesis of renal parenchymal and cyst infection in ADPKD usually results from retrograde spread of bacteria from bladder to kidney, rather than from haematogenous bacterial seeding. This opinion is based on the strong female preponderance for UTI in ADPKD with a preponderance of Gram-negative enterics as the causative organisms (Schwab *et al.* 1987). Thus, the vast majority of infections are caused by *E. coli*, Klebsiella, Pseudomonas, Proteus, and other Enterobacteriaceae, similar to organisms responsible for cystitis and pyelonephritis in the general population. Streptococcal (Schwab *et al.* 1987) and staphylo-coccal (Chapman *et al.* 1990) infections also occur rarely. The frequent absence of positive urine cultures, despite active cyst infection, deserves emphasis and probably reflects the fact that the majority of cysts become detached from their nephron segment of origin. Even when urine culture is positive, it does not in-variably predict the organism subsequently cultured from blood or cyst fluid (Waters *et al.* 1979). A few case reports document that renal cysts can become infected via the hematogenous route. These include reports of cyst infection by *Staphylococcus aureus* in an intravenous drug abuser (Chapman *et al.* 1990), by a staphylococcal species two years following staphylococcal peritonitis complicating peritoneal dialysis (Betan *et al.* 1988), and *Salmonella enteritidis* following enteric infection (Laing *et al.* 1993). The demonstration of low oxygen tension in some cysts (pO_2 < 40 mmHg) raises the possibility of anaerobic infection in some cysts. Indeed, anaerobic bacteria have occasionally been cultured from cyst fluid (Bennett 1985) and from a perinephric abscess (Sweet and Keane 1979). Fungal and tuberculous infections appear to be exceedingly rare. Gardner obtained eight positive cultures (organisms unspecified) from 69 cysts of four asymptomatic patients (Gardner and Evan 1984*b*), suggesting the possibility of subclinical cyst infection.

Therapy

Prompt and aggressive therapy of asymptomatic bacteriuria and cystitis is war-ranted in the ADPKD patient in order to prevent ascending involvement of renal parenchyma and cysts. Antibiotic selection should reflect the usual clinical considerations guiding the therapy of UTI in the general population. In the presence of concomitant advanced renal failure, bacteriological cure depends on the use of agents with effective delivery to the infected renal parenchymal and urinary tract sites (Bennett and Craven 1976). In this situation, drugs which are filtered, such as the highly polar aminoglycosides, are often ineffective. Gentamicin, when given in doses recommended for patients with severe renal failure, produces urinary drug concentrations lower than the desirable inhibitory concentrations, it would appear prudent to adopt a strategy of long-term anti-microbial prophylaxis similar to that shown to be efficacious in the general population of women with recurrent lower UTI, despite the lack of data on its value in persons with ADPKD. Instrumentation of the urinary tract, when un-avoidable, should be done under the cover of prophylactic antibiotics given before and for 24 hours after the procedure.

When upper UTI with cyst involvement occurs, eradication of the infection is often unsuccessful despite prolonged antibiotic therapy directed against infecting organisms known to be sensitive by *in vitro* assays (Rothermel *et al.* 1977; Sweet and Keane 1979; Schwab *et al.* 1987). In one series, 62 per cent of ADPKD pa-tients with presumed renal infection failed initial treatment with standard intra-venous antibiotic treatment for acute pyelonephritis (a beta-lactam and aminoglycoside) (Schwab *et al.* 1987). This high failure rate was shown by

Muther and Bennett (1981) to be due, in large part, to the failure of many commonly used antibiotics to achieve therapeutic concentrations within cyst fluid. This may result in the need for surgical drainage or nephrectomy.

According to current concepts, the primary route by which substances gain access to the cyst cavity is by transepithelial passage, with glomerular filtration playing little or no role. Cyst epithelium is capable of maintaining large gradients of sodium, creatinine, and hydrogen ions. These 'gradient' cysts are lined with epithelium that demonstrates functional and ultrastructural characteristics of distal nephron segments (Cuppage *et al.* 1980; Grantham *et al.* 1987). Such cysts, with their tight cell junctions, effectively prevent penetration of hydrophilic antibiotics (lipid-insoluble, polar) across the cyst epithelium. Included among these hydrophilic antibiotics with demonstrable poor penetration into cyst fluid are the aminoglycoside and the beta-lactam classes of antibiotic agents (Muther and Bennett 1981), which are commonly used for acute pyelonephritis because of their bactericidal activity against common pathogens. Schwab *et al.* (1983) showed that the concentration of the lipid-soluble antibiotic clindamycin, with its high pKa, increases as cyst fluid pH falls, whereas the similarly cationic, but lipophobic, aminoglycoside gentamicin, has low penetration at all cyst pH values from 5 to 8.

Most cysts are of the 'non-gradient' type and are lined with non-specific cells lacking distinctive features of any nephron segment. Some non-gradient cysts are lined with typical proximal tubular cells having villous brush borders (Grantham *et al.* 1987). Electrolyte concentrations in non-gradient cysts are typical of a plasma ultrafiltrate. Solute access to these more abundant cysts is probably by diffusion, either transcellular or though 'leaky' paracelluar channels, with a minor contribution, if any, from glomerular filtration. Conceivably, beta-lactam antibiotics may also gain entry into non-gradient cysts by an active organic anion transport pathway, as demonstrated for similar anionic molecules like PAH (Muther and Bennett 1981). However, may non-gradient cysts are lined with epithelium that lack the capacity to transport organic anions actively (Grantham *et al.* 1987).

Most therapeutic agents which are water soluble and ionized at physiological pH will penetrate the cyst fluid slowly and irregularly by diffusion, thereby achieving negligible or low, steady-state concentrations. Lipophilic agents, on the other hand, can penetrate both gradient and non-gradient type cyst epithelium. Additionally, those lipid-soluble drugs with a high pKa can theoretically accumulate in the acidic environment of the gradient cyst by the phenomenon of ion trapping, whereas the anionic beta-lactams, in addition to being hydrophilic, face an unfavourable electrical gradient.

Table 20.1 summarizes data concerning antibiotic penetration into cyst fluid. Bennett *et al.* (1985) sampled cyst fluid for antibiotic concentrations in 10 patients with ADPKD and found measurable concentrations of ampicillin, cefotaxime, erythromycin, metronidazole, and vancomycin in non-gradient cysts. Although absolute concentrations were low relative to serum values, nevertheless they were generally well above the minimum inhibitory concentrations of many

Table 20.1   Antibiotic penetration into cyst fluid

Antibiotic	Gradient cysts	Non-gradient cysts	Active against gram-negative enteric pathogens
Aminoglycosides	–	–[a]	Yes
Beta lactams	–	–/+[b]	Ampicillin/cephalosporins
Chloramphenicol	+[c]	+[c]	Yes
Clindamycin	++	+	No
Doxycycline	++	+/-	No
Erythromycin	+	NT	No
Fluoroquinolones	++	+[d]	Yes
Metronidazole	+	+	No
Trimethoprim-sulfamethoxazole	++[e]	+	Yes
Vancomycin	+	+/–	No

+, concentration greater than minimum inhibitory concentration (MIC) of likely infection organism; –, concentration less than MIC of likely infecting organism;
++, preferential accumulation demonstrated; NT not tested
[a]Isolated report of adequate concentration with amikacin. [b]Some cogeners such as ampicillin and cephalosporins achieve adequate levels with prolonged therapy (7–10 days).
[c]Based on clinical cures of cyst infection (cyst levels not measured). [d]Cliprofloxacin more effective than norfloxacin. [e]preferential accumulation trimethoprim only.

sensitive bacteria. However, with erythromycin, metronidazole, and vancomycin, the bacterial susceptibility profile is not favourable for likely infecting organisms. However, if staphylococcal infection resulting from a haematogenous source is documented or suspected, therapy with vancomycin has proven efficacy (Chapman *et al.* 1990). With the beta-lactams, prolonged administration (1–2 weeks) was necessary to achieve therapeutic levels in non-gradient cysts.

Based on observations of pH-dependent accumulation of clindamycin in cyst fluid Schwab *et al.* (1983) and Elzinga *et al.* (1987) studied 85 cyst fluids obtained by percutaneous aspiration or at surgery from ADPKD patients receiving trimethoprim-sulfamethoxazole (TMP-SMX) a lipid-soluble agent with an alkaline *p*Ka which, unlike clindamycin, has a favourable bacteriological spectrum against uropathogens. Mean ($\pm$ s.e.) cyst fluid TMP and SMX concentrations were 15 ± 3 μ/ml and 42 ± 2 μ/ml, respectively. Preferential accumulation of TMP, but not SMX, was observed in gradient cysts, exceeding serum levels more than eightfold. SMX penetrated both types of cysts to a lesser extent, with concentrations ranging from 10 to 70 per cent of the simultaneous serum concentration. Cyst fluid samples prior to TMP-SMX administration demonstrated no antibacterial activity against *E. coli*, *Proteus mirabilis*, and *Strept. faecalis*, whereas cyst fluid inhibitory and bactericidal following antibiotic administration were 1:32 or greater. These studies indicate the likely effectiveness of TMP-SMX in achieving bacteriological success in cyst infection.

Clinical experience, although limited, has shown cures in some patients with polycystic disease and refractory UTI (Schwab *et al.* 1987). One failure was associated in a gradient cyst with an amount of SMX inadequate to achieve antibacterial synergism with TMP (Schwab and Weaver 1986). Schwab and Weaver (1986) recommended withholding TMP-SMX unless the organism was sensitive to trimethoprim alone.

The quinolone class of antibiotics possess favourable antibacterial characteristics against likely pathogens in cyst infections. They also have relatively high lipid solubility, acting as zwitterions at physiological pH. Elzinga *et al.* (1988) sampled 70 cysts from 7 patients who were receiving oral ciprofloxacin. Ciprofloxacin accumulated in gradient cysts, exceeding serum concentrations by more than fourfold. The mean drug concentration in both types of cysts was 13 ± 2 μ/ml, a value well above the mean inhibitory concentration of the most likely pathogens. Indeed, post-treatment cyst fluid uniformly demonstrated high bactericidal activity against *E. coli* and *Proteus mirabilis* (1:32 or greater) with lesser activity against *Pseudomonas aeruginosa*, *Strept. faecalis*, and Gram-positive cocci. Similar studies with norfloxacin show preferential accumulation and bactericidal activity in gradient cysts, but unreliable penetration into the more plentiful non-gradient cysts (Bennett *et al.* 1989). Other congeners of this antibiotic class have not been evaluated.

In summary, the limited clinical experience with ciprofloxacin has been favourable. Patients with bacteraemia and persistent infection refractory to long courses of other antibiotics have been clinically cured within a week of receiving the drug (Elzinga *et al.* 1988; Laing *et al.* 1993; Rossi *et al.* 1993). Doxycycline, despite accumulating in gradient cysts on the basis of hydrophobicity and high *p*Ka, was unreliable at achieving concentrations above the minimum inhibitory concentration (MIC) for susceptible organisms in non-gradient cysts (Kohlhepp *et al.* 1990).

It should be noted that virtually all studies of antibiotic penetration into cysts have been carried out in patients who are clinically uninfected. Very few studies have been done in patients with actual cyst infections, and the permeability characteristics in this situation are not known. Amikacin has been found to penetrate non-gradient cysts and sterilize staphylococcal infections presumably because of infection-induced changes in cyst wall permeability to this usually impermeable aminoglycoside (Spiegel and Molitoris 1986).

In clinical practice, ADPKD patients with pyelonephritis can be managed with parenteral ampicillin and gentamicin. The absence of a clinical response to treatment with antibiotics that do not penetrate cysts supports a diagnosis of cyst infection. Localization of the specific infected cysts is often difficult, and when drainage is not possible, systemic antibiotics alone can be used. In this situation, the importance of selecting a therapeutic agent with documented ability to gain access to the cyst cavity is critical. Schwab *et al.* (1987) demonstrated the efficacy of a two-week course of parenteral chloramphenicol in eight patients who were refractory to five days of intravenous ampicillin and gentamicin. Presumably, these patients had pyogenic cyst infections. For patients who remain febrile after two to three weeks of appropriate cyst-penetrating antibiotics, percutaneous or surgical drainage should be considered if the purulent cyst can be identified. If fever recurs after initial response, obstruction, peripheric abscess, or nephrolithiasis should be ruled out. If antibiotics had been discontinued prior to onset of fever, reconstitution of a previously effective drug may produce clinical cure, although therapy may be required for several months.

Persistent or recurrent urinary infections are an indication for pre-transplant removal of polycystic kidneys.

Hepatic cyst infection

In contrast to renal cyst infection, infection of hepatic cysts is a rare event despite the high prevalence of liver cysts in patients with ADPKD. Infection of hepatic cysts may be more common in ADPKD patients treated by dialysis or renal transplantation than in those without renal failure (Grünfeld et al. 1985; Telenti et al. 1990).

The typical clinical and laboratory features of hepatic cyst infection include fever, right upper quadrant abdominal tenderness, and leucocytosis, often accompanied by mild elevations in alkaline phosphatase, serum bilirubin, or aspartate aminotransferase activity. The latter is particularly noteworthy since liver function tests are rarely abnormal in patients with uncomplicated polycystic involvement of the liver (Everson et al. 1988; Gabow et al. 1990; Gladziwa et al. 1993). Bacteraemia is frequently present, with Enterobacteriaceae as the predominant isolate from both blood and cyst fluid cultures. In contrast to the polymicrobial nature of non-cystic pyogenic liver abscesses, hepatic cyst infection usually involves a single bacterial species suggesting haematogenous seeding as the usual route of infection.

Accurate identification of infected cysts with the use of modern imaging techniques is essential for proper management. In most instance, this is best accomplished by computed tomography (CT) demonstrating thickened, indistinct cyst walls, and increased computed tomographic density of cyst contents. Contrast-enhancement may be helpful in indicating perifocal hyperaemia during the arterial phase (Oreopoulos et al. 1971). Telenti et al. (1990) reported accurate identification of infected hepatic cysts by ultrasound in four of eight cases and by CT in six of nine patients, while magnetic resonance imaging (two of two cases positive) and [^{111}In]-labelled leucocyte scanning (four of four cases positive) were also helpful and probably superior to [^{67}Ga] scintigraphy (one of three cases positive). Although nuclear scans may provide more specific evidence of infection, anatomical definition is less precise. Thus, combining the information derived from nuclear scintigraphy, and CT or ultrasound may prove useful.

Optimal management of hepatic cyst infection consists of a combination of drainage and antibiotic therapy. The high failure rate following antimicrobial therapy alone, without the benefit of cyst drainage, underscores the importance of accurate localization of the involved cyst (Telenti et al. 1990). Percutaneous cyst drainage can readily be accomplished under CT or ultrasound guidance and has the added benefit of providing material for microbiological assessment. Occasionally, surgical drainage or segmental hepatectomy is required.

The appropriate choice of antibiotics for the treatment of hepatic cyst infection is not well established. In contrast to kidney cysts in ADPKD, little information is available with respect to those antibiotics which effectively penetrate hepatic cysts. Although ciprofloxacin was shown to concentrate within hepatic cysts, chloramphenicol, another 'lipid-soluble' antibiotic, did not (Telenti *et al.* 1990), raising caution in extrapolating recommendations for infected renal cysts to hepatic cysts. Fortunately, if effective cyst drainage is provided, the need for an antibiotic which will gain entrance into the cyst fluid appears to be less critical. Clinical experience has indicated that successful therapeutic results can be achieved with drainage in combination with a wide variety of antibiotics (Telenti *et al.* 1990).

Nephrolithiasis

Renal and urinary calculi frequently complicate the course of ADPKD. The clinical manifestations are difficult to distinguish from other causes of abdominal and flank pains such as ruptured cysts, blood clot, or renal infection. Fifteen to 20 per cent of patients with ADPKD will manifest nephrolithiasis, although the calcifications can be difficult to localize in relation to the renal collecting system since parenchymal and cyst wall calcifications are common in these patients (Torres *et al.* 1993). CT scans and intravenous pyelograms are the most useful diagnostic imaging techniques for diagnosis of nephrolithiasis in ADPKD. In a study on 84 ADPKD patients regardless of stone history, 36 per cent had stones demonstrated (Levine and Grantham 1992).

Stones which form in ADPKD are largely composed of calcium oxalate and urate. In various ADPKD patients, metabolic factors leading to nephrolithiasis are hyperuricosuria, hyperuricaemia, and hypocitraturia. There may be also increases in urinary stasis from anatomical factors. This profile of factors involved in stone formation is more variable than in age-matched individuals from the general population who have a preponderance of calcium-containing urolithiasis (Torres *et al.* 1988). In a study examining ammonia excretion in ADPKD patients with a normal glomerular filtration rate (GFR), compared to age- and gender-matched controls, Torres and co-workers showed a reduction in ammonia excretion rate due to an impaired renal concentrating mechanism and reduced trapping of ammonia in a medulla distorted by cysts (Torres *et al.* 1994). Low urinary pH and low urinary citrate due to defective renal transport could increase the frequency of uric acid calculi. Compared to other patients with chronic renal failure, clinical gout and higher blood uric acid elevations are more frequent in ADPKD although fractional excretion of uric acid is similar (Mejias *et al.* 1989). A larger study failed to confirm this finding attributing hyperuricaemia to depressed GFR, independent of aetiology of renal insufficiency (Kaehny *et al.* 1990).

While diagnosis of stones in ADPKD is difficult, management of obstructing stones may be even more of a challenge because of concomitant anatomical abnormalities and infection. Extracorporeal shock wave lithotripsy can be used successfully for small (< 2 cm) stones lodged in the renal pelvis or collecting system but retained fragments are frequent (Torres *et al.* 1993).

Cardiovascular abnormalities unrelated to hypertension

Prolapse of the mitral and tricuspid valves and pulmonary valvular incompetence have been reported to be more frequent in patients with ADPKD than unaffected members of the same kindreds (Hossack *et al.* 1988). Over 25 per cent of patients with ADPKD can be shown to have mitral valve prolapse when cross-sectional surveillance is done by echocardiography (Hossack *et al.* 1988; Timio *et al.* 1990). Morbidity due to endocarditis and valvular incompetence (Timio *et al.* 1990) have been reported to contribute to cardiovascular death, although it is far more likely that coronary atherosclerosis and hypertension are responsible for cardiovascular death in the ADPKD population (Leier *et al.* 1984; Roscoe *et al.* 1993). This is confirmed in limited autopsy studies (Iglesias *et al.* 1983; Hida *et al.* 1984; Singh and Hariharan 1991). Left ventricular hypertrophy and hypertension, both together and independently, are risk factors for premature death in ADPKD (Timio *et al.* 1990). The valvular histology in ADPKD has shown myxoid degeneration with loss and disruption of collagen, features similar to Ehlers–Danlos' and Marfan's syndromes. A case of coexistent atrial myxoma and ADPKD has been reported but, of course, the association could be coincidental (Earle and Hoffbrand 1989).

Since aneurysm formation in the cerebral circulation complicates many ADPKD cases, there has been an attempt to survey the ADPKD population for aneurysms elsewhere. Abdominal aortic aneurysms have been associated with ADPKD, but there is some question about the causality of the relationship in an older population with known arterisclerotic and hypertensive cardiovascular disease (Chapman and Hilson 1980; Montoliu *et al.* 1980). Aortic root dilation and ectasia have also been noted (Leier *et al.* 1984; Nunez *et al.* 1986) as well as a greater than sevenfold increased frequency of thoracic aortic dissection at autopsy (Torres *et al.* 1985). Aortic aneurysms in the ADPKD population should be managed as in any other group of patients. An atrial septal aneurysm has been reported in a 6-year-old child with hypertension (Waz *et al.* 1994).

Coronary artery aneurysms are rare in the general population and when they occur, they are manifest as ectatic segments secondary to coronary atherosclerosis. A recent survey reviewed coronary angiograms in 32 ADPKD patients and found five patients with distinct saccular or fusiform aneurysms and another six patients with coronary ectasia associated with coronary artery disease. Two patients with coronary aneurysm but no associated atherosclerosis of the coronary vessels presented with ischaemic episodes and thrombus demonstrable in the aneurysms (Swan, personal communication).

Diverticular disease and GI complications

Colonic diverticulae are common in the general population, particularly in the elderly. In retrospective studies, colonic diverticulosis is virtually inevitable in ADPKD (Scheff *et al.* 1980), especially in patients on maintenance dialysis (Gabow 1993). Ruputre and inflammation of colonic diverticulae present a formidable array of clinical problems for the patient with ADPKD, particularly when they are on immunosuppression for a kidney transplant or are maintained on chronic dialysis (Carson *et al.* 1978; Starnes *et al.* 1985). The incidence and rupture rate of colonic diverticulae is higher than an age-matched non-ADPKD dialysis population or the general population (Scheff *et al.* 1980). In the general population, there is an increasing incidence of diverticulosis with age, approaching 50 per cent at age 80. The spectrum of diverticular rupture and sepsis must be kept in mind in any ADPKD with abdominal pain and fever.

There may be an increased prevalence of hiatal hernias in ADPKD (Scheff *et al.* 1980), although this has not been observed by others (Zeier *et al.* 1988). Inguinal hernias are up to five times more common than in the general population, possibly due to increased intra-abdominal pressure from enlarging liver and kidney cysts (Gabow *et al.* 1984; Zeier *et al.* 1988). Umbilical hernias may also occur, with incarceration of both types of hernia a distinct possibility.

Bleeding in ADPKD

Macroscopic and microscopic haematuria are extremely common in ADPKD with more than 60 per cent of individuals showing this sign at some time in their course (Delaney *et al.* 1985). Sometimes it is gross haematuria which brings the patient to medical attention and leads to the initial ADPKD dialysis. Patients may be asymptomatic or may present with colic. Rupture of a bleeding cyst into the retroperitoneal space with considerable loss of blood may occur. CT and MRI scans can be helpful. When cysts bleed which do not communicate with the urinary space, the major symptom is severe pain without haematuria (Levine and Grantham 1985, 1987). Hypertension and large kidneys appear to be the major risk factors. For haemorrhage, however, even then, the bleeding is usually not significant enough to require transfusion (Gabow *et al.* 1984). Neoplasm, stone, or infection should be considered in the differential diagnosis. Infection, stressful activity, or blunt trauma often precipitate episodes of gross haematuria (Gabow *et al.* 1992). Most episodes end spontaneously within 48 hours to 1 week (Milutinovic *et al.* 1984). Management consists of bed rest and analgesics.

When gross haematuria lasts more than a week following institution of conservative management, or if bleeding occurs first in a patient over the age of 50, urological evaluation to rule out neoplasia is indicated. In unusual circumstances, angiography with embolization of a bleeder can be useful (Harley *et al.* 1980; Sholder and Grayhack 1985). Rarely removal of part or all of a kidney is required for massive haemorrhage. Desmopressin acetate, epsilon-aminocaproic acid, and aprotinin have all met with success, although experience is limited (Zeier 1992). Episodes of haematuria may indicate a worse prognosis for renal functional deterioration vs. patients who do not bleed (Gabow *et al.* 1992). In black patients with end-stage renal disease (ESRD) due to ADPKD, the prevalence of associated sickle-haemoglobins is higher than in blacks with other causes of renal failure. Renal failure occurs earlier than in whites with ESRD and ADPKD. Whether sickling or intrarenal bleeding contributes to the early morbidity is unknown (Yium *et al.* 1993).

In patients on dialysis and those with advanced renal insufficiency, cryopre-cipitate or oestrogens may facilitate cessation of bleeding by correcting uraemic defects. If bleeding occurs, there should be an increase in the dialysis prescrip-tion. Care obviously must be given to tight control of intradialytic clotting parameters and anticoagulation.

Patients with ADPKD often start ESRD with higher haemoglobin and haematocrit than patients with other aetiologies of renal failure. This is due to a higher erythropoietin plasma level and perhaps local ischaemia stimulating inter-stitial cells to produce more erythropoietin (Eckardt *et al.* 1989). Five per cent of ADPKD patients have frank erythrocytosis when they are non-azotaemic (Gabow *et al.* 1992).

Neoplasm

There is a theoretical basis for a possible increased prevalence of malignant neo-plasia in ADPKD in view of the important role of cellular proliferation in exper-imental and clinical cyst pathogenesis. Many studies have shown, however, that the incidence is not increased over chance coincidence of two relatively common conditions (Iglesias *et al.* 1983; Hida *et al.* 1984; Singh and Hariharan 1991; Keith *et al.* 1993). Histology of tumours has been variable.

Diagnosis of renal tumours in enlarged cystic kidneys is difficult even with modern imaging techniques. Signs and symptoms of pain, haematuria, and renal masses are not helpful since ADPKD patients without neoplasm frequently have these clincal findings. [111In]-labelled white cell accumulation scans can give false positive tests in conditions where active neoplasia is present (Keith *et al.* 1993). CT scan with contrast with confirmatory angiography are probably the most helpful. In ADPKD, tumours are more apt to be bilateral than renal cell tumours in the population. Successful renal transplantation may cause regression of cyst and kidney volume. The effects of establishing normal renal function on incipient neoplasia in ADPKD is unknown. Hyperplastic polyps can be observed in over 90 per cent of ADPKD patients if kidneys are carefully examined (Gregoire *et al.* 1987).

In the largest series reported, Keith *et al.* (1993) confirms an earlier age of presentation (45 vs. 61 years), constitutional symptoms, metastasis at diagnosis, increased bilaterality, multicentricity, and sarcomatoid features of renal cell car-cinoma when compared to renal cell carcinoma in the general population (Keith *et al.* 1993). Thus, renal neoplasia, when it develops in a small subset of ADPKD patients, may have an accelerated biological behaviour. Papillary renal cell carcinoma, which makes up only about 10 per cent of all renal cell carcinomas in the general population (Mydlo and Bard 1987), have been observed in ADPKD kidneys (Sulser *et al.* 1993; Gatalica *et al.* 1994). Transitional cell tumours and non-neoplastic masses such as malacoplakia and xanthogranuloma-tous pyelonephtritis have been reported (Gregoire *et al.* 1987). Renal tumours should be anticipated in patients with increased sedimentation rate, severe anaemia, erythrocytosis, and abnormal liver function tests.

Extrarenal cysts

Other than the liver, other epithelial cysts are unusual. However, up to 10 per cent of patients have pancreatic involvement. In a recent autopsy study, ADPKD patients showed pancreatic cysts in six of 67 patients (9 per cent). Most were microscopic and of no clinical significance (Gabow, personal communication).

Ovarian cysts were incidental and noted in three of 18 autopsies. This is similar to post-menopausal women in the general population (Wolf *et al.* 1991). Furthermore, fertility is not compromised in women with ADPKD, although hypertensive pregnancies are more common relative to control women (Milutinovic *et al.* 1983). Fewer than 5 per cent of ADPKD patients have cysts in the spleen while there are rare case reports of cysts in the oesophagus, thyroid, endometrium, brain, seminal vesicle, and epididymis. These isolated cysts do not usually cause clinical problems.

References

Amesur, P., Castronuovo, J. J., and Chandramouly, B. (1988). Infected cyst localization with gallium SPECT imaging in polycystic kidney disease. *Clinical Nuclear Medicine*, **13**, 35–7.

Bennett, W. M. (1985). Evaluation and management of renal infection. In *Proceedings of the First International Workshop on Polycystic Kidney Disease*, (ed. J. J. Grantham and K. D. Gardner, Jr), pp. 98–105. Intercollegiate Press, Kansas City.

Bennett, W. M. and Craven, R. (1976). Ampicillin and trimethoprim-sulfamethoxazole treatment of urinary tract infections in patients with severe renal disease. *Journal of the American Medical Association*, **236**, 946–50.

Bennett, W. M., Hartnett, M. N., Craven, R., Gilbert, D. N., and Porter G. A. (1977). Gentamicin concentrations in blood, urine, and renal tissue of patients with end stage renal disease. *Journal of Laboratory and Clinical Medicine*, **90**, 389–93.

Bennett, W. M., Elzinga, L., Pulliam, J. P., Rashad, A. L., and Barry, J. M. (1985). Cyst fluid antibiotic concentrations in autosomal dominant polycystic kidney disease. *American Journal of Kidney Disease*, **6**, 400–4.

Bennett, W. M., Golper, T. A., and Elzinga, L. W. (1989). Fluoroquinolones in patients with polycystic kidney disease. *Kidney International*, **35**, 738.

Betan, P. N. Jr, Price, D. C., and McClure, R. D. (1988). Localization of abscess in adult polycystic kidney by indium-111 leukocyte scan. *Urology*, **32**, 169–171.

Carson, S. D., Krom, R. A. F., Uchida, K., Yokota, K., West, J. C., and Weil, R. (1978). Colon perforation after kidney transplantation. *Annals of Surgery*, **188**, 109–13.

Chapman, J. R. and Hilson, A. J. W. (1980). Polycystic kidneys and abdominal aortic aneurysms. *Lancet*, **1**, 646.

Chapman, A. B., Thickman, D., and Gabow, P. A. (1990). Percutaneous cyst puncture in the treatment of cyst infection in autosomal dominant polycystic kidney disease. *American Journal of Kidney Disease*, **16**, 252–5.

Cuppage, F. E., Huseman, R. A., Chapman, A., and Grantham, J. J. (1980). Ultrastructure and function of cysts from human adult polycystic kidneys. *Kidney International*, **17**, 372–81.

Dalgaard, O. Z. (1957). Bilateral polycystic disease of the kidneys: A follow-up of two hundred and eighty-four patients and their families. *Acta Medica Scandinavica* (Suppl.), **328**, 1–255.

De Bono, D. P. and Evans, D. B. (1977). The management of polycystic kidney disease with special reference to dialysis and transplantation. *Quarterly Journal of Medicine*, **183**, 353–63.

Delaney, V. B., Adler, S., Bruns F. J., Licinia, M., Segel D. P., and Fraley, D. S. (1985). Autosomal dominant polycystic kidney disease: Presentation, complications and prognosis. *American Journal of Kidney Disease*, **5**, 104–11.

Earle, K. and Hoffbrand, B. I. (1989). Adult dominant polycystic kidney disease and atrial myxoma. *Nephron*, **52**, 197.

Eckardt, K. U., *et al.* (1989). Erythropoietin in polycystic kidneys. *Journal of Clinical Investigation*, **84**, 1160.

Elzinga, L. W., Golper, T. A., Rashad, A. L., Carr, M. E., and Bennett, W. M. (1987). Trimethoprim-sulfamethoxazole in cyst fluid from autosomal dominant polycystic kidneys. *Kidney International*, **32**, 884–8.

Elzinga, L. W., Golper, T. A., Rashad, A. L., Carr, M. E., and Bennett, W. M. (1988). Ciprofloxacin activity in cyst fluid from polycystic kidneys. *Antimicrobial Agents and Chemotherapy*, **32**, 844–7.

Everson, G. T., Scherzinger, A., and Berger-Leff, N. (1988). Polycystic liver disease: Quantitation of parenchymal and cyst volumes from computed tomography images and clinical correlates of hepatic cysts. *Hepatology*, **8**, 1627–34.

Franz, K. A. and Reubi, F. C. (1983). Rate of functional deterioration in polycystic kidney disease. *Kidney International*, **23**, 526–9.

Gabow, P. (1993). Autosomal dominant polycystic kidney disease. *New England Journal of Medicine*, **329**, 332.

Gabow, P. A., Iklé, D. W., and Holmes, J. H. (1984). Polycystic kidney disease: Prospective analysis of nonazotemic patients and family members. *Annals of Internal Medicine*, **101**, 238–47.

Gabow, P. A., Johnson, A. M., and Kaehny, W. D. (1990). Risk factors for the development of hepatic cysts in autosomal dominant polycystic kidney disease. *Hepatology* **11**, 1033–7.

Gabow, P. A., Duley, I., and Johnson, A. M. (1992). Clinical profiles of gross hematuria in autosomal dominant polycystic kidney disease. *American Journal of Kidney Disease*, **20**, 140–3.

Gardner, K. D. and Evan, A. P. (1984*a*). Host-microbe interaction in nordihydro-guaiaretic acid induced renal cystic disease. *Kidney International*, **25**, 244–8.

Gardner, K. D. and Evan, A. P. (1984*b*). Cystic kidneys: An enigma evolves. *American Journal of Kidney Disease*, **3**, 403–13.

Gatalica, Z., Schwarting, R., and Petersen, R. O. (1994). Renal cell carcinoma in the presence of adult polycystic kidney disease. *Urology*, **43**, 102–5.

Gladziwa, U., Böhm, R., Malms, J., Krulers, P., Haase, G., and Sieberth, H. G. (1993). Diagnosis and treatment of a solitary infected hepatic cyst in two patients with adult polycystic kidney disease. *Clinical Nephrology*, **40**, 205–7.

Gregoire, J. R., Torres, V. E., Holley, K. E., and Farrow, G. M. (1987). Renal epithelial hyperplastic and neoplastic proliferation in autosomal dominant polycystic kidney disease. *American Journal of Kidney Disease*, **9**, 27–38.

Grantham, J. J., Geiser, J. L., and Evan, A. P. (1987). Cyst formation and growth in autosomal dominant polycystic kidney disease. *Kidney International*, **31**, 1145–52.

Grünfeld, J.-P., *et al.* (1985). Liver changes and complications in adult polycystic kidney disease. *Advanced Nephrology*, **14**, 1–20.

Harley, J. D., Shen, F. H., and Carter, S. J. (1980). Transcatheter infarction of a polycystic kidney for control of recurrent hemorrhage. *American Journal of Roentgenology*, **134**, 818–20.

Hida, M., Saitoh, H., and Satoh, T. (1984). Autopsy findings in dialysis patients with polycystic disease of the kidney. *Tokai Journal of Experimental and Clinical Medicine*, **9**, 389–94.

Hoddick, W., Jeffrey, R. B., Goldberg, H. I., Federle, M. P., and Laing, F. C. (1983). CT and ultrasonography of severe renal and perirenal infection. *American Journal of Roentgenology*, **140**, 517–20.

Hossack, K. F., Leddy, C. L., Johnson, A. M., Schrier, R. W., and Gabow, P. A. (1988). Echocardiographic findings in autosomal dominant polycystic kidney disease. *New England Journal of Medicine*, **319**, 907–12.

Iglesias, C. G., Torres, V. E., Offord, K. P., Holley, K. E., Beard, C. M., and Kurland, L. T. (1983). Epidemiology of adult polycystic kidney disease, Olmstead County, Minnesota: 1935–1980. *American Journal of Kidney Disease*, **2**, 630–9.

Kaehny, W. D., Tangel, D. J., Johnson, A. M., Kimberling, W. J., Schrier, R. W., and Gabow, P. A. (1990). Uric acid handling in autosomal dominant polycystic kidney disease with normal filtration rates. *American Journal of Medicine*, **89**, 49–52.

Keith, D. S., Torres, V. E., King, B. F., Zincki, H., and Farrow, G. M. (1994). Renal cell carcinoma in autosomal dominant polycystic kidney disease. *Journal of the American Society of Nephrology*, **4**, 1661–9.

Kime, S. W. Jr, McNamara, J. J., Luse, S., Farmer, S., Silbert, C., and Bricker, N. S. (1962). Experimental polycystic renal disease in rats: Electron microscopy, function and susceptibility to pyelonephritis. *Journal of Laboratory and Clinical Medicine*, **60**, 64–78.

Kohlhepp, S., Elzinga, L., Barry, J. M., and Bennett, W. M. (1990). Doxycycline and ceftazidine in cyst fluid from autosomal dominant polycystic kidneys. *Journal of the American Society of Nephrology*, **1**, 300.

Laing, R. B. S., Smith, F. W., and Douglas, J. G. (1993). *Salmonella enteritidis* urinary infection associated with polycystic renal disease. *Journal of Infection*, **27**, 71–3.

Leier, C. V., Baker, P. B., Kilman, J. W., and Wooley, C. F. (1984). Cardiovascular abnormalities associated with autosomal dominant polycystic kidney disease. *Annals of Internal Medicine*, **100**, 683–8.

Levine, E. and Grantham, J. J. (1981). The role of computed tomography in the evaluation of adult polycystic kidney disease. *American Journal of Kidney Disease*, **1**, 99–105.

Levine, E. and Grantham, J. J. (1985). High density renal cysts in autosomal dominant polycystic kidney disease demonstrated by CT. *Radiology*,**154**, 477–82.

Levine, E. and Grantham, J. J. (1987). Perinephric hemorrhage in autosomal dominant polycystic kidney disease: CT and MR findings. *Journal of Computer Assisted Tomography*, **11**, 108–11.

Levine, E. and Grantham, J. J. (1992). Calcified renal stones and cyst calcifications in autosomal dominant polycystic kidney disease: Clinical and CT study in 84 patients. *American Journal of Roentgenology*, **159**, 77–81.

Mejias, E., Navas, J., Lluberes, R., and Martinez-Maldonado, M. (1989). Hyperuricemia, gout, and autosomal dominant polycystic kidney disease.*American Journal of the Medical Sciences*, **297**, 145–8.

Milutinovic, J., Fialkow, P. J., Agodoa, L. Y. Phillips, P. A., and Bryant, J. I. (1983). *Obstetrics and Gynecology*, **61**, 566–70.

Milutinovic, J., Fialkow, P. J., Agodoa, L. Y, Phillips, P. A., Rudd, T. G., and Bryant, J. I. (1984). Autosomal dominant polycystic kidney disease symptoms and clinical findings. *Quarterly Journal of Medicine*, **212**, 511–22.

Mitcheson, H. D., Williams, G., and Castro, J. E. (1977). Clinical aspects of polycystic disease of the kidneys. *British Medical Journal*, **1**, 1196–9.

Montoliu, J., Torras, A., and Revert, L. (1980). Polycystic kidneys and abdominal aortic aneurysms. *Lancet*, **1**, 1133.

Muther, R. S. and Bennett, W. M. (1981). Cyst fluid antibiotic concentrations in polycystic kidney disease: Differences between proximal and distal cysts. *Kidney International*, **20**, 519–22.

Mydlo, J. H. and Bard, R. H. (1987). Analysis of papillary renal cell carcinoma. *Urology*, **30**, 529–34.

Nunez, L., O'Connor, L. F., Pinto, A. G., Gil-Aguado, M., and Gutierrez, M. (1986). Annuloaortic ectasia and adult polycystic kidney: A frequent association. *Chest*, **90**, 299–300.

Oreopoulos, D. G., Bell, T. K., and McGeown, M. G. (1971). Liver function and liver scan in patients with polycystic kidney disease. *British Journal of Urology*, **43**, 273–6.

Roscoe, J. M., Brissenden, J. E., Williams, E. A., Chery, A. L., and Silverman, M. (1993). Autosomal dominant polycystic kidney disease in Toronto. *Kidney International*, **44**, 1101–8.

Rossi, S. J., Healy, D. P., Savani, D. V., and Deepe, G. (1993). High-dose ciprofloxacin in the treatment of a renal cyst infection. *Annals of Pharmacotherapy*, **27**, 38–9.

Rothermel, F. J., Miller, F. J., Stanford, E., Drago, J., and Rohner, T. J. (1977). Clinical and radiographic findings of focally infected polycystic kidneys. *Urology* **9**, 580–5.

Scheff, R. T., Zuckerman, G., Harter, H., Delmez, J., and Koehler, R. (1980). Diverticular disease in patients with chronic renal failure due to polycystic kidney disease. *Annals of Internal Medicine*, **92**, 202–4.

Schwab, S. J. and Weaver, M. E. (1986). Penetration of trimethoprim and sulfamethoxazole into cysts in a patient with autosomal dominant polycystic kidney disease. *American Journal of Kidney Disease*, **6**, 434–8.

Schwab, S. J., Hinthorn, D., Diederich, D., Cuppage, F., and Grantham, J. (1983). pH-dependent accumulation of clindamycin in a polycystic kidney. *American Journal of Kidney Disease*, **3**, 63–6.

Schwab, S. J., Bander, S. J., and Klahr, S. (1987). Renal infection in autosomal dominant polycystic kidney disease. *American Journal of Medicine*, **82**, 714–18.

Simon, H. B. and Thompson, G. J. (1955). Congenital renal polycystic disease. A clinical and therapeutic study of three hundred sixty-six cases. *Journal of the American Heart Association*, **159**, 657–62.

Singh, S. and Hariharan, S. (1991). Renal replacement therapy in autosomal dominant polycystic kidney disease. *Nephron*, **57**, 40–4.

Sholder, A. J. and Grayhack, J. T. (1985). Management of pain and hemorrhage. In *Problems in diagnosis and management of polycystic kidney disease*, (ed. J. J. Grantham and K. D. Gardner Jr), pp. 111–20. Intercollegiate Press, Kansas City.

Sklar, A. H., Caruana, R. J., Lammers, J. E., and Strauser, G. D. (1987). Renal infections in autosomal dominant polycystic kidney disease. *American Journal of Kidney Disease*, **10**, 81–8.

Spiegel, D. and Molitoris, B. A. (1986). The role of percutaneous cyst aspiration in the management of polycystic kidney disease patients with cyst infections. *Clinical Research*, **34**, 85A.

Starnes, H. F. Jr., Lazarus, J. M., and Vineyard, G. (1985). Surgery for diverticulitis in renal failure. *Diseases of the Colon and Rectum*, **28**, 827–31.

Sulser, T., Fehr, J.-L., Hailemariam, S., Briner, J., and Hauri, D. (1993). Papillary renal cell carcinoma associated with autosomal dominant polycystic kidney disease. *Urologia Internationalis*, **51**, 164–6.

Sweet, R. and Keane, W. F. (1979). Perinephric abscess in patients with polycystic kidney disease undergoing chronic hemodialysis. *Nephron* **23**, 237–40.

Telenti, A., Torres, V. E., Gross, J. B. Jr, Van Scoy, R. E., Brown, M. L., and Hattery, R. R. (1990). Hepatic cyst infection in autosomal dominant polycystic kidney disease. *Mayo Clinic Proceedings*, **65**, 933–42.

Timio, M., Monarca, C., Pede, S., Gentili, S., Verdura C., and Lolli S. (1992). The spectrum of cardiovascular abnormalities in autosomal dominant polycystic kidney disease: a 10-year follow-up in a five-generation kindred. *Clinical Nephrology*, **37**, 245–51.

Torres, E. E., Holley, K. E., and Offord, K. P. (1985). General features of autosomal dominant polycystic kidney disease. A. Epidemiology. In *Problems in diagnosis and management of polycystic kidney disease. Proceedings of the First International Workshop on Polycystic Kidney Disease*, (ed. J. J. Grantham and K. D. Gardner), pp. 65–71. Intercollegiate Press, Kansas City.

Torres, V. E., Erickson, S. B., Smith, L. H., Wilson, D. M., Hattery, R. R., and Segura, J. W. (1988). The association of nephrolithiasis and autosomal dominant polycystic kidney disease. *American Journal of Kidney Disease*, **11**, 318–25.

Torres, V. E., Wilson, D. M., Hattery, R. R., and Segura, J. W. (1993). Renal stone disease in autosomal dominant polycystic kidney disease. *American Journal of Kidney Disease*, **22**, 513–19.

Torres, V. E., Keith, D. S., Offord, K. P., Kon, S. P., and Wilson, D. M. (1994). Renal ammonia in autosomal dominant polycystic kidney disease. *Kidney International*, **45**, 1745–53.

Waters, W. B., Hershman, H., and Klein, L. A. (1979). Management of infected polycystic kidneys. *Journal of Urology*, **122**, 383–5.

Waz W. R., Pieroni, D. R., Stapleton, F. B., and Feld L. G. (1994). Atrial septal aneurysm in a patient with autosomal dominant polycystic kidney disease. *American Journal of Kidney Disease*, **24**, 209–10.

Werder, A. A., Amoo, M. A., Nielson, A. H., and Wolfe, G. H. (1984). Comparative effects of germ-free and ambient environments on the development of cystic kidney disease in CFW_{WD} mice. *Journal of Laboratory and Clinical Medicine*, **103**, 399–407.

Wolf, S. I., *et al.* (1991). Prevalence of simple adnexal cysts in postmenopausal women. *Radiology*, **180**, 65–71.

Yium, J., Gabow, P., Johnson, A., Kimberling, W., and Martinez-Maldonado, M. (1993). Autosomal dominant polycystic kidney disease in blacks: Clinical course and effects of sickle-cell hemoglobin. *Journal of the American Society of Nephrology*, **4**, 1670–4.

Zeier, M. (1992). Treatment of gross hematuria in autosomal dominant polycystic kidney disease with aprotinin and desmopressin acetate. *Nephron*, **60**, 374.

Zeier, M., Geberth, S., Ritz, E., Jaeger, T., and Waldherr, R. (1988). Adult dominant polycystic kidney disease — clinical problems. *Nephron*, **49**, 177–83.

21

Polycystic liver disease

Vicente E. Torres

Definition

The term 'Polycystic liver disease' (PLD) is often used to describe a condition with numerous cysts scattered throughout the liver parenchyma (Poinso *et al.* 1954; Melnick 1955; Peltokallio 1970; Sanfelippo *et al.* 1974; Vauthey *et al.* 1991). Whether PLD exists as an entity independent from autosomal dominant polycystic kidney disease (ADPKD) has been controversial. In this chapter we will consider under PLD: (1) the association of hepatic cysts with ADPKD; (2) the familial aggregation of hepatic cysts with an autosomal dominant pattern of inheritance in the absence of renal cystic disease; and (3) the sporadic presentation of numerous hepatic cysts in patients without renal cysts and without a personal or a family history of other conditions associated with hepatic cysts. In addition to ADPKD, conditions associated with hepatic cysts include tuberous sclerosis complex (Torres *et al.* 1994*b*), von Hippel–Lindau disease (Horton *et al.* 1976), oro-facio-digital syndrome type 1 (Curry *et al.* 1992), acquired disorders associated with the development of cysts of the hepatic hilus, such as portal hypertension and biliary obstruction (Nakanuma *et al.* 1984), as well as parasitic and neoplastic cysts. Since simple hepatic cysts are common, trying to define PLD raises the issue of how many cysts are needed to support a diagnosis of PLD.

Frequency of simple hepatic cysts in the general population

Simple hepatic cysts are less common than simple renal cysts, and their frequency has not been as well studied (Ravine *et al.* 1993; Pedersen *et al.* 1993). This information is essential to assess the significance of one or several hepatic cysts in an individual, with or without a family history of ADPKD or PLD. Two recent studies in large numbers of patients with ultrasound examinations of the abdomen found simple hepatic cysts in 2.5 and 4.6 per cent of the patients (Gaines and Sampson 1989; Caremani *et al.* 1993). The frequency of the hepatic cysts increased with age from 0 per cent in patients less than 20 years old to 7 per cent in those over 80 years of age (Fig. 21.1). They were more common in women than in men. They were solitary in 61–74 per cent of the patients. A maximum of three cysts was observed in those patients with multiple lesions (Gaines and Sampson 1989). These observations suggest that conditions associ-

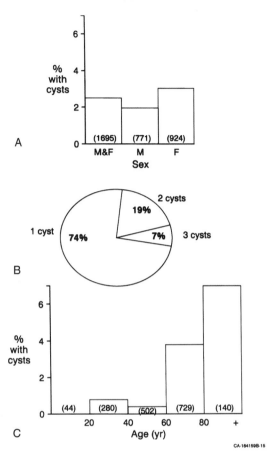

Fig. 21.1 Frequency of hepatic cysts by gender (A) and age (B), and number of hepatic cysts (C) in unselected patients who had sonographic evaluations of the abdomen (Adapted from Gaines, P. A. and Sampson, M. A. (1989). *British Journal of Urology*, **62**, 335–7.)

ated with the development of hepatic cysts, such as PLD, should be considered in the presence of four or more cysts, particularly in young individuals.

Genetics

ADPKD is a genetically heterogeneous disease with a locus in chromosome 16p13.3 (PKD1) (Reeders *et al.* 1985), a locus in chromosome 4q13-23 (Kimberling *et al.* 1993; Peters *et al.* 1993), and a third still unmapped locus (Daoust *et al.* 1993). PLD can occur in association with PKD1 and with non-PKD1. In one study, PLD was more frequent in non-PKD1, but the difference was not statistically significant (Wright *et al.* 1993). A preliminary observation that PLD occurs frequently in certain ADPKD families but not in others awaits confirmation (Simon *et al.* 1993). Whether exceptional families with autosomal dominant PLD without renal cystic disease (Torres *et al.* 1994*a*; Que *et al.* 1995) or with few renal cysts (Berrebi *et al.* 1982) have a different genotype is not known. Patients with PLD without renal cysts may have relatives with typical polycystic kidneys (Torres *et al.* 1994*a*; Dalgaard 1957). Sporadic cases of PLD may represent inherited disease with inadequate ascertainment of the families, new mutations, or true sporadic occurrences. A retrospective study of 33 700 medicolegal autopsies in Finland suggested the possibility that PLD may exist as an entity separate from ADPKD (Karhunen and Tenhu 1986). In this study, concurrent polycystic liver and kidneys were diagnosed in two, isolated polycystic livers with or without simple renal cysts in 10, and isolated polycystic kidneys with or without simple hepatic cysts in 10 autopsies.

Pathogenesis

PLD belongs to a family of liver diseases characterized by an overgrowth of biliary epithelium and supportive connective tissue, the hepatobiliary fibropolycystic diseases (Summerfield *et al.* 1986). These include dilatation of the extrahepatic and/or intrahepatic bile ducts, segmental dilatation of intrahepatic bile ducts (Caroli's disease), congenital hepatic fibrosis, autosomal recessive polycystic kidney disease, and PLD. Mixed presentations of these diseases can occur (Fig. 21.2) and are best explained by their overlapping pathogenesis. They result from an abnormal development and differentiation of the bile ducts which has been named the ductal plate malformation (Jorgensen 1973*a,b,c*; Jorgensen 1974). The bile ducts and the hepatic parenchyma derive from two primordia, the hepatic diverticulum and the septum transversum (Karpen and Suchy 1994; Desmet 1994) (Fig. 21.3). The hepatic diverticulum develops from the ventral floor of the distal foregut on the 18th day of gestation. Sprouts of endodermal cells extend from the the ventral and lateral surfaces of the hepatic diverticulum into

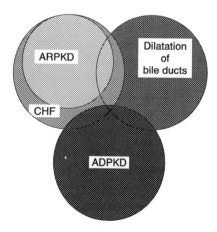

Fig. 21.2 Hepatobiliary fibropolycystic diseases.

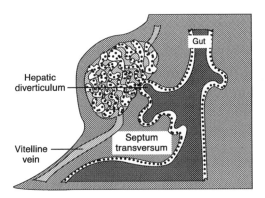

Fig. 21.3 Development of hepatic parenchyma from the hepatic diverticulum and the septum transversum.

the mesoderm of the septum transversum to form the hepatic anlage. The hollow portion of the hepatic diverticulum will develop into the gall bladder and extrahepatic bile ducts. At 7 weeks of gestation portal vein branches and surrounding mesenchyma start invading the hepatic anlage (Ruebner *et al.* 1990). The layer of hepatoblasts that enter in contact with the mesenchyma surrounding the portal vein branches divides and forms a double-walled cylinder with a slit-like lumen (ductal plate) and the cells gradually develop the immunohistochemical characteristics of bile duct epithelium (Van Eyken *et al.* 1988; Shah and Gerber 1990). The intrahepatic bile duct and ductules develop by centrifugal growth and remodelling of the ductal plate. This process continues during the whole pregnancy and the first year of post-natal life. Beyond the first year of life exposure to certain toxins, ischaemia, or liver injury may induce proliferation of bile ducts or ductular metaplasia from hepatocytes (Cruickshank and Sparshott 1971; Karhunen *et al.* 1986; Popövsky *et al.* 1979; Roskams *et al.* 1990, 1993). The hepatobiliary fibropolycystic diseases result from alterations in this normal centrifugal pattern of development and differentiation of the bile ducts (Fig. 21.4). The timing and severity of these alterations determine the distinctive features of these diseases. In Caroli's disease they occur early affecting the development of the large intrahepatic bile ducts. In congenital hepatic fibrous and autosomal recessive polycystic kidney disease they occur later and affect mainly the remodelling of the ductal plate and the development of the interlobular bile ducts in the portal tracts. In ADPKD the disease develops at an even later stage, and the interference with the developmental differentiation of the intralobular bile ductules results in the formation of biliary microhamartomas and cysts.

Pathology

Polycystic livers contain multiple cysts ranging in size from microscopic to occupying most of the abdominal cavity. The size of the liver may range from

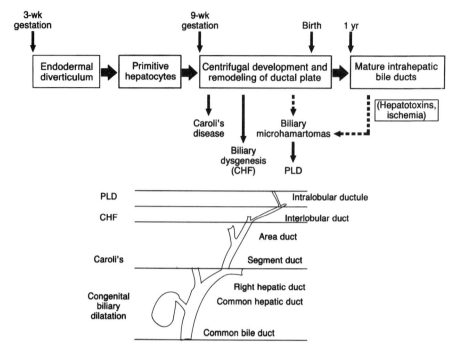

Fig. 21.4 Chronology, centrifugal pattern, and alterations of development and
differentiation of the bile ducts.

normal (1.2–1.5 kg) to enormously enlarged. The hepatomegaly produced by the
cysts causes relatively little compression atrophy of the uninvolved liver
parenchyma, and usually the liver parenchymal volume is well preserved
(Everson *et al.* 1988), even in patients with massive polycystic liver disease.
Often, the cystic disease involves more severely certain segments of the liver
while other segments are relatively spared (Nagorney *et al.* 1988). In addition to
cysts, other abnormalities of the bile ducts can be seen in patients with PLD or
ADPKD. These include biliary microhamartomas, biliary fibroadenomatosis,
cystic dilatation of the peribiliary glands, and rarely, dilatation of intrahepatic
and/or extrahepatic bile ducts.

Cysts

The cyst walls are usually thin and composed of a single layer of cuboidal or flat
epithelial cells and variable amounts of connective tissue (Watchi and Nezelof
1964). Flat or polypoid hyperplasia of the lining epithelial cells is observed in
less than 3 per cent of the cysts (Ramos *et al.* 1990). On serial sections the cysts
are often associated to biliary microhamartomas supporting the notion that
hepatic cysts derive from progressive dilatation of these structures (Watchi and
Nezelof 1964; Ramos *et al.* 1990). The epithelial cells lining the cysts stain positively for biliary specific epithelial markers (cytokeratin 7 and 19) (Jefferson

et al. 1992). The cyst fluid resembles the bile salt independent fraction of the bile (Fisher *et al.* 1974; Patterson *et al.* 1982; Everson *et al.* 1990). The electrolyte composition and osmolarity of the cyst fluids are similar to those in serum, whereas the concentrations of phosphorus, cholesterol, and glucose are lower (Patterson *et al.* 1982). The concentrations of bilirubin and bile salts are very low. Concentrations of aspartate aminotransferase, alanine aminotransferase, and alkaline phosphatase are lower, whereas that of gamma-glutamyl transferase is higher than in serum (Everson *et al.* 1990). The low glucose concentration and the presence of secretory IgA in the cyst fluids as well as the secretory responsiveness to the intravenous administration of secretin (Everson *et al.* 1990) strongly suggest that the epithelium lining the cysts is biliary epithelium.

Biliary microhamartomas

These are small clusters of bile ductules surrounded by fibrous tissue, which on serial sections and contrary to initial descriptions, are usually connected to the portal tracts (Watchi and Nezelof 1964; Ramos *et al.* 1990) (Fig. 21.5). They often contain bile, and their connection to the bile ducts has been demonstrated by microfilm injection (Grimm *et al.* 1990). Since the liver cysts, which are thought to be derived by progressive dilatation of biliary microhamartomas, do not contain bilirubin or bile salts and do not accumulate tracers secreted into the bile canaliculi, such as sulphobromophthalein sodium, cholic acid, and Tc-99n-hepatobiliary iminodiacetic acid-HIDA (Patterson *et al.* 1982; Fisher *et al.* 1974; Mishkin *et al.* 1986), it seems likely that as the biliary microhamartomas and microcysts enlarge they become disconnected from the bile ducts from which they derive. The presence of biliary microhamartomas is not pathognomonic of PLD. They have been found in 0.6 per cent of 2000 consecutive liver needle biopsies (Thommesen 1978). Biliary microhamartomas have been associated with liver damage produced by hepatotoxins, ischaemia, and other factors (Cruickshank and Sparshott 1971; Karhunen *et al.* 1986). Patients with simple hepatic cysts also have an increased frequency of biliary microhamartomas (Kida *et al.* 1992).

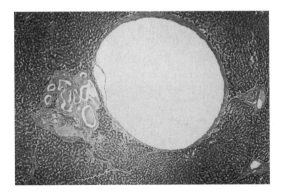

Fig. 21.5 Small hepatic cyst arising from a biliary microhamartoma.

Focal biliary fibroadenomatosis

This lesion is characterized by fibrosis and enlargement of the portal tracts with an apparent proliferation of bile ducts (Watchi and Nezelof 1964; Grünfeld *et al.* 1985). These are less diffuse and severe than those observed in biliary dysgenesis. Biliary dysgenesis is the characteristic lesion of idiopathic congenital hepatic fibrosis or congenital hepatic fibrosis associated with autosomal recessive polycystic kidney disease and a number of hereditary renal cystic displasias and tubulo-interstitial nephritis (Bernstein 1986, 1987). It is characterized by portal enlargement and fibrosis, absence of central bile ducts within the portal areas, apparent proliferation of bile ducts, and hypoplasia of portal veins frequently accompanied by portal hypertension. On the other hand, biliary fibroadenomatosis in ADPKD is usually localized and has no clinical consequence. Nevertheless, in a small number of families biliary dysgenesis or congenital hepatic fibrosis has been described in association with ADPKD (Gaisford and Bloor 1968; Bradford *et al.* 1986; Hoeffel *et al.* 1971; Tazelaar *et al.* 1984; Lee and Paes 1985; DeVos *et al.* 1988; Matsuda *et al.* 1990; Lipschitz *et al.* 1993; Cobben *et al.* 1990).

Dilatation of peribiliary glands

Numerous intramural and extramural peribilary glands surround and communicate with the extrahepatic and the large intrahepatic bile ducts (Terada *et al.* 1987; Ishida *et al.* 1989). Their function is not known. It has been suggested that they provide secretory IgA and contribute to local immunity against infectious agents in the bile (Terada *et al.* 1987). Certain pathological conditions, such as ascending cholangitis, biliary obstruction, and systemic infections, have been associated with inflammatory changes and cystic dilatation of these glands, and development of hilar cysts (Terada and Nakanuma 1990). Cystic dilatation of these glands and hilar cysts also develop in association with portal hypertension or portal vein obstruction (Terada and Nakanuma 1990). Dilatation of the intrahepatic peribilary glands occurs to a marked degree and to a broad extent in PLD (Kida *et al.* 1992). Epithelial cells of peribiliary glands and hilar cysts contain more neutral mucin, sialomucin, and sulphomucin than those of biliary microhamartomas and hepatic cysts (Terada *et al.* 1991). Because these cysts are located in the hepatic hilus, they are more likely to cause cholestasis and obstructive jaundice (Wanless *et al.* 1987). They may be responsible for the irregular filling of the intrahepatic ducts suggesting the presence of stones or sclerosing cholangitis on endoscopic retrograde cholangiopancreatography, which has been reported in PLD (Heather 1978; Howe *et al.* 1994).

Dilatation of extrahepatic and/or intrahepatic bile ducts

These lesions, which are more frequently associated with congenital hepatic fibrosis and autosomal recessive polycystic kidney disease, can also be seen in patients with ADPKD or PLD (Terada and Nakanuma 1988; Jordon *et al.* 1989; Grateau *et al.* 1990; Boudet *et al.* 1991). Caroli's disease, which can occur independently or associated with congenital hepatic fibrosis or autosomal recessive polycystic kidney disease (Caroli 1973), is characterized by cylindrical or cystic dilatations of segmental or area ducts with irregular lumens caused by bulbar protrusion and bridge formation of the duct walls due to an overgrowth of connective tissue. The dilatation of the extrahepatic and/or intrahepatic bile ducts seen in PLD lacks these bulbar protrusions and bridge formations suggesting some differences in pathogenesis (Terada and Nakanuma 1988).

Natural history

The natural history of PLD has been best described in patients with ADPKD (Grünfeld *et al.* 1985; Milutinovic *et al.* 1980; Levine *et al.* 1985; Gabow *et al.* 1990; Thomsen and Thaysen 1988). Therefore, the following observations contain an element of bias as they are based on patients selected because they had a diagnosis of ADPKD. Hepatic cysts are exceptionally rare in children with ADPKD (Milutinovic *et al.* 1989). In fact, the liver in biopsy specimens or autopsies of children with ADPKD usually appears macroscopically and microscopically normal (Milutinovic *et al.* 1989; Blyth and Ockenden 1971; Ross and Travers 1975; Bengtsson *et al.* 1975; Loh *et al.* 1977; Eulderink and Hogewind 1978; Proesmans *et al.* 1982; Rapola and Kääriäinen 1988). The frequency of cysts increases with age from approximately 20 per cent in the third to 75 per cent in the seventh decade of life (Grünfeld *et al.* 1985; Milutinovic *et al.* 1980; Levine *et al.* 1985; Gabow *et al.* 1990; Thomsen and Thaysen 1988) (Fig. 21.6). Women are more likely to have greater numbers of hepatic cysts and larger cysts at an earlier age than men (Grünfeld *et al.* 1985; Gabow *et al.* 1990). Women with ADPKD who had neither used oestrogens nor been pregnant are

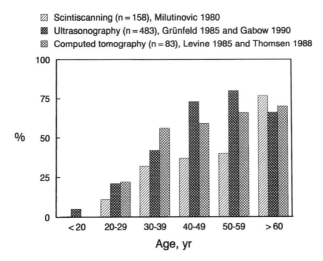

Fig. 21.6 Frequency of hepatic cysts in patients with ADPKD studied by scintiscanning, ultrasonography, or computer tomography.

less likely to have hepatic cysts than those who have used exogenous hormones, been pregnant, or both (Gabow *et al.* 1990). The number of hepatic cysts correlates with the number of pregnancies. In addition, the density of biliary microhamartomas and the extent of PLD correlate with the severity of renal functional impairment (Ramos *et al.* 1990; Gabow *et al.* 1990). This effect is independent of age. In a study of long-term outcome of renal transplantation for ADPKD, hepatic cysts were found in all the patients with a successful renal allograft for more than 10 years (Fitzpatrick *et al.* 1990).

Clinical manifestations

Most patients with PLD have no symptoms. A frequently quoted statement is that a polycystic liver is a 'huge, silent and durable liver' (Fiessinger, quoted by Dalgaard 1957 and by Grünfeld *et al.* 1985). More recently, symptoms caused by severe PLD have become more frequent as the life span of the patients with severe ADPKD has been prolonged by dialysis and renal transplantation. In one study, PLD was responsible for 10 per cent of the mortality of ADPKD patients on chronic hemodialysis (Grünfeld *et al.* 1985).

Symptoms in PLD may be due to abdominal distention caused by massive cystic livers or large dominant cysts, venous or biliary obstruction produced by severe cystic disease or strategically localized cysts, cysts complicated by haemorrhage, torsion, rupture, or infection, and conditions rarely associated with PLD such as congenital hepatic fibrosis, bile duct dilatation, and cholangiocarcinoma. Symptoms resulting from abdominal distention include fullness and abdominal discomfort; dyspnoea and orthopnoea associated with elevation of the diaphragm; early satiety, heartburn, and emesis; change in the bowel movement pattern and haemorrhoids; mechanical low-back pain, uterine prolapse, and even rib fractures (Que *et al.* 1995). Umbilical and ventral hernias are very frequently observed in patients with severe PLD. Intracystic haemorrhage occurs less frequently in the liver than in the kidney and may cause severe acute abdominal pain, extrinsic compression of bile ducts, and elevation of liver enzymes suggestive of acute cholecystitis (Schwed *et al.* 1993). The diagnosis of intracystic haemorrhage can be confirmed by ultrasound (internal echoes, irregular thick wall) or CT (high attenuation value, fluid–fluid levels) (Murphy *et al.* 1989; Barnes *et al.* 1981), but MR (hyperintense signal on both T-1 and T-2 weighted images) is the imaging modality most likely to differentiate a haemorrhagic hepatic cyst from a non-haemorrhagic cyst or other hepatic lesions (Wittenberg *et al.* 1988; Vilgrain *et al.* 1993). Torsion and spontaneous rupture (Orr and Thurston 1927; Sood and Watson 1976; Morgenstern 1959; Brunes 1974) of hepatic cysts are rare complications which present with acute, severe abdominal pain and ascites. Rupture of a haemorrhagic hepatic cyst causing a fatal haemoperitoneum has been reported only once (Fidas-Kamini and Busuttil 1986). Other complications and associations of PLD and their treatment will be discussed later in this chapter.

Because the volume of the liver parenchyma remains normal despite massive cystic enlargement, the hepatic function is well preserved even in patients with severe polycystic liver disease (Everson *et al.* 1988). In one study of a family with PLD the presence of the disease was associated with reduced antipyrine clearances and low serum HDL cholesterol, total cholesterol, and apoprotein A2 levels, suggesting that patients with PLD may have an impaired drug metabolizing capacity (Sotaniemi *et al.* 1979; Luoma *et al.* 1980). In another study of 12 patients with PLD, the hepatic metabolic functions measured by the galactose elimination capacity (a measure of functioning hepatocyte mass) and/or the salivary antipyrine clearance (a measure of the metabolic capacity of the cytochrome P450 system in the liver) were normal (Que *et al.* 1995). Slight elevations in serum alkaline phosphatase, gamma-glutamyltransferase, aspartate aminotransferase, and bilirubin levels can occur in patients with severe PLD (Que *et al.* 1995). Patients with severe PLD may also have low levels of total and HDL cholesterol, triglycerides, and serum albumin, probably reflecting a poor nutritional status (Que *et al.* 1995).

Treatment

As the symptoms of PLD are related to the mass effect of the hepatic cysts, the goal of therapy is to reduce the volume of the cysts. Non-invasive options to achieve this goal are limited. Since alcohol or drug abuse and certain hepatotoxins (Cruickshank and Sparshott 1971; Karhunen *et al.* 1986; Popövsky *et al.* 1979; Lambruschi and Rudolf 1979) have been reported to induce the development of biliary microhamartomas or cysts, the potential role of exogenous factors should be considered, particularly in patients with severe PLD. Epidemiological observations suggesting that oestrogens may have an effect on the development of hepatic cysts (Gabow *et al.* 1990; Grünfeld *et al.* 1985) have practical implications on the counselling of patients with significant PLD in relation to safety of future pregnancies or use of oral contraceptives or postmenopausal oestrogens. If the administration of oestrogens cannot be avoided, transdermic preparations without a first pass effect on the liver may be safer in these patients. The effect of oestrogen antagonists in patients with severe PLD has not been studied. No significant benefit on liver volume was detected in one of our patients with massive PLD who was treated with tamoxifen for six months. The sensitivity of the epithelium lining the hepatic cysts to hormones that have an effect on the biliary system, such as secretin, suggests that the growth of these cysts may be influenced pharmacologically. It has been shown in one patient that the administration of an H_2-blocker can reduce the secretion rate of unroofed hepatic cysts, possibly by inhibiting gastric acidity and secretion of secretin (Paliard and Partensky 1980). Since the action of secretin is mediated by intracellular cAMP (Kaminski *et al.* 1979) and cAMP plays a role in the secretion of fluid by intact cysts isolated from polycystic kidneys (Ye and Grantham 1993), avoidance of excessive amounts of caffeine and other cAMP agonist seems prudent. The administration of somatostatin markedly inhibits the secretion of secretin and may be accompanied by a reduction in the rate of drainage following surgical unroofing of cysts in PLD (unpublished observation).

Surgical options for the treatment of severe symptomatic PLD range from interventions with minimal morbidity, such as cyst aspiration and sclerosis, to those with significant morbidity and possible mortality, such as surgical fenestration, resection fenestration, and transplantation. Interventions such as portosystemic shunts, peritoneal venous shunts, cavocaval or cavoatrial shunts, and stenting of the inferior vena cava are indicated only in exceptional situations which will be discussed later in the chapter. The treatment of choice is dictated by the size and distribution of the symptomatic cysts and by the particular features of each patient.

Cyst aspiration followed by instillation of a sclerosing agent is indicated when the symptoms are caused by one or few dominant or strategically located cysts. Aspiration alone is almost always followed by re-accumulation of cyst fluid (Saini *et al.* 1983). Several sclerosing agents have been used to treat hepatic cysts, including pantopaque (Goldstein *et al.* 1976), minocycline (Hagiwara *et al.* 1992), doxycycline (Tokunaga *et al.* 1994; vanSonnenberg *et al.* 1994), tetracycline (vanSonnenberg *et al.* 1994), and 95 per cent alcohol (Bean and Rodan 1985). Ninety-five per cent alcohol has been the most extensively used and probably provides the best results (vanSonnenberg *et al.* 1994; Bean and Rodan 1985; Trinkl *et al.* 1985; Kairaluoma *et al.* 1989; Anderson *et al.* 1985; Buckenham and Teele 1990; McCullough 1993). The sclerosing effect of tetracycline solutions is due to their acidic pH and can be used when instillation of 95 per cent alcohol is too painful (Hagiwara *et al.* 1992; Tokunaga *et al.* 1994; vanSonnenberg *et al.* 1994). The standard technique involves trocar insertion of a catheter, removal of the cyst fluid, instillation of contrast material to rule out leakage into the peritoneum or communication with bile ducts, removal of the contrast material, instillation of 95 per cent alcohol or another sclerosing agent, frequent turning of the patient to assure adequate contact of the sclerosing agent with the entire inner wall of the cyst, and complete removal of the sclerosing agent and the catheter after 30 minutes (Fig. 21.7). There is no agreement on the volume of 95 per cent alcohol instillated into the cyst which can range from 5 to 10 ml to one-quarter of the cyst volume. While most interventional radiologists remove the catheter after draining the alcohol, some leave the catheter to gravity drainage into a bag to allow re-sclerosis 1–2 days later if continued drainage is significant (more than 10–15 ml/day) (vanSonnenberg *et al.* 1994). In our centre, the primary success rate has been 69 per cent of 13 patients (Welch, unpublished). The secondary success rate after repeated sclerosis has been 23 per cent, while 8 per cent has failed repeated treatments. The main complication of alcohol sclerosis is transient local pain. It has been suggested that this pain can be successfully ameliorated or prevented by intracavitary instillation of lidocaine or bupivacaine hydrochloride before or after the alcohol infusion (vanSonnenberg *et al.* 1994). A potential problem when large volumes of alcohol are used is systemic absorption, and patients should be discouraged from driving a vehicle after this treatment. Other reported complications include pleural effusion, pneumothorax, haemothorax, cyst infection, and arteriovenous fistula.

Several new applications of laparoscopic surgery have been recently developed. Symptomatic, large, superficial hepatic cysts are accessible to this type of

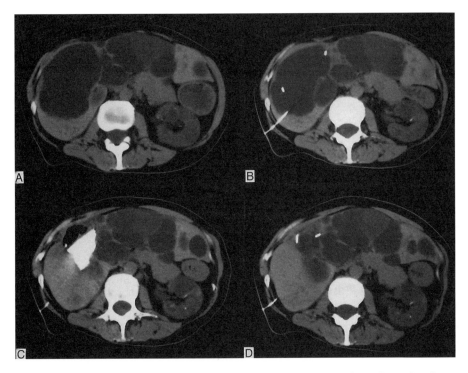

Fig. 21.7 Alcoholic sclerosis of a dominant hepatic cyst (A): insertion of catheter (B), aspiration of cyst fluid and instillation of contrast material (C), aspiration of contrast material and instillation of 95 per cent alcohol with turning of patients to ensure adequate contact with the entire inner wall of the cyst (D). The alcohol is aspirated and the catheter removed after 30 minutes.

treatment (Z'graggen *et al.* 1991; Paterson-Brown and Garden 1991; Moritz 1992; Lange *et al.* 1992; Klotz *et al.* 1993). Cyst walls can be laparoscopically excised using scissors (Klotz *et al.* 1993), electrocautery (Z'graggen *et al.* 1991), or laser scalpel (Paterson-Brown and Garden 1991). The latter has been recommended when the cyst wall is thick and vascular (Paterson-Brown and Garden 1991). Because of the limited experience, the role of laparoscopic surgery in the treatment of symptomatic PLD is still uncertain. It may become the treatment of choice for very large cysts, which are more likely to recur after alcohol sclerosis, and replace surgical fenestrations for large dominant cysts.

Cyst aspiration sclerosis and laparoscopic fenestration are of very limited value in patients with massive polycystic livers without large symptomatic dominant cysts. Extended surgical fenestrations have been used in some of these patients. Lin and co-workers reported extensive fenestration procedures in three patients with PLD in whom successively deeper cysts were unroofed and drained through more superficial ones, resulting in significantly decreased hepatic symptoms (Lin *et al.* 1968). Van Erpecum *et al.* reported nine patients who underwent a Lin fenestration procedure (van Erpecum *et al.* 1987). Although one patient died from haemorrhagic shock, abdominal complaints resolved in seven of the eight surviving patients. Furthermore, obstructive jaundice and oesophageal varices resolved in three of these patients. Turnage *et al.* reported one patient with diffuse PLD who died from surgical complications following the Lin procedure (Turnage *et al.* 1988). Howard *et al.* reported resolution of biliary obstruction in one patient after Lin decompression (Howard *et al.* 1976). Bensa *et al.* also reported good results with this surgery in 11 patients with symptomatic PLD, five of them without severe hepatomegaly (Bensa *et al.* 1989). In practice, this surgery is limited by the extent of the cysts, access to central cysts, post-operative walling off of cysts, and the rigid architecture of the fenestrated liver, which does not completely collapse. Thus, this surgery can result in relief of symptoms, but rarely a documented reduction in abdominal girth.

Combined hepatic resection and cyst fenestration for the treatment of massive polycystic liver disease was first reported by Armitage and Blumgart (1984). Successive fenestration along a projected plane between diffusely cystic and spared liver parenchyma allowed safe resection of non-functioning symptomatic cystic mass with preservation of liver function. Thus the extent of fenestration was reduced and diffusely cystic volume was excised (Figs 21.8 and 21.9). Because two or more adjacent liver segments are often relatively spared even in patients with massive PLD (Nagorney *et al.* 1988), combined hepatic resection and cyst fenestration is anatomically feasible in most patients with highly symptomatic disease (Newman *et al.* 1990). Que and co-workers have reported the result of this surgery in 31 patients treated between 1985 and 1993 (Que *et al.* 1995). The mean liver volume of these patients was 9357 cc before and 3567 cc after the surgery. There was one death from post-operative intracerebral bleed. Eighteen patients experienced complications, usually transient pleural effusions or transient ascites. Twenty-eight of 29 surviving patients with adequate follow-up have experienced a sustained relief of symptoms and improvement in the quality of life. After a median follow-up of 2.4 (range 0.2–7.9) years, the majority of patients have not had clinically significant enlargement of the liver. Sequential CT scans of the abdomen before and after surgery suggest that the hepatic enlargement in the age range of the patients in the study mainly results from the expansion of the existing cysts rather than from the development of new cysts. Thus, the extent of hepatic resection and fenestration is important for the long-term effectiveness of this procedure. The mortality rate of 3 per cent and the high morbidity rate is consistent with those reported in smaller series. Three of 22 patients in seven combined reports died after the surgery (Iwatsuki and Starzl 1988; Sanchez *et al.* 1991; Vauthey *et al.* 1992; Ambrosetti *et al.* 1992; Henne-Bruns *et al.* 1993; Johnstone *et al.* 1993). The morbidity rate in the larger of these series including eight patients was 37.5 per cent (Henne-Bruns *et al.* 1993). Combined hepatic resection and cyst fenestration is an effective treatment with an acceptable surgical risk when performed by an experienced liver surgeon for patients with highly symptomatic PLD who cannot be adequately treated using less invasive procedures.

A small number of patients with severe PLD have been treated by liver transplantation (Sanchez *et al.* 1991; Kwok and Lewin 1988; Starzl *et al.* 1990; Pirsch

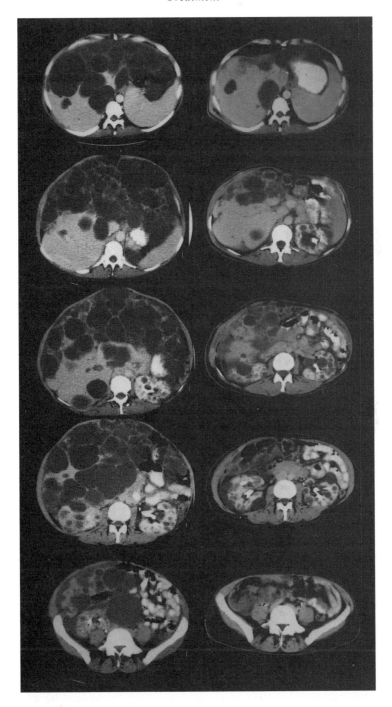

Fig. 21.8 CT scan of the abdomen before (left panels) and after (right panels) combined hepatic resection and cyst fenestration for massive polycystic liver disease.

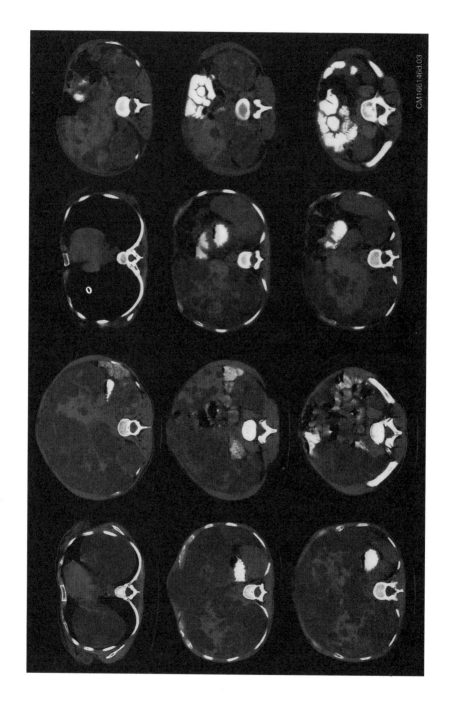

Fig. 21.9 CT scan of the abdomen before (left panels) and after (right panels) combined hepatic resection and cyst fenestration for massive polycystic liver disease.

CM166146d.03

et al. 1991; Taylor *et al.* 1991). Three of eight patients with a reported outcome have died. Primary hepatic transplantation for PLD should be used preferably in patients without spared liver segments or in rare patients with liver failure.

Special complications of PLD

Hepatic cyst infection

Infected hepatic cysts are an unusual complication of PLD (Robson and Fenster 1964; Clinicopathological Conference 1965; Parneix *et al.* 1978; Gesundheit *et al.* 1982; Bourgeois *et al.* 1983; Abascal *et al.* 1984; Du Toit *et al.* 1985; London *et al.* 1988; Desir *et al.* 1986; Telenti *et al.* 1990; Dofferhoff *et al.* 1990; Gladziwa *et al.* 1993). Possible risk factors include a history of recent abdominal surgery, renal transplantation, and chronic dialysis (Telenti *et al.* 1990; Gladziwa *et al.* 1993). The clinical and laboratory features of hepatic cyst infections are fairly consistent: a febrile illness with new onset of right abdominal pain, leucocytosis, and a high erythrocyte sedimentation rate (Telenti *et al.* 1990). Increased serum levels of alkaline phosphatase are found in nearly half of the patients. Elevations in the serum levels of aspartate aminotransferase or bilirubin occur more rarely. Infected cysts are frequently associated with bacteraemia and positive blood cultures. Cultures of undrained cyst fluids are also usually positive despite several days of antibiotic therapy. In contrast to patients with non-cystic hepatic abscesses in whom polymicrobial infections are common, monomicrobial infections with Enterobacteriaceae seem to predominate in hepatic cyst infections in patients with PLD (Telenti *et al.* 1990). Localizing infected cysts in patients with PLD may be difficult and necessitate assistance from imaging techniques. Computed tomography provides the best anatomic resolution, but the choice of imaging techniques should depend on the availability of local expertise in these techniques and the features particular to each case. The presence of infection, haemorrhage, calcification, or abnormal protein content within the cyst or group of cysts can cause a non-specific alteration of computed tomographic density, ultrasound echogenicity, or magnetic resonance signal intensity. The finding of gas bubbles within hepatic cysts on computed tomography is considered an indication of infection, but gas can also be seen if cysts were previously punctured or communicate with bile ducts that contain air. Air may appear on ultrasonograms as echogenic fluid with shadowing and may be overlooked on magnetic resonance scans. Other changes in cyst walls, such as nodularity, thickening, indistinct margins, contour enhancement of the cyst wall in a contrast-enhanced CT scan, and calcification, or a dominant cyst that shows enlargement on serial examination, might also suggest infection. Magnetic resonance imaging may be the most sensitive technique to differentiate a complicated from non-complicated cyst in PLD. [111In]-labelled leukocyte scans may also be helpful in locating an infected cyst and are probably superior to [67Ga]-citrate scans (Telenti *et al.* 1990; Dofferhoff *et al.* 1990) (Fig. 21.10). Gallium scanning with single photon imagers and computed tomography has also been used to locate infected cysts

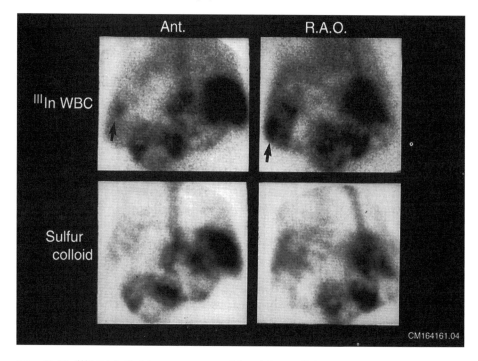

Fig. 21.10 [¹¹¹In]-labelled leucocyte scan with sulphur colloid subtraction. Note uptake of [¹¹¹In]-labelled leukocytes in an infected cyst in the right lobe of the liver (arrows).

in polycystic organs (Amesur *et al.* 1988). Indium or gallium studies may not be positive early in the course of the infection, and repeat studies may be necessary. Any cyst with unusual appearance on any imaging study in a clinical setting suggesting a cyst infection should be aspirated for diagnostic purposes. The best management for infected hepatic cysts is drainage in combination with antibiotic therapy (Telenti *et al.* 1990). Percutaneous drainage is usually effective and safe, but surgical drainage may become necessary if the percutaneous drainage is inadequate. Long-term oral antibiotic suppression or prophylaxis should be reserved for those patients with substantiated relapses or recurrences. Orally administered antibiotics that concentrate in the biliary tree and the cysts, such as trimethoprim-suphamethoxazole or ciprofloxacin (Telenti *et al.* 1990; Parry *et al.* 1988; Rieder 1973) should be used. Increasing numbers of patients with this complication are being seen due to the improved survival on dialysis or after renal transplantation.

Hepatic venous outflow obstruction

Hepatic venous outflow obstruction (HVOO) is an uncommon condition characterized by hepatomegaly, abdominal pain, and ascites (Mitchell *et al.* 1982;

Rectro *et al.* 1985; Wang *et al.* 1989; Kohli *et al.* 1993). Causes of HVOO include hepatic vein thrombosis (Budd–Chiari), cardiac disease (constrictive pericarditis), congenital webs of the inferior vena cava, and veno-occlusive disease (Ludwig *et al.* 1990). Hepatic vein thrombosis is associated with hypercoagulable states such as pregnancy, use of oral contraceptives, polycythaemia vera, paroxysmal nocturnal haemoglobinuria, and myeloproliferative disorders. Polycystic liver disease is an unusual cause of HVOO. Ten cases have been reported between 1990 and 1994 (Yaqoob *et al.* 1990; Bhupalan *et al.* 1992; Ambrosetti *et al.* 1992; Clive *et al.* 1993; Johnstone *et al.* 1993; Torres *et al.* 1994*c*). All the patients had severe extrinsic compression of the intrahepatic inferior vena cava by cysts and four had proven superimposed thrombosis of the inferior vena cava and/or hepatic veins. Possible predisposing factors included recent abdominal surgery, which in three cases was a bilateral nephrectomy (Clive *et al.* 1993; Torres *et al.* 1994*c*). The development of HVOO following bilateral nephrectomy has been attributed to the possible haemodynamic effect of the spatial changes caused by the removal of large polycystic kidneys. The hypercoagulable state associated with abdominal surgery and, possibly in one case, administration of cyclosporine might have also played a role. Severe ascites was the presenting feature in every case (Yaqoob *et al.* 1990; Bhupalan *et al.* 1992; Ambrosetti *et al.* 1992; Clive *et al.* 1993; Johnstone *et al.* 1993; Torres *et al.* 1994*c*). The presentation can be insidious in patients with extrinsic compression of the vena cava only or acute in patients with superimposed thrombosis. Hepatomegaly and abdominal pain are common but less likely to suggest a diagnosis of hepatic outflow obstruction in the presence of massive PLD. Dilated thoraco-abdominal collateral veins are helpful in the diagnosis. Standard liver tests may be normal or non-specific and of limited value. Liver biopsy shows centrilobular congestion in acute cases, but this may be less prominent in chronic cases (Rectro *et al.* 1985). HVOO may have been unrecognized in patients with severe PLD. It is possible that some of the patients with fatal PLD or PLD associated with portal hypertension of undetermined aetiology might have had HVOO (Katzen 1964; DelGuercio *et al.* 1973; Ratcliffe *et al.* 1984; Iannuccilli and Yu 1981; McGarrity *et al.* 1986) In the past it has been assumed, without convincing evidence, that the portal hypertension in these patients resulted from extrinsic compression of the portal veins or from compression and collapse of the hepatic sinusoids (McGarrity *et al.* 1986). A diagnosis of HVOO can now be reliably established with current non-invasive imaging techniques (Torres *et al.* 1994*c*). Most patients with severe PLD have a CT scan of the abdomen. If HVOO is suspected, MRI, should be performed for further evaluation. MRI with spin echo and gradient echo images is particularly useful in establishing the patency and direction of flow in the IVC, hepatic, and portal veins, and in detecting abnormal collateral veins. If thrombosis in the IVC or hepatic vein is suspected by MRI, inferior vena cavogram and hepatic venograms should be performed. HVOO is often fatal and requires aggressive surgical decompression of the congested liver (Mitchell *et al.* 1982; Rectro *et al.* 1985; Wang *et al.* 1989; Kohli *et al.* 1993). The damage to the liver results finally from the marked increase in venous pressure. In the absence of hepatic vein thrombosis the treatment should be directed at relieving the obstruction of the intrahepatic IVC. If the obstruction is caused by a large dominant cyst, this may be accomplished by alcohol sclerosis or laparoscopic fenestration. If the obstruction is caused by an enlarged cystic liver without dominant cysts, combined hepatic resection and cyst fenestration is the only practical alternative (Torres *et al.* 1994*c*). When hepatic venous flow cannot be reestablished because of hepatic vein thrombosis, non-selective portosystemic shunting with or without decompression of the inferior vena cava should be performed or liver transplantation should be considered. The outcome of patients with PLD and HVOO with superimposed thrombosis is worse than that of the patients without thrombosis (Torres *et al.* 1994*c*). Of four patients with HVOO and superimposed thrombosis, one patient treated by a portocaval shunt recovered with disappearance of the ascites, while the remaining three patients died. On the other hand, five of six patients without proven thrombotic occlusion of the hepatic veins were initially treated with alcohol sclerosis (one patient), surgical fenestration (one patient), or combined hepatic resection and cyst fenestration (three patients). These five patients had resolutions of the HVOO although the patient treated by surgical fenestration later required a partial hepatic resection because of recurrence of the ascites. Treatment alternatives with very limited reported experience include peritoneo-venous shunting (McGarrity *et al.* 1986) and inferior vena cava stenting (Sawada *et al.* 1992).

Obstructive jaundice

Obstructive jaundice caused by cysts is a rare complication of PLD and should be diagnosed only after other aetiologies have been excluded (Peltokallio 1970; Cryer and Kissane 1977). In the series by Peltokallio, for example, jaundice occurred in nine patients but it was attributed to the cysts in only three (Peltokallio 1970). The cysts causing the obstruction are usually located in the porta hepatis (Wittig *et al.* 1978; Ergün *et al.* 1980; Salem and Keeffe 1989; Lerner *et al.* 1992; Garber *et al.* 1993) and may be of biliary or peribilary gland origin. Cysts of peribiliary gland origin have been reported to cause obstructive jaundice in patients without PLD (Wanless *et al.* 1987). Ultrasound and computed tomography may demonstrate intrahepatic biliary ductal dilatation, but differentiation from multiple small cysts may be difficult. Endoscopic retrograde cholangioran-creatography (ERCP) is essential to confirm the diagnosis and establish the level of obstruction (Salem and Keeffe 1989; Lerner *et al.* 1992). Irregularities in the walls of the bile ducts caused by small cysts may mimic the appearance of bile duct stones or sclerosing cholangitis (Heather 1978; Howe *et al.* 1994). A CT examination immediately following ERCP may be especially helpful in separating cysts from dilated bile ducts and in identifying the obstructing cysts (Lerner *et al.* 1992). Cyst aspiration, alcohol sclerosis, and surgical fenestration have been used successfully to treat these patients (vanErpecum *et al.* 1987; Howard *et al.* 1976; Wittig *et al.* 1978; Ergün *et al.* 1980; Lerner *et al.* 1992; Garber *et al.* 1993).

Bile duct dilatation

Dilatation of the intra- and extrahepatic bile ducts is rarely seen in association with PLD. In a prospective study of 40 patients studied by ultrasonography it was found in only one patient (Grateau *et al.* 1990). The appearance of the dilation is different from the segmental cystic dilatation characteristic of Caroli's disease. It may be accompanied by a moderate degree of portal and periportal fibrosis and lymphocytic infiltration (Terada and Nakanuma 1988; Jordan *et al.* 1989; Grateau *et al.* 1990; Boudet *et al.* 1991). It causes no symptoms or liver function abnormalities unless it becomes complicated by ascending cholangitis. Except for the treatment of the episodes of ascending cholangitis, no other therapy is necessary. Chronic antimicrobial prophylaxis with antibiotics with good penetration into the bile such as trimethoprim-sulphamethoxazole or ciprofloxacin, may be indicated in patients with recurrent episodes of cholangitis.

Congenital hepatic fibrosis

Congenital hepatic fibrosis has been reported in 22 patients from 13 families with ADPKD (Gaisford and Bloor 1968; Bradford *et al.* 1968; Hoeffel *et al.* 1971; Tazelaar *et al.* 1984; Lee and Paes 1985; DeVos *et al.* 1988; Matsuda *et al.* 1990; Lipschitz *et al.* 1993; Cobben *et al.* 1990). Two or more siblings were affected in eight of these families. Contrary to the cystic disease, the transmission of congenital hepatic fibrosis in these families does not occur in an autosomal dominant pattern suggesting the coexistence of modifying alleles or genes. Interestingly, 18 of these 22 patients with ADPKD and congenital hepatic fibrosis had inherited the cystic disease from their mothers and only 4 from their fathers. The age at the time of diagnosis of the congenital hepatic fibrosis ranged from birth to 24 years. All the patients had splenomegaly and signs of portal hypertension. Nearly half of the patients developed bleeding oesophageal varices. Hepatomegaly was common, but only two patients had small hepatic cysts. Three patients had ascending cholangitis or bilestones. Eight patients underwent a successful portocaval or splenorenal shunt, and one patient was treated with sclerotherapy of oesophageal varices and administration of propranolol.

Cholangiocarcinoma

Cholangiocarcinoma is a vary rare complication of PLD (Willis 1943; Azizah and Paradinas 1980; Landis *et al.* 1984; Levine *et al.* 1985). Cholangiocarcinoma is a rare tumour in Europe and North America and is usually not associated with other liver pathology. Few cases have been associated with congenital hepatic fibrosis, Caroli's disease, choledochal cysts, biliary microhamartomas, and simple hepatic cysts (Daroca *et al.* 1975; Chen 1981; Dayton *et al.* 1983; Dekker *et al.* 1989). The association of cholangiocarcinoma and well-documented cases of PLD or ADPKD is extremely rare (Willis 1943; Aziazh and Paradinas 1980; Landis *et al.* 1984; Levine *et al.* 1985). One case of cholangiocarcinoma in a patient with ADPKD has been diagnosed at the Mayo Clinic between 1965 and 1990. The diagnosis is difficult and requires a high index of suspicion. The clinical presentation is with systemic symptoms such as fever, anorexia, and weight loss, hepatomegaly, right upper quadrant pain, obstructive jaundice, and superficial or deep vein thrombophlebitis. An elevation of the alkaline phosphatase, gamma-glutamyltransferase, bilirubin, and aspartate aminotransferase may be present at presentation. The prognosis is extremely poor, and death supervenes in most patients within six months after presentation (Willis 1943; Aziazh and Paradinas 1980; Landis *et al.* 1984; Levine *et al.* 1985).

References

Abascal, J., Moya, M., and Martin, F. (1984). Infection of hepatic cysts in polycystic disease (Letter to the editor). *World J. Surg.*, **8**, 424–5.

Ambrosetti, P., Widmann, J. J., Robert, J., and Rohner, A. (1992). Acute Budd-Chiari's syndrome after surgical treatment of polycystic liver disease. *Gastroenterol. Clin. Biol.*, **16**, 894–6.

Amesur, P., Castronuovo, J. J., and Chandramouly, B. (1988). Infected cyst localization with gallium SPECT imaging in polycystic kidney disease. *Clin. Nucl. Med.*, **13**, 35–7.

Anderson, R., Jeppsson, B., Lunderquist, A., and Bengmark, B. (1985). Alcohol sclerotherapy of nonparasitic cysts of the liver. *Br. J. Surg.*, **76**, 254–5.

Armitage, N. C. and Blumgart, L. H. (1984). Partial resection and fenestration in the treatment of polycystic liver disease. *Br. J. Surg.*, **71**, 242–4.

Azizah, N. and Paradinas, F. J. (1980). Cholangiocarcinoma coexisting with developmental liver cysts: a distinct entity different from liver cystadenocarcinoma. *Histopathology*, **4**, 391–400.

Barnes, P. A., Thomas, J. L., and Bernardino, M. E. (1981). Pitfalls in the diagnosis of hepatic cysts by computed tomography. *Radiology*, **141**, 129–33.

Bean, W. J. and Rodan, B. A. (1985). Hepatic cysts: Treatment with alcohol. *AJR*, **144**, 237–41.

Bengtsson, U., Hedman, L., and Svalander, C. (1975). Adult type of polycystic kidney disease in a newborn child. *Acta Med. Scand.*, **197**, 447–50.

Bensa, P., Haas, O., Rat, P., Dia, A., and Favre, J. P. (1989). Polycystic liver. Is Lin's operation still justified? *Ann. Chir.*, **43**, 720–3.

Bernstein, J. (1986). Hepatic and renal involvement in malformation syndromes. *Mt. Sinai. J. Med.*, **53**, 421–8.

Bernstein, J. (1987). Hepatic involvement in hereditary renal syndromes. In *Genetic aspects of developmental pathology*, (ed. E. F. Gilbert and J. M. Opitz), pp. 115–30. Liss, New York.

Berrebi, G., Erickson, R. P., and Marks, B. W. (1982). Autosomal dominant polycystic liver disease: A second family. *Clin. Genet.*, **21**, 342–7.

Bhupalan, A., Talbot, K., Forbes, A., Owen, M., Samson, D., and Murray-Lyon, I. M. (1992). Budd-Chiari syndrome in association with polycystic disease of the liver and kidneys. *J. Roy. Soc. Med.*, **85**, 296–7.

Blyth, H. and Ockenden, B. G. (1971). Polycystic disease of kidneys and liver presenting in childhood. *J. Med. Genet.*, **8**, 257–84.

Boudet, R., Gerardin, A., Leitchnam, P. A., and Honore, P. (1991). Biliary tract dilatation associated with polycystic kidney disease in adults (Letter to the editor). *Presse Méd.*, **20**, 917.

Bourgeois, N., Kinnaert, P., Vereerstraeten, P., Schoutens, A., and Toussaint, C. (1983). Infection of hepatic cysts following kidney transplantation in polycystic kidney disease. *World J. Surg.*, **7**, 629–31.

Bradford, W. D., Bradford, J. W., Porter, F. S., and Sidbury, J. B. Jr (1968). Cystic disease of liver and kidney with portal hypertension. *Clin. Pediatr.*, **7**, 299–306.

Brunes, L. (1974). Rupture of a solitary non-parasitic cyst of the liver: Report of a case. *Acta Chir. Scand.*, **140**, 159–60.

Buckenham, T. M. and Teele, R. (1990). Percutaneous therapy for hepatic cysts: Case report and review of literature. *Austral. Radiol.*, **34**, 159–61.

Caremani, M., Vincenti, A., Benci, A., Sassoli, S., and Tacconi, D. (1993). Ecographic epidemiology of non-parasitic hepatic cysts. *J. Clin. Ultrasound*, **21**, 115–18.

Caroli, J. (1973). Diseases of the intrahepatic biliary tree. *Clin. Gastroenterol.*, **2**, 147–61.

Chen, K. T. (1981). Adenocarcinoma of the liver: association with congenital hepatic fibrosis and Caroli's disease. *Arch. Pathol. Lab. Med.*, **105**, 294–5.

Clinicopathological Conference (1965). A case of polycystic disease of the liver and kidneys (clinicopathological conference). *Br. Med. J.*, **2**, 1356–8.

Clive, D. M., Davidoff, A., and Schweizer, R. T. (1993). Budd-Chiari syndrome in autosomal dominant polycystic kidney disease: A complication of nephrectomy in patients with liver cysts. *Am. J. Kidney Dis.*, **21**, 202–5.

Cobben, J. M., Bruening, M. H., Schoots, C., ten Kate, L. P., and Zerres, K. (1990). Congenital hepatic fibrosis in autosomal-dominant polycystic kidney disease. *Kidney Int.*, **38**, 880–5.

Cruickshank, A. H. and Sparshott, S. M. (1971). Malignancy in natural and experimental hepatic cysts: Experiments with aflatoxin in rats and the malignant transformation of cysts in human livers. *J. Pathol.*, **104**, 185–90.

Cryer, P. E. and Kissane, J. M. (1977). Obstructive jaundice in a patient with polycystic disease. *Am. J. Med.*, **62**, 616–26.

Curry, N. S., Milutinovic, J., Grossnickle, M., and Munden, M. (1992). Renal cystic disease associated with orofaciodigital syndrome. *Urol. Radiol.*, **13**, 153–7.

Dalgaard, O. Z. (1957). Bilateral polycystic disease of the kidneys: A follow-up of two hundred and eighty-four patients and their families. *Acta Med. Scand.* (Suppl. 328), 1–255.

Daroca, P. J., Tuthill, R., and Reed, R. J. (1975). Cholangiocarcinoma arising in congenital hepatic fibrosis. *Arch. Pathol. Lab. Med.*, **99**, 592–5.

Daoust, M. C., Bichet, D. G., and Somlo, S. (1993). A French-Canadian family with autosomal dominant polycystic kidney disease (ADPKD) (Abstract No. 91P). *J. Am. Soc. Nephrol.*, **4**, 262.

Dayton, M. T., Longmire, W. P., and Tompkins, R. K. (1983). Caroli's disease: A premalignant condition? *Am. J. Surg.*, **145**, 41–8.

Dekker, A., F. J. W., ten Kate, L. P., and Terpstra, O. T. (1989). Cholangiocarcinoma associated with multiple bile-duct hamartomas of the liver. *Dig. Des. Sci.*, **34**, 952–8.

DelGuercio, E., Greco, J., Kim, K. E., Chinitz, J., and Swartz, C. (1973). Esophageal varices in adult patients with polycystic kidney and liver disease. *N. Engl. J. Med.*, **289**, 678–9.

Desir, G., Helman, D., Herlick, M., Turka, L., and Johnson, B. M. (1986). *Haemophilus parainfluenzae* liver abscess in a recipient of a renal transplant who had polycystic disease (Letter to the editor). *JAMA*, **255**, 1878.

Desmet, V. J. (1994). The cholangiopathies. In *Liver disease in children*, (ed. F. J. Suchy), pp. 145–65. Mosby Year Book, St. Louis, LA.

De Vos, M., Barbier, F., and Cuvelier, C. (1988). Congenital hepatic fibrosis. *J. Hepatol.*, **6**, 222–8.

Dofferhoff, A. S. M., Sluiter, H. E., Geerlings, W., and de Jong, P. E. (1990). Complications of liver cysts in patients with adult polycystic kidney disease. *Nephrol. Dial. Transplant.*, **5**, 882–5.

Du Toit, D. F., van Schalkwyk, P., and Laker, L. (1985). Hepatic abscess in a patient with polycystic liver disease: A case report. *S. Afr. Med. J.*, **67**, 559–60.

Ergün, H., Wolf, B. H., and Hissong, S. L. (1980). Obstructive jaundice caused by polycystic liver disease. *Radiology*, **136**, 435–6.

Eulderink, F. and Hogewind, B. L. (1978). Renal cysts in premature children. Occurrence in a family with polycystic kidney disease. *Arch. Pathol. Lab. Med.*, **102**, 592–5.

Everson, G. T. *et al.* (1988). Polycystic liver disease: Quantitation of parenchymal and cyst volumes from computed tomography images and clinical correlates of hepatic cysts. *Hepatology*, **8**, 1627–34.

Everson, G. T., Emmett, M., Brown, W. R., Redmond, P., and Thickman, D. (1990). Functional similarities of hepatic cystic and billiary epithelium: Studies of fluid constituents and *in vivo* secretion in response to secretin. *Hepatology*, **11**, 557–65.

Fidas-Kamini, A. and Busuttil, A. (1986). Fatal intraperitoneal haemorrhage of hepatic origin. *Postgrad. Med. J.*, **62**, 1097–1100.

Fisher, J., Mekhjian, H., Pritchett, E. L. C., and Charme, L. S. (1974). Polycystic liver disease: Studies on the mechanisms of cyst fluid formation: A Case report. *Gastroenterology*, **66**, 423–8.

Fitzpatrick, P. M., Torres, V. E., Charboneau, J. W., Offord, K. P., Zincke, H., and Holley, K. E. (1990). Long-term outcome of renal transplantation in autosomal dominant polycystic kidney disease. *Am. J. Kidney Dis.*, **15**, 535–43.

Gabow, P. A., Johnson, A. M., Kaehny, W. D., Manco-Johnson, M. L., Duley, I. T., and Everson, G. T. (1990). Risk factors for the development of hepatic cysts in autosomal dominant polycystic kidney disease. *Hepatology*, **11**, 1033–7.

Gaines, P. A. and Sampson, M. A. (1989). The prevalence and characterization of simple haptic cysts by ultrasound examination. *Br. J. Radiol.*, **62**, 335–7.

Gaisford, W. and Bloor, K. (1968). Congenital polycystic disease of kidneys and liver. Portal hypertension — portacaval anastomasis. *Proc. R. Soc. Med.*, **61**, 304.

Garber, S., Mathieson, J., and Cooperberg, P. L. (1993). Percutaneous sclerosis of hepatic cysts to treat obstructive jaundice in a patient with polycystic liver disease. *Am. J. Roentgenol.*, **161**, 77–8.

Gesundheit, N., Kent, D. L., Fawcett, H. D., Effron, M. K., and Maffly, R. H. (1982). Infected liver cyst in a patient with polycystic kidney disease. *West. J. Med.*, **136**, 246–9.

Gladziwa, U., Böhm, R., Malma, J., Keulers, P., Haase, G., and Sieberth, H.-G. (1993). Diagnosis and treatment of a solitary infected hepatic cyst in two patients with adult polycystic kidney disease. *Clin. Nephrol.*, **40**, 205–7.

Goldstein, H. M., Carlyle, D. R., and Nelson, R. S. (1976). Treatment of symptomatic hepatic cyst by percutaneous instillation of pantopaque. *Am. J. Roentgenol.*, **127**, 850–3.

Grateau, G., *et al.* (1990). Dilatation of bile ducts in polycystic kidney disease in adults. *Presse Méd.*, **19**, 1669–71.

Grimm, P. C., Crocker, J. F. S., Malatjalian, D. A., and Ogborn, M. R. (1990). The microanatomy of the intrahepatic bile duct in polycystic disease: Comparison of the cpk mouse and human. *J. Exp. Pathol.*, **71**, 119–31.

Grünfeld, J.-P., *et al.* (1985). Liver changes and complications in adult polycystic kidney disease. In *Advances in Nephrology*, (ed. J.-P. Bach, J. Crosnier, J.-L. Frunck-Brentano, and J. -P. Grünfeld), Vol. 14, pp. 1–20. Year Book Medical, Chicago.

Hagiwara, H., *et al.* (1992). Successful treatment of a hepatic cyst by one-shot instillation of minocycline chloride. *Gastroenterology*, **103**, 675–7.

Heather, B. (1978). Choledochoscopic appearance of hepatic ducts in polycystic disease of the liver. *J. Roy. Soc. Med.*, **71**, 526–9.

Henne-Bruns, D., Klomp, H. J., and Kremer, B. (1993). Non-parasitic liver cysts and polycystic liver disease: Results of surgical treatment. *Hepatogastroenterology*, **40**, 1–5.

Hoeffel, J.-C., Jacottin, G., and Bourgeois, J.-M. (1971). A propos d'une famille associant des cas de polykystose rénale de type juvénile et de type adulte. *Ann. Radiol.*, **14**, 205–9.

Horton, W. A., Wong, V., and Eldridge, R. (1976). Von Hippel-Lindau disease: Clinical and pathological manifestations in nine families with 50 affected members. *Arch. Intern. Med.*, **136**, 769–77.

Howard, R. J., Hanson, R. F., and Delaney, J. P. (1976). Jaundice associated with polycystic liver disease: Relief by surgical decompression of the cysts. *Arch. Surg.*, **111**, 816–17.

Howe, C. D., Hill, D. B., and Gubbins, G. (1994). Polycystic liver disease mimicking sclerosing cholangitis during endoscopic retrograde cholangiopancreatography. *AJG*, **89**, 128–9.

Iannuccilli, E. A. and Yu, P. P. (1981). Adult fibropolycystic liver disease and symptomatic portal hypertension. *Rhode Island Med. J.*, **64**, 551–4.

Ishida, F., Terada, T., and Nakanuma, Y. (1989). Histologic and scanning electron microscopic observations of intrahepatic peribiliary glands in normal human livers. *Lab. Invest.*, **60**, 260–5.

Iwatsuki, S., and Starzl, T. E. (1988). Personal experience with 411 hepatic resections. *Ann. Surg.*, **208**, 421–34.

Jefferson, D. M., Grubman, S. A., Cox, L. J., Torres, V. E., Toth, I., Perrone, R. D. (1992). Immortalized epithelial cell lines: A model for the study of ADPKD-assicuated kuver disease. *Proceedings of the Fifth International Workshop on Polycystic Kidney Disease*, (ed. P. A. Gabow and J. J. Grantham). Polycystic Kidney Research Foundation, Kansas City.

Johnstone, A. J., Turnbull, L. W., Allan, P. L., and Garden, O. J. (1993). Cholangitis and Budd-Chiari syndrome as complications of simple cystic liver disease. *HPB Surg.*, **6**, 223–8.

Jordon, D., Harpaz, N., and Thung, S. N. (1989). Caroli's disease and adult polycystic disease: A rarely recognized association. *Liver*, **9**, 30–35.

Jorgensen, M. (1973a). A sterological study of intrahepatic bile ducts. 1. Method and application to normal livers. *Acta Pathol. Microbiol. Scand.*, A, **81**, 657–62.

Jorgensen, M. (1973b). A stereological study of intrahepatic bile ducts. 2. Bile duct proliferation in some pathological conditions. *Acta Pathol. Microbiol. Scand.*, A, **81**, 663–69.

Jorgensen, M. (1973c). A stereological study of intrahepatic bile ducts. 3. Infantile polycystic disease. *Acta Pathol. Microbiol. Scand.*, A, **81**, 670–5.

Jorgensen, M. (1974). A stereological study of intrahepatic bile ducts. 4. Congenital hepatic fibrosis. *Acta Pathol. Microbiol. Scand.*, *A*, **82**, 21–9.

Kairaluoma, M. I., Leinonen, A., Stahlberg, M., Paivansalo, M., Kiviniemi, H., and Siniluoto, T. (1989). Percutaneous aspiration and alcohol scherotherapy for symptomatic hepatic cysts: An alternative to surgical intervention. *Ann. Surg.*, **210**, 208–15.

Kaminski, D. L., Ruwart, M. J., and Deshpande, Y. G. (1979). The role of cyclic AMP in canine secretin-stimulated bile flow. *J. Surg. Res.*, **27**, 57–61.

Karhunen, P. J. and Tenhu, M. (1986). Adult polycystic liver and kidney diseases are separate entities. *Clin. Genet.*, **30**, 29–37.

Karhunen, P. J., Penttila, A., Liesto, K., Männikkö, A., and Möttönen, M. (1986). Benign bile duct tumours, non-parasitic liver cysts and liver damage in males. *J. Hepatol.*, **2**, 89–99.

Karpen, S. and Suchy, F. J. (1994). Embryology and structural development of the liver. In *Liver disease in children*, (ed. F. J. Suchy) pp. 3–10. Mosby Year Book, St. Louis.

Katzen, N. G. (1964). Fatal hepatic polycystic disease (Letter to the editor). *Br. Med. J.*, **1**, 839–40.

Kida, T., Nakanuma, Y., and Terada, T. (1992). Cystic dilatation of peribiliary glands in livers with adult polycystic disease and livers with solitary nonparasitic cysts: An autopsy study. *Hepatology*, **16**, 334–40.

Kimberling, W. J., Kumar, S., Gabow, P. A., Kenyon, J. B., Connolly, C. J., and Somlo, S. (1993). Autosomal dominant polycystic kidney disease: Localization of the second gene to chromosome 4q13-q23. *Genomics*, **18**, 467–72.

Klotz, H. P., Schlumpf, R., Weder, W., and Largiadèr, F. (1993). Minimal invasive surgery for treatment of enlarged symptomatic liver cysts. *Surg. Lapar. Endo.*, **3**, 351–3.

Kohli, V., Pande, G. K., Dev, V., Reddy, K. S., Kaul, U., and Nundy, S. (1993). Management of hepatic venous outflow obstruction. *Lancet*, **342**, 718–22.

Kwok, M. K. and Lewin, K. J. (1988). Massive hepatomegaly in adult polycystic liver disease. *Am. J. Surg. Pathol.*, **12**, 321–4.

Lambruschi, P. G. and Rudolf, L. E. (1979). Massive unifocal cyst of the liver in a drug abuser. *Ann. Surg.*, **189**, 39–43.

Landis, P., *et al.* (1984). Cholangiocellular carcinoma in polycystic kidney and liver disease. *Arch. Intern. Med.*, **144**, 2274–6.

Lange, V., Meyer, G., Rau, H., and Schildberg, F. W. (1992). Minimally invasive interventions in solitary liver cysts. *Chirurg.*, **63**, 349–52.

Lee, F. I. and Paes, A. R. (1985). Congenital hepatic fibrosis and adult-type autosomal dominant polycystic kidney disease in a child. *Postgrad. Med. J.*, **61**, 641–2.

Lerner, M. E., Roshkow, J. E., Smithline, A., and Ng, C. (1992). Polycystic liver disease with obstructive jaundice: Treatment with ultrasound-guided cyst aspiration. *Gastrointest. Radiol.*, **17**, 46–8.

Levine, E., Cook, L. T., and Grantham, J. J. (1985). Liver cysts in autosomal dominant polycystic kidney disease: Clinical and computed tomographic study. *AJR*, **145**, 229–33.

Lin, T.-Y., Chen, C.-C., and Wang, S.-M. (1968). Treatment of non-parasitic cystic disease of the liver: A new approach to therapy with polycystic liver. *Ann. Surg.*, **168**, 921–7.

Lipschitz, B., Berdon, W. E., Defelice, A. R., and Levy, J. (1993). Association of congenital hepatic fibrosis with autosomal dominant polycystic kidney disease. Report of a family with review of literature. *Pediatr. Radiol.*, **23**, 131–3.

Loh, J. P., Haller, J. O., Kassner, E. G., Aloni, A., and Glassberg, K. (1977). Dominantly-inherited polycystic kidneys in infants: Association with hypertrophic pyloric stenosis. *Pediatr. Radiol.*, **6**, 27–31.

London, R. D., Malik, A. A., and Train, J. S. (1988). Infection in a patient with polycystic kidney and liver disease: Noninvasive localization and treatment. *Am. J. Med.*, **84**, 1082–5.

Ludwig, J., Hashimoto, E., McGill, D. B., and van Heerden, J. A. (1990). Classification of hepatic venous outflow obstruction: Ambiguous terminology of the Budd–Chiari syndrome. *Mayo Clin. Proc.*, **65**, 51–5.

Luoma, P. V., Sotaniemi, E. A., and Ehnholm, C. (1980). Low high-density lipoprotein and reduced antipyrine metabolism in members of a family with polycystic liver disease. *Scand. J. Gastroenterol.*, **15**, 869–73.

Marchal, G. J., *et al.* (1986). Caroli disease: High-frequency US and pathologic findings. *Radiology*, **158**, 507–11.

Matsuda, O., *et al.* (1990). Polycystic kidney of autosomal dominant inheritance, polycystic liver and congenital hepatic fibrosis in a single kindred. *Am. J. Nephrol.*, **10**, 237–41.

McCullough, K. M. (1993). Alcohol sclerotherapy of simple parenchymal liver cysts. *Austral. Radiol.*, **37**, 177–81.

McGarrity, T. J., Koch, K. L., and Rasbach, D. A. (1986). Refractory ascites associated with polycystic liver disease Treatment with peritoneovenous shunt. *Dig. Dis. Sci.*, **31**, 217–20.

Melnick, P. J. (1955). Polycystic liver. *AMA Arch. Pathol.*, **59**, 162–72.

Milutinovic, J., Fialkow, P. J., Rudd, T. G., Agodoa, L. Y., Phillips, L. A., and Bryant, B. A. (1980). Liver cysts in patients with autosomal dominant polycystic kidney disease. *Am. J. Med.*, **68**, 741–4.

Milutinovic, J., Schabel, S. I., and Ainsworth, S. K. (1989). Autosomal dominant polycystic kidney disease with liver and pancreatic involvement in early childhood. *Am. J. Kidney Dis.*, **13**, 340–4.

Mishkin, J., Makler, T. Jr, Velchik, M. G., and McCarthy, K. (1986). Technetium-99m DISIDA imaging in autosomal-dominant polycystic kidney. *Clin. Nucl. Med.*, **11**, 368.

Mitchell, M. C., Boitnott, J. K., Kaufman, S., Cameron, J. L. and Maddrey, W. C. (1982). Budd-Chiari syndrome: Etiology, diagnosis and management. *Medicine*, **61**, 199–218.

Morgenstern, L. (1959). Rupture of solitary nonparasitic cysts of the liver. *Ann. Surg.*, **150**, 167–71.

Moritz, E. (1992). Laparoscopic fenestration of solitary giant cysts of the liver. *Chirurgie*, **63**, 379–80.

Murphy, B. J., Casillas, J., Ros, P. R., Morillo, G., Albores-Saavedra, J., and Rolfes, D. B. (1989). The CT appearance of cystic masses of the liver. *Radiographics*, **9**, 307–21.

Nagorney, D. M., Torres, V. E., Rakela, J., and Welch, T. J. (1988). Surgical anatomy of the liver in adult polycystic kidney disease (Abstract). *Kidney Int.*, **33**, 202.

Nakanuma, Y., Terada, T., Ohta, G., Kurachi, M., and Matsubara, F. (1982). Caroli's disease in congenital hepatic fibrosis and infantile polycystic disease. *Liver*, **2**, 346–54.

Nakanuma, Y., Kurumaya, H., Ohta, G. (1984). Multiple cysts in the hepatic hilum and their pathogenesis. A suggestion of periductal gland origin. *Virchows Archiv A*, **404**, 341–50.

Newman, K. D., Torres, V. E., Rakela, J., and Nagorney, D. M. (1990). Treatment of highly symptomatic polycystic liver disease. *Ann. Surg.*, **212**, 30–7.

Orr, T. G. and Thurston, J. A. (1927). Strangulated non-parasitic cyst of the liver. *Ann. Surg.*, **86**, 901–4.

Paliard, P. and Partensky, C. (1980). Traitment par fenestration iterative d'une from douloureuse, puis cholestatique de polykystose hépatique. *Gastroenterol. Clin. Biol.*, **4**, 854–7.

Parneix, M., Lotte, P., Barandon, E., and Amouretti, M. (1978). Polycystic disease of the liver. Three complicated forms. *Chirurgie*, **104**, 284–94.

Parry, M. F., Smego, D. A., and Digiovanni, M. A. (1988). Hepatobiliary kinetics and excretion of ciprofloxacin. *Antimicrob. Agents Chemother.*, **32**, 982–5.

Paterson-Brown, S. and Garden, O. J. (1991). Laser-assisted laparoscopic excision of liver cyst. *Br. J. Surg.*, **78**, 1047.

Patterson, M., Gonzalez-Vitale, J. C., and Fagan, C. J. (1982). Polycystic liver disease: A study of cyst fluid constituents. *Hepatology*, **2**, 475–8.

Pedersen, J. F., Emamian, S. A., and Nielsen, M. B. (1993). Simple renal cyst: Relations to age and arterial blood pressure. *Br. J. Radiol.*, **66**, 581–4.

Peltokallio, V. (1970). Non-parasitic cysts of the liver A clinical study of 117 cases. *Ann. Chirurg. Gynaec. Fenn.*, (Suppl. 174), **59**, 1–63.

Peters, D. J. M., *et al.* (1993). Chromosome 4 localization of a second gene for autosomal dominant polycystic kidney disease. *Nature Genetics*, **5**, 359–62.

Pirsch, J. D., *et al.* (1991). Orthotopic liver transplantation in patients 60 years of age and older. *Transplantation*, **51**, 431–3.

Poinso, R., Monges, H., and Payan, H. (1954). *La maladie kystique du foie*. Expansion Scientifique Française, Champagne, France.

Popövsky, J. A., Costa, J. C., and Doppman, J. L. (1979). Meyenburg complexes of the liver and bile cysts as a consequence of hepatic ischemia. *Hum. Pathol.*, **10**, 425–32.

Proesmans, W., Van Damme, B., Casaer, P., and Marchal, G. (1982). Autosomal dominant polycystic kidney disease in the neonatal period: Association with a cerebral arteriovenous malformation. *Pediatrics*, **70**, 971–5.

Que, F., Nagorney, D. M., Gross, J. B. Jr, and Torres, V. E. (Submitted). Liver resection and cyst fenestration in the treatment of severe polycystic liver disease. *Gastroenterology*, **108**, 487–94.

Ramos, A., Torres, V. E., Holley, K. E., Offord, K. P., Rakela, J., and Ludwig, J. (1990). The liver in autosomal dominant polycystic kidney disease. *Arch. Pathol. Lab. Med.*, **114**, 180–4.

Rapola, J. and Kääriäinen, H. (1988). Morphological diagnosis of recessive and dominant polycystic kidney disease in infancy and childhood. *APMIS*, **96**, 68–76.

Ratcliffe, P. J., Reeders, S., and Theaker, J. M. (1984). Bleeding esophageal varices and hepatic dysfunction in adult polycystic kidney disease. *Br. Med. J.*, **288**, 1330–1.

Ravine, D., Gibson, R. N., Donlan, J., and Sheffield, L. J. (1993) An ultrasound renal cyst prevalence survey: Specificity data for inherited renal cystic diseases. *Am. J. Kidney Dis.*, **22**, 803–7.

Rectro, W. G. Jr, Xu, Y., Goldstein, L., Peters, R. L., and Reynolds, T. B. (1985). Membranous obstruction of the inferior vena cava in the United States. *Medicine*, **64**, 134–43.

Reeders, S. T., *et al.* (1985). A highly polymorphic DNA marker linked to adult polycystic kidney disease on chromosome 16. *Nature*, **317**, 542–4.

Rieder, J. (1973). Excretion of sulfamethoxazole and trimethoprim into human bile. *J. Infect. Dis.*, **128** (Suppl.), S574.

Robson, G. B. and Fenster, L. F. (1964). Fatal liver abscess developing in a polycystic liver. *Gastroenterology*, **47**, 82–4.

Roskams, T., van den Oord, J. J., De Vos, R., and Desmet, V. J. (1990). Neuroendocrine features of reactive bile ductules in cholestatic liver disease. *Am. J. Pathol.*, **137**, 1019–25.

Roskams, T., Campos, R. V., Drucker, D. J., and Desmet, V. J. (1993). Reactive human bile ductules express parathyroid hormone-related peptide. *Histopathology*, **23**, 11–19.

Ross, D. G. and Travers, H. (1975). Infantile presentation of adult-type polycystic kidney disease in a large kindred. *J. Pediatr.*, **87**, 760–3.

Ruebner, B. H., Blankenberg, T. A., Burrows, D. A., Soohoo, W., and Lund, J. K. (1990). Development and transformation of the ductal plate in the developing human liver. *Pediatr. Pathol.*, **10**, 55–68.

Saini, S., Mueller, P. R., Ferrucci, J. R., Jr, Simeone, J. F., Wittenberg, J., and Butch, R. J. (1983). Percutaneous aspiration of hepatic cysts does not provide definitive therapy. *AJR*, **141**, 559–60.

Salem, M. and Keeffe, E. B. (1989). Liver cysts associated with polycystic kidney disease: Role of Tc-99m hepatobiliary imaging. *Clin. Nucl. Med.*, **14**, 803–7.

Sanchez, H., Gagner, M., Rossi, R. L., Jenkins, R. L., Lewis, W. D., Munson, J. L., and Braasch, J. W. (1991). Surgical management of nonparasitic cystic liver disease. *Am. J. Surg.*, **161**, 113–18.

Sanfelippo, P. M., Beahrs, O. H., and Weiland, L. H. (1974). Cystic disease of the liver. *Ann. Surg.*, **179**, 922–5.

Sawada, S., *et al.* (1992). Application of expandable metallic stents to the venous system. *Acta Radiologica*, **33**, 156–9.

Schwed, D. A., Edoga, J. K., and Stein, L. B. (1993). Biliary obstruction due to spontaneous hemorrhage into benign hepatic cyst. *J. Clin. Gastroenterol.*, **16**, 84–6.

Shah, K. D. and Gerber, M. A. (1990). Development of intrahepatic bile ducts in humans. *Arch. Pathol. Lab. Med.*, **114**, 597–600.

Simon, P., Ang, K. S., Cam, G., Charasse, C., and Houitte, H. (1993). Epidemiological data favouring genetic heterogeneity in adult polycystic liver and kidney diseases (Abstract No. 9P). *J. Am. Soc. Nephrol.*, **4**, 266.

Sood, S. C. and Watson, A. (1976). Solitary cyst of the liver presenting as an abdominal emergency. *Postgrad. Med. J.*, **550**, 48–50.

Sotaniemi, E. A., Luoma, P. V., Järvensivu, P. M., and Sotaniemi, K. A. (1979). Impairment of drug metabolism in polycystic non-parasitic liver disease. *Br. J. Clin. Pharmacol.*, **8**, 331–5.

Starzl, T. E., Reyes, J., Tzakis, A., Mieles, L., Todo, S., and Gordon, R. (1990). Liver transplantation for polycystic liver disease. *Arch. Surg.*, **125**, 575–7.

Summerfield, J. A., Nagafuchi, Y., Sherlock, S., Cadafalch, J., and Scheuer, P. J. (1986). Hepatobiliary fibropolycystic disease: a clinical and histological review of 51 patients. *J. Hepatol.*, **2**, 141–56.

Taylor, J. E., Calne, R. Y., and Stewart, W. K. (1991). Massive cystic hepatomegaly in a female patient with polycystic kidney disease treated by combined hepatic and renal transplantation. *Q. J. Med.*, **80**, 771–5.

Tazelaar, H. D., Payne, J. A., and Patel, N. S. (1984). Congenital hepatic fibrosis and asymptomatic familial adult-type polycystic kidney disease in a 19-year-old woman. *Gastroenterology*, **86**, 757–60.

Telenti, A., Torres, V. E., Gross, J. B., Jr, Van Scoy, R. E., Brown, M. L., and Hattery, R. R. (1990). Hepatic cyst infection in autosomal dominant polycystic kidney disease. *Mayo Clin. Proc.*, **65**, 933–42.

Terada, T. and Nakanuma, Y. (1988). Congenital biliary dilatation in autosomal dominant adult polycystic disease of the liver and kidneys. *Arch. Pathol. Lab. Med.*, **112**, 1113–16.

Terada, T. and Nakanuma, Y. (1990). Pathological observations of intrahepatic peribiliary glands in 1,000 consecutive autopsy livers. III. Survey of necroinflammation and cystic dilatation. *Hepatology*, **12**, 1229–33.

Terada, T. and Nakanuma, Y. (1993). Development of human intrahepatic peribiliary glands. Histological, keratin immunohistochemical, and mucus histochemical analyses. *Lab. Invest.*, **68**, 261–9.

Terada, T., Nakanuma, Y., and Ohta, G. (1987). Glandular elements around the intrahepatic bile ducts in man: their morphology and distribution in normal livers. *Liver*, **7**, 1–8.

Terada, T., *et al.* (1991). Mucin-histochemical and immunohistochemical profiles of epithelial cells of several types of hepatic cysts. *Virchows Archive A*, **419**, 499–504.

Thommesen, N. (1978). Biliary hamartomas (von Meyenburg complexes) in liver needle biopsies. *Acta Pathol. Microbiol. Scand. A*, **86**, 93–9.

Thomsen, H. S. and Thaysen, J. H. (1988). Frequency of hepatic cysts in adult polycystic kidney disease. *Acta Med. Scand.* **224**, 381–4.

Tokunaga, K., Teplick, S. K., and Banerjee, B. (1994). Simple hepatic cysts. First case report of percutaneous drainage and sclerosis with doxycycline, with a review of literature. *Dig. Dis. Sci.*, **39**, 209–14.

Torres, V. E., Gross, J. B., and Nagorney, D. N. (1994*a*). The liver in ADPKD. In *Proceedings of the Fifth International Workshop on Polycystic Kidney Disease*, (ed. P. A. Gabow and J. J. Grantham), pp. 45–50. Polycystic Kidney Research Foundation, Kansas City.

Torres, V. E., King, B. F., Holley, K. E., Blute, M. L., and Gomez, M. R. (1994*b*). The kidney in the tuberous sclerosis complex. *Adv. Nephrol.*, **23**, 43–70.

Torres, V. E., Rastogi, S., King, B. F., Stanson, A. W., Gross, J. B., and Nagorney, D. M. (1994*c*). Hepatic venous outflow obstruction in autosomal dominant polycystic kidney disease. *Journal of the American Society of Nephrology*, **5**, 1186–92.

Trinkl, W., Sassaris, M., and Hunter, F. M. (1985). Nonsurgical treatment for symptomatic nonparasitic liver cyst. *Am. J. Gastroenterol.*, **80**, 907–11.

Turnage, R. H., Eckhauser, F. E., Knol, J. A., and Thompson, N. W. (1988). Therapeutic dilemmas in patients with symptomatic polycystic liver disease. *Am. Surg.*, **54**, 365–72.

vanErpecum, K. J., Janssens, A. R., Terpstra, J. L., Tjon, A., and Tham, R. T. O. (1987). Highly symptomatic adult polycystic disease of the liver: A report of fifteen cases. *J. Hepatol.*, **5**, 109–17.

van Eyken, P., Sciot, R., Callea, F., Van der Steen, K., Moerman, P., and Desmet, V. J. (1988). The development of the intrahepatic bile ducts in man: A keratin-immunohistochemical study. *Hepatology*, **81**, 1586–95.

vanSonnenberg, E., *et al.* (1994). Symptomatic hepatic cysts: Percutaneous drainage and sclerosis. *Radiology*, **190**, 387–92.

Vauthey, J. N., Maddern, G. J., and Blumgart, L. H. (1991). Adult polycystic disease of the liver. *Br. J. Surg.*, **78**, 524–7.

Vauthey, J. N., Maddern, G. J., Kolbinger, P., Baer, H. U., and Blumgart, L. H. (1992). Clinical experience with adult polycystic liver disease. *Br. J. Surg.*, **79**, 562–5.

Vilgrain, V., Silbermann, O., Benhamou, J.-P., and Nahum, H. (1993). MR imaging in intracystic hemorrhage of simple hepatic cysts. *Abdom. Imaging*, **18**, 164–7.

Wang, Z., *et al.* (1989). Recognition and management of Budd-Chiari syndrome: Report of one hundred cases. *J. Vasc. Surg.*, **10**, 149–56.

Wanless, I. R., Zahradnik, J., and Heathcote, E. J. (1987). Hepatic cysts of periductal gland origin presenting as obstructive jaundice. *Gastroenterology*, **93**, 894–8.

Watchi, J.-M. and Nezelof, C. (1964). Les maladies polykystiques hepato-renales. *Rev. Internal. Hepatol.*, **14**, 489–538.

Willis, R. A. (1943). Carcinoma arising in congenital cysts of the liver. *J. Pathol. Bacteriol.*, **LV**, 492–9.

Wittenberg, J., *et al.* (1988). Differentiation of hepatic metastases from hepatic hemangiomas and cysts by using MR imaging. *AJR*, **151**, 79–84.

Wittig, J. H., Burns, R., and Longmire, W. P. Jr (1978). Jaundice associated with polycystic liver disease. *Am. J. Surg.*, **136**, 383–6.

Wright, G. D., Hughes, A. E., Larkin, K. A., Doherty, C. C., and Nevin, N. C. (1993). Genetic linkage analysis, clinical features and prognosis of autosomal dominant polycystic kidney disease in Northern Ireland. *Q. J. Med.*, **86**, 459–63.

Yaqoob, M., Saffman, C., Finn, R., and Carty, A. T. (1990). Inferior vena caval compression by hepatic cysts: An unusual complication of adult polycystic kidney disease. *Nephron*, **54**, 89–91.

Ye, M. and Grantham, J. J. (1993). The secretion of fluid by renal cysts from patients with autosomal dominant polycystic kidney disease. *N. Engl. J. Med.*, **329**, 310–13.

Z'graggen, K., Metzger, A., and Klaiber, C. (1991). Symptomatic simple cysts of the liver: Treatment by laparoscopic surgery. *Surg. Endosc.*, **5**, 224–5.

Intracranial aneurysms in autosomal dominant polycystic kidney disease

Yves Pirson and Dominique Chauveau

Introduction

Intracranial aneurysm (ICA) rupture entails a 30 to 50 per cent mortality rate in the general population. The association of ICA and autosomal dominant polycystic kidney disease (ADPKD) has been established for many years. Although it remains a rare manifestation of ADPKD, ICA rupture is part of the spectrum of extrarenal features that may occur at any time in the ADPKD patient. (Pirson and Grünfeld 1992)

In recent years several groups interested in ADPKD have shed some light on the epidemiology and outcome of ICA rupture in ADPKD patients. In addition, they documented that ICA occurence aggregates in some ADPKD families, thus suggesting genetic determination.

In view of the poor prognosis of ruptured ICA, the question of screening for asymptomatic ICA in ADPKD patients has been considered over the last decade.

In the meantime, there have been substantial advances in neuroradiology, both to screen for silent ICA and to treat some ruptured ICA by the endovascular route. Concomitantly, neurosurgeons have clarified the natural history of unruptured aneurysms in the general population. The timing of surgery for ruptured ICA has been modified and there have been improvements in the prevention and treatment of cerebral vasospasm, a major risk of severe morbidity after subarachnoid haemorrhage. Do these advances apply to ADPKD patients? There is room for a critical survey of this topic. This review retraces these developments, highlights pending questions, and attempts to provide guidance for nephrologists and neurosurgeons facing ADPKD-associated ICA.

Pathogenesis

The mechanisms leading to the formation of ICA in ADPKD are yet to be defined. As in non-ADPKD patients, ICA mainly develop at bifurcation sites of the circle of Willis. In non-ADPKD patients, the internal elastic lamina is thought to be the crucial structure which is first damaged before an ICA forms (Yong-Zhong and van Alphen 1990). Disruption of this layer is a constant feature of saccular ICA. Surprisingly, whether or not ADPKD-associated ICA has a distinct histological picture remains, unknown.

A genetic basis for ADPKD-associated ICA is supported by both the young age of some affected patients and the (although inconstant) familial aggregation of the association (Chauveau *et al.* 1994). Alteration of the extracellular matrix would best explain the diversity of clinical manifestatons of ADPKD including ICA. It should be noted that ICA are known to develop in a variety of inherited connective tissue disorders such as Marfan syndrome and the vascular form of Ehler–Danlos syndrome. Once the protein coded by the mutated PKD gene(s) is identified, its expression in the arterial wall will be sought.

Not suprisingly, linkage of ADPKD to PKD1 was demonstrated in two families including at least two members with ICA (Chauveau *et al.* 1994). ICA could also be associated with the PKD2 form of the disease. ICA was indeed recognized in one member of the large PKD2 family reported by Kimberling *et al.* (1988, 1993) and in two members of another PKD2 family recently studied by Breuning (personal communication). Whether specific mutations of the PKD genes favour the development of ICA will need to be investigated.

As a congenital vessel wall defect should be expressed throughout the body, one may wonder why aneurysms are essentially confined to the brain. This could be due to the unique fragility of intracranial arteries resulting from the virtual absence of a well-developed external elastic lamina (Yong-Zhong and van Alphen 1990).

In the addition to the PKD mutation, other genetic and non-genetic factors could play a role in the development of ICA. They could explain the frequent discordance for ICA within ADPKD families, even in monozygotic twins (Chauveau *et al.* 1994). Although variable in ADPKD patients with ICA (see below), hypertension, whenever present, could stimulate the growth of ICA (Chauveau *et al.* 1994). In a case-control study among non-ADPKD patients, the development of saccular ICA was indeed correlated with arterial hypertension (de la Monte *et al.* 1985).

In summary, the PKD mutation is likely to account for the formation of ICA through an arterial wall defect. However, other factors, such as hypertension are also involved, at least in ICA growth.

Prevalence

The wide variation in the prevalence of asymptomatic ICA in ADPKD reported up to 1990 — from zero to 60 per cent at autopsy or with conventional angiography (reviewed by Chapman *et al.* 1993) — most probably reflects selection bias and small sample size. In the largest, carefully conducted autopsy study, unruptured ICA were found in 4 per cent of ADPKD patients in whom the cause of death was not a ruptured ICA. This indicates a rate twice as high as (but not significantly different from) that of a control-matched population (Schievink *et al.* 1992).

The development of high-resolution computed tomography (CT) and magnetic resonance imaging (MRI) has recently allowed non-invasive detection of ICA. These new techniques are especially welcome in ADPKD subjects who seem to be at increased risk of complications from conventional cerebral angiography. Among 32 ADPKD subjects undergoing this investigation, 25 per cent experienced various neurovascular complications, a rate 2.5 times higher than that found among the general population at the same institution (Chapman *et al.* 1992).

Using either CT with 3 mm slices or first-generation MRI, Torres *et al.* (1990) found no definite ICA but an indeterminate vascular image in 11 out of 96 ADPKD subjects. Refinements in both methods have now improved their accuracy. High-resolution CT with 1.5 mm slices has allowed the detection of 74 (97 per cent) of 76 angiographically or autopsy-verified ICA in a series of non-ADPKD patients; the two ICA undetected by CT were < 6 mm in size (Schmid *et al.* 1987). This method is, however, not sufficiently specific: angiography confirmed the presence of an ICA in only two out of seven ADPKD patients with a suspicious CT result (Chapman *et al.* 1992). Moreover, CT imaging requires contrast medium injection, a matter of concern in ADPKD patients with renal failure. Recently, advances in MRI techniques have allowed better — and safer, as no contrast agent is needed — imaging of intracranial vascular structures including ICA. Using MR angiography (MRA) in non-ADPKD patients, Horikoshi *et al.* (1994) detected 79 per cent of 28 angiographically proven ICA; the six ICA escaping MRA were also < 6 mm in size. The specificity of the method was 92 per cent. Using MRA in a large group of ADPKD subjects, Huston *et al.* (1993) and Ruggieri *et al.* (1994) found an ICA prevalence of about 10 per cent (Table 22.1). This rate may have been slightly overestimated as patients with a family history of ICA (see below) were apparently over-represented, accounting for 32 and 29 per cent of the patients investigated by Huston and Ruggieri, respectively.

Combining the three large prospective series using thin-section CT or MRA (Table 22.1), asymptomatic ICA are detected in 7.9 per cent of ADPKD patients, a rate definitely higher than the 1.2 per cent found with angiography in the general Western population (Atkinson *et al.* 1989). Just as in the general

Table 22.1 Prevalence of asymptomatic saccular intracranial aneurysms in autosomal dominant polycystic kidney disease

	Chapman *et al.* (1992)	Huston *et al.* (1993)	Ruggieri *et al.* (1994)	Total
Method	Angio or CT	MRA	MRA	
Subjects (*n*)	88	85	93	266
Mean age (yrs)	36	45	48	43
Subjects with ICA (*n*)	4 (4.5%)	9 (10.6%)	8 (8.6%)	21 (7.9%)
ICA (*n*)	8	9	11	28
6–10 mm	0	2	2	4
3–5	7	2	5	14
< 3	1	5	4	10

Angio, conventional angiography; CT, thin-section high-resolution contrast-enhanced computerized tomography; MRA, magnetic resonance angiography.

population, 90 per cent of the ICA in ADPKD patients were found in the anterior circulation (Atkinson *et al.* 1989). Of note, all detected ICA were small: none were > 10 mm in diameter and only four ICA in three patients (i.e. 14 per cent of the detected ICA and 1 per cent of the investigated patients) were 6–10 mm in diameter, a finding to be taken into account when the usefulness of screening is discussed (see below).

Huston *et al.* (1993) and Ruggieri *et al.* (1994) have tried to identify clinical features associated with the presence of occult ICA in ADPKD patients. No significant association was found between ICA and age, gender, prevalence of hypertension, or abnormal renal function. In the Mayo Clinic series, there was trend for an association between ICA and severe polycystic liver disease (Huston *et al.* 1993). The only characteristic clearly associated with the presence of ICA was a family history of ICA. In the combined three series mentioned above, the relative risk for harbouring ICA was indeed 2.6 times higher among patients with a definite family history of ICA or subarachnoid haemorrhage than in those without (Table 22.2).

In summary, about 8 per cent of ADPKD patients have asymptomatic ICA. Only 14 per cent have ICA of ≥ 6 mm in diameter. The prevalence reaches 16 per cent in ADPKD patients with a family history of ICA.

Symptomatic ICA

As symptoms arising from ICA are virtually always due to its rupture, the following section will focus on this aspect of the problem.

ICA rarely becomes symptomatic through another mechanism. Focal findings, such as cranial nerve palsy (particularly oculomotor and optic nerves) or seizures, may result from compression by a large ICA. Transient ischaemic attack may result either from an embolus from an ICA or from direct compression of adjacent vessels.

Rupture entails a 35–55 per cent risk of combined mortality and morbidity (Schievink *et al.* 1992; Chauveau *et al.* 1994) in ADPKD patients. This is close to the corresponding figures reported in non-ADPKD patients (Säveland *et al.* 1986; Sarti *et al.* 1991). These high rates of mortality and morbidity are attrib-

Table 22.2 Prevalence of asymptomatic ICA* among 263 ADPKD patients according to the existence of a definite family history of ICA or subarachnoid haemorrhage

Study	Positive family history		Negative family history
Chapman *et al.* (1992)	2/29		2/59
Huston *et al.* (1993)	6/27		3/56
Ruggieri *et al.* (1994)	4/21		6/71
Total	12/77	$P < 0.05$	11/186
	(15.6%)		(5.9%)

*21 were saccular, 2 were fusiform.

uted mainly to brain damage from initial bleeding, re-bleeding, and delayed cerebral ischaemia. It is hoped that early diagnosis and judicious management might improve this dismal prognosis.

Epidemiology

Incidence

The risk of suffering an ICA rupture in ADPKD patients is not well defined. On the basis of the population data of Rochester Minnesota, this risk in ADPKD patients was calculated to be about 1/2000 person-year overall, and 1/1000 person-year in patients over the age of 30 years (Schievink *et al.* 1992). The mortality from cerebrovascular accident is higher in ADPKD than in non-ADPKD end-stage renal disease patients, 11 vs. 5 per cent in the Toronto Registry (Roscoe *et al.* 1993) and 13 vs. 10 per cent in the EDTA Registry (Ritz *et al.* 1994). However, ICA rupture accounts for only a minority of fatal neurological events in ADPKD patients. In the Heidelberg autopsy series, while cerebral complications were observed in 20 per cent of ADPKD patients, ICA rupture was found in only 12 per cent of them (Zeier *et al.* 1988). Also, in the general population, subarachnoid haemorrhage represents only 11 per cent of all strokes (Sarti *et al.* 1991). The epidemiological evalution of ICA rupture among ADPKD patients therefore requires unequivocal demonstration of a ruptured ICA. Three such studies were recently reported: a critical review by Lozano and Leblanc (1992) of 79 cases gathered from the literature, a report of 41 cases seen at the Mayo Clinic (Schievink *et al.* 1992), and our multicentre European Study including 71 cases (Chauveau *et al.* 1994). These data allow the development of a clinical profile of ADPKD patients presenting with ICA rupture.

Patient characteristics

Age. The mean age at rupture is lower in ADPKD patients (39 years in Lozano and Leblanc 1992, 47 years in Schievink *et al.* 1992, 39 years in Chauveau *et al.* 1994) than in the general population (51 years), but close to that found in the subset with the familial form of ICA (42 years) (Lozano and Leblanc 1987). In our series, age at rupture ranged from 15 to 69 years; it is noteworthy that 10 per cent of the patients were aged less than 21 years (Chauveau *et al.* 1994).

Renal and blood pressure status. As expected from the mean age at rupture, a substantial proportion of patients had normal renal function at that time: 50 per cent in Chauveau's series, and 60 per cent in Schievink's series. More strikingly, 25–29 percent (Lozano and Leblanc 1992; Schievink *et al.* 1992; Chauveau *et al.* 1994) had normal blood pressure before rupture, demonstrating that established hypertension is not a prerequisite for the development of ICA. This does not exclude a role for episodes of hypertension among otherwise normotensive patients and does not detract from the fact that chronic hypertension is a recognized risk factor for ICA rupture, at least in the general population (see discussion in Pirson, in press).

Clinical markers. We found no predictive clinical feature identifying ADPKD patients with ruptured ICA (Chauveau *et al.* 1994). Just as for asymptomatic ICA (see above), the only characteristic associated with ruptured ICA was a family history of ICA: such a history was indeed found to be five times more often in patients with ruptured ICA than in a control group of ADPKD patients without ruptured ICA (Chauveau *et al.* 1993).

Clinical features

As cerebral arteries are contained within arachnoidal cisterns, ICA rupture results in subarachnoid haemorrhage (SAH). Blood tracks into cerebrospinal fluid and may extend into brain (cerebral haematoma) and ventricles (ventricular haemorrhage). The location and extent of the haemorrhage determine the severity of the neurological clinical presentation.

Many neurologists have emphasized that in the general population ICA rupture is preceded in up to 40 per cent of cases by headaches (due to a minor leak from the ICA) a few hours to two weeks before rupture (Leblanc 1987). On the other hand, only 25 per cent of patients seen by general practitioners for sudden and severe headache proved to have SAH (Linn *et al.* 1994). Nevertheless, the nephrologist should be alerted by headaches of sudden onset and unusual character or severity in an ADPKD patient. Recognizing a warning symptom of headache is important, since delay in diagnosis of ICA rupture may seriously affect patient outcome (Kopitnik and Samson 1993).

When significant rupture occurs, the patient generally complains of excruciating headache often described as an 'explosion in the head'. The pain then radiates into occipital or cervical region. It should be known that neck stiffness takes four to six hours to develop and even remains occasionally absent. Other symptoms of SAH include nausea and vomiting, photophobia, focal neurological deficit, seizures, lethargy, and loss of consciousness. ICA rupture may also mimic an acute psychiatric illness.

Investigations (Fig. 22.1)

This first-line procedure is CT scanning, which is able to confirm the diagnosis of SAH if it is obtained within five days after the haemorrhage. Haemorrhage appears as areas of high or isodensity in superficial subarachnoid spaces and in the basal cisterns. The bleeding pattern may indicate the site of the ICA. Coexisting intracerebral haematoma or intraventricular blood may be seen. The total amount of subarachnoid blood is thought to predict delayed cerebral ischaemia (see below) (Hijdra *et al.* 1988).

In the 15 per cent of the cases in whom diagnosis remains in question following CT, lumbar puncture should be performed (Kopitnik and Samson 1993). If both CT scan and lumbar puncture are normal, the episode should be attributed to an unusually severe bout of 'ordinary headache' and not to SAH. Up to

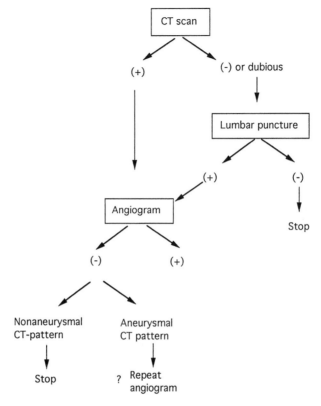

Fig. 22.1   Approach to the ADPKD patient with clinical suspicion of subarachnoid haemorrhage.

20 per cent of the ADPKD population report frequent, common headache (Gabow *et al.* 1984). Since follow-up of such (non-ADPKD) patients with negative CT scan and lumbar puncture was proven to be reassuring with little risk of a subsequent SAH, the risk of angiography does not seem justified in this setting (van Gijn 1992).

Once the diagnosis of SAH has been established, further investigations should be made under the guidance of a neurosurgeon. Four-vessel angiography with multiple views is usually performed as soon as possible, with the aim of localizing the ruptured ICA, delineating its size and neck, assessing the degree of vasospasm, and detecting unruptured ICA. Angiography may be postponed in some comatose patients. If ICA are multiple, the location of SAH on CT scan and the lobular contour of ICA will help identify the ruptured ICA. In our series, 91 per cent of the ruptured ICA are found in the anterior circulation (as expected from the location of the unruptured ICA), and 50 per cent are located on the middle cerebral artery (Chauveau *et al.* 1994). Lozano and Leblanc (1992) also found an over-representation of this site in ADPKD patients compared to non-ADPKD patients. The second most frequent location is the anterior communicating artery. Of note, intracerebral haematomas are not uncommon with ruptured ICA at those sites. The size distribution of 27 ruptured ICA in ADPKD patients was as follows: < 5 mm, 19 per cent; 5–9 mm, 33 per cent; 10–24 mm, 26 per cent; > 25 mm, 22 per cent. All were saccular (Schievink *et al.* 1992). As in non–ADPKD patients, multiplicity of ICA is not uncommon in ADPKD. In our series, 31 per cent of the patients with a ruptured ICA had at least one additional intact ICA, 12 per cent had at least two and one patient had seven.

In about 15 per cent of non–ADPKD patients with proven SAH, angiography will not detect ICA. According to van Gijn (1992), two subsets of those patients should be distinguished on the basis of the location of the haemorrhage on CT: (1) those with accumulation of blood in the cisterns aground the midbrain ('perimesencephalic' pattern) have an excellent prognosis; whereas (2) those with a blood distribution indistinguishable from that seen in proven ICA bleeds ('aneurysmal pattern') may suffer re-bleeding and other complications. The search for an undetected ICA by magnetic resonance or repeated angiography should thus be pursued in the latter category but not in the former (Rinkel *et al.* 1991). The proportion of ADPKD patients with angiogram-negative SAH is not known.

Management

The ADPKD patient with ICA rupture should be managed in a neurosurgical unit. If the patient is in chronic renal failure or on renal replacement therapy, the referral unit will be chosen so as to have access to appropriate renal treatment. As the neurosurgeon may be unfamiliar with these conditions (and sometimes unduly worried about them), he will welcome the assistance of the nephrologist for prescribing medical treatment and taking decisions about surgery. Guidelines generally applied to ICA rupture roughly apply to the ADPKD patient and will be summarized. Besides nursing, treatment is aimed at preventing both cerebral ischaemia and re-bleeding and includes a medical and a surgical approach.

Medical therapy

Headaches can sometimes be alleviated by mild analgesics such as paracetamol or dextropropoxyphene; most cases will respond to codeine; aspirin should be avoided (van Gijn 1992).

Up to 25 per cent of patients with ICA rupture will have cerebral ischaemia, mainly between day 5 and 14 after rupture (van Gijn 1992) thought to be due, at least in part, to vasospasm of large arteries. Vasospasm usually involves vessels adjacent to the ruptured ICA but also those surrounding thick blood clots. Clinical manifestations include increased headaches, decreased consciousness, focal neurological deficits, and even cerebral infarction if blood flow is severely impaired. As vasospasm is exacerbated by both hypotension and dehydration, the patient should be kept normotensive and normovolaemic. In the face of established severe cerebral vasospasm, and provided the aneurysm has been clipped (see below) some neurosurgeons will even recommend 'hyperdynamic therapy' (i.e. the induction of hypertension and hypervolaemia). Particular attention should thus be paid in this setting to the ADPKD patient on periodic dialysis. As the calcium antagonist nimodipine (in a 60 mg dose every four hours) was found to reduce by 34 per cent the incidence of cerebral infarction (Pickard *et al.* 1989), this treatment is now routinely administered prophylactically by most neurosurgeons.

Surgical therapy

The mainstay of ruptured ICA surgery is ICA exclusion. Parent vessel preservation and clot removal are also warranted. Surgical clipping of the ruptured ICA at its neck is the standard method. Uncomplicated operation entails morbidity and mortality rates of approximately 10 per cent. Despite appropriate anaesthetic and surgical techniques, intra-operative ICA rupture may sometimes occur, doubling the morbidity and mortality rates (Kopitnik and Samson 1993). Asymptomatic ICA accessible during the surgical exposure must also be clipped. Details of surgical management are beyond the scope of this chapter, but have been recently reviewed (Kopitnik and Samson 1993). Although the timing of surgery is still a matter of debate among neurosurgeons, there is currently a trend to perform surgery as early as possible, preferably within the first three days after SAH. The main reason is that about 35 per cent of non-operated patients are threatened by re-bleeding, with an attendant mortality rate of 50 per cent, within four weeks after initial haemorrhage (van Gijn 1992). Moreover, early clipping allows for the 'hyperdynamic' therapy of vasospasm (see above). Surgery will, however, be postponed in patients with poor neurological condition and in those with technically demanding ICA. Waiting 10 to 14 days appears appropriate with most of these patients (Heros 1990). In this category of patients, the newer techniques of endovascular treatment might soon represent a valuable alternative to surgery.

Endovascular treatment was initially limited to permanent balloon occlusion of the parent artery. The results of this technique on the internal carotid artery for treatment of unclippable ICA of the cavernous carotid artery have compared favourably with surgical ligation of the common carotid or internal carotid artery (Nichlos *et al.* 1994). Advances in catheter and imaging technology have made it possible to achieve selective occlusion of the ICA while preserving the parent artery. Detachable balloons were first used. Because of several disadvantages (incomplete occlusion, deflation, etc.) this technique has now been largely abandoned (Nichols *et al.* 1994). A detachable platinum coil system has been developed by Guglielmi *et al.* (1992); application of an electric current allows detachment of the coil and promotes thrombosis around it within the ICA. Despite remaining technical difficulties, Casasco *et al.* (1993) reported impressive results using fibred platinum coils in 67 patients with ICA rupture. At six month follow-up evaluation, 84 per cent of the patients had a good recovery, 4 per cent had disability, and 11 per cent had died; 84 per cent of the ICA were demonstrated to be completely occluded. If long-term effectiveness of the coils can be established, it is expected that endovascular therapy will play a major role in the treatment of ruptured ICA (Nichols 1993) in the near future.

Outcome

In our series of ADPKD patients with ICA rupture, four (24 per cent) of 17 non-operated, but only three (6 per cent) of 54 operated patients died within three months after rupture (i.e. an overall mortality rate of 10 per cent Chauveau *et al.* 1994). Our inclusion criteria may have underestimated the true mortality of ICA rupture in ADPKD patients: since ICA rupture had to be proven, the most severe forms, leading to death before any investigation and even hospital admission, may indeed have been missed. In the combined autopsy-angiography Mayo Clinic Study including 41 patients, mortality rate at 6 months following rupture was as high as 55 per cent (Schievink *et al.* 1992). Morbidity is also serious: in our series 27 (43 per cent) of 62 patients surviving beyond three months after ICA rupture had severe neurological disability (Chauveau *et al.* 1994).

In the long term, survivors are threatened by recurrent haemorrhage. Not surprisingly, four (31 per cent) out of the 13 non-operated patients surviving the first week after the first haemorrhage re-bled from the same ICA during the follow-up (4 months to 29 years later). It is of interest that four (9 per cent) out of the 47 patients surviving successful clipping beyond three months experienced rupture of another ICA 6 to 14 years later. In three cases, this ICA was not de-tectable retrospectively on the four-vessel angiography performed at the time of the first rupture (Chauveau *et al.* 1990). The fourth patient had seven ICA on initial arteriography, only two of which were clipped. The multiplicity and the new development of ICA suggest that, at least in a subset of ADPKD patients, ICA reflects a diffuse and progressive disease of the cerebral arterial tree. This also justifies regular screening for another ICA of ADPKD patients surviving a first rupture (see below).

In summary, ADPKD-associated ICA may rupture also in young and nor-motensive patients. SAH is frequently preceded by 'warning' headaches. Suspicion of SAH warrants emergency evaluation. Surgical clipping is the current standard treatment; endovascular occlusion might soon become an alter-native. Survivors should be regularly screened for development of another ICA.

Natural history of unruptured ICA

The natural history of unruptured ICA in ADPKD remains largely unknown. Reference, therefore, must be made to current knowledge of the course of un-ruptured ICA in the general population, recognizing the limitations of such extrapolation.

Overall risk of rupture

Available epidemiological data in ADPKD populations suggest that a significant fraction of ICA never rupture. Assuming in ADPKD patients an incidence of ICA rupture of about 1/2000 person-year (Schievink *et al.* 1992) and a lifespan of 64 years (Roscoe *et al.* 1993), this event should occur in about 3 per cent of

ADPKD patients, whereas asymptomatic ICA is found in about 8 per cent (see above). This proportion (37 per cent) of ADPKD patients harbouring an ICA who will suffer rupture could be slightly lower than the corresponding figure in the general population (62 per cent): assuming, in the latter, an incidence of ICA rupture of 1/10.000 person-year and a lifetime of 75 years, rupture would indeed affect 0.75 per cent of the general population, for an ICA prevalence of 1.2 per cent (Atkinson *et al.* 1989). It should be emphasized, however, that these estimates rely on figures still awaiting confirmation (especially the annual incidence of ICA rupture in ADPKD patients).

As stated above, the mean age at rupture is lower in ADPKD patients than in the sporadic form of ICA, but close to that of the familial form of ICA (Lozano and Leblanc 1987), an observation supporting the pathogenic role of congenital factors in ADPKD-associated ICA.

Risk factors for rupture

In the general population, the natural history of unruptured ICA might not be the same among patients without history of (another) ICA rupture and those with such a history (Wiebers and Torres 1992).

The first category has been best studied by Wiebers *at al.* (1987). They followed, over an eight year period, 130 patients (mean age: 56 years) with 161 unruptured ICA, discovered fortuitously or because of symptoms unrelated to intracranial haemorrhage. Rupture occurred in 15 patients, giving an average annual incidence of 1.4 per cent. No relationship was found between rupture and age, sex, number, and location of ICA, and presence of hypertension. The only significant variable was ICA size: all ruptures occurred among the 51 ICA of $\geq$ 10 mm in diameter whereas none of the 102 ICA < 10 mm ruptured. In the same institution, however, ICA discovered at the time of rupture had a mean diameter of 8 mm. Two possible explanations for this discrepancy are offered by the authors. First, the size of ICA may decrease after rupture. Secondly, many ICA may rupture soon after their formation when they are still small, thus being more likely to escape detection. A similar longitudinal study in ADPKD patients is lacking. As in non-ADPKD patients, the size of ADPKD-associated ICA discovered at the time of rupture may be small: 52 per cent were < 10 mm in diameter in the Mayo Clinic series (Schievink *et al.* 1992).

The natural history of unruptured ICA among the second category of non-ADPKD patients (i.e. those with a history of ICA rupture), has been best studied by Juvela *et al.* (1993). They followed, for a median period of 14 years, 131 patients (median age: 42 years) with multiple ICA of which the ruptured lesion was clipped at the beginning of the study. Interestingly, both ruptured and unruptured ICA were most often located on the middle cerebral artery, just as in both ADPKD-associated (Chauveau *et al.* 1994) and familial ICA (Lozano and Leblanc 1987). Twenty-four episodes of haemorrhage from a previously un-ruptured ICA occured, giving an average annual rupture incidence of 1.3 per cent. The risk of bleeding was nearly constant over the three decades following diagnosis. The only variable that tended to predict rupture was age, the risk of rupture being inversely associated with it. Size did not predict rupture: 17 (71 per cent) of the 24 ICA that later ruptured were ≤ 6 mm in diameter at the begining of study. Angiographic monitoring of 31 patients showed an increase in size of all 17 ICA which ruptured compared with only two of the largest ICA in 14 patients without rupture. In addition, a new ICA was found in six patients. Thus, in the general population, as compared with patients with no history of ICA rupture, those with such a history had a similar incidence of further ICA rupture, but rupture was not predicted by ICA size.

We followed, during a period of eight years, the course of 52 ADPKD patients after clipping of a ruptured ICA (Chauveau *et al.* 1994). Further rupture occured in six, giving an average annual incidence of 1.4 per cent. Among the 48 patients in whom a four-vessel angiography was available, two ruptures occured in the subgroup of nine patients with multiple ICA diagnosed at time of clipping (annual incidence: 4 per cent), and the three others in the subgroup of 39 patients without detectable intact ICA at clipping (annual incidence: 1.2 per cent).

In summary, in the general population with ICA and no history of rupture, ICA size is the best predictor of first rupture. In the ADPKD population without history of ICA rupture, the natural history of unruptured ICA remains unknown. In the general population with a history of ICA rupture, rupture of another ICA is not predicted by ICA size but inversely correlated with age. In ADPKD patients successfully operated for a first ICA rupture, the annual incidence of another ICA rupture is 1.4 per cent.

Screening for unruptured ICA

Given both the severe prognosis of ICA rupture and the possibility to detect and repair ICA before rupture, screening for ICA in ADPKD patients has been considered. The value of screening was assessed by Levey *et al.* (1983) using decision analysis. Using a one-year difference in life expectancy as threshold, the authors concluded that routine screening by cerebral angiography was warranted only in patients younger than 25 years provided the prevalence of ICA exceeded 30 per cent. Since then, several authors, including Levey (Levey 1990; Wiebers and Torres 1992; Chapman *et al.* 1993; Black 1994) considered whether new information on the baseline probabilities founding the original analysis would alter their conclusions.

Four main issues need to be re-examined: prevalence of ICA, accuracy of new non-invasive screening tests, outcome of prophylactic clipping (screening arm of the analysis), and probability of rupture (observation arm).

Prevalence. The above mentioned 8 per cent overall prevalence of ICA in ADPKD is far below the 30 per cent prevalence assumed by Levey *et al.* (1983), although, as already stated, prevalence reached 15 per cent among patients with a family history of ICA.

Non-invasive screening tests. MRA emerges as the best non-invasive screening test (Fig. 22.2). As mentioned above, the sensitivity is 100 per cent for ICA

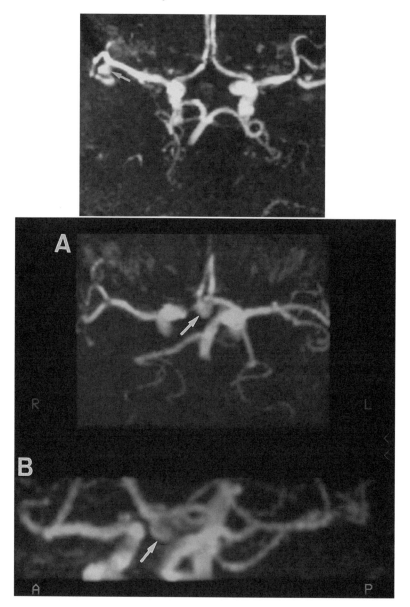

Fig. 22.2 (Top), Cerebral MRA screening of a 31-year-old woman with ADPKD, showing an aneurysm (arrow) of 6 mm in diameter on the right middle cerebral artery. This patient was admitted for massive polycystic liver disease requiring surgery. Her mother, also affected by ADPKD, died at the age of 45 from rupture of an aneurysm of the anterior communicating artery. (Bottom), Cerebral MRA of a 65-year-old woman with ADPKD and massive polycystic liver disease, showing an aneurysm (arrow) of 8 mm in diameter on the anterior communicating artery: (A) anteroposterior view; (B) oblique view.

≥ 6 mm, which is appropriate if this is also the size threshold for surgical repair (see below). The current specificity of 92 per cent (Horikoshi *et al.* 1994) also seems excellent at first glance. However, as a result of the relatively low prevalence of ICA, routine screening with MRA would result in false positive MRA in 42 per cent of the patients — and thus in a useless conventional angiography, with its attendant risks in ADPKD patients (see above), an often omitted consideration. The existence of renal failure should also be taken into account, as it worsens the risks of arteriography (Earnest *et al.* 1984) and surgery.

Outcome of prophylactic clipping. Among 167 non-ADPKD patients with a mean age of 49 years (range: 16–75) surgically treated for an unruptured ICA, there was no operative mortality and a morbidity rate of only 2.4 per cent (Rice *et al.* 1990), which is nevertheless slightly higher than the 1 per cent rate described by Levey *et al.* (1993). The prognosis notably depends on the ICA size: in a recent series of 202 prophylactic interventions, excellent or good outcome (defined as minor neurological deficit) was achieved in 100 per cent of patients with < 10 mm ICA, 95 per cent with 11 to 25 mm ICA, and 70 percent with > 25 mm ICA (Solomon *et al.* 1994).

Probability of rupture. Levey had assigned a 2 per cent annual rupture rate to all unruptured ICA. As stated above, no information is available among ADPKD patients without history of SAH. By analogy with available data in the general population, the risk is thought to be related to the ICA size. Among ADPKD patients with a history of SAH, we calculated an annual incidence rate of 1.4 per cent (see above).

Taken together, these new pieces of information should not change Levey's original conclusions substantially in favour of screening. Recently reassessing his own analysis, Levey (1990) maintained that routine screening is not justified. However, he suggested screening patients who have a family history of ICA. Wiebers and Torres (1992) recommended adding to this category patients who undergo major elective surgery with anticipated haemodynamic instability, those in high-risk occupations, and those who want the reassurance that screening can provide. No age threshold was mentioned. Using revised estimates of Levey's analysis, Chapman *et al.* (1993) calculated that screening with non-invasive techniques patients younger than 35 years of age with a positive family history would add 3.1 years of life; methodological details were not provided. In contrast, Black (1994) advised against screening ADPKD patients in general, essentially because of the uncertainties about the natural course of ICA. With respect to Levey's decision model, he rightly suggests subdividing ICA according to size, as this variable strongly affects ICA prevalence, risk of surgery, and, most probably, the natural course.

In summary, it seems reasonable today to screen with MRA 18–35 year old ADPKD patients with a family history of ICA. As long as data on the natural history of unruptured ICA in ADPKD are not available, it seems wise to rely on the guidelines for surgery used in the general population (Chapman

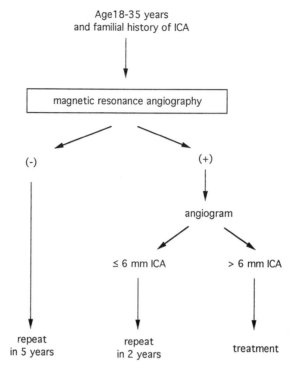

Fig. 22.3   Screening occult intracranial aneurysm in ADPKD patients.

et al. 1993) (Fig. 22.3). If screening is accepted, it remains to be determined how frequently at-risk patients with a negative MRA should be re-evaluated; we now recommend MRA every five years. Patients surviving a first ICA rupture warrant MRA re-screening every 2 to 3 years; ICA size threshold for surgery could be lower in this subset.

Conclusions

Several recent studies in ADPKD patients have provided an accurate assessment of the prevalence of ICA and a comprehensive description of the clinical consequences of ICA rupture. ADPKD patients have benefited from advances in the diagnosis of asymptomatic ICA and the management of ruptured ICA. The currently debated issue of screening for occult ICA could soon be enlightened by more precise identification of at-risk patients and better knowledge of the natural history of ICA in ADPKD.

Acknowledgements

To Drs B. Bolland, T. Duprez, G. Lot, and G. Stroobandt for helpful advice and Mrs R. Jacobs and D. Broneer for secretarial assistance.

References

Atkinson, J. L. D., Sundt, T. M., Houser, O. W., and Whisnant, J. P. (1989). Angiographic frequency of anterior circulation intracranial aneurysms. *Journal of Neurosurgery*, **70**, 551–5.

Black, W. C. (1994). Intracranial aneurysm in adult polycystic kidney disease: is screening with MR angiography indicated? *Radiology*, **191**, 18–20.

Casasco, A. E., *et al.* (1993). Selective endovascular treatment of 71 intracranial aneurysms with platinum coils. *Journal of Neurosurgery*, **79**, 3–10.

Chapman, A. B., *et al.* (1992). Intracranial aneurysms in autosomal dominant polycystic disease. *New England Journal Of Medicine*, **327**, 916–20.

Chapman, A. B., Johnson, A. M., and Gabow, P. A. (1993). Intracranial aneurysms in patients with autosomal dominant polycystic kidney disease: how to diagnose and who to screen. *American Journal of Kidney Diseases*, **22**, 526–31.

Chauveau, D., Sirieix, M. E., Schillinger, F., Legendre, C., and Grünfeld, J. P. (1990). Recurrent rupture of intracranial aneurysms in autosomal dominant polycystic kidney disease. *British Medical Journal*, **301**, 966–7.

Chauveau, D., Joly, D., Bonaiti-Pellié, C., and Grünfeld, J. P. (1993). Family clustering of intracranial aneurysm (ICA) rupture in autosomal dominant polycystic kidney disease (ADPKD). *Journal of American Society of Nephrology*, **4**, 261.

Chauveau, D., Pirson, Y., Verellen-Dumoulin, C., Macnicol, A., Gonzalo, A., and Grünfeld, J. P. (1994). Intracranial aneurysms in autosomal dominant polycystic kidney disease. *Kidney International*, **45**, 1140–6.

de la Monte, S. M., Moore, G. W., Monk, M. A., and Hutchins, G. M. (1985). Risk factors for the development and rupture of intracranial berry aneurysms. *American Journal of Medicine*, **78**, 957–64.

Earnest, F., *et al.* (1984). Complications of cerebral angiography: prospective assessment of risk. *American Journal of Radiology*, **142**, 247–53.

Gabow, P. A., Iklé, D. W., and Holmes, J. H. (1984). Polycystic kidney disease: prospective analysis of nonazotemic patients and family members. *Annals of Internal Medicine*, **101**, 238–47.

Gulglielmi, G., *et al.* (1992). Endovascular treatment of posterior circulation aneurysms by electrothrombosis using electrically detachable coils. *Journal of Neurosurgery*, **77**, 515–24.

Heros, R. C. (1990). Intracranial aneurysms: a review. *Minnesota Medicine*, **73**, 27–32.

Hijdra, A., van Gijn, J., Nagelkerke, N. J. D., Vermeulen, M., and van Crevel, H. (1988). Prediction of delayed cerebral ischemia, rebleeding and outcome after aneurysmal subarachnoid hemorrhage. *Stroke*, **19**, 1250–6.

Horikoshi, T., Fukamachi, A., Nishi, H., and Fukasawa, I. (1994). Detection of intracranial aneurysms by three-dimensional time-of-flight magnetic resonance angiography. *Neuroradiology*, **36**, 203–7.

Huston, J., Tores, V. E., Sulivan, P. P., Offord, K. P., and Wiebers, D. O. (1993). Value of magnetic resonance angiography for the detection of intracranial aneurysms in autosomal dominant polycystic kidney disease. *Journal of the American Society of Nephorology*, **3**, 1871–7.

Juvela, S., Porras, M., and Heiskanen, O. (1993). Natural history of unruptured intracranial aneurysms: a long-term follow-up study. *Journal of Neurosurgery*, **79**, 174–82.

Kimberling, W. J., Fain, P. R., Kenyon, J. B., Goldgar, D., Sujansky, E., and Gabow, P. A. (1988). Lingkage heterogeneity of autosomal dominant polycystic kidney disease. *New England Journal of Medicine*, **319**, 913–18.

Kimberling, W. J., Kumar, S., Gabow, P. A., Kenyon, J. B., Connolly, C. J., and Somlo, S. (1993). Autosomal dominant polycystic kidney disease: localization of the second gene to chromosome 4q13-q23. *Genomics*, **18**, 467–72.

Kopitinik, T. A. and Samson, D. S. (1993). Management of subarachnoid haemorrhage. *Journal of Neurology*, **56**, 947–59.

Leblanc, R. (1987). The minor leak preceding subarachnoid hemorrhage. *Journal of Neurosurgery*, **66**, 35–9.

Levey, A. S. (1990). Screening for occult intracranial aneurysms in polycystic kidney disease: interim guidelines. *Journal of the American Society of Nephrology*, **1**, 9–12.

Levey, A. S., Pauker, S. G., and Kassirer, J. P. (1983). Occult intracranial aneurysms in polycycstic kidney disease. When is cerebral arteriography indicated? *New England Journal of Medicine*, **308**, 986–94.

Linn, F. H. H., Wijdicks, E. F. M., van der Graaf, Y., Weerdesteyn-van Vliet, F. A. C., Bartelds, A. I. M., and van Gijn J. (1994). Prospective study of sentinel headache in aneurysmal subarachnoid haemorrhage. *Lancet*, **344**, 590–3.

Lozano, A. M. and Leblanc, R. (1987). Familial intracranial aneurysms. *Journal of Neurosurgery*, **66**, 522–8.

Lozano, A. M. and Leblanc, R. (1992). Cerebral aneurysms and polycystic kidney disease: a critical review. *Canadian Journal of Neurological Sciences*, **19**, 222–7.

Nichols, D. A. (1993). Endovascular treatment of the acutely ruptured intracranial aneurysm. *Journal of Neurosurgery*, **79**, 1–2.

Nichols, D. A., Meyer, F. B., Piepgras, D. G., and Smith, P. L. (1994). Endovascular treatment of intracranial aneurysms. *Mayo Clinic Proceedings*, **69**, 272–5.

Pickard, J. D., *et al.* (1989). Effect of oral nimodipine on cerebral infarction and outcome after subarachnoid haemorrhage: British aneurysm nimodipine trial. *British Medical Journal*, **298**, 636–42.

Pirson, Y. (in press). Ruptured and occult intracranial aneurysms in autosomal dominant polycystic kidney disease. *Nephron*,

Pirson, Y. and Grünfeld, J. P. (1992). Autosomal-dominant polycystic kidney disease. In *Oxford Textbook of Clinical Nephrology*, (ed. J. S., Cameron, A. M., Davison, J. P., Grünfeld, D. N. S., Kerr, and E. Ritz), pp. 2171–88. Oxford University Press.

Rice, B. J., Peerless, S. J., and Drake, C. G. (1990). Surgical treatment of unruptured aneurysms of the posterior circulation. *Journal of Neurosurgery*, **73**, 165–73.

Rinkel, G. J. E., *et al.* (1991). Outcome in patients with subarachnoid haemorrhage and negative angiography according to pattern of haermorrhage on computed tomography. *Lancet*, **338**, 964–8.

Ritz, E., Zeier, M., Scheider, P., and Jones, E. (1994). Cardiovascular mortality of patients with polycystic kidney disease on dialysis; is there a lesson to learn? *Nephron*, **66**, 125–8.

Roscoe J. M., Brissenden, J. E., Williams, E. A., Chery, A. L., and Silverman, M. (1993). Autosomal dominant polycystic kidney disease in Toronto. *Kidney International*, **44**, 1101–8.

Ruggieri, P. M., *et al.* (1994). Occult intracranial aneurysms in polycystic kidney disease: screening with MR angiography. *Radiology*, **191**, 33–9.

Sarti, C., *et al.* (1991). Epidemiology of subarachnoid hemorrhage in Finland from 1983 to 1985. *Stroke*, **22**, 848–53.

Säveland, H., *et al.* (1986). Outcome evaluation following subarachnoid hemorrhage. *Journal of Neurosurgery*, **64**, 191–6.

Schievink, W. I., Torres, V. E., Piepgras, D. G., and Wiebers, D. O. (1992). Saccular intracranial aneurysms in autosomal dominant polycystic kidney disease. *Journal of the American Society of Nephrology*, **3**, 88–95.

Schmidt, U. D., Steiger, H. J., and Huber, P. (1987). Accuracy of high resolution computed tomography in direct diagnosis of cerebral aneurysms. *Neuroradiology*, **29**, 152–9.

Solomon, R. A., Fink, M. E., and Pile-Spellman, J. (1994). Surgical management of unruptured intracranial aneurysms. *Journal of Neurosurgery*, **80**, 440–6.

Torres, V. E., Wiebers, D. A., and Forbes, G. S. (1990). Cranial computed tomography and magnetic resonance imaging in autosomal dominant polycystic kidney disease. *Journal of the American Society of Nephrology*, **1**, 84–90.

van Gijn, J. (1992). Subarachnoid haemorrhage. *Lancet*, **339**, 653–8.

Wiebers, D. O. and Torres, V. E. (1992). Screening for unruptured intracranial aneurysms in autosomal dominant polycystic kidney disease. *New England Journal of Medicine*, **327**, 953–5.

Wiebers, D. O., Whisnant, J. P., Sundt, T. M., and O'Fallon, W. M. (1987). The significance of unruptured intracranial saccular aneurysms. *Journal of Neurosurgery*, **66**, 23–9.

Yong-Zhong, G. and van Alphen, H. A. M. (1990). Pathogenesis and histopathlogy of saccular aneurysms: review of the literature. *Neurological Research*, **12**, 249–55.

Zeier, M., Geberth, S., Ritz, E., Jaeger, T., and Waldherr, R. (1988). Adult dominant polycystic kidney disease — clinical problems. *Nephron*, **49**, 177–83.

23

Particular problems in childhood and adolescence in autosomal dominant polycystic kidney disease

Arlene B. Chapman

Introduction

The original nomenclature for Autosomal dominant polycystic kidney disease (ADPKD) was 'adult polycystic kidney disease' due to the usual age of presentation. However, the disease is autosomal dominantly inherited and the number of neonates, infants, and children diagnosed with ADPKD has increased dramatically during the past 20 years. The increased recognition of ADPKD in the paediatric age group is due to a number of factors. With increased awareness of the genetic nature of ADPKD (i.e. dominant, non-sex-linked inheritance), affected families are having asymptomatic offspring screened for the presence of ADPKD. In addition, clinical, radiographic, and pathological characteristics of ADPKD are more clearly defined so that differentiation of ADPKD from other neonatal or childhood cystic disorders is being made with more certainty. Finally, due to research efforts, ADPKD is being extensively studied in asymptomatic children who are obligate gene carriers. In the past, ADPKD diagnosed *in utero* or within the first year of life was difficult to differentiate from other genetic renal cystic disorders. However, with the chromosomal and gene locations of the common genetic renal cystic disorders, such as ADPKD and autosomal recessive polycystic kidney disease (ARPKD), differentiation between the two can now be made more easily. The purpose of this chapter is to characterize ADPKD in the paediatric and adolescent age groups with special attention to diagnostic evaluation. Information regarding the use of the identified ADPKD1 gene as well as the changing role of gene linkage analysis is included. In addition, the clinical characteristics of very early onset ADPKD (presenting less than one year of age) and childhood or adolescent ADPKD are discussed in detail.

Cystic disease in childhood

Simple cysts are rare in children. A recent prospective report (Ravine *et al.* 1993) demonstrated a 9.5 per cent overall prevalence rate of simple cysts in 729 individuals in the general population aged between 15 and 70 years of age. No cysts were found in 120 individuals less than 29 years of age. Others (Ahmed 1972; Kramer *et al.* 1982; Yamagishi *et al.* 1988) have demonstrated a slightly greater frequency of simple cysts in children up to 20 years of age ranging from 1 to 4 per cent. In all, 45 cases of simple renal cysts had been reported in the paediatric age group by 1982 (Kramer *et al.* 1982). The aetiology of simple cysts in children is not well understood. However, they appear to be calyceal diverticuli that have lost communication with the collecting system (Gordon *et al.* 1979). Importantly, simple cysts may have clinical consequences including flank pain, haematuria, and hypertension. Given the low frequency of simple cysts in the paediatric age group, cysts found *in utero* or childhood are most likely due to a primary renal disorder, either genetic or syndromal, or part of multiple malformations and deserve further evaluation (Table 23.1). In particular, simple cysts found in off-spring of ADPKD patients most likely indicate the presence of ADPKD.

Acquired cystic disease is well known in adult dialysis patients and those with chronic renal insufficiency prior to entry into end-stage renal disease (ESRD). Although not common, acquired cystic disease has been reported in children undergoing long-term dialysis (Leichter *et al.* 1988) as well as those with chronic renal insufficiency with non-cystic disorders prior to entry into ESRD (Querfeld *et al.* 1990; Hogg 1992).

Table 23.1 Cystic diseases of the kidney found in childhood and adolescence

Genetic cystic disorders Disease	Genetics	Chromosome	Gene
ARPKD	Recessive	6	Unknown
ADPKD	Dominant	4, 16	16.13p
Tuberous sclerosis	Dominant	9, 16	16.13p, tumour suppressor
Nephronopthisis	Recessive	2	Unknown
von Hippel–Lindau	Dominant	3	Unknown
Glomerulocystic disease	?	?	?

Congenital and syndromal cystic disorders
Zellweger syndrome
Meckel syndrome
Jeune syndrome
Bardet–Biedl syndrome
Beckwith–Wiedemann syndrome
Ivemark syndrome
Congenital hypernephronic nephromegaly with tubular dysgenesis
Trisomy 9 and 13

Acquired cystic disorders
Transient nephromegaly
Nephroblastomatosis
Pyelonephritis
Glomerulonephritis
Bilateral Wilms' tumour

A recent autopsy series of 6521 paediatric patients under 16 years of age demonstrated 136 (2.1 per cent) individuals with renal cysts (Mir *et al.* 1983). Half of these individuals died within the first year of life. Of the patients with renal cysts, the most common disease was renal dysplasia (Table 23.2). Only one of 136 had ADPKD, most likely because ADPKD is not commonly lethal, even when presenting *in utero*.

Both American and European Registries of ESRD in paediatric patients show 16–18 per cent of patients requiring renal replacement therapy due to renal cystic disease. Paediatric patients account for 1–2.5 per cent of the entire ESRD population (Brunner *et al.* 1992) and ADPKD is not the most common renal cystic disease in paediatric patients, accounting at most for only 4.3 per cent of American and European paediatric ESRD population (USRDS 1993). The majority of children receiving dialysis with renal cystic disease suffer from renal dysplasia (12–15 per cent). Importantly, when children with renal cystic disease including those not yet on dialysis are evaluated, ADPKD is common and accounts for 28 per cent of such children (99 of 350) (Zerres *et al.* 1992). Therefore, although ADPKD may be present in childhood and may be a common renal cystic disorder in the general population, it does not appear to be a common cause of death or renal failure in childhood (Alexander *et al.* 1993).

Diagnosis of ADPKD in childhood and *in utero*

Although the gene for ADPKD1 has recently been identified (EPKDC 1994), the complexity of the gene and the heterogeneic nature of ADPKD (Kimberling

Table 23.2 Distribution of renal cystic disease in 136 autopsy cases under the age of 16 years

	Number	Per cent
Renal dysplasia		
Bilateral	28	20
Unilateral	23	17
Segmental	14	10
Hereditary polycystic kidneys		
ARPKD	15	11
ADPKD	1	1
FJN*	3	2
Hereditary		
Meckel syndrome	3	2
Malformation		
Cortical cysts	33	31
Simple cysts	7	5

*FJN, familial juvenile nephronopthisis. Adapted from Mir *et al.* (1983).

et al. 1988) indicate that gene-specific therapy may not be available for some time. Furthermore, after screening more than 150 unrelated affected individuals, only four different mutations responsible for ADPKD have been found, so that until the entire gene is cloned and all mutations identified, the gene responsible for ADPKD1 will not identify 100 per cent of ADPKD1 individuals (EPKDC 1994). Therefore, the gene will be most useful in the immediate future in increasing the accuracy of gene linkage analysis.

In families where information is available on multiple affected members, gene linkage analysis is useful for identification of obligate gene carriers for ADPKD1 on chromosome 16 and ADPKD2 on chromosome 4. At least two affected persons are needed to determine which alleles of the DNA probes are travelling with the gene in a given family (Kimberling *et al.* 1991). Flanking markers both distal and proximal to the gene are available and with identification of the gene, the tail portion of the gene can now be used in gene linkage analysis in families. The availability of gene linkage analysis for diagnosing asymptomatic individuals, particularly *in utero* or childhood, makes it important to review carefully the indications for screening for the disease. In addition, it is necessary to conduct genetic counselling before putting gene linkage analysis into practical application.

Attitudes of affected and at-risk individuals informed about the nature of their disease who would consider gene linkage analysis to test potential offspring *in utero* either by chorionic villous sampling (Reeders *et al.* 1986; Turco *et al.* 1992) or amniocentesis (Gabow and Wilkins-Haug 1991) show little indication for prenatal diagnosis (Sujansky *et al.* 1990; Hodgkinson *et al.* 1990). Although 65 per cent of 141 individuals questioned were interested in determining if their offspring were gene carriers for ADPKD, only 4 per cent would alter the course of their pregnancy based on the outcome of gene linkage analysis (Sujansky *et al.* 1990). In this same cohort, 25 per cent stated they would terminate a pregnancy for a very serious medical problem. Given that medical action would not be changed based on the test outcome, and that both amniocentesis and chorionic villous sampling carry some risk, gene linkage analysis has not been routinely used prenatally in the United States or Europe (Zerres 1992). Given that most gene carriers can be identified by ultrasound at an early asymptomatic age (see below), gene linkage has been reserved clinically for potential adult kidney donors who are at risk for the disease or in those who would alter family planning based on the test outcome (Gabow *et al.* 1989a; Zerres 1992).

The diagnosis of ADPKD in an asymptomatic child has a psychological impact on both child and parent as well as an effect on medical insurability (Fick *et al.* 1992). Also, the ethical concerns of carrying out a diagnostic procedure on a child without the child's ability to participate fully in informed consent are real. Therefore, the decision to proceed with gene linkage analysis should not be undertaken without appropriate support and counselling prior to testing.

Identification of gene carriers by phenotypic expression of the disease is done primarily by abdominal ultrasound (Berger *et al.* 1980; Han and Babcock 1985; Walker *et al.* 1984). Ultrasound (US) is considered the radiographic diagnostic procedure of choice in children, as there is no radiation exposure or invasive manoeuvre involved. Clearly, in symptomatic, complicated cases where there is an abrupt onset of pain or change in renal function, other imaging modalities, such as a computed tomography (CT) scan may be more useful (Grantham 1993).

Previous reports of at-risk individuals suggest that there is suboptimal sensitivity of US in screening young individuals with high false negative rates for diagnosis (Milutinovic *et al.* 1980; Bear *et al.* 1984). This has been a concern most often in children under 10 years of age. In a small study of 11 children shown by gene linkage analysis to have ADPKD, US was negative in 4 of 4 children less than 10 years of age and positive in 6 of 7 children between 10 and 14 years of age (De Paoli *et al.* 1987). Bear *et al.* (1984) studied 371 individuals from 17 families and ultrasonographically diagnosed 11 per cent of at-risk individuals less than 10 years of age and 33 per cent of at-risk individuals between ages 10 and 20 years. This indicates a non-detection rate of affected individuals of 39 per cent in those less than 10 years of age and 17 per cent in those between 10 and 20 years.

More recently, diagnostic US findings defined as the presence of one cyst in an at-risk individual have been found in 92–100 per cent of estimated potential gene carriers under 30 years of age (Bear *et al.* 1992; Taitz *et al.* 1987; Gabow *et al.* 1984). In these studies estimation of at-risk individuals was determined as 50 per cent of individuals studied. These findings suggest that US may be a sensitive screening technique for at-risk children, particularly in those older than 10 years of age. Most recently, series using gene linkage analysis have determined sensitivity and specificity of US in diagnosing ADPKD in at-risk children (Ravine *et al.* 1994; Gabow *et al.* 1994). Both studies demonstrate 100 per cent positive predictive value of US when one cyst is found in individuals under the age of 20. Specificity in both studies was 96 per cent in those under the age of 20. Negative US in children predicted to be positive by gene linkage analysis were found in 22 per cent of children under the age of 10 (Gabow *et al.* 1994) giving a specificity of 78 per cent and a negative predictive value of 71 per cent in those screened under the age of 10 years. In longitudinal studies of at-risk individuals without gene linkage analysis available, no child over the age of 10 who was negative at initial screening was positive at future US evaluations (Fick *et al.* 1994; Sedman *et al.* 1987). Therefore, positive US findings in any at-risk children support the diagnosis of ADPKD, with negative US in children over the age of 10 most likely indicating a negative gene carrier state. These data support a much earlier age of phenotypic presentation of ADPKD than previously thought, where it was estimated that 11–24 per cent of positive gene carriers would be phenotypically negative for ADPKD by US prior to age 30 (Parfrey *et al.* 1990).

With improved US technology and the high frequency of pre-natal US, ADPKD is being increasingly diagnosed *in utero* (Lawson *et al.* 1981). In 24 cases available for review, the most common US findings were enlarged kidneys in 23 of 24, increased echogenicity in 15 of 24, cysts in seven of 24 and oligohydramnios in 2 of 24 individuals (Fick *et al.* 1993; Romero *et al.* 1984). Unfortunately, these US findings are not specific for ADPKD unless found in an offspring of an affected parent and are also present in Meckels' syndrome and ARPKD as well as other disorders (Reilly *et al.* 1979; Stapleton *et al.* 1983), (Table 23.1). To clarify the diagnosis of enlarged echogenic kidneys found *in utero*, the most helpful information is clinical, based on the presence of renal cystic disease in a parent indicating an autosomal dominant disorder or ADPKD. Importantly, between 30 and 70 per cent of ADPKD patients diagnosed *in utero* have parents who were unaware that they had ADPKD until follow-up US was performed (Fick *et al.* 1993; Gagnodoux *et al.* 1989; Pretorius *et al.* 1987). Therefore, screening parents is extremely important in establishing a diagnosis of ADPKD. When both parents are negative for the presence of cysts by US and are older than 30 years of age, the question of non-paternity should also be raised. In a minority of cases (< 5 per cent) more sensitive imaging with CT scanning may be helpful. If the parents are less than 30 years of age and negative by US and another affected family member exists, such as an aunt or uncle, gene linkage analysis may still be helpful. To demonstrate the difficulty in obtaining an accurate diagnosis of the cause of cystic disease in childhood, as recently as 1987, retrospective reports were unable to classify the cause of cystic disease in 18 of 48 (37 per cent) children (Cole *et al.* 1987). In addition, new-borns with cystic disease are often classified as having ARPKD erroneously until screening of the parents is performed (Cole *et al.* 1987; Gagnadoux *et al.* 1989). Given the significantly worse patient prognosis associated with a diagnosis of ARPKD, it is important to make a correct diagnosis in order to guide families in medical decision-making. With identification of the location of the ARPKD gene to chromosome 6 without evidence of genetic heterogeneity (Zerres *et al.* 1994), and identification of the ADPKD1 gene (EPKDC 1994), genetic analysis will be more helpful in differentiating ADPKD from ARPKD in informative families. However, this approach is still limited in that two other affected relatives are necessary to perform such analyses. Occasionally, in cases with incomplete parental information or where genetic analysis is not informative, liver and kidney biopsies are necessary in determining the presence of ARPKD as congenital hepatic fibrosis is invariably associated with ARPKD (McDonald and Avner 1991) and only rarely reported in adults with ADPKD (Matsuda *et al.* 1990).

The earliest US diagnosis of ADPKD supported with gene linkage analysis *in utero* has been at 14 weeks' gestation (Ceccherini *et al.* 1989). However, the majority of positive US findings have been identified between 26 and 38 weeks' gestation. Importantly, the majority of ADPKD individuals diagnosed *in utero* survive and no structural predictors of patient or renal survival can be found by US other than findings of severe oligohydramnios and Potter facies (Journel *et al.* 1989). Therefore, positive US findings *in utero* supported by a positive family history of ADPKD or gene linkage analysis only provide diagnostic information. Ultrasonographic appearance and disappearance of simple cysts over time *in utero* have been documented (Musiani and Villani 1984) and developing medullary units or rays have been mistaken for renal cysts (Haller 1980). Screening at-risk fetuses for the presence of ARPKD has resulted in the decision to discontinue a pregnancy based on 'abnormalities' found on US and have resulted in the death of an otherwise healthy fetus (Luthy and Hirsch 1985). Therefore, prenatal US lacks both sensitivity and specificity in diagnosing ADPKD and cannot be used in isolation when diagnosing ADPKD.

Clinical characteristics of ADPKD diagnosed in the first year of life and in childhood

ADPKD diagnosed prior to adulthood appears to have a bimodal presentation, at birth and later in childhood. Although this is not an official classification for ADPKD found in childhood, those with very early onset ADPKD diagnosed *in utero* or the first year of life have a different clinical course carrying a different prognostic importance and will be discussed separately from children diagnosed after the first year of life.

ADPKD diagnosed *in utero* or the first year of life

Although the ADPKD gene is present from the time of conception, ADPKD diagnosed *in utero* or in the first year of life depicts a subgroup of ADPKD patients who have more severe renal cystic disease with a worse perinatal and long-term renal outcome. Microdissection of kidneys from a fetus aborted for reasons unrelated to ADPKD but found to have ADPKD pathologically (Lundin and Olow 1961) as well as kidneys from fetuses identified as gene carriers by gene linkage analysis but without ultrasonographic evidence of ADPKD (Waldherr *et al.* 1989) demonstrate the presence of microcysts in approximately 2–5 per cent of nephrons. This number of cysts is all that is required in adult ADPKD kidneys to result in ESRD. Therefore, the more aggressive form of very early onset ADPKD suggests that an alteration either in the gene or the environment has occurred to allow for the development of severely enlarged and echogenic kidneys *in utero* (Fick *et al.* 1993; Kääriäinen 1987; Kääriäinen *et al.* 1988; Taitz *et al.* 1987). Many hypotheses have been proposed to explain this distinct group of patients with very early onset of disease and include: the presence of the ADPKD gene in both parents, inheritance of both ADPKD and ARPKD genes in the affected individual, the presence of modifying alleles at the same gene locus (Zerres and Propping 1987), anticipation (Fick *et al.* 1993), gender-related issues in the affected parent and/or the offspring (Taitz *et al.* 1987; Sedman *et al.* 1987; Zerres and Stephan 1986; Fick *et al.* 1993), environmental issues, and finally, that very early onset ADPKD represents one end of the spectrum of clinical severity in a disorder that is highly variable in its clinical presentation (Zerres and Propping 1987).

Evidence for transmission of the ADPKD gene from both parents of affected offspring has not been found (Kääriäinen 1987; Fick *et al.* 1993). In addition, ARPKD and ADPKD are not allelic, and the presence of both ARPKD and

ADPKD in affected offspring has not been found (Zerres *et al.* 1985; Kääriäinen *et al.* 1988). In one family with four very early onset ADPKD offspring, paternity was different for two offspring indicating that a comorbid allele from the unaffected parent is not important in all cases (Kääriäinen *et al.* 1987).

Familial clustering of early onset ADPKD is reported (Blyth and Ockenden 1971; Ceccherini *et al.* 1989; Eulderink and Hogewind 1978; Farrell *et al.* 1984; Fick *et al.* 1993; Fryns and Van Den Berghe 1979; Fryns *et al.* 1986; Gal *et al.* 1989; Kääriäinen 1987; Loh *et al.* 1977; Ross and Travers 1975; Sedman *et al.* 1987; Taitz *et al.* 1987; Zerres *et al.* 1985) and is also reported in diseases where congenital onset in a typical adult-onset autosomal disorder has been observed such as in myotonic dystrophy (Harper and Dyken 1972). This form of clinical anticipation has shown a relationship to genetic anticipation in both fragile X syndrome (Rousseau *et al.* 1991) and myotonic dystrophy (Harley *et al.* 1992). Genetic anticipation has been shown to be due to an increasing number of triplet repeats within the gene corresponding to an earlier age of onset and more severe form of the disorder (Brook *et al.* 1992; Harley *et al.* 1992). Although evidence for unstable triplet repeats within the ADPKD1 gene have not been found, genetic anticipation may play a role in the presentation of ADPKD *in utero* or infancy. With the cloning of the ADPKD1 gene, the role of genetic anticipation in this group of patients will be clarified. The presence of spontaneous mutation was reported in three of eight parents of 11 early diagnosed ADPKD infants (Fick *et al.* 1993). This may represent a situation where the parent has developed a postzygotic mutation with somatic mosaicism. The offspring will manifest a more severe disorder where all cells have a mutation. In a similar fashion, the occurrence of more severe disease in an offspring has been described in osteogenesis imperfecta (Cohn *et al.* 1990).

Reports have suggested both a predominance of father-to-son (Zerres *et al.* 1982) and mother-to-daughter transmissions in very early onset ADPKD patients (Fick *et al.* 1993). When available information was compiled (71 cases) 27 mother-to-daughter transmissions, 15 mother-to-son transmissions, 14 father-to-daughter transmissions, and 15 father-to-son transmissions were found without significant differences between groups.

Finally, in the limited number of pregnancies where complete information was available involving an offspring diagnosed with ADPKD *in utero* or in the first year of life, ($n = 28$), the pregnancy was complicated either by the presence of twins ($n = 8$), ovulatory induction therapy ($n = 1$), or pre-eclampsia in the mother ($n = 10$), suggesting that an altered fetal environment may contribute to the development of enlarged or echogenic kidneys in an affected offspring.

At present, there are 79 cases from 58 families of APDKD diagnosed *in utero* or in the first year of life that are available for review to understand better the clinical features and natural history of very early onset ADPKD. Although follow-up was not available in nine cases, five (6 per cent) were aborted, four (5 per cent) were stillbirths, 21 (32 per cent) died within the first month of life, five of whom were in ESRD, six (8 per cent) died in the first year, and 34 (49 per cent) were alive. The majority of those who died in the perinatal period were born prematurely. In neonatal cases, the most common symptom at presentation was bulging abdominal flanks or an abdominal mass. Asymmetrical or single kidney involvement has been reported in a number of infants (Bengtsson *et al.* 1975; Blyth and Ockenden 1971; Edwards and Baldinger 1989; Farrell *et al.* 1984; Fellows *et al.* 1976; Fick *et al.* 1993; McLean *et al.* 1980; Proesmans *et al.* 1982; Sheu *et al.* 1991) which led to nephrectomy or renal biopsy in many cases for the presumptive diagnosis of Wilms' tumour, multicystic dysplasia, or congenital hydronephrosis.

When those children who survive the first year of life are studied separately, a more aggressive form of ADPKD, with regard to renal function and hypertension, is found (Begleiter *et al.* 1977; Bengtsson *et al.* 1975; Blyth and Ockenden 1971; Ceccherini *et al.* 1989; Chavalier *et al.* 1981; Cole *et al.* 1987; Edwards and Baldinger 1989; Eulderink and Hogewind 1978; Farrell *et al.* 1984; Fellows *et al.* 1976; Fick *et al.* 1993; Fryns *et al.* 1986; Gal *et al.* 1989; Garel *et al.* 1983; Hayden *et al.* 1984; Journel *et al.* 1989; Kääriäinen *et al.* 1988; Kaye and Lewy 1974; Loh *et al.* 1977; Main *et al.* 1983; McClean *et al.* 1980; Mehrizi *et al.* 1964; Milutinovic *et al.* 1989; Novelli *et al.* 1989; Pretorius *et al.* 1987; Proesman *et al.* 1982; Ross and Travers 1975; Sedman *et al.* 1987; Sheu *et al.* 1991; Shokeir 1978; Smedley and Bailey 1987; Stickler and Kelalis 1975; Taitz *et al.* 1987; Zerres *et al.* 1985). On physical examination palpable abdominal masses or bulging flanks were reported in 6 of 16 cases (Cole *et al.* 1987; Fick *et al.* 1993; Kääriäinen *et al.* 1988). Hypertension was present in the majority of diagnosed fetuses at birth with temporary improvement in blood pressure in some during the first year of life. In affected children older than one year of age, chronic persistent hypertension was documented in 16 of 20 (80 per cent) (Cole *et al.* 1987; Fick *et al.* 1993; Kääriäinen *et al.* 1988).

In the 34 children who survived the first year of life, 9 of 34 (26 per cent) had chronic renal insufficiency (three), or had entered ESRD (six). Those who required renal replacement therapy all entered ESRD before the age of five with the exception of one patient who was 15 years of age (Cole *et al.* 1987; Fick *et al.* 1993; Gagnadoux *et al.* 1989).

Thus, very early onset ADPKD is a more severe disorder than in adult onset ADPKD, and may be similar to, or more severe than, ARPKD children who survive childbirth.

Clinical characteristics of ADPKD diagnosed in childhood and adolescence

Information concerning the natural history of ADPKD diagnosed in childhood is derived from a combination of both retrospective and prospective studies with and without unaffected control populations. Therefore, the literature carries information about both symptomatic or more severely affected individuals, as well as asymptomatic individuals diagnosed as part of a family screening or research programme.

For the most part, diagnosed ADPKD children are asymptomatic, although there are a significant portion who have signs and symptoms of the disease (usually 25–30 per cent) leading to the diagnosis of ADPKD. The most common presenting signs and symptoms included abdominal pain, palpable kidneys, increased blood pressure, urinary tract infections, or intermittent haematuria and proteinuria (Fick *et al.* 1994; Gagnadoux *et al.* 1989; Kääriäinen *et al.* 1988; Kaplan *et al.* 1989; Sedman *et al.* 1987). Those who are evaluated because of a specific complaint tend to be younger than those who are asymptomatic (6 vs. 10 years of age, $P < 0.05$) (Fick *et al.* 1994), indicating that symptomatic children tend to have a more aggressive form of ADPKD. Importantly, when 'asymptomatic' at-risk children are screened for the presence of ADPKD approximately 30–60 per cent have signs and symptoms of flank pain, hypertension, urinary tract infections, or proteinuria (Fick *et al.* 1994; Ravine *et al.* 1991). This suggests that value is obtained by screening at-risk 'asymptomatic' children for the presence of ADPKD in hopes of early therapy for hypertension or urinary tract infections.

If one evaluates ADPKD children with regard to renal involvement or cyst number, those with more severe involvement have significantly more symptoms than their unaffected or more mildly affected counterparts. In a carefully designed study with unaffected, well-matched family members used as a control group, Fick *et al.* (1994) compared severely affected children (those with > 10 cysts, $n = 25$) with mildly affected children (those with < 10 cysts, $n = 37$) and unaffected age matched family members ($n = 78$). Importantly, the severely affected children in this study accounted for only 18 per cent of the study group and were significant older (13 vs. 10 years, $P < 0.05$) than mildly affected children. Symptoms of flank and back pain were more frequent in the severely affected (Table 23.3) and urinary frequency was significantly more common in both mildly and severely affected compared to unaffected children. Interestingly, other signs and symptoms of extrarenal involvement were more common in severely affected children including palpitations (usually associated with mitral valve prolapse) and inguinal hernias. Headaches, nausea, nocturia, haematuria,

Table 23.3 Symptoms found more commonly in SADPKD ($n = 25$) and/or MADPKD ($n = 37$) children as compared to NADPKD children ($n = 78$) ($P < 0.05$)

Symptom	Frequency (%)		
	SADPKD	MADPKD	NADPKD
Flank pain	28	0	5
Back pain	32	5	4
Palpitations	8	0	0
Frequency	36	16	8
Inguinal hernia	16	5	1

SAPKD, severely affected; MADPKD, mildly affected; NADPKD, unaffected. Adapted from Fick *et al.* (1994).

and history of urinary tract infections were not more frequent in ADPKD children (data not shown). Renal volumes were significantly greater in the severely affected as compared to the mildly affected children (210 ± 23 vs. 103 ± 7 cm^3, $P < 0.05$) even when adjusted for age. These data suggest that children with more severe renal involvement manifest more symptoms, similar to adults with ADPKD (Gabow 1993), and that more clinical evidence of the systemic nature of the disease is present with regard to extrarenal manifestations.

Preliminary longitudinal data is available in 22 ADPKD children, including those who were diagnosed due to symptoms and not part of a family screening programme (Fick *et al.* 1994; Sedman *et al.* 1987). The mean time interval for follow-up was 3.7 years, during which time 19 out of 22 demonstrated progressive renal structural involvement determined by increased renal volume, cyst number, and cyst size. Four children initially found to have unilateral renal involvement developed bilateral disease, whereas three children demonstrated a decreased number of cysts at follow-up. Thirteen children showed increased cyst number resulting in a mean increase of 5.3 cysts. Maximum cyst size changed at a rate of 0.16 ± 0.6 cm/year, increasing on average from 1.9 to 2.5 cm. Finally, renal volume increased 13 ± 3 cm^3/year in the ADPKD children compared to 6 ± 1 cm^3/year in unaffected age-adjusted children ($P < 0.05$). Therefore, at a very early, usually asymptomatic stage of ADPKD, renal cyst growth and enlargement can be easily and accurately detected by ultrasound and those with aggressive courses identified.

Glomerular filtration rate and urinary concentrating ability have been studied in both symptomatic ADPKD children (Gabow *et al.* 1984; Kääriäinen *et al.* 1988; Martinez-Maldonado *et al.* 1972) and asymptomatic children who are part of a screening or research programme (Fick *et al.* 1994). Glomerular filtration rate (GFR) is typically normal in the majority of children where it is determined using serum creatinine concentration and the formula of Schwartz *et al.* (1987). In those children diagnosed due to the presence of signs and symptoms, serum creatinine concentrations are normal (Fick *et al.* 1994; Gagnadoux *et al.* 1989; Kääriäinen *et al.* 1988). Importantly, Fick *et al.* (1994) demonstrated significantly greater GFRs in severely affected, compared to unaffected children (123 ± 7 vs. 112 ± 4 ml/min/1.73 m^2) with 16 per cent of all ADPKD children having glomerular hyperfiltration (GFR > 150 ml/min/1.73 m^2). Although the number of children in this study is small and serum creatinine concentrations were used for determining renal function, the increased GFR found in the severely affected children is similar to the increased GFR found in insulin-dependent diabetics with incipient nephropathy (Mogenson and Christiansen 1984). Glomerular hyperfiltration has been reported early in the course of adult ADPKD (Chapman *et al.* 1989). Larger numbers of children are needed to determine if a rise in GFR is part of the natural history of ADPKD children when cyst number is increasing.

ADPKD children do not report an increased frequency of polydypsia or polyuria when compared to their unaffected counterparts (Fick *et al.* 1994). Therefore, as in adults, the concentrating defect found in children is mild and usually asymptomatic (Gabow 1993). Following 12 hours of water deprivation, Kääriäinen *et al.* (1988) demonstrated abnormal urinary concentrating ability in 5 out of 10 ADPKD children with the lowest urinary osmolality being 500 mmol/kg/H_2O in a 5-year-old. Martinez-Maldonado *et al.* (1972) also demonstrated decreased urinary concentrating ability in 3 out of 4 ADPKD individuals under the age of 20 years, although the most severe concentrating defect was in a child with sickle-cell disease as well. Fick *et al.* (1994) systematically showed a relationship between structure and function with regard to urinary concentrating ability in ADPKD children as has been shown in adults (Gabow *et al.* 1989*b*). Severely affected children demonstrated significantly lower maximum urinary concentrating ability compared to both mildly and unaffected children (Severe, 823 ± 54 vs. mild, 940 ± 22 vs. unaffected, 945 ± 21 mmol/kg/H_2O; $P < 0.05$).

Extrarenal manifestations in children and adolescents with ADPKD

Hypertension

Hypertension is common in adult ADPKD patients occurring in approximately 60 per cent prior to loss of renal function (Gabow *et al.* 1990). Hypertension also occurs frequently in ADPKD children (Chapman *et al.* 1991; Parfrey *et al.* 1989) occurring in up to 33 per cent of affected individuals depending on the diagnostic criteria used. Most recently, Fick *et al.* (1994) reported a 15 per cent incidence of hypertension in 62 ADPKD children where more than 50 per cent of 12 in-house readings were greater than the 95th percentile for age- and gender-matched children (Task Force 1987). As with other signs and symptoms in children with more structural involvement, those children with more than 10 cysts demonstrated a higher incidence of hypertension (Fick *et al.* 1994).

Young normotensive ADPKD adults (Harrap *et al.* 1991), as well as hypertensive ADPKD adults with normal renal function (Chapman *et al.* 1990), demonstrate activation of the renin-angiotensin-aldosterone axis. Decreased effective renal plasma flow and increased exchangeable sodium has been shown in young normotensive ADPKD adults (Harrap *et al.* 1991), suggesting that sodium retention in the setting of activation of the renin-angiotensin-aldosterone axis is responsible for the development of hypertension in ADPKD.

The effect of elevated blood pressure is apparent in normotensive ADPKD adolescents between 15 and 25 years of age where increased evening blood pressures during 24-hour ambulatory blood pressure monitoring and increased left ventricular mass index were found. Increases in left ventricular mass index were due primarily to increased posterior wall thickness and end-diastolic diameter of the left ventricle compared to age- and gender-matched unaffected controls (Zeier *et al.* 1993). Ivy *et al.* (1995) have found a correlation ($r = 0.44$, $P < 0.001$) between left ventricular mass index and systolic blood pressure in normotensive ADPKD children. These data suggest that end-organ damage (increased left ventricular mass index) is occurring early in ADPKD children or adolescents due to small, clinically insignificant increases in blood pressure. In support of these findings, there have been a number of reports of endocardial fibroelastosis in ADPKD children presumably due to the presence of un-controlled hypertension (de Chadarevian and Kaplan 1981; Easterly and Oppenheimer 1967; Mehrizi *et al.* 1964).

Mitral valve prolapse

Mitral valve prolapse, which occurs in 26 per cent of ADPKD adults (Hossack *et al.* 1988), also appears to be more common in ADPKD children (Ivy *et al.* 1995). Ivy *et al.* (1995) reported a 12 per cent incidence of mitral valve prolapse in ADPKD children as compared to 3 per cent of unaffected family members ($P = 0.08$). ADPKD children with mitral valve prolapse were older than ADPKD children without mitral valve prolapse suggesting an age-related appearance of this condition in APDKD. Palpitations were more common in ADPKD children with severe renal involvement (> 10 cysts bilaterally). However, whether this correlates with the presence of mitral valve prolapse is yet to be determined. Finally, ADPKD children have a 5 per cent incidence of congenital heart defects as compared to 1 per cent of unaffected family members (Ivy *et al.* 1995)

Extrarenal cysts

The extrarenal features of ADPKD seen commonly in adults are very rarely seen in paediatric patients. Hepatic cysts typically present in adulthood (Grunfeld *et al.* 1985), however, they have been reported to occur before one year of age in a child with ADPKD (Milutinovic *et al.* 1989). In our own data-base, two children, aged 15 and 16, demonstrate multiple liver cysts (un-published observations). In another child, a single liver cyst was seen at autopsy, at the age of seven months. Pancreatic cysts are unusual in ADPKD patients (less than 10 per cent of patients); however, two reports of ADPKD children with pancreatic cysts can be found in the literature (Blythe and Ockenden 1971, Porch *et al.* 1986).

Intracranial aneurysms

Similarly, intracranial aneurysms have rarely been reported in ADPKD chil-dren. However, there are two reports of intracranial aneurysms occurring in ADPKD children (Anton and Abramowsky 1982; Proesmans *et al.* 1982) and one fatal case known to our group, occurring in a 20-year old ADPKD woman who had undergone renal transplantation at the age of 18 and was screened for the presence of aneurysms at that time (unpublished observations).

Nephrolithiasis

No paediatric ADPKD patients have been reported to have nephrolithiasis, although this occurs in 20–25 per cent of adult patients (Gabow 1993). Similarly, although diverticular disease is a problem in adult ADPKD patients on dialysis, (Scheff *et al.* 1986), it has not been reported in the ADPKD paediatric population.

Conclusion

ADPKD can commonly present *in utero*, infancy, or childhood. Differentiation of ADPKD from other renal cystic disease is often difficult and supportive information from family screening is paramount in making a diagnosis. Although the gene for ADPKD1 has been located, gene linkage analysis is still the method for diagnosing phenotypically negative at-risk individuals. Diagnosis in asymptomatic young individuals should only be done with extreme care and with pre-test genetic counselling. Those children diagnosed ultrasonographically *in utero* or in the first year of life have a more severe form of ADPKD with a significant perinatal mortality rate and a high frequency of hypertension and chronic renal insufficiency.

Patients diagnosed later in childhood have a more benign course. Those children with more severe renal involvement have more signs and symptoms including flank and back pain, as well as renal functional abnormalities such as decreased urinary concentrating ability. Importantly, children with more severe renal cystic involvement also appear to demonstrate more extrarenal manifestations, such as inguinal hernias and palpitations, which are consistent with mitral valve prolapse. These findings, overall, indicate more severe systemic disease process. Finally, associated conditions, such as hypertension and urinary tract infections, are often present even in 'asymptomatic ADPKD children', which are treatable, suggesting that early intervention may help long-term outcome in this disorder.

Acknowledgements

This research was supported by Grant 5 PO1 DK34039, Human Polycystic Kidney Disease (PKD), awarded by the Department of Health and Human Services, Public Health Service, NIDDK, and the Clinical Research Center, Grant MORR-00051 from the General Clinical Research Centers Research Program of the Division of Research Resources, National Institutes of Health.

References

Ahmed, S. (1972). Simple renal cysts in childhood. *British Journal of Urology*, **44**, 71–5.

Alexander, S. R., Sullivan, E. K., Harmon, W. E., Stablein, D. M., and Tejani, A. (1993). Maintenance dialysis in North American children and adolescents: A preliminary report. *Kidney International*, **44**, S104–9.

Anton, P. A. and Abramowsky, C. R. (1982). Adult polycystic kidney disease presenting in infancy: A report emphasizing the bilateral involvement. *Journal of Urology*, **128**, 1290–1.

Bear, J. C., Parfrey, P. S., Morgan, J. M., Martin, C. J., and Cramer, B. C. (1992). Autosomal dominant polycystic kidney disease: New information for genetic counseling. *American Journal of Medical Genetics*, **43**, 548–53.

Bear, J. C., *et al.* (1984). Age at clinical onset and at ultrasonographic detection of adult polycystic kidney disease: Data for genetic counseling. *American Journal of Medical Genetics*, **18**, 45–53.

Begletiter, M. L., Smith, T. H., and Harris, D. J. (1977). Ultrasound for genetic counseling in polycystic kidney disease (Letter). *Lancet*, **2**, 1073–4.

Bengtsson, U., Hedman, L., and Svalander, C. (1975). Adult type of polycystic kidney disease in a new-born child. *Acta Medica Scandinavica*, **197**, 447–50.

Berger, P. E., Menschauer, R. W., and Kuhn, J. P. (1980). Computed tomography and ultrasound of renal and perirenal diseases in infants and children. *Pediatric Radiology*, **9**, 91–9.

Blyth, H. and Ockenden, B. G. (1971). Polycystic disease of kidneys and liver presenting in childhood. *Journal of Medical Genetics*, **8**, 257–84.

Brook, D. *et al.* (1992). Molecular basis of myotonic dystrophy. Expansion of a trinucleotide (CTG) repeat at the 3' end of a transcript encoding a protein kinase family member. *Cell*, **68**, 799–808.

Brunner, F. P. and Selwood, N. H. (1992). Profile of patients on RRT in Europe and death rates due to major causes of death groups. *Kidney International*, **42**, S4–15.

Ceccherini, I., *et al.* (1989). Autosomal dominant polycystic kidney disease: Prenatal diagnosis by DNA analysis and sonography at 14 weeks. *Prenatal Diagnosis*, **9**, 751–8.

de Chadarevian, J-P. and Kaplan, B. S. (1981). Endocardial fibroelastosis, myocardial scarring and polycystic kidneys. *International Journal of Pediatric Nephrology*, **2**, 273–5.

Chapman, A. B., Johnson A., Kaehny, W., Schrier, R., and Gabow, P. (1989). Glomerular hyperfiltration: An early manifestation of autosomal dominant polycystic kidney disease (Abstract). *Kidney International*, **35**, 203.

Chapman, A. B., Johnson, A., Gabow, P. A., and Schier, R. W. (1990). The renin-angiotensin-aldosterone system and autosomal dominant polycystic kidney disease. *New England Journal of Medicine*, **323**, 1091–6.

Chapman, A., Johnson, A., Duley, I., and Gabow, P. (1991). Hypertension (HBP) occurs frequently in children with autosomal dominant polycystic kidney disease (ADPKD) (Abstract). *Journal of the American Society of Nephrology*, **2**, 251.

Chavalier, R. L., Garland, T. A., and Buschi, A. J. (1981). The neonate with adult-type autosomal dominant polycystic kidney disease. *International Journal of Pediatric Nephrology*, **2**, 73–7.

Cohn, D. H., Starman, B. J., Blumberg B., and Byers, P. H. (1990). Recurrence of lethal osteogenesis imperfecta due to parental mosaicisim for a dominant mutation in a human type I collagen gene (COLIAI). *American Journal of Human Genetics*, **46**, 591–601.

Cole, B. R., Conley, S. B., and Stapleton, F. B. (1987). Polycystic kidney disease in the first year of life. *Journal of Pediatrics*, **111**, 693–9.

De Paoli, V. E., *et al.* (1987). Adult polycystic kidney disease in northern Italy: Use of a DNA-marker for presymptomatic diagnosis. *Nephrology, Dialysis, Transplantation*, **2**, 409–16.

Easterly, J. R. and Oppenheimer, E. H. (1967). Some aspects of cardiac pathology in infancy and childhood. IV. Myocardial and coronary lesions in cardiac malformations. *Pediatrics*, **39**, 896–903.

Edwards, O. P. and Baldinger, S. (1989). Prenatal onset of autosomal dominant polycystic kidney disease. *Urology*, **34**, 265–70.

EPKDC (European Polycystic Kidney Disease Consortium) (1994). The polycystic kidney disease 1 gene encodes a 14 kb transcript and lies within a duplicated region on chromosome 16. *Cell*, **77**, 881–94.

Eulderink, F. and Hogewind, B. L. (1978). Renal cysts in premature children: Occurrence in a family with polycystic kidney disease. *Archives Pathology and Laboratory Medicine*, **102**, 592–5.

Farrell, T. P., Boal, D. K., Wood, B. P., Dagen, J. E., and Rabinowitz, R. (1984). Unilateral abdominal mass an unusual presentation of autosomal dominant polycystic kidney disease in children. *Pediatric Radiology*, **14**, 349–52.

Fellows, R. A., Leonidas, J. C., Beatty, E. C. Jr (1976). Radiologic features of 'adult type' polycystic kidney disease in the neonate. *Pediatric Radiology*, **4**, 87–92.

Fick, G., Johnson, A., and Gabow, P. (1992). Health Insurance and life insurance in patients with autosomal dominant polycystic kidney disease (Abstract). *Journal of the American Society of Nephrology*, **3**, 295.

Fick, G. M., et al. (1993). Characteristics of very early onset autosomal dominant polycystic kidney disease. *Journal of the American Society of Nephrology*, **3**, 1863–70.

Fick, G. M., Duley, I. T., Johnson, A. M., Strain, J. D., Manco-Johnson, M. L., and Gabow, P. A. (1994). The spectrum of autosomal dominant polycystic kidney disease in children. *Journal of the American Society of Nephrology*, **4**, 1654–60.

Fryns, J. P. and Van Den Berghe, H. (1979). "Adult" form of polycystic kidney disease in neonates. *Clinical Genetics*, **15**, 205–6.

Fryns, J. P., Vandenberghe, K., and Moerman, F. (1986). Mid-trimester ultrasonographic diagnosis of early manifesting "adult" form of polycystic kidney disease. *Human Genetics*, **74**, 461.

Gabow, P. A. (1993). Autosomal dominant polycystic kidney disease. *New England Journal of Medicine*, **329**, 332–42.

Gabow, P. A., Ikle, D. W., and Holmes, J. H. (1984). Polycystic kidney disease: Prospective analysis of nonazotemic patients and family members. *Annals of Internal Medicine*, **101**, 238–47.

Gabow, P. A., et al. (1989a). Gene testing in autosomal dominant polycystic kidney disease: Results of National Kidney Foundation Workshop. *American Journal of Kidney Disease*, **13**, 85–7.

Gabow, P. A., et al. (1989b). The clinical utility of renal concentrating capacity in polycystic kidney disease. *Kidney International*, **35**, 675–80.

Gabow, P. A., et al. (1990). Renal structure and hypertension in autosomal dominant polycystic kidney disease. *Kidney International*, **38**, 1177–80.

Gabow, P. A. and Wilkins-Haug, L. (1991). Prediction of likelihood of polycystic kidney disease in the fetus when a parent has autosomal dominant polycystic disease. In *International Year Book of Nephrology* (ed. V. E. Andreucci and L. G. Fine), pp. 199–207. Springer-Verlag, London

Gabow, P. A., Johnson, A., Kimberling, W., Velidi, M., Fowler, T., and Strain, J. (1994). Utility of ultrasonography (US) in children in families with chromosome 16 autosomal dominant polycystic kidney disease (ADPKD1) (Abstract). *Journal of the American Society of Nephrology*, **7**, 646.

Gagnadoux, M-F., Habib R., and Levy, M. (1989). Cystic renal diseases in children. *Advances in Nephrology*, **18**, 33–58.

Gal, A., *et al.* (1989). Childhood manifestation of autosomal dominant polycystic kidney disease *Clinical Genetics*, **35**, 13–19.

Garel, L., Sauvegrain, J., and Filiatrault, D. (1983). Dominant polycystic disease of the kidney in a newborn child: Report of one case. *Annals of Radiology*, **26**, 183–6.

Gordon, R. L., Pollack, H. M., Popky, G. L., and Duckett, J. W. Jr (1979). Simple serious cysts of the kidney in children. *Pediatric Radiology*, **131**, 357–61.

Grantham, J. J. (1993). Polycystic kidney disease: Hereditary and acquired. *Advances in Internal Medicine*, **38**, 409–20.

Grunfeld, J. G., Albouze, G., and Jungers, P. (1985). Liver changes and complications in adult polycystic kidney diseases. *Advances in Nephrology*, **14**, 1–20.

Haller, J. O. (1980). Urinary tract and adrenal glands. In *Pediatric ultrasound*, (1st edn), (ed. J. O. Heller and M. Schneider), pp. 84–104. Year Book Medical, Chicago.

Han, B. K. and Babcock, D. S. (1985). Sonographic measurements and appearance of normal kidneys in children. *American Journal of Roentgenology*, **145**, 611–16.

Harley, H. G., *et al.* (1992). Unstable DNA sequence in myotonic dystrophy. *Lancet*, **339**, 1125–8.

Harper, P. S. and Dyken, P. R. (1972). Early-onset dystrophia myotonica. Evidence supporting a maternal environmental factor. *Lancet*, **2**, 53–5.

Harrap, S. B., *et al.* (1991). Renal, cardiovascular and hormonal characteristics of young adults with autosomal dominant polycystic kidney disease. *Kidney International*, **40**, 501–8.

Hayden, C. K. Jr, Swischuk, L. E., Davis, M., and Brouhard, B. H. (1984). Puddling: A distinguishing feature of adult autosomal dominant polycystic kidney disease in the neonate. *American Journal of Radiology*, **142**, 811–12.

Hossack, K. F., Leddy, C. L., Johnson, A. M., Schrier, R. W., and Gabow, P. A. (1988). Echocardiographic findings in autosomal dominant polycystic kidney disease. *New England Journal of Medicine*, **319**, 907–12.

Hodgkinson, K. A., Kerzin-Storrar, L., Watters, E. A., and Harris, R. (1990). Adult polycystic kidney disease: knowledge, experience, and attitudes to prenatal diagnosis. *Journal of Medical Genetics*, **27**, 552–8.

Hogg, R. J. (1992). Acquired renal cystic disease in children prior to the start of dialysis. *Pediatric Nephrology*, **6**, 176–8.

Ivy, D., *et al.* (1995). Cardiovascular abnormalities in children with autosomal dominant polycystic kidney disease. *Journal of the American Society of Nephrology*, **5**, 2032–6.

Journel, H., Guyot, C., Barc, R. M., Belbeoch, P., Quemener, A., and Jouan, H. (1989). Unexpected ultrasonographic prenatal diagnosis of autosomal dominant polycystic kidney disease. *Prenatal Diagnosis*, **9**, 663–71.

Kääriäinen, H. (1987). Polycystic kidney disease in children: a genetic and epidemiological study of 82 Finnish patients. *Journal of Medical Genetics*, **24**, 474–81.

Kääriäinen, H., Koskimies, O., and Norio, R. (1988). Dominant and recessive polycystic kidney disease in children: evaluation of clinical features and laboratory data. *Pediatric Nephrology*, **2**, 296–302.

Kaplan, B. S., Kaplan, P., Rosenberg, H. K., Lamothe, E., and Rosenblatt, D. S. (1989). Polycystic kidney diseases in childhood. *Journal of Pediatrics*, **115**, 867–80.

Kaye, C. and Lewy, P. R. (1974). Congenital appearance of adult-type (autosomal dominant) polycystic kidney disease: Report of a case. *Journal of Pediatrics*, **85**, 807–10.

Kimberling, W. J., Fain, P. R., Kenyon, J. B., Goldgar, D., Sujansky, E., and Gabow, P. A. (1988). Linkage heterogeneity of autosomal dominant polycystic kidney disease. *New England Journal of Medicine*, **319**, 913–18.

Kimberling, W. J., Pieke-Dahl, S. A., and Kumar, S. (1991). The genetics of cystic diseases of the kidney. *Seminars in Nephrology*, **11**, 596–606.

Kramer, S. A., Hoffman, A. D., Aydin, G., and Kelalis, P. P. (1982). Simple renal cysts in children. *Journal of Urology*, **128**, 1259–61.

Lawson, T. L., Foley, W. D., Berland, L. L., and Clark, K. E. (1981). Ultrasonic evaluation of fetal kidneys: Analysis of normal size and frequency of visualization as related to stage of pregnancy. *Radiology*, **138**, 153–6.

Leichter, H. E., *et al.* (1988). Acquired cystic disease in children undergoing long-term dialysis. *Pediatric Nephrology*, **2**, 8–11.

Loh, J. P., Haller, J. O., Kassner, E. G., Aloni, A., and Glassberg, K. (1977). Dominantly-inherited polycystic kidneys in infants: Association with hypertrophic pyloric stenosis. *Pediatrics Radiology*, **6**, 27–31.

Lundin, P. M. and Olow, I. (1961). Polycystic kidneys in newborns, infants and children: A clinical and pathological study. *Acta Paediatrica*, **50**, 185–200.

Luthy, D. A. and Hirsch, J. H. (1985). Infantile polycystic kidney disease: Observation from attempts at prenatal diagnosis. *American Journal of Medical Genetics*, **20**, 505–17.

Main, D., Mennuti, M. T., Cornfeld, D., and Coleman, B. (1983). Prenatal diagnosis of adult polycystic kidney disease. *Lancet*, **2**, 337–8.

Matsuda, O., *et al.* (1990). Polycystic kidney of autosomal dominant inheritance, polycystic liver and congenital hepatic fibrosis in a single kindred. *American Journal of Nephrology*, **10**, 237–41.

Martinez-Maldonaldo, M., Yium, J. J., Eknoyan, G., and Suki, W. N. (1972). Adult polycystic kidney disease: Studies of the defect in urine concentration. *Kidney International*, **2**, 107–13.

McDonald, R. A. and Avner, E. D. (1991). Inherited polycystic kidney disease in children. *Seminars in Nephrology*, **11**, 1–11.

McLean, R. H., Goldstein, G., Gonard, F. U., Radoulpour, M., and Crawford, B. (1980). Autosomal dominant (adult) polycystic kidney disease in childhood. *Connecticut Medical*, **44**, 690–92.

Mehrizi A., Rosenstein, B. H., and Pusch, A. (1964). Myocardial infarction and endocardial fibroelastosis in children with polycystic kidneys. *Bulletin Johns Hopkins Hospital*, **115**, 95–8.

Milutinovic, J., *et al.* (1980). Autosomal dominant polycystic kidney disease: Early diagnosis and data for genetic counselling. *Lancet*, **1**, 1203–5.

Milutinovic, J., Schabel, S. I., and Ainsworth, S. K. (1989). Autosomal dominant polycystic kidney disease with liver and pancreatic involvement in early childhood. *American Journal of Kidney Diseases*, **12**, 340–4.

Mir, S., Rapola, J., and Koskimies, O. (1983). Renal cysts in pediatric autopsy material. *Nephron*, **33**, 189–95.

Mogensen, C. E. and Christiansen C. K. (1984). Predicting diabetic nephropathy in insulin-dependent patients. *New England Journal of Medicine*, **311**, 89–93.

Musiani, U. and Villani, U. (1984). Spontaneous disappearance and successive reappearance of renal cyst. *Urology*, **24**, 366–7.

Novelli, G., *et al.* (1989). Prenatal diagnosis of adult polycystic kidney disease with DNA markers on chromosome 16 and the genetic heterogeneity problem. *Prenatal Diagnosis*, **9**, 759–67.

Parfrey, P. S., Morgan, J., Singh, M., Cramer, B., and Bear, J. (1989). Autosomal dominant polycystic kidney disease in children (Abstract). *Kidney International*, 35, 206.

Parfrey, P. S., *et al.* (1990). The diagnosis and prognosis of autosomal dominant polycystic kidney disease. *New England Journal of Medicine*, 323, 1085–90.

Porch, P., Noe, H. N., and Stapleton, F. B. (1986). Unilateral presentation of adult-type polycystic kidney disease in children. *Journal of Urology*, 135, 744–5.

Pretorius, D. H., Lee, M. E., Manco-Johnson, M. L., Weingast, G. R., Sedman, A. B., and Gabow, P. A. (1987). Diagnosis of autosomal dominant polycystic kidney disease in utero and in the young infant. *Journal of Ultrasound in Medicine*, 6, 249–55.

Proesmans, W., Van Damme, B., Casaer, P., and Marchal, G. (1982). Autosomal dominant polycystic kidney disease in the neonatal period: Association with a cerebral arteriovenous malformation. *Pediatrics*, 70, 971–5.

Querfeld, U., *et al.* (1990). Acquired cystic kidney disease in paediatric patients with chronic renal insufficiency (Abstract). (EDTA-ERA 27 Annual Congress, Vienna). *Nephrology Dialysis Transplant*, 5, 656.

Ravine, D., Walker, R. G., Gibson, R. N., Sheffield, L. J., Kincaid-Smith, P., and Danks, D. M. (1991). Treatable complications in undiagnosed cases of autosomal dominant polycystic kidney disease. *Lancet*, 337, 127–9.

Ravine, D., Gibson, R. N., Donlan, J., and Sheffield, L. J. (1993). An ultrasound renal cyst prevalence survey: Specificity data for inherited renal cystic diseases. *American Journal of Kidney Diseases*, 22, 803–7.

Ravine, D., Gibson, R. N., Walker, R. G., Sheffield, L. J., Kincaid-Smith, P., and Danks, D. M. (1994). Evaluation of ultrasonographic diagnostic criteria for autosomal dominant polycystic kidney disease 1. *Lancet*, 343, 824–7.

Reeders, S. T., *et al.* (1986). Prenatal diagnosis of autosomal dominant polycystic kidney disease with DNA probe. *Lancet*, 2, 6–8.

Reilly, K. B., Ribin, S. P., Blanke, B. G., and Yeh, M-N. (1979). Infantile polycystic kidney disease: A difficult antenatal diagnosis. *American Journal of Obstetrics and Gynecology*, 133, 580–1.

Romero, R., *et al.* (1984). The diagnosis of congenital renal anomalies with ultrasound: Infantile polycystic kidney disease. *American Journal of Obstetrics and Gynecology*, 150, 259–62.

Ross, D. G. and Travers, H. (1975). Infantile presentation of adult-type polycystic kidney disease in a large kindred. *Journal of Pediatrics*, 87, 760–3.

Rousseau, F., Heitz, D., and Biancalana, V. (1991). Direct diagnosis by DNA analysis of the fragile X syndrome of mental retardation. *New England Journal of Medicine*, 325, 1673–81.

Scheff, R. T., Zuckerman G., Harter, H. T., Delmez, J., and Koehler, R. (1986). Diverticular disease in patients with chronic renal failure due to polycystic kidney disease. *Annals of Internal Medicine*, 92, 202–4.

Schwartz, G. J., Brion, L. P., and Spitzer A. (1987). The use of plasma creatinine concentration for estimating glomerular filtration rate in infants, children and adolescents. *Pediatric Nephrology*, 34, 571–90.

Sedman, A., *et al.* (1987). Autosomal dominant polycystic kidney disease in childhood: A longitudinal study. *Kidney International*, 31, 1000–5.

Sheu, J-N., Chen, C-H., Tsau, Y-K., Wu, T-T., Chien, C-T., and Shy, S-W. (1991). Autosomal dominant polycystic kidney disease: An unusual presentation as unilateral renal mass in the infant. *American Journal of Nephrology*, 11, 252–6.

Shokeir, M. H. K. (1978). Expression of 'adult' polycystic renal disease in the fetus and newborn. *Clinical Genetics*, **14**, 61–72.

Smedley, M. G. and Bailey, R. R. (1987). Autosomal dominant polycystic kidney disease diagnosed *in utero* using ultrasonography. *New Zealand Medical Journal*, **100**, 606.

Stapleton, F. B., Magill, H. L., and Kelly, D. R. (1983). Infantile polycystic kidney disease: An imaging dilemma. *Urologic Radiology*, **5**, 89–94.

Stickler, G. B. and Kelalis, P. P. (1975). Polycystic kidney disease: Recognition of the 'adult form' (autosomal dominant) in infancy. *Mayo Clinic Proceedings*, **50**, 547–8.

Sujansky, E., Kreutzer, S. B., Johnson, A. M., Lezotte, D. C., Schrier, R. W., and Gabow, P. A. (1990). Attitudes of at-risk and affected individuals regarding presymptomatic testing for autosomal dominant polycystic kidney disease. *American Journal of Medical Genetics*, **35**, 510–15.

Taitz, L. S., Brown, C. B., Blank, C. E., and Steiner, G. M. (1987). Screening for polycystic kidney disease: importance of clinical presentation in the newborn. *Archives of Disease in Childhood*, **62**, 45–9.

Task Force (Task Force on Blood Pressure Control in Children) (1987). Report of the second task force on blood pressure control in children. *Pediatrics*, **79**, 1–25.

Turco, A., Peissel, B., Quaia, P., Morandi, R., Bovicelli, L., and Pignatti, F. (1992). Prenatal diagnosis of autosomal dominant polycystic kidney disease using flanking DNA markers and the polymerase chain reaction. *Prenatal Diagnosis*, **12**, 513–24.

U.S. Renal Data System, USRDS, Annual Data Report (1993) Bethesda, MD. The National Institutes of Health, National Institute of Diabetes, Digestive and Kidney Diseases.

Waldherr, R., Zerres, K., Gall, A., and Enders, H. (1989). Polycystic kidney disease in the fetus. *Lancet*, 274–5.

Walker, F. C., Loney, L. C., Root, E. R., Melson, G. L., McAlister, W. H., and Cole, B. R. (1984). Diagnostic evaluation of adult polycystic kidney disease in childhood. *American Journal of Roentgenology*, **142**, 1273–7.

Yamagishi, F., Kitahara, N., Mogi, W., and Itoh, S. (1988). Age-related occurrence of simple renal cysts studied by ultrasonography. *Klinische Wochen-Schrift*, **66**, 385–7.

Zeier, M., Geberth, S., Schmidt, K. G., Mandelbaum, A., and Ritz, E. (1993). Elevated blood pressure profile and left ventricle mass in children and young adults with autosomal dominant polycystic kidney disease. *Journal of the American Society of Nephrology*, **4**, 1451–7.

Zerres, K. (1992). Polycystic kidney disease: Thoughts on the meaning of prevention. *Contributions to Nephrology*, **97**, 7–14.

Zerres, K. and Propping, P. (1987). Autosomal dominant polycystic kidney disease in children (Correspondence). *Archives of Diseases in Childhood*, **62**, 870–1.

Zerres, K. and Stephan, M. (1986). Attitudes to early diagnosis of polycystic kidney disease. *Lancet*, **i**, 1395.

Zerres, K., Weiss, H., Bulla, M., and Roth, B. (1982). Prenatal diagnosis of an early manifestation of autosomal dominant adult-type polycystic kidney disease. *Lancet*, **2**, 988.

Zerres, K., Hansmann, M., Knopfle, G., and Stephan, M. (1985). Prenatal diagnosis of genetically determined early manifestation of autosomal dominant polycystic kidney disease? *Human Genetics* **71**, 368–9.

Zerres, K., Rudnik-Schöneborn, S., and Deget, F. (1992). Routine examination of children at risk of autosomal dominant polycystic kidney disease. *Lancet*, **339**, 1356–7.

Zerres, K., *et al.* (1994). Mapping of the gene for autosomal recessive polycystic kidney disease (ARPKD) to chromosome 6p21-cen. *Nature Genetics*, **7**, 429–32.

24

Counselling and ethical considerations in autosomal dominant polycystic kidney disease

Anne M. Macnicol and Alan F. Wright

Introduction

Autosomal dominant polycystic kidney disease (ADPKD) is a common and serious genetic disorder with onset of symptoms generally after the reproductive age resulting in the propagation of the disease over many generations. It therefore presents an important opportunity to genetic counsellors to inform affected and 'at-risk' family members about the nature of the disorder and the treatment options, the recurrence risks to offspring and the advantages and disadvantages of pre-symptomatic testing. Advances in treatment have gradually led to an improved prognosis. Specific treatment is not available in ADPKD but early diagnosis leading to the prevention of hypertension is beneficial. Even if medical intervention is rejected until a late stage, end-stage renal disease can be treated by dialysis or transplantation so that patients can, perhaps, justifiably accept or reject the treatment option itself. As a result, attitudes to the disease vary widely and difficult choices increasingly accompany options such as pre-symptomatic or antenatal diagnosis.

Advances in molecular genetics have led to the development of accurate predictive tests and more recently to the isolation of the PKD1 gene itself (EPKDC 1994). Genetic studies have also demonstrated an unexpected complexity, since there are now known to be at least two ADPKD loci, making the task of the counsellor more difficult. The most common form of the disease, PKD1, is located in chromosomal region 16p13.3 (Reeders *et al.* 1985) and a second locus, PKD2, is located in chromosomal region 4q13-q23 (Kimberling *et al.* 1993; Peters *et al.* 1993), each of which is capable of producing similar or identical phenotypes. In the comparatively small number of families where genetic markers are requested for early diagnosis, considerable caution is therefore required in their application.

How is this rather complex picture conveyed to at-risk or affected family members? Patients are inevitably influenced not only by the information itself but also by the way in which it is conveyed by the counsellor, even with the most non-directive approach. Are there effective ways in which to educate patients, both about the natural history of the disease and its mode of inheritance? How are the often complex ethical issues and decisions presented in the counselling situation? What is the evidence that the provision of genetic counselling is actually effective? These questions are not easily answered since they deal with subtle interactions between patients and physicians or counsellors. The long-term genetic effects of a counselling programme, which could be monitored by observing changes in the incidence of disease, will be negligible if patients choose not to alter their reproductive plans, and yet the programme could be highly effective. The cost effectiveness of a counselling programme in health economic terms is another aspect of the picture but it is not a primary concern of the counsellor. What then is the role of the counsellor? He or she has many roles, the first of which is to convey basic information on the disease, its mode of inheritance, and the risks to other family members.

Basic principles of counselling in ADPKD

When patients are diagnosed as having ADPKD, their perception of the disease may already have been influenced by previous experiences of the condition in other family members. The condition is extremely variable, complicating the relay of information to these patients. The first task facing the counsellor is to give the patient clear information about the clinical implications of the disorder and available therapy. The most important clinical aspects of ADPKD and their implications for counselling are listed in Table 24.1.

The mode of inheritance of the disease should be clarified since patients often have confused ideas, either exaggerating or showing unawareness of the genetic risks. Studies of patients' knowledge and attitudes to the disease often reveal poor understanding of the potential to transmit the disorder to offspring and difficulty in understanding that asymptomatic individuals may be gene carriers (Sahney *et al.* 1982; Milutinovic *et al.* 1980; Hodgkinson *et al.* 1990; Macnicol *et al.* 1990). The disorder is inherited as an autosomal dominant trait. The carrier status of an individual can be clarified most simply by renal ultrasonography, which is both sensitive and non-invasive (Bear *et al.* 1992). Ultrasound scans, which normally include liver, spleen, and pancreas, as well as the kidney, therefore provide a sound basis for establishing the diagnosis, at least in those over the age of 30 years.

There are a number of situations where counselling in ADPKD is less clear-cut. The first is when there is no family history of the disorder. In most cases, this is due to lack of information about previous generations but the occurrence of new mutations has been reported and should be considered. Non-paternity is another possibility, which, if discovered is not discussed with the patient. The recurrence risk for siblings of an isolated patient, when the parents have normal renal ultrasound scans, is very low but this is quite uncommon and alternative diagnostic possibilities, such as acquired or drug-induced cystic disease, must be considered (Gardner 1988). More common is the situation of an isolated patient with parents who have died or are unavailable so that there is no good data on their clinical status. In this situation, the lack of a family history should at least raise some doubts about the diagnosis. This group would potentially benefit

Table 24.1   ADPKD: Clinical aspects and counselling

Clinical	Basic facts	Implications for counselling
Age at clinical presentation	Usually between 30–50 years with more severe manifestations in childhood and milder diseases in late adulthood.	Considerable variation among members of one family, with earlier and later onset cases. In families with early onset, there is a high recurrence risk for early manifestation in siblings of about 50% of gene carrier.
Natural history	77% probability that ADPKD patients will be alive without replacement therapy at age 50.	Individual prognosis can be different within members of a family. Counselling strategies are best tailored to each individual.
MAIN CLINICAL SYMPTOMS		
Flank pain	50% (19–78%)[a]	Patients should be warned
Abdominal pain	65% (60–75%)	about the possibility of their
Haematuria	35% (13–56%)	symptoms to reduce anxiety.
Headache	27% (15–50%)	
Gastrointestinal complaints	15%	
Hypertension		Indicate the reason for attempts at
Urinary tract infection		early detection and treatment.
Nephrolithiasis	20%	
Hepatic cysts	Common manifestations in two-thirds of patients.	Liver cysts do not usually present a threat to liver function in the long term.
Palpable hepatomegaly	30%	
Cardiac manifestations	Mitral valve prolapse can be found in about 25%. Other cardiac manifestations possible.	Routine cardiological examination should be performed in ADPKD patients.
Intracranial aneurysms	9% of ADPKD patients die from rupture of berry aneurysm.	Routine screening for berry aneurysms has been a matter for debate (see Chapter 22).
ADPKD and pregnancy	Can have an adverse effect on renal function if > 4 pregnancies. Onset of hypertension during pregnancy is a common complication.	Besides the possibility of transmitting the disease to children and the uncertainty about their own future, the question of children is an important issue with respect to the self-esteem of women with ADPKD.

Table 24.1 *Continued*

Clinical	Basic facts	Implications for counselling
Pre-symptomatic testing	Until the age of 20 years about 90% of all gene carriers can be identified and nearly all by the age of 30 years.	Ultrasound is usually a reliable method for the identification of a gene carrier but debatable whether at-risk children should be screened before 18 years of age.

[a]Range of studies.

most from a means of efficiently scanning the gene itself for mutations. This may be some way off, due to the large size of the PKD1 gene and the likelihood of at least several distinct mutations. In some cases, there is diagnostic doubt due to the presence of atypical cysts or non-renal manifestations when alternative diagnoses again need to be considered (see Chapter 7).

Counselling strategy

How can counselling be made effective? An outline strategy is presented below which has been in use for several years in Edinburgh and provides a pragmatic approach, similar to many others throughout the world except that it has some novel features designed to facilitate the comprehension and reinforcement of counselling information (Macnicol *et al.* 1986).

The diagnosis is first established by the appropriate medical specialist. The proband and at-risk relatives are given counselling which includes the following:

1. Discussion about the clinical aspects of the disease.

2. The showing and loan of a video tape explaining the mode of inheritance as well as the clinical implications of ADPKD, which assist the reinforcement process and provides consistency.

3. Establishing with the patient whether at-risk family members would like to have counselling. The proband is encouraged to make this initial contact with family members.

4. The primary care physician (general practitioner) is asked if he has any objection to the at-risk relative receiving counselling.

5. The at-risk individual is given the option to contact the counsellor directly.

6. If the relative agrees, he/she is counselled and renal ultrasound scanning is organized. Ultrasound scans can be combined with pre-symptomatic DNA screening in young adults who wish accurate information on which to base reproductive decisions.

7. A repeat counselling session is arranged following screening, irrespective of the result, to ensure that the individual fully understands his/her situation.

8. Clients are encouraged to organize further appointments with the counsellor in the event of changed circumstances. No matter how well a patient has been counselled, there may be doubts and uncertainties that merit further discussion. The counsellor can then obtain feedback on how well the counsellee has understood and coped with earlier sessions.

If the patient agrees, his/her name is entered on a computer database (ADPKD register) to facilitate regular follow-up. This depends on close co-operation between the counsellor, the hospital, and the primary care service. All patients are contacted once a year to remind them to attend their primary care physician for a blood pressure check and renal function tests. The results are sent to the specialist renal physician and the computer information is updated. Information is requested on any changes of address. If renal function or blood pressure has been found to deteriorate, then referral to a specialist renal clinic can be organized. Unaffected relatives under the age of 30 can also be followed up in this way.

Psychological impact of counselling

Although counselling is essentially an educational process, a sensitive and informed counsellor can recognize the psychological processes experienced by patients, which allows for more effective communication. The stages of the 'coping process' have to be recognized and counselling tailored accordingly. The sequence of responses of individuals under stress as described by Falek and de la Cruz (1977) are:

(1) shock or denial;

(2) anxiety;

(3) anger or guilt;

(4) depression; and

(5) psychological homeostasis or acceptance.

During the denial stage, the patient usually absorbs little new information so that a full explanation at the time of diagnosis usually proves ineffective.

Case study I

This case study illustrates the processes as experienced by a newly diagnosed patient.

A trainee pilot, aged 26 was diagnosed as having ADPKD, subsequent to his brother having a positive ultrasound scan. His initial response in *Phase (1)* (*shock or denial*) was:

(a) 'This is a mistake. I've undergone countless medicals as part of my training programme and nothing was found to be wrong.'

(b) 'I'd like a second opinion.'

Phase (2) (anxiety)

He experienced panic attacks and doubted his ability to fly a plane again. He began to feel that his body was unreliable. As an individual who had relied on having events strictly controlled, he reacted badly to the uncertainty he now faced. He was frequently upset and tearful at his inability to control the possible implications of having this condition. His feelings were compounded by the detection of asymptomatic hypertension.

Phase (3) (anger or guilt)

He focused his developing anger on the medical staff who had not informed him about the possible implications of a positive diagnosis. When he informed the American Civil Aviation Authority about the result of his scan he was suspended from training for three months.

Phase (4) (depression)

The patient experienced a period of hopelessness and inadequacy. At this point, counselling was commenced to help provide insight into the processes he was experiencing.

Phase (5) (acceptance)

Two months later, the patient felt confident enough to return to America to complete his training course. His antihypertensive medication was acceptable to the Civil Aviation Authority.

It is important for the counsellor to recognize that, depending on the age at which a patient is diagnosed as having ADPKD, there will be different worries to deal with. In older family members, these may include:

(1) anxiety about children and the condition;

(2) worries about developing end-stage renal failure;

(3) concern about the presence of cerebral aneurysms, especially when there is a family history;

(4) increased apprehension and vulnerability in those with end-stage renal failure; and

(5) concern about effects on existing relationships.

Younger family members may be frightened by the prospect of developing the disease, especially when they may have seen severe effects on another family member. Guilt feelings in the parent commonly inhibit communication about the disease leading either to complete ignorance or to increased apprehension as a result of misconceptions within younger family members. Medical contact may also be avoided as a means of denial. Finally, worries about how ADPKD might prejudice pre-marital relationships may be perceived as a significant problem by young persons.

Case study II

The following case study illustrates how the incidence of cerebral aneurysms in a family can have a profound psychological effect, especially when it is not recognized or acknowledged by patients.

KM who is 40 years old, came for a clinical follow-up visit. She was diagnosed as having the condition 15 years ago, and has required antihypertensive medication for the past seven years. She was extremely tearful and expressed feelings of hopelessness and that 'nothing in life seemed worthwhile'. She was puzzled as to why she should feel so depressed when she was unable to pin-point any contributory factors. She was offered a series of counselling sessions, in which the following were discussed:

(a) The effect of an inherited illness on the family.

(b) Her mother had an aneurysm rupture which caused paralysis at the age of 40 years. KM made the connection with the fact that in two months time she would be the same age as her mother when the aneurysm ruptured.

(c) KM, when she was 16 years old, had to take responsibility for the care of her mother and two younger sisters. This meant leaving school and giving up plans for college. Her father opted out of contributing to the care of his wife and began drinking heavily as a means of further distancing himself from the situation.

(d) The impact of past events and their relationship to behaviour and attitudes in the present. For example, KM was forever 'testing' her husband to prove to herself that he would be supportive of her if she was ever ill and helpless.

The result of these sessions was that KM gained new insights into where her feelings of hopelessness originated and felt 'as if a huge weight had been lifted from me'. Magnetic resonance image scanning for cerebral microaneurysms was organized and was negative, but will be repeated at regular intervals.

Pre-symptomatic testing

It is extremely important that at-risk relatives understand both the advantages and disadvantages of pre-symptomatic screening. The ethical issues regarding the testing of children for 'adult' genetic disease have been highlighted since DNA testing became available to ADPKD families (Harper and Clarke 1990). Assessment of children by ultrasound scanning is of limited value because of a significant false negative rate (Bear *et al.* 1984). It seems reasonable in the case of ADPKD, where there is a low frequency of serious complications in child-hood, to wait until the child is at least 18 years old before suggesting ultrasound scanning. By this age, at-risk relatives can make their own decisions, and can more easily assimilate the information on which to base that choice. However even after this age, the pros and cons of pre-symptomatic testing remain a complex issue.

In order to make an informed choice about pre-symptomatic testing, individuals require information about the advantages of early screening. Early diagnosis would allow the possibility of identification and management of treatable complications (see Table 24.1) such as hypertension. A study by Ravine *et al.* (1991) demonstrated that one third of previously undiagnosed patients had hypertension. Since hypertension tends to develop early in the course of the illness (Watson *et al.* 1986), early and effective blood pressure control is potentially of great value. ADPKD patients also have a higher risk of cerebral haemorrhage as

a consequence of ruptured cerebral microaneurysms or other arterial malformations. Screening of affected patients by cerebral angiography to identify such abnormalities is probably not justified (Levey *et al.* 1983), but a reduced incidence
of rupture might be expected from early, aggressive treatment of hypertension.
Since not all adult polycystic kidney disease patients progress to end-stage renal
failure, early control of hypertension may delay or avoid this progression.
Patients may be more amenable to the idea of pre-symptomatic screening if it
can be shown that intervention, such as control of hypertension or restriction of
dietary protein, have a beneficial effect on progression to renal failure. It is important, when counselling patients, to be realistic and to convey information in a
way that is understood, without alarming the patient unnecessarily.

Perhaps the most important factor in the use of genetic tests for early diagnosis is the availability and adequacy of counselling both at the time of testing and
as required afterwards. Family members are vulnerable and need to obtain a balanced view of the advantages and disadvantages of genetic testing. Once a decision has been made to proceed with testing, adequate support and follow-up is
essential, since the process of testing, regardless of the outcome, generates great
anxiety. Even a negative test result can alter a person's world view quite
significantly, and requires talking through and adjustment. For example, there
are a surprising number of individuals who just assume that they will develop
the parent's disease because the condition is familial. A negative test can have a
significant emotional impact on individuals with such an attitude. Similarly, a
positive test results can have a devastating effect on an unprepared individual.
Counselling and support is therefore mandatory for any form of early diagnostic
testing, whether using genetic methods, renal function tests, or ultrasound
scanning.

Impact of accurate genetic markers on counselling

The evidence is quite clear that very little use has been made of the availability
of accurate markers for predictive testing to date. Surveys of patients' and family
members' attitudes show that while most are in favour of predictive testing, few
wish to make use of such tests (Sujansky *et al.* 1990). How is the recent isolation
of the PKD1 gene likely to affect predictive counselling in ADPKD? It is ar-
guable that it will have very little impact on counselling until it leads to new
forms of treatment. Predictive tests will only become simpler if common mutations are found in certain populations. The evidence to date suggest that most
populations have several independent mutations (Snarey *et al.* 1994) and scanning a large gene, such as PKD1, for mutations is not likely to be routinely
available until new and more efficient methods of mutation scanning become
available. In the meantime, early diagnosis by means of linkage with flanking
markers will probably remain the mainstay of genetic testing other than by renal
ultrasonography.

Stephan and Zerres (1988) highlighted the fears commonly expressed by patients undergoing predictive testing for ADPKD. They include:

(1) lack of a cure;

(2) insurance consequences;

(3) intense wish to have children;

(4) fear of the future;

(5) career problems;

(6) coming to terms with dialysis and an early death;

(7) loss of self-worth/esteem;

(8) burdening of partner and family.

Zerres investigated the effects of a positive pre-symptomatic test on a group of 58 patients and noted that, of these, 20 changed their sporting activities, 19 had insurance problems (either loaded or refused), 11 modified their career plans (either by changing career or having employment refused), and 43 felt that they had suffered adverse social and psychological changes after their results.

As highlighted by Marteau (1989), screening inevitably has psychological costs. A positive result in any screening programme invariably causes anxiety. In some studies, telling patients that they had hypertension led to absenteeism, reduced self-esteem, and impaired marital relationships (Haynes *et al.* 1978; Mossey 1981; Alderman *et al.* 1981). These problems were reduced by regular supportive follow-up in a controlled trial (Mann 1984). Marteau suggests that counselling before screening is important, but comments 'there are few data to show what information participants should be given to ensure informed uptake and minimized adverse emotional and behavioural consequences of participation'.

The uncertainty of not knowing the diagnosis can also be extremely stressful to some individuals. The counsellor can at least provide a forum for that person to explore the many issues involved. It may be inappropriate however to screen an individual who is about to leave home, start a university course or new employment. Too many changes at one time may mean that none are dealt with adequately. Many patients have expressed the view that following a positive renal ultrasound scan, the problem is not so much for those in established employment, but relates to the discrimination experienced, whether real or imagined, in the open labour market.

Reproductive plans

A study by Sujansky *et al.* (1990) suggests that pre-symptomatic testing will not substantially modify the incidence of adult polycystic kidney disease, since it rarely alters reproductive plans. These individuals had sufficient knowledge about the genetic and clinical implications of the disease to make an informed decision. In contrast, 46 per cent of a group of affected individuals studied by Stephan and Zerres (1988) stated that they would not have had children had they been aware of their status. This difference may be explained by the fact that many in the latter group were on haemodialysis, whereas in the Sujansky study, the majority of patients were under 50 years of age and were for the most part not requiring renal replacement therapy. These differences suggest that, despite adequate counselling, patients' attitudes can change once they have experienced the most severe effects and therapies associated with advanced disease. It would appear that attitudes regarding reproduction can be affected by the reality of life on dialysis. There is much evidence to show that patients are influenced as much by the implications of 'the burden' of the disease as by the actual genetic risks involved.

DNA markers in predictive testing

The availability of DNA markers that flank the PKD1 gene has led to the development of an accurate and relatively straightforward means of prenatal or pre-symptomatic diagnosis (Breuning *et al.* 1987). Reeders *et al.* (1986) used a single highly polymorphic genetic marker (3′ HVR) for prenatal diagnosis of ADPKD in a chorionic villus sample from a 9-week-old fetus at a 1 in 2 risk of carrying the gene. The fetus inherited the high (96 per cent) risk allele and the mother elected to terminate the pregnancy. Microscopic examination of the kidneys from the aborted fetus showed multiple glomerular and tubular cysts in the renal cortex. Error rates of less than 1 per cent are possible using markers that flank the gene, since double recombinants are extremely rare in small genetic intervals. This has been used to exclude the disease in some at-risk family members (Dalgaard and Norby 1989).

One complication in the use of DNA markers for early diagnosis arises from genetic heterogeneity. This is a common problem in human genetic disease and it is now the exception rather than the rule when a disorder is found to be genetically homogeneous. The analysis of linkage in the presence of heterogeneity is a problem however (Cavalli-Sforza and King 1986). The relative frequencies of the PKD1 and PKD2 forms may vary in different populations but in a large collaborative study of linkage data from 328 European ADPKD families, 86 per cent (95 per cent confidence interval 79–91 per cent) were estimated to be due to mutation at the PKD1 locus (Peters and Sandkuijl 1992). It now appears that at least a significant proportion of non-PKD1 families have mutations at the PKD2 locus on chromosome 4 (Peters *et al.* 1993), although these two loci do not appear to account for all ADPKD families. Others have estimated the frequency of PKD1 vs. non-PKD1 mutations in specific populations without finding significant evidence of linkage heterogeneity in some cases (Reeders *et al.* 1987; Mandich *et al.* 1990), while others detected a minority of unlinked families. Detailed haplotype analysis using 14 markers spanning the PKD1 region in a set of 35 Scottish ADPKD families showed that 30 were linked to PKD1 (87 per cent) (Wright *et al.* 1993; Snarey *et al.* 1994). It is clear from these studies that the power to detect heterogeneity is dependent on the informativeness of markers *on each side* of the disease locus; studies using a single highly informative marker were not able to reliably detect heterogeneity.

Finally, the families ascertained in most of the above linkage studies generally showed clinically severe forms of ADPKD, identified through medical renal units or dialysis registers, which may systematically under-represent patients with reduced penetrance, late age of onset, or mild disease. The true proportion of PKD2 families, if the phenotype is indeed milder, may therefore be higher than expected.

Prediction in the presence of genetic heterogeneity

How is a pre-symptomatic diagnosis made in the presence of genetic heterogeneity? The 'common sense' approach is to determine whether the family shows linkage to PKD1 but not to PKD2 or vice versa. If the results are consistent with mutation at one or other locus, then it is safe to apply the markers in a predictive context. This approach is endorsed by one of the first analyses of genetic linkage heterogeneity by Morton (1956) who separated families with elliptocytosis into linked and unlinked groups and demonstrated linkage to the Rh locus on chromosome 1p. This was later confirmed by finding a defective protein 4.1 near Rh in one group and defective alpha-spectrin (unlinked to Rh, on chromosome 1q) in the other group (Conboy *et al.* 1986). The problem with this method arises when the size, structure, or informativeness of the family is such that it is not clear whether a family is linked or not. The situation therefore needs to be quantified and other information has to be entered into the equation, namely the frequency of the two forms in the population. The standard way of doing this is by a Bayesian analysis, in which prior probabilities (the relative frequencies of the two forms of disease) are combined with conditional probabilities (based on the analysis of recombinants with PKD1 and PKD2 markers) to produce joint (prior × conditional) and final or posterior probabilities for linkage to PKD1 and PKD2 (Narod 1991; Young 1991). There are reasonable data in many populations on which to base the prior probabilities of linkage, as discussed above. Computer programs written for analysis of linkage heterogeneity are also available to compute the conditional probabilities of linkage to each locus, based on the lod scores (Ott 1991; Maclean *et al.* 1992; Terwilliger and Ott 1994). Conditional risk estimates based on linkage data with markers for PKD1, PKD2 or preferably both loci are simply obtained provided that the linkage phase and recombination frequencies between marker and disease are known but in more complex situations they are easily computed using programs such as MLINK (Ott 1991). These conditional risk can be combined using the Bayesian approach, essentially by averaging the risks for each locus weighted by the prior probabilities of mutation at each locus (Narod 1991).

Ethics and counselling

The prevention of ADPKD has significant implications for health economics, which is an area of growing importance to governments and health authorities (Mooney 1986; Chapple *et al.* 1987). Prevention could occur either by more accurate predictive tests and improved counselling or by the use of antenatal diagnosis and selective termination of pregnancies. On the other hand, early diagnosis has major social and ethical implications for ADPKD family members, for whom the benefits have to be clearly set against the disadvantages. Is it acceptable to families to terminate pregnancies which are predicted to have a late-manifesting and in many cases treatable condition, and when the primary pathological effect of the ADPKD gene, progressive renal failure due to cyst expansion, may even become completely treatable within the next decade? The majority of patients and families have already answered this question by not making use of DNA-based diagnostic tests for antenatal diagnosis (Watson *et al.* 1986). On the other hand, ADPKD families tend to willingly participate in the use of improved ultrasound scanning methods for early diagnosis in adults since the potential benefits in terms of prevention of hypertension and infection are clear. Nevertheless, probably only a minority of all at-risk family members are currently screened. Pre-symptomatic diagnosis for those under the age of about 18 years has few advocates, since parental curiosity to know the diagnosis may not be in the child's best interest and in terms of disease prevention, monitoring of blood pressure and renal function may be all that is required until that age (Macnicol *et al.* 1990; Harper and Clarke 1990). After the age of 18 years, there may also be a cost attached to a pre-symptomatic diagnosis. First, insurance premiums are routinely increased even for those with a negative ultrasound scan until the age of 30–35 years, but a positive result more than doubles the loading (NRG, underwriting notes). Insurers can justify this by the actuarial evidence that even with good blood pressure control and normal renal function, an extra mortality of at least 200–300 per cent is found in this group of young gene carriers. Once elevated creatinine concentrations are present, individuals are, in general, not insurable, since renal insufficiency is evident (Brackenridge 1992). In the light of recent evidence regarding the severity of disease in PKD1 families, insurers might soon insist on negative DNA tests as well as normal ultrasound scans and renal function in order to offer normal premiums. A balanced view would suggest that if the disease is milder, then although routine scanning is less sensitive, the risk of renal failure is correspondingly reduced. The advent of DNA tests for early diagnosis of adult genetic disorders is certainly having an impact on insurance strategies (Alexander 1988).

Screening for ADPKD in high-risk and other populations

Would there be a case for introducing genetic testing for PKD1 mutations on a large scale if it was to become feasible? Population screening is considered cost-effective in the prevention of severe, high prevalence disorders for which testing is relatively straightforward and cheap. Recently introduced carrier testing programmes for cystic fibrosis and long-established neonatal screening for metabolic disorders are typical examples. The gene frequency of PKD1 is relatively high (~ 1 in 1200) and the morbidity is significant both in personal and economic terms. Since antenatal diagnosis is not an acceptable option for most ADPKD families, the case could only be made for large-scale screening if improved treatment options become available. This could become a reality in the medium term, since improved understanding of the mechanism of cyst expansion may follow from the identification of PKD1 gene product, suggesting new ways of pharmacological intervention. Under these circumstances the most cost-effective way of screening would be to confine it to the 'high-risk' group, such as the families of known affected individuals, since the majority of patients have a family history of ADPKD.

Why are ADPKD families generally disinterested in antenatal diagnosis? Even if the parents consider the disease serious enough to warrant antenatal intervention in principle, prenatal diagnosis is unacceptable to many ethnic and religious groups as well as to a significant proportion of highly educated individuals in more secular Western societies (Bundey 1978). Despite this, in some instances the prevailing religious ethic has not prevented the widespread use of antenatal diagnosis within high-risk groups for the prevention of severe disorders such as thalassaemia (Weatherall 1985). Is it possible that an alternative means of prevention could become acceptable in ADPKD such as *in vitro* fertilization and testing prior to embryo transfer. At present, this is a costly and inefficient procedure but advances in this field could transform it into a much more acceptable form of prevention than antenatal diagnosis and termination of pregnancy.

Conclusion

The provision of counselling in ADPKD is an essential but uncertain process. The disease is theoretically one of the most suitable for the partial prevention of long-term and costly morbidity either by early diagnosis and treatment of complications, such as hypertension, or by means of antenatal diagnosis. It has a high population prevalence so that an effective means of preventing morbidity would be socially and economically important. Accurate means of carrying out pre-symptomatic diagnoses have been available for more than 10 years, despite all of which there is little or no evidence to show that prevention of ADPKD is actually occurring at all. One possible reason is that the counselling and long-term management of patients is frequently split between different services such as primary care, genetics, and nephrology. Genetic registers and specialist ADPKD clinics are the exception so that monitoring the effects of improved counselling and care is difficult. It is possible that counselling in ADPKD is in many cases very effective but it will not be reflected in a declining incidence and morbidity for many years because of the slow progression and late onset. Alternatively, the impact of antenatal diagnosis has undoubtedly been small and the perception of the disease as a late-onset and relatively treatable disorder is increasing, with the result that ADPKD families are not altering their reproductive plans. Morbidity may be declining but incidence is likely to be relatively constant. This situation may change following the recent identification of the PKD1 gene but only if new therapeutic strategies become available as a result. In theory, this could have a dysgenic effect with a slow increase in the number of PKD1 mutations in the population, but this is unlikely since there is little evidence to show that ADPKD families significantly restrict their size at the present time. There is, however, a sparsity of systematic evidence on the consequences of counselling over long time periods.

Recent advances in ADPKD, with the identification of PKD1 and mapping of PKD2 genes, will gradually lead to an increased understanding of these disorders and there is now a reasonable prospect of improved treatment in the future. Counselling provides the interface between the often complex realities of a rapidly changing genetics and the patient who must make pragmatic choices and decisions. The need for informed counselling is therefore likely to increase in the next decade so that provision of adequate services, perhaps involving joint genetic/nephrologist clinics and disease registers within specialist centres, requires careful consideration and planning.

References

Alderman, M., Charlson, M., and Melchier, L. (1981). Labelling and absenteeism: The Massachusetts mutual experience. *Clinical Investigative Medicine*, **4**, 165–71.

Alexander, W. H. (1988). Insurance and genetics. *Journal of Insurance Medicine*, **20**, 35–41.

Bear, J., *et al.* (1984). Age at clinical onset and at ultrasonographic detection of adult polycystic kidney disease: data for genetic counselling. *American Journal of Medical Genetics*, **18**, 45–53.

Bear, J. C., Parfrey, P. S., Morgan, J. M., Martin, J. C., and Cramer, B. C. (1992). Autosomal dominant polycystic kidney disease: new information for genetic counselling. *American Journal of Medical Genetics*, **43**, 548–53.

Brackenridge, R. D. (1985). *Medical selection of life risks*, (2nd edn). Macmillan, Bath. (A comprehensive guide to life expectancy for underwriters and clinicians.)

Breuning, M. H., *et al.* Improved early diagnosis of adult polycystic kidney disease with flanking DNA markers. *Lancet*, **ii**, 1359–61.

Bundey, S. (1978). Attitudes of 40 year old college graduates towards amniocentesis. *British Medical Journal*, **ii**, 1475–7.

Cavalli-Sforza, L. L. and King, M. (1986). Detecting linkage for genetically heterogeneous diseases and detecting heterogeneity with linkage data. *American Journal of Human Genetics*, **38**, 599–616.

Chapple, J. C., Dale, R., and Evans, B. G. (1987). The new genetics: will it pay? *Lancet*, (i), 1189–92.

Churchill, D., Bear, J., Moran, J., Payne, R., McManamon, P., and Gault, H. (1984). Prognosis of adult onset polycystic kidney disease re-evaluated. *Kidney International*, **26**, 190–3.

Conboy, J. N., Mohandas, G., Tchernia, G., and Kan, Y. W. (1986). Molecular basis of hereditary elliptocytosis due to protein 4.1 deficiency. *New England Journal of Medicine*, **315**, 680–5.

Dalgaard, Z. and Norby, S. (1989). ADPKD in the 1980's. *Clinical Genetics*, **36**, 320–5.

EPKDC (European Polycystic Kidney Disease Consortium) (1994). The polycystic disease 1 gene encodes a 14 Kb transcript and lies within a duplicated region on chromosome 16. *Cell*, **77**, 881–94.

Falek, A. and de la Cruz, F. (ed.) (1977). Use of the coping process to achieve psychological homeostatis in genetic counselling. *Genetic counselling*, Vol. 2, p. 179, Raven, New York.

Gardner, K. D. (1988). Cystic kidneys. *Kidney International*, **33**, 610–21.

Harper, P. and Clarke, A. (1990). Should we test children for 'adult' genetic disease? *Lancet*, **335**, 1205–6.

Haynes, R., Sackett, D., Taylor, D., Gibson, E., and Johnston, A. (1978). Changes in absenteeism and psychosocial function due to hypertension screening and therapy among working men. *New England Journal of Medicine*, **299**, 741–4.

Hodgkinson, K. A., Kerzin-Storrar, L., Watters, E. A., and Harris, R. (1990). Polycystic kidney disease: knowledge, experience and attitudes to diagnosis. *Journal of Medical Genetics*, **27**, 552–8.

Kimberling, W. J., Kumar, S., Gabow, P. A., Kenyon, J. B., Connolly, C. J., and Somlo S. (1993). Autosomal dominant polycystic kidney disease: localization of the second gene to chromosome 4q13-q23. *Genomics*, **18**, 467–72.

Levey, A., Parker, S., and Kassirer, J. (1983). Occult intracranial aneurysms in polycystic kidney disease. When is cerebral arteriography indicated? *New England Journal of Medicine*, **308**, 986–94.

Maclean, C. J., Ploughman, L. M., Diehl, S. R., and Kendler, K. S. (1992). A new test for linkage in the presence of locus heterogeneity. *American Journal of Human Genetics*, **50**, 1259–66.

Macnicol, A. M., Watson, M. L., and Wright, A. F. (1986). Implications of a genetic screening programme for polycystic renal disease. *Aspects of Renal Care*, **1**, 219–22.

Macnicol, A. M., Watson, M. L., and Wright, A. F. (1990). Adult polycystic kidney disease. Many advances in diagnosis, assessment and counselling. *British Medical Journal*, **300**, 62–3.

Mandich, P., Restagno, G., Novelli, G., Bellone, E., and Potenza, L. (1990). Autosomal dominant polycystic kidney disease: a linkage evaluation of heterogeneity in Italy. *American Journal of Medical Genetics*, **35**, 579–81.

Mann, A. (1984). Hypertension: psychological aspects and diagnostic impact in a clinical trial. *Psychological Medicine*, **15** (Suppl. 5), 3–35.

Marteau, T. (1989). Psychological costs of screening. *British Medical Journal*, **299**, 527.

Milutinovic, J., Fialkow, P. J., Rudd, T. G., Agodoa, L. Y., Phillips, L. A., and Bryant, J. I. (1980). Liver cyst patients with autosomal dominant polycystic kidney disease. *American Journal of Medicine*, **68**, 741–4.

Mooney, G. H. (1986). *Economics, medicine and health care*. Wheatsheaf, Brighton.

Morton, N. E. (1956). The detection and estimation of linkage between the genes for elliptocytosis and the Rh blood type. *American Journal of Human Genetics*, **8**, 80–96.

Mossey, J. (1981). Psychosocial consequence of labelling in hypertension. *Clinical Investigations in Medicine*, **4**, 201–7.

Narod, S. (1991). Counselling under genetic heterogeneity: a practical approach. *Clin. Genet.* **39**, 125–31.

Ott, J. (1991). *Analysis of human genetic linkage*. Johns Hopkins University Press, Baltimore.

Peters, D. J. and Sandkuijl, L. A. (1992). Genetic heterogeneity of polycystic kidney disease in Europe. *Contributions to Nephrology*, **97**, 128–39.

Peters, D. J., *et al.* (1993). Chromosome 4 localization of a second gene for autosomal dominant polycystic kidney disease. *Nature Genetics*, **5**, 359–62.

Ravine, D., Walker, R., Gibson, R., Sheffield, L., Smith, P., and Dansk, D. (1991). Treatable complications in undiagnosed cases of ADPKD. *Lancet*, **337**, 127–9.

Reeders, S. T., *et al.* (1985). A highly polymorphic DNA marker linked to adult polycystic kidney disease on chromosome 16. *Nature*, **317**, 542–4.

Reeders, S. T., *et al.* (1986). Prenatal diagnosis of autosomal dominant polycystic kidney disease with a DNA probe. *Lancet*, 2, 6–8.

Reeders, S. T., *et al.* (1987). A study of genetic linkage heterogeneity in adult polycystic kidney disease. *Human Genetics*, 76, 348–51.

Sahney, S., Weiss, L., and Levin, N. W. (1982). Genetic counselling in adult polycystic kidney disease. *American Journal of Medical Genetics*, 11, 461–8.

Scientific Advisory Board of the National Kidney Foundation (1989). Gene testing for autosomal dominant polycystic kidney disease: Results of the National Kidney Foundation Workshop. *American Journal of Kidney Disease*, 13, 85–7.

Snarey, A., *et al.* (1994). Linkage disequilibrium in the region of the autosomal dominant polycystic kidney disease gene (PLD1). *American Journal of Human Genetics*, 55, 365–71.

Stephan, M. and Zerres, K. (1988). ADPKD — Attitudes of affected persons to early diagnosis. *Medical Psychology*, 38, 251–8.

Sujansky, E., Kreutzer, S., Johnston, A., Lezotte, D., Schrier, R., and Gabow, P. (1990). Attitudes of at risk and affected individuals regarding presymptomatic testing for ADPKD. *American Journal of Medical Genetics*, 35, 510–15.

Terwilliger, J. D. and Ott, J. (1994). *Handbook of human genetic linkage*. Johns Hopkins, University Press, Baltimore.

Watson, M., Macnicol, A., Allan, P., Clayton, J., Reeders, S., and Wright, A. (1986). Genetic markers for polycystic kidney disease and their implications for detection of hypertension. *Journal of Hypertension*, 4 (Suppl. 6), S40–1.

Weatherall, D. J. (1985). *The new genetics and clinical practice*. (2nd edn). Oxford University Press, Oxford.

Wright, A. F., *et al.* (1993). A study of genetic linkage heterogeneity in 35 adult-onset polycystic kidney disease families. *Human Genetics*, 90, 569–71.

Young, I. D. (1991). *Introduction to risk calculation in genetic counselling*, pp. 1–160. Oxford University Press.

Index